BSAVA Manual of Canine and Feline Shelter Medicine: Principles of Health and Welfare in a Multi-animal Environment

T0203389

Editors:

Rachel Dean
BVMS PhD MSc(EBHC) DipSAM(Feline) SFHEA MRCVS
Recognised Specialist in Feline Medicine
VetPartners Ltd, Leeman House, Station Business Park,
Holgate Park Drive, York YO26 4GB, UK

Maggie Roberts
BVM&S MRCVS
Cats Protection, National Cat Centre, Chelwood Gate,
Haywards Heath, Sussex RH17 7TT, UK

Jenny Stavisky
BVM&S PhD FHEA MRCVS
University of Nottingham, Nottingham NG7 2RD, UK

Published by:

British Small Animal Veterinary Association
Woodrow House, 1 Telford Way,
Waterwells Business Park, Quedgeley,
Gloucester GL2 2AB

A Company Limited by Guarantee in England
Registered Company No. 2837793
Registered as a Charity

Figures 6.11, 12.4 and the drawings in Quick Reference Guide 19.5 were drawn by S.J. Elmhurst BA Hons (www.livingart.org.uk) and are printed with her permission.

A catalogue record for this book is available from the British Library.

978 1 905319 84 8

The publishers, editors and contributors cannot take responsibility for information provided on dosages and methods of application of drugs mentioned or referred to in this publication. Details of this kind must be verified in each case by individual users from up to date literature published by the manufacturers or suppliers of those drugs. Veterinary surgeons are reminded that in each case they must follow all appropriate national legislation and regulations (for example, in the United Kingdom, the prescribing cascade) from time to time in force.

Printed by Cambrian Printers, Aberystwyth, UK
Printed on ECF paper made from sustainable forests

Titles in the BSAVA Manuals series

Manual of Avian Practice: A Foundation Manual
Manual of Canine & Feline Abdominal Imaging
Manual of Canine & Feline Abdominal Surgery
Manual of Canine & Feline Advanced Veterinary Nursing
Manual of Canine & Feline Anaesthesia and Analgesia
Manual of Canine & Feline Behavioural Medicine
Manual of Canine & Feline Cardiorespiratory Medicine
Manual of Canine & Feline Clinical Pathology
Manual of Canine & Feline Dentistry and Oral Surgery
Manual of Canine & Feline Dermatology
Manual of Canine & Feline Emergency and Critical Care
Manual of Canine & Feline Endocrinology
Manual of Canine & Feline Endoscopy and Endosurgery
Manual of Canine & Feline Fracture Repair and Management
Manual of Canine & Feline Gastroenterology
Manual of Canine & Feline Haematology and Transfusion Medicine
Manual of Canine & Feline Head, Neck and Thoracic Surgery
Manual of Canine & Feline Musculoskeletal Disorders
Manual of Canine & Feline Musculoskeletal Imaging
Manual of Canine & Feline Nephrology and Urology
Manual of Canine & Feline Neurology
Manual of Canine & Feline Oncology
Manual of Canine & Feline Ophthalmology
Manual of Canine & Feline Radiography and Radiology: A Foundation Manual
Manual of Canine & Feline Rehabilitation, Supportive and Palliative Care:
    Case Studies in Patient Management
Manual of Canine & Feline Reproduction and Neonatology
Manual of Canine & Feline Shelter Medicine: Principles of Health and Welfare in a Multi-animal Environment
Manual of Canine & Feline Surgical Principles: A Foundation Manual
Manual of Canine & Feline Thoracic Imaging
Manual of Canine & Feline Ultrasonography
Manual of Canine & Feline Wound Management and Reconstruction
Manual of Canine Practice: A Foundation Manual
Manual of Exotic Pet and Wildlife Nursing
Manual of Exotic Pets: A Foundation Manual
Manual of Feline Practice: A Foundation Manual
Manual of Ornamental Fish
Manual of Practical Animal Care
Manual of Practical Veterinary Nursing
Manual of Psittacine Birds
Manual of Rabbit Medicine
Manual of Rabbit Surgery, Dentistry and Imaging
Manual of Raptors, Pigeons and Passerine Birds
Manual of Reptiles
Manual of Rodents and Ferrets
Manual of Small Animal Practice Management and Development
Manual of Wildlife Casualties

For further information on these and all BSAVA publications, please visit our website: **www.bsava.com**

Contents

Section 3: Working with people in the shelter environment

Appendix

Quick reference guides

Contributors

Wendy Adams
BVSc BSc CertVA PhD MRCVS
Eastfield Veterinary Clinic Ltd,
Station Road, North Thoresby, Grimsby,
Lincolnshire DN36 5QU, UK

Maria Afonso
DVM MScVet MRCVS
University of Liverpool,
Leahurst Campus, Chester High Road,
Neston, Wirral CH64 7TE, UK

Zoe Belshaw
MA VetMB PhD CertSAM DipECVIM-CA MRCVS
Recognised Specialist in Small Animal Medicine
School of Veterinary Medicine and Science,
University of Nottingham, Sutton Bonington campus,
Loughborough LE12 5RD, UK

Gemma Bourne
BVSc PGDip(CABC) MPhil MRCVS
Foxhall Veterinary Clinic,
Brookside close, Ruskington,
Lincolnshire NG34 9GB, UK

Paula Boyden
BVetMed MRCVS
Dogs Trust, 17 Wakley Street, London EC1V 7RQ, UK

Alexandra Brower
DVM DipACVP
Midwestern University College of Veterinary Medicine,
5725 West Utopia Road, Glendale, AZ 85308, USA

Tim Browning
MA VetMB MRCVS
PDSA Pet Aid Hospital,
10 Tuxford Close, Wolverhampton WV10 0JQ, UK

Joe Brownlie
CBE BVSc PhD FRCPath DipECVP DSc FRASE LLD h.c. FRAgS FRCVS
Royal Veterinary College,
Hawkshead Lane, North Mymms,
Hatfield, Hertfordshire AL9 7TA, UK

Sarah Caney
BVSc DipSAM(Feline) PhD MRCVS
RCVS Recognised Specialist in Feline Medicine
Vet Professionals Ltd,
Midlothian Innovation Centre,
Roslin, Midlothian EH25 9RE, UK

Rachel Casey
BVMS PhD MRCVS RCVS
Recognised Specialist in Veterinary Behavioural Medicine
Bristol Veterinary School, Langford House,
Langford, Bristol BS40 5DU, UK

Trevor Cooper
Cooper and Co Solicitors, The Old Boiler House,
Menzies Rd, Whitfield, Dover CT16 2HQ, UK

Victoria Crossley
BVM&S BSc MRCVS
Bristol Veterinary School,
Langford House, Langford, Bristol BS40 5DU, UK

Rachel Dean
BVMS PhD MSc(EBHC) DipSAM(Feline) SFHEA MRCVS
Recognised Specialist in Feline Medicine
VetPartners Ltd,
Leeman House, Station Business Park,
Holgate Park Drive, York YO26 4GB, UK

Nathalie Dowgray
BVSc MRCVS
Institute of Ageing and Chronic Disease,
University of Liverpool, William Henry Duncan Building,
6 West Derby Street, Liverpool L7 8TX, UK

Sarah Ellis
BSc(Hons) PGDip(CABC) PhD
International Cat Care,
Place Farm, Tisbury SP3 6LW, UK

Rebecca Elmore
BVMS MRCVS
Amical Veterinary Centre,
90 High Street, March, Cambridgeshire PE15 9LQ, UK

Sally Everitt
BVSc MRCVS
Vine Tree Vets,
Walford Road, Ross-on-Wye,
Herefordshire HR9 5RS, UK

Allison German
BVSc MSc PhD MRCVS
ACG Veterinary Consultancy,
Heswall, Wirral CH60 7RJ, UK

Andy Gibson
BVetMed(Hons)
Mission Rabies,
4 Castle Street, Cranborne, Dorset BH21 5PZ, UK

Steve Goward
Dogs Trust,
17 Wakley Street, London EC1V 7RQ, UK

Tim Gruffydd-Jones
BVetMed PhD MRCVS
Bristol Veterinary School,
Langford House, Langford, Bristol BS40 5DU, UK

Vicky Halls
RVN DipCouns
PO Box 269, Faversham ME13 3AZ, UK

Runa Hanaghan
BVSc PGDip SSRM MRCVS
Dogs Trust, 17 Wakley Street, London EC1V 7RQ, UK

Sarah Heath
BVSc DipECAWBM(BM) CCAB MRCVS
RCVS and EBVS European Recognised Specialist in Veterinary Behavioural Medicine
Behavioural Referrals Veterinary Practice,
10 Rushton Dr, Upton, Chester CH2 1RE, UK

John Helps
BVetMed CertSAM MRCVS
Companion Animal Business Unit, MSD Animal Health,
Walton Manor, Walton, Milton Keynes MK7 7AJ, UK

Karen Hiestand
BVSc MSc BSc MA MRCVS
University of Surrey, Guildford, Surrey GU2 7XH, UK

Virginia Luis Fuentes
MA VetMB CertVR DVC PhD DipACVIM DipECVIM-CA MRCVS
RCVS Recognised Specialist in Veterinary Cardiology
Royal Veterinary College, Hawkshead Lane,
North Mymms, Hatfield, Hertfordshire AL9 7TA, UK

Ian MacFarlaine
RVN
Inspectorate Department Bermuda SPCA,
32 Valley Road, Paget, Bermuda

Dorothy McKeegan
BSc(Hons) MSc PhD
Institute of Biodiversity, Animal Health and Comparative Medicine, University of Glasgow,
Bearsden Road, G61 1QH, UK

Lila Miller
BS DVM
American Society for the Prevention of Cruelty to Animals, 520 8th Avenue, New York, NY 10018-4100, USA

Lisa Morrow
DipAppChemBiol BMLSc DVM MSc(VetEpi) DLSHTM MRCVS
School of Veterinary Medicine and Science,
University of Nottingham, Sutton Bonington campus,
Loughborough LE12 5RD, UK

Emily Newbury
VetMB MRCVS
School of Veterinary Medicine and Science,
University of Nottingham, Sutton Bonington campus,
Loughborough LE12 5RD, UK

Shaun Opperman
BVSc MRCVS
Battersea Dogs and Cats Home,
4 Battersea Park Road, London SW8 4AA, UK

Jessie Rose Payne
BVetMed MVetMed DipACVIM PhD MRCVS
Langford Small Animal Referral Hospital,
University of Bristol, Langford House, Langford,
Bristol BS40 5DU, UK

Alan Radford
BVSc BSc PhD MRCVS
Institute of Infection and Global Health,
University of Liverpool, Leahurst Campus,
Chester High Road, Neston, Wirral CH64 7TE, UK

Maggie Roberts
BVM&S MRCVS
Cats Protection, National Cat Centre, Chelwood Gate,
Haywards Heath, West Sussex RH17 7TT, UK

Janet M. Scarlett
DVM MPH PhD
Cornell University, Ithaca, New York 14853, USA

Steve Shaw
BVetMed PhD DVD MRCVS
UK VetDerm, 16 Talbot Street, Whitwick,
Coalville, Leicestershire LE67 5AW, UK

Beth Skillings
BVSc MRCVS
Cats Protection, National Cat Centre, Chelwood Gate,
Haywards Heath, West Sussex RH17 7TT, UK

Jenny Stavisky
BVM&S PhD FHEA MRCVS
School of Veterinary Medicine and Science,
University of Nottingham, Sutton Bonington Campus,
Loughborough LE12 5RD, UK

Dominic Sullivan
LLB(Hons) Solicitor
Cats Protection, National Cat Centre, Chelwood Gate,
Haywards Heath, West Sussex RH17 7TT, UK

Séverine Tasker
BSc BVSc DipSAM PhD DipECVIM-CA FHEA MRCVS
Bristol Veterinary School, Langford House,
Langford, Bristol BS40 5DU, UK

Nicky Trevorrow
BSc(Hons) PG Dip(CABC) RVN
Cats Protection, National Cat Centre, Chelwood Gate,
Haywards Heath, West Sussex RH17 7TT, UK

Carri Westgarth
BSc MPH PhD
Institute of Infection and Global Health,
University of Liverpool, Leahurst Campus,
Chester High Road, Neston, Wirral CH64 7TE, UK

Kate White
MA VetMB DVA DipECVAA MRCVS
School of Veterinary Medicine and Science,
University of Nottingham, Sutton Bonington Campus,
Loughborough LE12 5RD, UK

Rebecca Willby
BVSc BSc MRCVS
RSPCA Birmingham Animal Centre and Hospital,
Newbrook Farm, Frankley Green Lane, Frankley,
Birmingham B32 4AX, UK

David Yates
BVSc MRCVS
RSPCA Greater Manchester Animal Hospital,
411 Eccles New Road, Salford,
Manchester M5 5NN, UK

James Yeates
BVSc BSc DWEL DipECAWBM PhD FRCVS
RSPCA,
Wilberforce Way,
Horsham, West Sussex RH13 9RS, UK

Helen Zulch
BVSc(Hons) DipECAWMB MRCVS
RCVS Recognised Specialist in Veterinary Behavioural Medicine
Dogs Trust, 17 Wakley Street, London EC1V 7RQ, UK

Foreword

I was very honoured to be asked to write the foreword for the first edition of the *BSAVA Manual of Canine and Feline Shelter Medicine: Principles of Health and Welfare in a Multi-animal Environment*. As veterinary surgeons (veterinarians) in the USA began to work more closely with shelters in the 1980s, it quickly became clear that shelter medicine is much more than disease control, and that the knowledge gained from a traditional veterinary education alone was not broad enough to truly improve the welfare of the innumerable homeless animals being cared for. The unique medical, behavioural, organizational and emotional challenges faced by shelters dealing with limited resources, and an increasing awareness of and responsiveness to the human animal bond, necessitated the development of innovative, science-based approaches to best serve this often neglected population.

When I co-edited the Shelter Medicine for Veterinarians and Staff textbook that was published in 2004, shelter medicine was still in its infancy and faced an uncertain future. However, the field matured and the creation of a board certified specialty in shelter medicine in the USA in 2014, along with several educational programmes at veterinary colleges and conferences, confirmed the need for specialised training to help animals in shelters. Veterinary experts created special wellness and disease prevention protocols for animals in the USA shelters and, while some disease control principles are universal, veterinary surgeons working with shelters in the UK must ensure that their protocols reflect an understanding of the different laws and the distinct challenges regarding stray population control, shelter design, neutering programmes, rehoming strategies, euthanasia and countless other subjects.

BSAVA has assembled an impressive array of international experts to cover all these topics in this comprehensive manual. This excellent resource is an essential addition to any veterinary surgeon's library, whether employed by a shelter or not, and I am very proud to have been asked to be a contributing author.

Lila Miller BS DVM
Vice President, Shelter Medicine,
American Society for the Prevention of Cruelty to Animals

Preface

Shelter medicine is a newly emerging clinical discipline in veterinary medicine. It is a recognized speciality in the United States and interest is growing across the rest of the world. Shelter medicine encompasses vital aspects of physical and psychological health and welfare, infectious disease management, epidemiology, diagnostic testing and population control. The challenge of being a good shelter medicine clinician is balancing the health and welfare needs of the individual with that of the larger population from which it originates. Simultaneously, it is essential to be cognisant of the culture, ethos, polices and resources of the organization which shelters the animal. The clinical setting is vastly different to that of private practice, requiring a different set of skills and an informed and pragmatic approach.

Our aim with this manual is not to provide an exhaustive textbook on all aspects of shelter medicine. Instead, we want to introduce the reader to a new way of thinking when approaching cases in this environment; each chapter has a number of Quick Reference Guides that provide specific practical information on a number of subjects. There is an extensive resources section in the Appendix 1, which supports the manual content.

The manual is divided into three sections:
The first section covers the principles of shelter medicine, describing how to approach problems and be an effective decision maker within the shelter context. It includes the concepts of 'herd health' and epidemiology, which are usually applied in a large animal context. In addition, different perceptions and definitions of ethics and animal welfare are covered, and how to incorporate them into clinical decision-making, including population control and euthanasia.

The second section covers the prevention, management and control of infectious diseases and the management of behaviour in the shelter environment. The major infectious disease syndromes are presented by affected body system, rather than by pathogen, for ease of use in clinical situations. The second half of this section focuses on the psychological and emotional effects of caring for large numbers of cats and dogs within a single environment. The importance of socialization of young animals and environmental enrichment is covered, and an approach to training fearful cats and dogs is included.

The third section of the manual encompasses the 'people aspect' of shelter medicine. Providing clinical care for animals in shelters has to be done alongside the people working there and with an understanding of the objectives, policies and values of the individual organization that runs the shelter. Some organizations focus on rehoming, while others face the challenges of dealing with problematic situations, such as hoarding and non-accidental injury; an introduction to these aspects of shelter medicine is included.

We are delighted to have been given the opportunity to create and edit the first edition of the *BSAVA Manual of Canine and Feline Shelter Medicine* and feel this will provide useful information for anyone who undertakes clinical work, whether it be in private practice or in a charity setting.

We would like to thank the many contributors to this manual for their knowledge, insight, wisdom, hard work, humour, inspiration and patience during the production of this book. Many of them work in hugely challenging clinical environments and they work tirelessly to protect the health and welfare of thousands of animals in their care. Their expertise shines through in the content of this manual and will go further to impact and improve the care of many more cats and dogs. We would also like to thank the BSAVA publication team for their unwavering support of our contributors and us, the editorial team. Finally, we wish to thank our family, friends and colleagues who have continued to support us as we realized our ambition to create a manual of shelter medicine, and have remained patient and supportive through the long nights and weekends of work. In particular we would like to thank Rachel's family, Jamie, Michael and Christopher, Maggie's Cats Protection family and Jenny's family, Chris and Sam.

We are very proud of the manual and we sincerely hope you will find it a useful and practical aid to your clinical work in the charity setting.

Rachel Dean, Maggie Roberts and Jenny Stavisky
October 2018

Chapter 1

What is shelter medicine?

Rachel Dean, Jenny Stavisky and Janet M. Scarlett

Shelter medicine is a newly emerging discipline of veterinary medicine. The clinical focus for veterinary professionals working in this field is the population of unowned animals cared for by charities or individuals until they find new homes. Shelter medicine encompasses all the health and welfare needs of these animals and involves working closely with the organizations that care for them. The term describes a way of thinking and a clinical style that is applicable not only to 'shelters' in the traditional sense or those using a network of fosterers, but also to other types of charity-based medicine, including low-cost veterinary hospitals, high-throughput neutering, work in field clinics with free-living or community-owned animals, and dealing with hoarding and other emergency situations.

Even within organizations primarily concerned with rehoming animals, the term 'shelter' can be controversial. Some organizations avoid using this term, as they feel it inaccurately suggests that they aim to provide a permanent home for their animals. Descriptions such as 'rehoming centre' and 'rescue' are often used instead. The choice of identity may reflect the values and principles of the organization involved. Each organization is different, and, even within a given organization, different branches may function very differently. Some organizations are very pragmatic and aim to rehome animals in a very business-like way, focusing on the best overall outcome for the greatest possible number; whereas others take the approach that every animal can be saved and may focus on the needs of each individual. Euthanasia policy is often a decisive – and sometimes divisive – issue. Some shelters have a strong 'no-kill' ethos; others will euthanase animals only if they have severe physical or psychological health problems, while some may feel forced to euthanase animals, sometimes in high numbers, as a result of an overwhelming demand for space.

Some large shelters have a dedicated team of veterinary surgeons (veterinarians) and veterinary nurses based permanently on site who undertake all the veterinary work required. Similarly, some providers of low-cost veterinary care run hospitals with dedicated veterinary professionals providing a tailored service. This is far from universally the case, however, and in the UK the majority of shelters engage the services of private veterinary practitioners. Additionally, many thousands of animals are treated in private veterinary clinics every year under the auspices of schemes run by a number of charities, including the RSPCA (Royal Society for the Prevention of Cruelty to Animals), Blue Cross and PDSA (People's Dispensary for Sick Animals). These schemes provide subsidized care via private practices to stray and injured animals, and subsidize veterinary, preventive care and neutering for owners unable to meet costs.

A survey carried out by the charity Cats Protection (www.cats.org.uk) in 2008 found that 94.8% of veterinary practices in the UK did some form of work with charities. It is estimated that around 90,000 dogs and 130,000 cats pass through shelters and rescue centres each year, although the true figure is likely to be much higher (Stavisky et al., 2012). It has been estimated that around one-third of the 8 million pet dogs and 10 million cats in the UK are obtained from a rehoming charity (Pet Food Manufacturers Association, 2008). It is, therefore, clear that even when veterinary practices do not deal with shelter clients directly, a proportion of their pet owners will have acquired their animals from a charitable organization. Animals that have been rehomed from a shelter still require this aspect of their origin to be considered, particularly in the immediate post-adoption period.

In contrast to the situation in the UK, the number of veterinary surgeons in the USA specializing in shelter medicine is growing rapidly and, at the time of writing, 80% of veterinary schools in the USA have some form of shelter medicine programme. This increase has been fuelled by the sheer number of homeless animals requiring care, societal expectations, the growth of shelter medicine courses and post-DVM training programmes in veterinary colleges, and the newly recognized specialty in shelter medicine. Many shelters in the USA still receive veterinary services from private practitioners, but a growing number have full-time or part-time shelter medicine specialists on their staff. These specialist veterinary surgeons have training beyond that of the traditional small animal practitioner, encompassing infectious disease management at the population level, preventive medicine, behavioural health, veterinary forensics, shelter metrics, staff training, shelter-oriented protocols (such as those relating to vaccination, treatments, sanitation and facility design) and other topics. The need for this additional training has led to the formal recognition of shelter medicine as a boarded specialty under the aegis of the American Board of Veterinary Practitioners.

In the future, other countries may follow this path, and shelter medicine may become a specialization internationally. Whether or not this occurs – and even though there are many differences between shelters in the USA and elsewhere – the skills and expertise of veterinary surgeons working at shelters in the USA represent valuable experiences to draw on that can be adapted for use by their counterparts around the world.

Clinical approach: herd health for companion animals

Shelter medicine requires a different approach to the care of cats and dogs than that used in the care of owned animals. This is because in a shelter the treatment of one individual may affect the potential health and treatment options of a much larger population. In many situations, the veterinary care and management of these animals bears more resemblance to farm animal practice, where animals often present in herds (Figure 1.1), than to companion animal practice, where they more commonly present singly or in small numbers. It is essential that the health and welfare needs of each individual patient are met but, at the same time, it is crucial that this does not compromise the needs of the shelter population considered as a whole. This is the case whether the veterinary surgeon is working directly for a shelter or seeing shelter animals within the context of private practice.

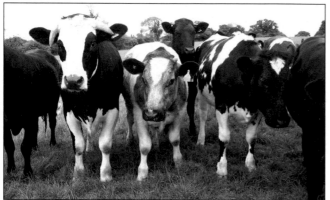

1.1 Principles of herd health, including consideration of the entire group of animals, awareness of husbandry and monitoring of key performance indicators, are transferable from farm animal practice to shelter medicine.
(Courtesy of M Brennan)

A dynamic population

When veterinary surgeons practice shelter medicine, they need to think about some heterogeneous sub-populations of animals (Figure 1.2). The whole pet population is divided into two groups – the unowned and the owned populations. The unowned population can be subdivided further into animals that are housed in a shelter and those that are

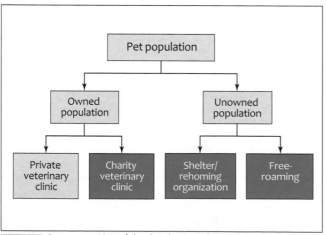

1.2 Representation of the distribution of the pet population and where the principles of shelter medicine apply (shown in green).

free-roaming (e.g. feral or stray cats and dogs). The owned population can be subdivided into animals that receive healthcare from private veterinary clinics and those that receive subsidized care via charitable organizations. Of course, more widely, there are also many animals that never receive veterinary care.

Within an animal's lifetime, it may move – sometimes several times – between these populations, depending on its ownership status and the circumstances of the owner. The challenges to the health and welfare of each individual animal will vary depending on the population it is in at any given time. However, experiences and diseases acquired in one phase of life can be carried forward and remain relevant lifelong. For example, puppies that do not receive appropriate socialization and reassurance while in a shelter may remain fearful after adoption, and kittens infected with high concentrations of coronavirus may be at increased risk of feline infectious peritonitis (FIP) as they age.

Application of the principles of shelter medicine to charity practice

The basic principles of considering the whole picture, the whole population and the most efficient targeting of resources apply equally well to a shelter, a charity hospital or when seeing shelter or charity clients within private practice. Even when patients are seen individually, they should always be regarded as inextricably part of a larger population. Pragmatic decisions about care must still be made. For example, choosing to perform a pre-anaesthetic biochemistry profile on a healthy patient before elective neutering may be considered ideal in some circumstances, but may represent the cost of vaccinating several other animals in a shelter situation.

Application of the principles of shelter medicine to private practice

Many of the basic principles of shelter medicine are applicable to any clinical situation, whether within a charity or a private practice and across species. The core principle of the veterinary profession is advocacy for the patient, tempered by respect for the owner or carer. However, when resources are constrained and repercussions may occur at a population level, it becomes particularly important to make decisions with clarity, good evidence and a deep understanding of the needs of each stakeholder, while remaining the advocate for the animals.

As for any new discipline, a consensus definition of 'shelter medicine' has not yet been achieved. The Association of Shelter Veterinarians in the USA defines shelter medicine as 'a field of veterinary medicine dedicated to the care of homeless animals in shelters or other facilities dedicated to finding them new homes'. Even in the USA, however, some practitioners find this definition restrictive, and would include in their definition the care of owned animals seized because of neglect or cruelty, those temporarily separated from their owner by disaster, and high-volume, high-quality neutering of owned and unowned animals. However, most shelter medicine specialists in the USA do not consider the provision of charity (subsidized) care for owned animals to fall under the purview of shelter medicine. Some animal shelters in the USA do operate full-service veterinary hospitals or wellness clinics, but services are delivered to individual owned animals where the primary decision-maker is the owner, analogous to the situation in private practice. In light of this, shelters that operate veterinary clinics often employ both shelter medicine specialists to deliver care to animals in the shelter population, and traditionally trained veterinary surgeons to deliver care to owned animals presented to the clinics.

In contrast, in the UK, the division between charity and private practice is less clearly defined. Indeed, many private practitioners will carry out some kind of shelter medicine or charitable treatment, whether on an occasional or regular basis. In this situation, the distinction between shelter medicine and private practice becomes one of context more than clinical specialization.

The decision-making process

Decision-making is the cornerstone of any kind of veterinary practice. Scientists and medical professionals tend towards a belief in making balanced, logical decisions. However, many studies have shown that, far from this idealized picture, humans are highly intuitive and often make decisions at a subconscious level based on pattern recognition. These heuristics (or 'rules of thumb') evolved to enable early humans to make decisions – such as whether to run away from a dangerous predator – very quickly. This tendency has been passed down through the generations, and is responsible for many aspects of how we see the world, from mistakenly 'recognizing' strangers in the street to responding to a placebo pill (and even responding better to two placebo pills than one). However, in our world of complex and multifaceted decision-making, heuristics can fail quite spectacularly. Therefore, it is helpful to break down the components of decision-making and consider separately the major factors that feed into the choices veterinary surgeons make when practising shelter medicine.

The difficulty in many of the decisions made in this context is often created by the challenge of balancing conflicting needs and wants. Prominent points of conflict include the distribution of resources between individuals and groups, and societal and personal concerns, norms and perceptions.

Individuals *versus* groups

No matter how big or small, every shelter will have limitations on money, time, human resources and space. Deciding how to distribute these resources is critical. This requires a thorough appreciation of the ethical standpoint of the organization caring for the animals in question, as well as a clear understanding of what we are personally and professionally prepared to do.

For example, some shelters will invest time, money and emotional commitment to intensively nurse kittens with cat 'flu. Other organizations take the decision to euthanase even quite mildly affected kittens in order to limit the infectious burden within the population and reduce the risk of infection to other cats. The eventual consequences of a decision can sometimes be unexpectedly disproportionate to what might be expected. For example, dermatophytosis (ringworm) is common, not life-threatening, and typically self-resolves over a few weeks. However, due to the zoonotic risk and potential for long-term environmental contamination, some shelters will euthanase animals with ringworm. The consequences of an outbreak of ringworm could, in extreme cases, involve closing temporarily some or all of a shelter, in which case many more animals could lose the opportunity to be rehomed and potentially be euthanased as a result.

Societal concerns, norms and perceptions

Societal norms form the unspoken context of veterinary medicine. However, these norms can differ substantially between organizations and, on a wider scale, when working with different populations of animals. For example, in the USA, procedures such as declawing, ear cropping and testicular implants are considered to be 'the norm' by many, whereas in the UK they would be considered to be unethical mutilations or unnecessary cosmetic procedures. In contrast, in Scandinavia, prophylactic neutering of dogs is considered to be an unnecessary mutilation, whereas it is routine (and often seen as a sign of responsible pet ownership) in the UK and USA. Within society, pet ownership, veterinary care and surgery can carry a weight of cultural expectation, which varies from a highly utilitarian perspective to viewing animals as family members.

The public perception of shelters and animal welfare is also often highly coloured by emotion, particularly with regard to the euthanasia of animals considered potentially rehomeable. It is intuitively shocking to many veterinary professionals to consider euthanasing animals for what would, in a different context, be treatable conditions. For the pet-owning public, the ethical stances of different animal welfare organizations often prove to be an emotive subject, possibly bolstered by a lack of overview on the sources of these problems. It can be easier to blame particular organizations for 'not really trying' than to recognize the complex social reasons underlying overpopulation of companion animal species. The strong societal component is underlined by the fact that in some northern European countries, such as Norway (where prophylactic neutering of dogs is prohibited), there is effectively no dog overpopulation problem.

The challenges of shelter medicine

Working with different stakeholders

One of the great challenges, and positive aspects, of shelter medicine is the vast number of different organizations and individuals with which veterinary surgeons can work. The shelter may be anything from a national government-run organization to a single individual sheltering a very small number of animals. Some organizations will have strict and rigorous policies that need to be adhered to, whereas others may have very little in the way of structured guidance or policy (see Chapter 20). The experience and/or knowledge of the individuals working within organizations can also be very variable, as the veterinary team may be working with an experienced shelter manager one moment and a new volunteer the next (Figure 1.3) (see Chapters 22 and 23 for further details).

Difficulties can arise in a number of situations. Possibly, the most frequent challenge will be animals with conditions that need time and resources spent on them and which, therefore, slow the 'flow' of animals through the shelter. As the aim of many organizations is to rehome each animal as quickly as possible, this can lead to conflict between the veterinary surgeon/team and the operational side of the organization. This is inevitable no matter what type of organization the veterinary surgeon is working with.

Another potential, but common, difficulty arises when the policies or beliefs of the people working within the

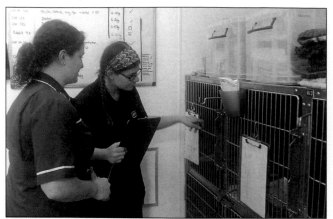

1.3 Effective communication between the veterinary team and all members of staff is essential to ensure the best possible care for animals in a shelter.
(Courtesy of J Toner)

shelter organization are different from those of the veterinary surgeon undertaking the clinical work. Euthanasia of animals can be a frequent point of contention, either when a veterinary surgeon wants to euthanase an animal but the organization does not agree, or, conversely, when a veterinary surgeon is asked to euthanase a number of healthy animals. Both parties will always want what is 'best' for the animals, but opinions on what is best may differ on the basis of personal and professional experience.

Such issues are often tied to underlying ethical principles, which may not be consciously considered (Mullan and Main, 2001). Some practitioners hold absolutist ethics, which consider causing harm to any individual animal to be an unacceptable violation of its rights (see Chapter 2). This is also a relatively common approach among workers in shelter organizations. In the field of shelter medicine, the most common approach among veterinary professionals is a pragmatic utilitarian approach, whereby we strive to do the greatest good (or the least harm) for the greatest number – even if that is at a cost to the welfare of some individuals. This principle, which is reflected in much of the content of this manual, is simply due to the overwhelming size of the population of animals with which we are faced in shelter medicine. Some readers may find this approach challenging, uncomfortable or even unacceptable. However, by mapping the points on our own moral compass, we can each more fully understand our own decision-making process.

Balancing physical and psychological health

The time spent in a shelter by any animal has the potential to compromise both its physical and its psychological health. Shelter populations are at increased risk of disease. Infectious diseases are common, owing to close mixing of a heterogeneous population of animals exchanging pathogens. Stress can also be a factor, both in perpetuating disease and also as a primary causative agent, for example, diarrhoea and feline lower urinary tract disease. A clinically ill animal is likely to take longer to be rehomed, exposing it to further risk of stress-related physical disease as well as psychological or behavioural problems. Animals that have behavioural problems are harder to rehome, increasing their length of stay and risk of physical and psychological health problems. This is a vicious cycle that is expensive in terms of both time and financial resources and can be very hard to break. In addition, what

might be a good physical environment to reduce stress (e.g. group housing of dogs) may make the control of infectious disease and management of the population impossible. This is true of all shelters, even where significant interventions are in place to reduce stress (see Chapter 19).

Stress, welfare and behaviour

Most shelters represent a relatively stressful environment for cats and dogs. In the shelter environment, life is full of new and potentially unwelcome experiences for the animals. The resident animals may have been free-roaming or in a home before entering the shelter. In either case, they are likely to have more restrictions on their physical space and to be in close proximity to a large number of conspecifics (and potentially other species) to which they have not previously been socialized. In some situations, even prey and predator species may be housed near each other. The animals may be habituated to humans to a variable degree, and their caregivers in the shelter are almost inevitably unfamiliar and can change frequently. The smells, sights and sounds are new. The animals have little ability to control their own environment and may find it fear-inducing and unpredictable, at least at first. Following a period of adaptation, animals will often acclimatize to some extent to the shelter environment. Stress falls during this period, but in many animals it subsequently rises again (e.g. due to barrier frustration, boredom, disease), along with an increase in frustration-related behaviours, such as spinning, vocalizing and obsessively soliciting attention.

It is, therefore, important to consider the psychological impact of any intervention in a shelter. It is inevitable that trade-offs will occur. For example, careful isolation of a litter of puppies in a shelter where parvovirus infection is endemic is clearly a sensible clinical decision. However, depriving the same litter of social and environmental stimuli during a critical period of development could lead to the development of severe behavioural problems later in life, potentially even resulting in euthanasia. In fact, unacceptable behaviour is one of the most commonly stated reasons for relinquishing animals to a shelter (Salman et al., 1998; Diesel et al., 2009). Therefore, care must be taken to balance best clinical practice with the recognition of the psychological needs of the animal, as these factors can often be in conflict.

Balancing conflicting needs can be extremely difficult and complex, and different aspects of animal welfare may be weighted differentially, according to the perspective of the various stakeholders (see Chapter 19). For example, some feral cat workers will weigh the importance of a secure home and regular access to food much more highly than the importance of freedom to perform natural behaviours, resulting in these essentially wild animals being kept in cages in a constant state of severe stress (Figure 1.4). When assessing decisions made in such circumstances, the key tenet, as stated in Chapter 2, is simply that 'No animal's welfare should be made worse by the organization's work'.

Gathering consistent clinical information about individuals and the population

Some organizations may rely extensively on volunteers to care for animals, foster them, raise funds and carry out many other tasks – sometimes including transporting animals to the veterinary surgery, for shelters that do not

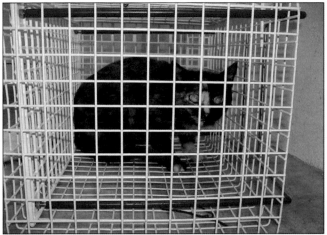

1.4 Even brief periods of captivity can be stressful for feral cats. This cat was placed in a crush cage prior to being anaesthetized for neutering as part of a trap-neuter-return programme. The programme organizers balanced the relatively short period of stress and discomfort for each individual against the improvement in welfare for the population of cats.
(© Jenny Stavisky)

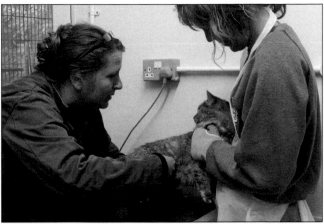

1.5 Veterinary surgeon examining a cat and discussing its history during a shelter visit.
(© Jenny Stavisky)

have an on-site veterinary team. The animal's primary caregiver, the main decision-maker and the person presenting the animal for treatment may therefore all be different people. This can make history taking quite challenging, particularly when seeing an animal presented at the surgery, away from the shelter, and also means that decisions about diagnostic work-up and treatment options must all be confirmed with the person with authority for making such decisions. This may be complicated by a lack of prior information, or inconsistent information, about the animal. Having different caregivers can lead to difficulties in obtaining an accurate case history and deciding which procedures or treatments provide the best option overall. As with any patient, a thorough history is essential. Obtaining this may also necessitate identifying the animal's primary caregiver, in order to obtain the best possible information when following the clinical progression of cases.

Principles and skills needed to meet the challenges

Know your shelter

Frequent visits to the shelter for private practitioners who provide veterinary services to a shelter, or regular site examinations of the non-veterinary areas of shelters that have a veterinary team *in situ*, will help to deal with many of the challenges listed above. Only by seeing the animals in their everyday environment and working directly alongside the people who care for them, can the pressures on the shelter be understood (Figure 1.5). Basic information that a veterinary surgeon will need to understand the environment is outlined in Figure 1.6.

Epidemiology and shelter metrics to aid decision-making

A survey of shelters in the USA found that only 36% had a disease outbreak plan, and only 6% had a veterinary surgeon in charge of infectious disease control; 90% of respondents said they would like further training on infectious disease control (Steneroden *et al.*, 2011). While

- **Where do the animals come from?**
  - Are they predominantly stray or owner-relinquished? What is their body condition/nutrition/potential immunity to disease?
  - Are many litters born on site?
  - Is intake controlled (e.g. waiting list, taking only certain types of animal) or is the organization open intake?
- **What biosecurity measures are in place?**
  - Is there a quarantine period? Many shelters will aim to keep animals quarantined for a variable period on entry, where possible in a separate block or building
  - Do animals stay in the same pen throughout their time in the shelter? If they are moved, what happens to their bedding/scratching post/litter tray?
  - Are cleaning and feeding materials shared between pens and between blocks?
  - Is the housing appropriate (size, materials, single or multi-animal occupancy) and are there sufficient trained staff to clean, disinfect and provide enrichment?
  - What preventive healthcare is already in place (vaccination, treatment for endoparasites and ectoparasites)? When is it given, by whom and to which animals?
- **What is the contingency plan?**
  - Is there a previous history of infectious disease?
  - Is there an isolation facility?
  - If so, is it separate from the main population? How are animals in this facility cared for? Are its resources shared with other housing areas?
- **What is the euthanasia policy?**
  - Is it clearly defined?
  - Are all staff aware of it and comfortable with it?

1.6 Basic information needed when visiting a shelter.

there are many differences between the situation in the USA and the UK, there is an opportunity for veterinary surgeons to become more actively involved in proactive 'herd health' programmes for shelters, rather than the reactive 'firefighting' approach that has been traditionally used.

To deal with populations of animals, as opposed to individuals, a small animal veterinary surgeon needs the following skill set:

- A basic understanding of the epidemiology of the diseases encountered, with a particular focus on the ways in which each disease spreads
- A good understanding of the social behaviours and population dynamics of the animals concerned
- An ability to think about the 'big picture'
- A basic understanding of shelter metrics
- An ability to work within the different ethical frameworks, environments, resources and pressures that are particular to each individual organization.

'Shelter metrics' (see Chapter 7) describes the systematic measurement of the performance of a shelter using data generated within the shelter environment (Hurley, 2004; Hurley and Miller, 2009; Scarlett, 2012; Newbury and Hurley, 2013). Many shelters put huge amounts of time, energy, emotion and money into their work, but shy away from systematically monitoring many of their outcomes. Veterinary surgeons make preventive medicine-related recommendations to minimize the frequency of disease in shelters, but rarely monitor the effects of those recommendations. At best, shelter workers might say, 'It seems as if we have less disease' or, 'The isolation ward appears to contain fewer cats' after the implementation of the veterinary surgeon's recommendations, but rarely quantitate the incidence of disease before and after the changes were made. Similarly, shelters often know their overall yearly rehoming statistics, but fail to link those statistics to their programmes aimed at reducing intake. Shelters are animal welfare organizations, but they are also businesses with the goal of rehoming homeless animals. As both an animal welfare organization and a business, they have an obligation to take all possible actions to ensure that the health and welfare of the animals they care for is constantly improving and that their resources are being wisely spent on behalf of the animals.

Creative thinking

In many shelters, the buildings, number of staff and financial constraints mean that it is not possible to create an ideal disease-free and stress-free environment. Shelters vary greatly in terms of the way they are designed and managed, so a change that will help to reduce stress in one shelter may not be possible in another. However, with some creative thinking, small but effective differences can be made. For example, all cats ideally need space where they can be alone and out of sight of other cats. This can be very difficult in an overcrowded cat shelter. In such situations, placing a blanket over the front of the cage or hanging it over a chair, or providing cardboard boxes for the cats to hide in, are inexpensive solutions (Figure 1.7). Similarly, in many dog shelters there is not enough outdoor space for all dogs to have their own exercise area. Identifying groups of dogs that can be exercised in a paddock together, or finding volunteers to walk dogs, will take the pressure off the shelter staff.

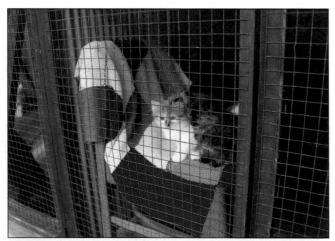

1.7 These kittens have chosen to sit on the comfortable blanket near the door of their enclosure, where they are on view to the public. The overhanging blanket also provides a potential hiding place below the chair.
(© Jenny Stavisky)

Pragmatic decision-making

Pragmatism is the cornerstone of clinical shelter medicine; what is appropriate for a private client may not always be the option of choice for a shelter client (see Chapter 3). For example, a complex and costly orthopaedic surgery may offer limb-sparing treatment for an individual animal, but for a shelter, a better option might be to proceed with an amputation and use the money saved to neuter another 15–20 animals, preventing many potentially unwanted litters.

Thinking about what is best for the shelter population can also mean 'thinking outside the box' with regard to veterinary interventions. For example, for kittens and puppies, initial vaccination is generally recommended at 6–9 weeks of age, with a second vaccination 2–5 weeks later, depending on the vaccine and species. However, in a shelter situation, particularly where there is a high disease burden or an active outbreak, off-label use of vaccines may be considered in order to protect the animals at highest risk. This can include vaccinating puppies and kittens from 4 weeks of age, and repeating doses at 2-week intervals until 16–18 weeks of age (Rickard et al., 1977; Schultz, 2006).

Another common question is whether all animals should be vaccinated on entry to a shelter, even if they are already compromised by poor condition or concurrent injury or disease. Each shelter's policies must be carefully considered to determine what is appropriate for that environment, and management practices such as appropriate use of isolation or fostering are also important. However, a risk–benefit calculation indicates that a vaccine is unlikely to harm the individual animal (although adjuvanted vaccines may on occasion cause fever and malaise) and may at least partially protect it from disease and reduce shedding of pathogens, thereby better protecting the shelter population. Studies in feral cats have shown that vaccination at the time of neutering induces a protective antibody response in the majority of cases (Fischer et al., 2007). This suggests that stress and surgery may not significantly inhibit the immune response to vaccines.

Evidence-based veterinary medicine

As shelter medicine is a new discipline, much remains to be learned about the optimal care of animals in shelters. Engagement with the principles of evidence-based veterinary medicine is essential in order to improve knowledge, understanding and practice (see Chapter 3). As well as providing veterinary care, the veterinary team has a role to play in understanding and improving the science behind the decisions made around the healthcare and management of animals in shelters. Many practitioners lack the skills to evaluate the value of published studies pertaining to shelter medicine, and information is accumulating rapidly. Unfortunately, peer-review and continuing education presentations cannot be counted on to ensure the validity of information. Therefore, in this rapidly expanding field, it is particularly incumbent on interested practitioners to evaluate much of the primary literature themselves. Similarly, while individual practitioners may not have the time or skills to initiate research projects themselves, they have a role to play in increasing the evidence base. A number of universities now have shelter medicine programmes, which are able to work with shelters and their veterinary teams to generate good data to aid decision-making.

Cruelty, forensics and the law

For some veterinary surgeons, there is a requirement to become involved in legal aspects of veterinary work.

Cruelty, hoarding and neglect are probably much more frequently encountered by those involved in charity practice. Dealing with these cases requires highly specialized knowledge of the legal system and of veterinary forensics. Although, some introductory material is presented within this manual (see QRGs 23.1 and 23.2), for more detailed information readers are referred to the British Veterinary Forensic and Law Association and the International Veterinary Forensic Science Association. Even outside these relatively specialized aspects of veterinary care, an awareness of the laws surrounding everyday practices, such as the use of medications (in particular those also used in humans), definitions of consent, data protection and animal ownership, is essential. Further detail of the current situation is provided in Chapter 21.

Conclusion

This clinical area is highly multidisciplinary and requires excellent communication skills, including a willingness to consider and concede to others' points of view. It is not a field that rewards the solo pioneer making unilateral decisions; instead, it demands listening, understanding, negotiation, compromise and, above all, teamwork. The veterinary team also has a responsibility to teach veterinary undergraduates about shelter medicine, to provide continuing professional development for practising veterinary surgeons and nurses and to support the education of lay shelter workers. A thorough understanding of the special needs of the groups of animals cared for by shelters, and the pressures of husbandry and management in these environments, will aid the practice of the demanding – but exceptionally rewarding – evolving discipline of shelter medicine.

References and further reading

Diesel G, Brodbelt D and Pfeiffer DU (2009) Characteristics of relinquished dogs and their owners at 14 rehoming centers in the United Kingdom. *Journal of Applied Animal Welfare Science* **13**, 15–30

Fischer SM, Quest CM, Dubovi EJ *et al.* (2007) Response of feral cats to vaccination at the time of neutering. *Journal of the American Veterinary Medical Association* **230**, 52–58

Hurley K (2004) Implementing a population health plan in an animal shelter: Goal setting, data collection and monitoring, and policy development. In: *Shelter Medicine for Veterinarians and Staff*, ed. L Miller and S Zawistowski, pp. 211–234. Wiley-Blackwell, Iowa

Hurley K and Miller L (2009) Introduction to disease management in animal shelters. In: *Infectious Disease Management in Animal Shelters*, ed. L Miller and K Hurley, pp. 13–15. Wiley-Blackwell, Iowa

Mullan S and Main D (2001) Ethical decision-making in veterinary practice. *Veterinary Record* **149**, 339–340

Newbury S and Hurley K (2013) Population management. In: *Shelter Medicine for Veterinarians and Staff, 2nd edn*, ed. L Miller and S Zawistowski, pp. 93–113. Wiley-Blackwell, Iowa

Pet Food Manufacturers Association (2008) *Pet Food Manufacturers Association Annual Report 2008*. www.pfma.org.uk

Rickard MD, Coman BJ and Cannon RM (1977) Age resistance and acquired immunity to *Taenia pisiformis* infection in dogs. *Veterinary Parasitology* **3**, 1–9

Salman M, New J, Scarlett J *et al.* (1998) Human and animal factors related to relinquishment of dogs and cats in 12 selected animal shelters in the United States. *Journal of Applied Animal Welfare Science* **1**, 207–226

Scarlett JM (2012) *Magical Metrics and Dazzling Data: How Medical Fact-Finding Guides Shelters to Improved Animal Health*. www.maddiesfund.org/Maddies_Institute/Webcasts/Magical_Metrics_and_Dazzling_Data.html

Schultz RD (2006) Feline vaccination programs in the shelter environment. *Proceedings of the North American Veterinary Conference* **20**, 1353–1354

Stavisky J, Brennan M, Downes M and Dean R (2012) Demographics and economic burden of unowned cats and dogs in the UK: results of a 2010 census. *BMC Veterinary Research* **8**, 163

Steneroden KK, Hill AE and Salman MD (2011) A needs-assessment and demographic survey of infection-control and disease awareness in western US animal shelters. *Preventive Veterinary Medicine* **98**, 52–57

Useful websites

Association of Shelter Veterinarians:
www.sheltervet.org

British Veterinary Forensic and Law Association:
www.bvfla.org.uk

International Veterinary Forensic Science Association:
www.ivfsa.org

QRG 1.1: Top 10 tips for shelter medicine vets

by Rachel Dean and Jenny Stavisky

1 Visit the shelter regularly: Every shelter is different. Knowledge of the layout, husbandry and available facilities is essential to understand how diseases can be acquired, transmitted, controlled and treated.

2 Engage with and respect the decision-making team: The funders, managers, animal carers, volunteers and public are all stakeholders in the health and welfare of animals in shelters. Running a shelter is a team effort – and it is important to be part of the team. Often, the views expressed by other members of the team may differ from your own. By respecting and engaging with all members of the team, no matter what their philosophy and viewpoint, the common priority of maximizing the health and welfare of animals in the shelter can be achieved.

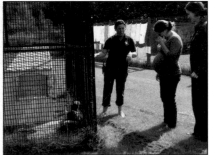

Engage with the shelter team.
(© Jenny Stavisky)

3 Think of many when faced with one: The animal presented to you needing treatment, preventive medicine or surgery needs individual care. However, every single shelter animal is part of a wider population, and decisions made for one member of that population will inevitably affect the others directly or indirectly.

4 Manage resources when making clinical decisions: Time, money and space are critical and limited resources in shelters, and must be used wisely and in keeping with the values/goals of the organization involved. Have clear reasons for making decisions, and ensure ➡

QRG 1.1 *continued*

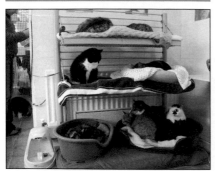

Resources are often limited and decisions on how to distribute them can be complex.
(© Jenny Stavisky)

that the long-term consequences, including the possibility of setting a precedent, are considered every time.

5 **Pragmatism is the key:** In an ideal situation, every animal would have care perfectly tailored to its needs. However, when resources are limited and a large population of animals needs to be considered, pragmatism and a utilitarian ethical stance are the cornerstone of shelter medicine. Retaining a vision for the future while dealing with the present often remains a personal challenge for many working in the field.

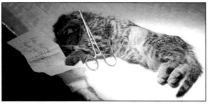

Pragmatic decision-making is essential – early neutering can reduce the need for euthanasia where overpopulation exists. This feral kitten has been neutered as part of a trap-neuter-return population control programme.
(© Jenny Stavisky)

6 **Face the challenge of bad news:** If a hard and unpopular decision needs to be made, check it is the right one and then carry it out quickly. Difficult decisions, such as euthanasing an individual animal or a

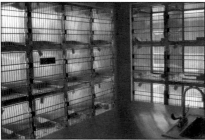

Sometimes difficult decisions must be made. This shelter opted to depopulate in order to control an outbreak of panleukopenia.
(© Rachel Dean)

group of animals, implementing time-consuming biosecurity measures or shutting a shelter, will never be easy or pleasant. However, if these decisions must be made, delaying them will not make them easier or more successful.

7 **Vaccinate and disinfect:** Infectious diseases are endemic to shelters. Constant vigilance is required to protect vulnerable populations of animals. Vaccines and excellent cleaning and disinfection (with due regard to balancing these with enrichment; see point 9) are the biggest weapons we have against these diseases. Take the time to engage with the shelter team, watch their cleaning routine and ask questions. Look for simple solutions such as colour-coded cleaning equipment, which can really help as a visual reminder and motivator of good biosecurity. Vaccinate judiciously and with a good consideration of the risks and benefits.

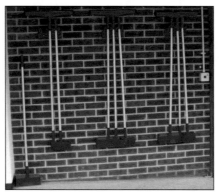

Colour-coding cleaning equipment can be useful in helping to maintain biosecurity within a shelter. The red equipment will only be used in the isolation block, and use of out of place equipment will be obvious.
(© Jenny Stavisky)

8 **Be sure of why you are undertaking a diagnostic test:** Diagnostic tests (beyond a history and clinical examination, which are the most important tests of all) need to be applied judiciously. They are expensive and, if not used with a clear rationale, can complicate a clinical picture as easily as they can simplify it. Ask yourself, 'What will I do if this

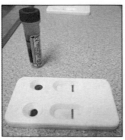

Diagnostic tests should be undertaken only where there is a clear rationale and the result will affect decision-making.
(© Jenny Stavisky)

test is positive? What will I do if it is negative?' If the answer to both questions is the same, do not undertake the test.

9 **Consider psychological health:** Clinicians often focus on the physical health of an animal, but sometimes find it harder to assess psychological health. Encourage the use of enrichment; a simple cardboard box placed in a cat's cage can transform the animal's welfare by giving it a place to hide. Balance the need for good hygiene with the need for an animal to have a stable olfactory environment. Engage with other animal care professionals with knowledge and understanding of animal behaviour. Be prepared to respect their opinion and take on their recommendations – they may be much more aware of aspects of animal welfare than most veterinary surgeons.

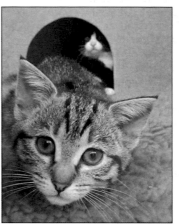

Where possible and appropriate, enrichment, which may be as simple as a hiding place, should be provided.
(© Jenny Stavisky)

10 **Make it a short stay:** However much we try to improve shelter environments, few are ideal places for animals to live in the long term. The ultimate goal is always to decrease the length of stay and increase throughput.

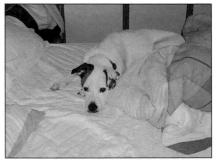

However well managed a shelter is, most animals will have better welfare in a home environment.
(Courtesy of Christopher Hawke)

Chapter 2

Ethics and animal welfare

James Yeates and Dorothy McKeegan

A wide range of animal shelters exist, from small single-site operations to nationwide organizations, and have a variety of operational constraints, ideological starting points and specific strategies. Despite these differences, they often share similar aims and face common welfare issues and ethical challenges. Shelters are usually not-for-profit organizations funded by charitable donations. They need to consider multiple animals, whose welfare and treatment can interact and whose presenting problems are often the result of factors external to the shelter. In addition, the work of shelters is set against a background of societal failures and public demands.

Decisions in shelter veterinary medicine differ from treatment choices for individual owned animals, primarily because of the interactions between different animals in a shelter. These interactions are essentially that:

* Animals can affect each other (e.g. noise, transmission of infection)
* Each animal can use up resources that could be spent on other animals (e.g. space or carer time).

These interactions raise critical ethical and welfare issues and require in particular that shelter medicine veterinary surgeons (veterinarians) should almost never consider a single animal in isolation (see also Chapter 1).

This chapter introduces specific welfare and ethical issues that are faced in shelter medicine and outlines the factors that give rise to them. It will focus on two key issues that are the source of many welfare and ethical concerns: the challenges of resource distribution and euthanasia. The discussion of how to meet these challenges will introduce the concept of ethical reasoning and consideration of further strategies that can be used to make appropriate, consistent individual, team and policy decisions. As the chapter aims to give a framework for each veterinary surgeon's own views, it adopts a pluralistic approach to ethics, accommodating a range of positions. While the principles are outlined here, it is important to recognize that real-life challenges often involve a more complex combination of many ethical concerns. Nevertheless, where appropriate, some prescriptive comments are given where the authors have found them to be helpful. Readers may choose to adopt these or utilize the tools provided to clarify their own ethical standpoint to draw appropriate conclusions. Different people involved, or supporting shelter work, may have a range of ethical views. As well as each ensuring our work is consistent with their own values, we should speak to others to enrich our views and be respectful of one another's.

Key welfare and ethical concepts

Welfare concepts

Animal welfare has been defined in various ways relating to an animal's health, ability to cope with challenges and opportunity to exhibit natural behaviour. Ultimately, animal welfare is about mental state, which can be unpleasant ('suffering') or pleasant ('enjoyment') (Figure 2.1). While veterinary medicine often focuses on removing or preventing negative states, there is increasing emphasis on the presence of positive states to ensure a good quality of life (Yeates and Main, 2009).

Unpleasant mental states
• Hunger and thirst
• Pain, pruritus, malaise, nausea and discomfort
• Distress, confusion and fear
• Frustration and boredom

Pleasant mental states
• Gustatory pleasure and satiety
• Play and comfort
• Contentment and control
• Satisfaction and interest

2.1 Key pleasant and unpleasant mental states that an animal may experience.

An animal's mental state depends on the balance and character of sensory and other inputs from within the animal's body and from its environment. For example, hunger depends on the animal's metabolism, its appetite, the availability of food and the animal's food intake. Fear depends on the animal's environment and its previous experiences. Many feelings, both unpleasant and pleasant, are related to the five welfare needs (Figure 2.2); in the UK these needs are set out in the Animal Welfare Act 2006. Veterinary surgeons can play a major role in the 'diagnosis' or identification of welfare problems and in treating them (Yeates, 2013).

• Need for a suitable environment
• Need for a suitable diet
• Need to be able to exhibit normal behaviour patterns
• Need to be housed with, or apart from, other animals
• Need to be protected from pain, suffering, injury and disease

2.2 The five welfare needs of animals.
(Adapted from the Animal Welfare Act 2006)

Assessing how animals feel can be difficult, but different mental states can reveal themselves in various physiological and behavioural states (i.e. signs). For example, animals in shelters may try to escape or bite their human caregivers (suggesting unpleasant associations with the environment or the presence of humans), have increased heart rates (suggesting fear, excitement or cardiovascular pathology), have raised plasma glucose concentrations (suggesting stress or diabetes), perform repetitive behaviours (suggesting frustration or boredom) or may be inactive (suggesting malaise, boredom or fear).

Each sign has a number of differential feelings that can be diagnosed. Often it is the combination of signs that needs to be considered to reach a diagnosis. In turn, these signs can cause further mental or physical states to be triggered; for example, excessive pacing may lead to footpad damage or excessive licking to granuloma formation.

It is well recognized that animals have a range of needs. Many of these are fundamentally linked to the biology of the species – often related to obtaining a particular resource or responding to a particular environmental or bodily stimulus. The most basic needs are encapsulated in the 'Five Freedoms' (which are closely related to the five welfare needs), while key opportunities for positive welfare are included in the corresponding 'Five Opportunities' (Figure 2.3). While basic, these are always helpful to consider as ways to promote good animal welfare and avoid negative mental states.

Five Freedoms		Five Opportunities	
Freedom	Provision required	Opportunity	Provision required
Freedom from hunger and thirst	By ready access to fresh water and a diet to maintain full health and vigour	Opportunity for selection of dietary inputs	By provision of a diet that has been preferentially selected
Freedom from discomfort	By providing an appropriate environment and a comfortable resting area	Opportunity for control of the environment	By allowing the achievement of motivations
Freedom from pain, injury and disease	By prevention or rapid diagnosis and treatment	Opportunity for pleasure, development and vitality	By maintaining and developing beneficial inputs
Freedom to express normal behaviour	By providing sufficient space, proper facilities and the company of the animal's own kind	Opportunity to express normal behaviour	By providing sufficient space, a good quality environment and group housing for social animals
Freedom from fear and distress	By ensuring conditions and treatment that avoid mental suffering	Opportunity for interest and confidence	By providing conditions and treatment that lead to mental enjoyment

2.3 The Five Freedoms and Five Opportunities.
(Adapted from FAWC (1993) and Yeates (2013))

Ethical concepts

Ethics is about what is right and wrong, good and bad. Therefore, ethics is (partly) about mental states as well, because it is reasonable to argue that suffering is intrinsically bad and should be avoided in all humans and animals that are able to suffer. From this, it follows that causing suffering is generally wrong and preventing suffering is right (depending on the circumstances). In this context,

ethical decisions should be partly animal welfare-based decisions. These ethical decisions are important to determine how practitioners should turn welfare assessments into actions. Less clear is whether death is intrinsically 'bad' or neutral, what 'rights' animals have, and whether it is acceptable to harm one animal to benefit another.

Various ethical theories provide frameworks to help determine the ethically correct actions to take. Under one such framework, veterinary surgeons could aim to maximize the 'greater good' by weighing up the costs and benefits of an action for all animals and humans who might be affected, and then choosing the option that provides the greatest overall net benefit. In this scenario, it may be considered justifiable to cause a certain amount of suffering if it is outweighed by sufficiently good consequences. This is relatively uncontroversial when the harms and benefits are for the same animal – many veterinary interventions involve minor and short-term suffering (e.g. those caused by an injection; Figure 2.4), but this is outweighed by greater long-term benefits to the animal (e.g. protection from parvovirus).

However, this 'adding-up' method also allows the suffering to be borne by one group and the benefit to go to another group, as long as the overall benefits outweigh the harms. It can even be used to justify extreme harms being caused in order to benefit other individuals. For example, it could be used to defend research on animals (or even on humans), lying, stealing or even murder if they provide greater benefits than the suffering caused. Some people would deem such actions unfair or simply wrong, whatever the benefits.

A different approach to deciding what is ethically justified is based on applying fixed ethical rules, which contend that certain actions are always unjustified, regardless of their consequences. These can be described in terms of actions that are considered ethically or morally wrong, such as killing, lying or stealing. They can also be described in terms of outcomes that should never be caused or allowed when they can be avoided, for example, extreme suffering, death, captivity or physical mutilations. Arguably, these different descriptions are two sides of the same coin.

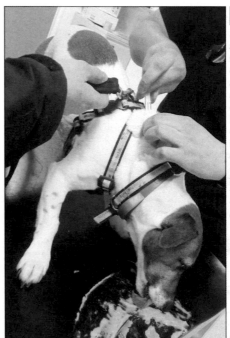

2.4 Most people would agree that the momentary discomfort of having a vaccine administered is outweighed by the benefits the vaccine confers to that individual. In this case, a dog is distracted by a food treat (peanut butter) while undergoing vaccination.
(© Jenny Stavisky)

Veterinary surgeons – and all people – often combine the different types of argument when considering ethical problems. In some situations they will 'weigh up' the options and decide what to do based on the likely consequences, but, at the same time, they may use the 'rules' basis to reject certain possibilities outright as being inherently 'wrong', probably because they transgress an important ethical principle.

Welfare and ethical challenges

Unfulfilled needs

In general, it is understood that shelters may not be able to offer ideal conditions to the animals they care for. Considering the Five Freedoms (Farm Animal Welfare Council (FAWC), 1993; see Figure 2.3) in turn, welfare needs may not be completely met in various ways:

- Nutritional needs
  - May be limited by competition between animals in group housing
- Comfort needs
  - May be limited by concrete kennelling, insufficient bedding and noise levels
- Veterinary needs
  - Animals may present with painful or unpleasant diseases, which may have been left untreated by previous owners (Figure 2.5)
  - Infectious disease control can be very difficult where the density of animals is high
  - Resources may limit expenditure on individual animals
- Normal behaviour
  - Behavioural problems may result from physical restrictions and lack of appropriate social contact or, conversely, from the inability to escape large numbers of unfamiliar conspecifics outside the social group
- Fear and distress (Figure 2.6)
  - Animals may struggle to cope with the challenges of a multi-animal environment
  - Animals that are fearful of humans may be exposed to close contact with caregivers and visitors
  - The process of rehoming may create stress through relocation to their new home after adoption (particularly for cats).

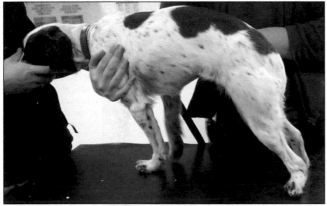

2.5 Animals may present with long-standing injuries that have been left untreated. This dog was presented at a shelter with a deformed leg, which had resulted in difficulty walking and chronic damage to the wearing surface of the paw.
(© Jenny Stavisky)

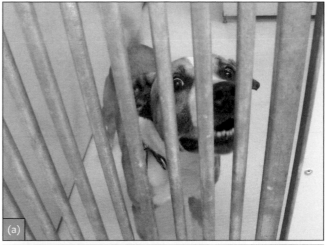
(a)

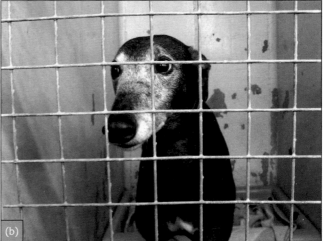
(b)

2.6 Stress can be expressed in varying ways. (a) This dog is showing the whites of its eyes, panting, quivering its tail and has a tense facial expression. (b) This dog appears withdrawn.
(© Jenny Stavisky)

Some of these welfare compromises are considered to be acceptable in the context of temporary holding and rehabilitation of animals. Effectively, the short-term harms may be outweighed by the long-term benefits of rehoming. At the same time, these compromises place a duty on veterinary surgeons to help shelters to minimize the welfare impact of their activities, for example, by promoting practices such as providing environmental enrichment.

However, this does not mean that these compromises are acceptable in the longer term. While the needs of the animal may be met by fostering them into homes (effectively a short-term form of adoption), long-term or permanent kennelling is not acceptable, unless the accommodation in the shelter is made so lavish that it could not be accurately described as kennels (Figure 2.7). It may sound harsh, but permanent kennelling in most kennels for most animals would be a 'life worse than death'.

Welfare assessment

Veterinary surgeons may find it particularly difficult to assess the welfare of animals in shelters. The primary factors causing this difficulty are:

- No history
  - Do not know what is normal for that individual animal

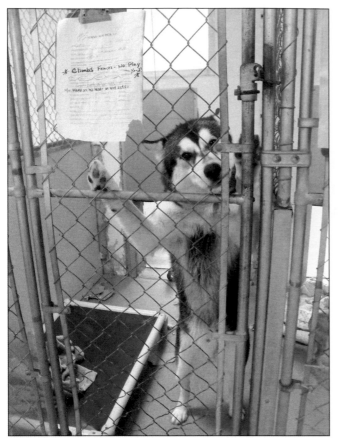

2.7 In most circumstances, long-term kennelling does not provide an adequate quality of life for most animals.
(© Jenny Stavisky)

- Do not know if a clinical sign has commenced recently or has been present for a long time, and whether it has progressed slowly or rapidly
- In some cases even basic signalment is lacking, particularly age and neuter status
- No owner
  - Shelters may have a primary caregiver who has become familiar with the individual animal and any idiosyncratic characteristics it has, but this rarely replaces the insights of a knowledgeable and empathetic owner who has kept the animal for many years
- Abnormal context (e.g. stressors make it hard to assess behaviour)
- Limited time and resources available, particularly for diagnostic tests.

Resource distribution

Any resources spent on one animal in a shelter may effectively deprive another. No shelter has unlimited funds; most are dependent on donations from individuals or government support, both of which are limited. Few shelters have only a few animals in need of help – there are always more kittens and puppies being born, more animals straying or being relinquished or abandoned, and more people maltreating their pets. Consequently, all shelters must make decisions about which animals to help and how much to help them.

In particular, all shelters face several questions relating to decisions that often – and perhaps always – interact with one another. These questions are:

- How many animals?
- How much per animal?
- Which types of animals?
- How much per particular animal?
- How much per area of work?
- How much now *versus* later?

For example, a shelter may be considering a programme to promote neutering (Figure 2.8) or deciding whether to implement a 'no-kill' policy (Figure 2.9). In each case, the proposed action will need to be considered both from an ethical point of view (see above) and in terms of its likely use of resources (see Chapter 20).

- Diverts resources from rehoming efforts
- Requires additional resources to neuter particular unneutered animals
- Prevents future welfare compromises due to stray animals and unsuitable ownership
- Reduces future demands on resources through reducing overpopulation

2.8 Effects of promoting neutering.

- Attracts donations
- Avoids public censure
- Necessitates a policy of 'unlimited' resource allocation per animal
- Reduces the ability to help other animals because the shelter is forced to limit intake
- Reduces the ability to help other animals because the shelter may use resources providing long-term care for one individual that could better help more animals
- The shelter may provide treatment not in the interests of an individual, whose welfare would be better served by euthanasia (e.g. in situations of long-term kennelling, overcrowding or overtreatment)

2.9 Effects of a 'no-kill' policy.

How many animals?

All shelters face a decision about intake. Intake policies can range from having an unlimited intake (e.g. taking all strays), through to limiting intake by linking it to space in the shelter and throughput (e.g. refusing intake when full). In addition, intake can be active (e.g. collecting stray animals), passive (e.g. taking animals that are relinquished or through contracts with local government to accommodate stray animals) or linked to another area of active work (e.g. cruelty investigations). An unlimited intake may mean that more animals are sheltered than in limited intake schemes, although this does not necessarily mean that more animals are helped (e.g. if more animals are kept in poor conditions that do not meet their welfare needs). Having a policy of active intake may increase a shelter's control over its intake. The dilemma is whether to help a set of animals very well but effectively 'ignore' the others, or to help as many as possible but less well.

How much per animal?

A related question is how much of the available resources should be used to help each animal. If resources are limited overall, then this can limit the average resources available to help each animal.

> **Mean resources per animal (£) =**
> **Overall resources for helping animals (£)**
> **Total number of animals**

In general, this means that for a fixed amount of resources, the intake is inversely proportional to the resources per animal (i.e. if more animals are taken in, there are fewer resources available to help each one). In some situations, this equation can be avoided by linking intake to a provision of resources per animal. For example, some shelters may levy a financial charge to each owner who wants to relinquish an animal or those shelters that have contracts with the local authorities to deal with stray animals may charge the government a fixed fee per animal. However, even in these situations there is a question as to whether the shelter should go beyond that set-up and help other animals.

Which types of animals?

Given that shelters cannot help every animal, all shelters face the challenge of deciding which animals to help (and which not to help). Again, this decision is linked to intake – unless a shelter has a policy of completely unlimited intake, it has to decide, on some kind of basis, which animals to take.

Many shelters focus on particular species (e.g. cats) or breeds (e.g. Labrador Retrievers). This may be based on prioritization of the most important welfare needs in the area, may be a deliberate attempt to find a 'unique selling point' or may simply reflect the personal preferences and facilities of the charity's founders or governors. Other shelters may focus on animals in particular situations:

* Relinquished pets
* Relinquished working animals (e.g. ex-military dogs, racing Greyhounds or guide dogs)
* Animals rescued from cruelty cases
* Stray animals
* Feral animals
* Animals involved in human abuse cases (e.g. domestic abuse)
* Animals from a geographical area (e.g. the local region or a particular country).

Such a focus allows specialization, which may help those animals better. For example, a specialist breed rescue may increase the availability of potential adopters of that breed (and may also help discourage potential owners from buying puppies from other sources). However, this type of specialization could be considered to unfairly discriminate against other animals that also need help. At the very least, ignoring some animals can create an 'assistance lottery' whereby the help an animal receives depends on its geographical location or breed. Furthermore, such specialism may disadvantage other animals. For example, potential adopters might go to a non-specialist shelter with the aim of rehoming a purebred dog, but while there fall in love with a crossbreed; if all purebred dogs are taken in by specialist breed rescues, then adopters might preferentially go to these rescues and the crossbreeds may be less likely to be rehomed.

How much per particular animal?

The formula above represents average resource allocation. It could be applied so that the same amount of resources (e.g. in financial terms) is expended on each and every animal. However, it still allows that, in practice, greater resources are expended on some animals than others.

Different animals may simply cost more to care for; for example, a dog with hyperadrenocorticism (Figure 2.10) is

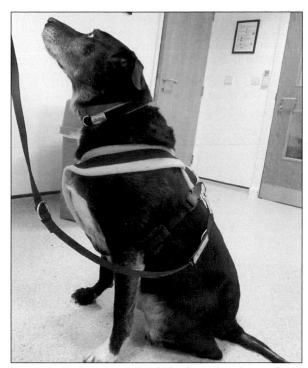

2.10 This dog presented with the classic clinical signs of hyperadrenocorticism (Cushing's disease), including excessive thirst, a pot belly and hair loss on the ventrum and tail. This type of case can be expensive both for the shelter and for the new owner, and can cause debate regarding resource allocation.
(© Jenny Stavisky)

likely to be more expensive to rehabilitate than an animal with a small wound. In addition, some animals may benefit more than others; for example, a young, rehomeable animal may arguably benefit more from very expensive curative treatment than an older animal, which would be better off given palliative care. More controversially, different animals may be perceived as having a greater or lower value (e.g. one animal may be especially beloved by the shelter staff or prominent in the media).

Several approaches can potentially be used to allocate resources per animal (Figure 2.11). Some of these approaches lead to the same amount of resources being allocated to every animal, while others allocate more to

Type of resource allocation	Description	Example
Unlimited	Whatever the animal needs	Giving an animal a hip replacement or chemotherapy if required
Set	Identical expenditure for every animal	Giving every animal £300 worth of treatment
Limited	A maximum amount of resources per animal	Giving animals treatment as needed up to a cost of £500 only
Animal-based formulaic	Based on a set calculation that takes into account the attributes of the animal	Treating animals more if they are a dog rather than a cat, or if they are younger or considered easier to rehome
Context-based formulaic	Based on a set calculation that takes into account the context	Providing more resources per animal during winter when there are fewer needy animals

2.11 Approaches to resource allocation.

some animals than others depending on their characteristics. Differential expenditure on different animals can be very difficult for staff and volunteers to accept, and the perceived unfairness can potentially lead to criticism.

How much per area of work?

Shelters face a much wider decision when they have to set budgets across multiple areas of work. Some decisions must balance multiple operational areas. For example, shelters may provide other 'direct' help to animals, such as veterinary treatment, microchipping and neutering. Some shelters may also engage in educational, campaigning and lobbying activities. Other decisions must balance operational activities with fundraising efforts, which also take up resources, either financial (e.g. investment in the production of appeal leaflets) or time (e.g. volunteers 'shaking tins').

How much now *versus* later?

Some decisions can be considered in terms of when to help different animals. Shelters need to decide how much to devote to preventing problems rather than remedying them. For example, rehoming and remedial treatment aim to alleviate current welfare compromises, whereas neutering, vaccination, education and political campaigning may be expected to reduce future welfare problems through reducing overpopulation, infectious diseases, owner ignorance and unaccountability (Yeates, 2013).

Euthanasia

Shelter veterinary surgeons are likely to face difficult decisions concerning euthanasia. Veterinary surgeons base these decisions on animal welfare assessments – that is, whether an animal is (or will be) suffering, on the grounds that the suffering is worse than death. Such decisions may be made more complicated in several ways:

- The animal's future welfare may be affected by the stress of kennelling
- The animal's future welfare may be affected by the stress of rehoming
- The prediction of suffering may depend on 'non-clinical' guesses about the individual animal, such as how likely it is to be rehomed, the duration of kennelling and the stress of kennelling and rehoming
- Treatment may not be available due to resource limitations (e.g. money for veterinary care)
- Limitations may mean that resources are not available for other animals (e.g. space)
- Treatment may make adoption more difficult (e.g. if it would require an adopter to have specialist skills, such as for a cat with behavioural problems, or to spend significant sums of money for ongoing treatment, such as on a dog with hyperadrenocorticism)
- Treatment may present risks to other animals in the shelter (e.g. through feline herpesvirus transmission)
- Treatment may present risks to other animals after adoption (e.g. through feline leukaemia virus transmission)
- Treatment may present risks to adopters (e.g. through zoonotic disease transmission)
- Rehoming may be illegal (e.g. of types restricted by the Dangerous Dogs Act 1991 (as amended) in Great Britain) or risk litigation (e.g. of dogs that are known to have previously bitten a human)

- There may be strong duties to humans that rule out certain options
- Caregivers may become particularly attached to individual animals
- Individual animals may receive special interest from the media or donors.

Meeting the challenges

Welfare assessment

It is vital to undertake regular welfare assessment of the animals in the shelter. This can be informal or formal, ranging from completely subjective observation of the animals to sophisticated recordings of both animal-based and resource-based welfare indicators. It is important to recognize that welfare assessment is really useful only when it contributes to the perception of a problem, prompts evaluation of its cause and leads to attempts to solve the problem with some action; without these steps, it is simple measurement.

Welfare assessment should include evaluation of 'inputs' and pathophysiological and behavioural 'outcomes'. Some examples of inputs and outcomes are listed in Figure 2.12; however, these are merely suggestions that serve to illustrate that both input and output measures can be useful, and that welfare assessment should go beyond a narrow focus on health. All assessments should ultimately focus on the mental states and feelings that animals are experiencing, which the observable signs represent. The scoring system used should consider the intensity (i.e. how bad/good the outcome is) for each animal affected, the duration of any signs of pleasure or suffering, and the frequency and probability of those mental states occurring.

Input	Outcomes
Diet	Body condition scores
Hiding places	Hiding
Toy enrichment	Repetitive behaviours
Exercise	Apathy
Human company (good and bad)	Aggression Approach/avoidance of human caregivers
Animal company (good and bad)	Vocalization, body language Conflict Affiliative or play behaviours
Routine veterinary care, hygiene and biosecurity	Signs of infectious disease
Remedial veterinary care	Signs of non-infectious disease

2.12 Key inputs and outcomes for shelter welfare assessment.

Particular problems to look out for, which are perhaps more pertinent in a shelter than for owned animals, include:

- Signs of overcrowding (which may occur with just two animals) (Figure 2.13)
- Boredom and frustration
- Fear (including aggression and hiding)
- Infectious diseases
- Lack of exercise
- Lack of human company.

Assessments must consider the animals as they came into the shelter – many may have been neglected and

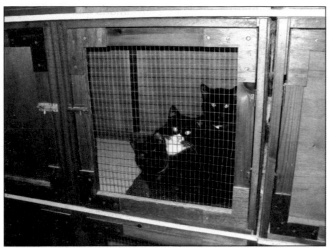

2.13 Overcrowding can occur even with a small number of animals. (Courtesy of L Gosling)

pathological or behavioural sequelae can persist while they are in kennels. Assessment should pay particular attention to whether animals are getting better or worse, especially if their psychological health or wellbeing is being affected by kennelling.

Ethical reasoning

Veterinary work is ethically challenging and shelter medicine gives rise to specific morally difficult situations. Dealing with these complex scenarios is a significant challenge and, as outlined above, decisions should not be taken in isolation, as the outcome of one dilemma may impact on another. Unfortunately, many veterinary surgeons (those who qualified before the inclusion of formal ethics tuition in veterinary curricula) may have not had any training in ethical reasoning.

This is problematic not only from the point of view that poor decision-making may have a negative effect on animal welfare or the reputation of the organization, but also because repeated exposure to challenging ethical conflicts is known to cause an erosion of emotional wellbeing and even a state of 'moral distress'. Moral distress (defined as painful feelings and/or psychological disequilibrium) may result from lack of confidence in a decision, or from recognizing an ethically appropriate action yet not taking it because of obstacles, such as lack of time, reluctance on the part of a supervisor, policy or legal considerations.

In the face of these challenges, there is a risk that veterinary professionals might take refuge in the assumption of a professional moral absolutism, dependence on 'gut feeling', or a risky and impotent moral relativism (the view that no decision or action is objectively right or wrong). Although ethical reasoning is something everyone does regularly (in making decisions regarding other parts of life), applying ethical skills in veterinary work can seem daunting, and the ethical reasoning behind decisions is often not obvious.

An additional complication in veterinary ethics is that the competing views surrounding animal ethics can give rise to disagreements about crucial questions, such the role of animals in society, whether animals have 'rights' and whether an animal's painless death is a moral problem. Unlike medical ethics (where the value of human life *per se* is rarely disputed), veterinary ethical decisions are not made against the background of a solid conceptual

consensus. Therefore, it is easy to imagine how differing views in relation to animal ethics could give rise to conflicts within a veterinary team. This highlights the need for a culture of respect for different ethical starting positions, open ethical discussion and transparent decision-making.

An important first step is to be able to recognize an ethical conflict when faced with one. Usually, this will be obvious, as ethical conflicts may be simply defined as occasions when it is not clear which is the right course of action to take – where competing actions or outcomes may seem equally good, or equally bad. Dealing with these decisions requires 'moral judgement', which, broadly speaking, involves defining what the moral issues are, deciding how conflicts are to be settled and generating the rationale for adopting a particular course of action.

Advice on ethical reasoning is wide-ranging, but informal feedback from veterinary professionals suggests that a structured, stepwise approach is attractive and can help the individual or team to avoid feeling overwhelmed by a complex situation. As for all clinical decisions, information, reflection and communication are vital. One approach to consider is:

* Preparation
* Describe the situation and question
* Identify and weight the ethical principles
* Apply them to reach a decision
* Reflect further on the process and decision reached for the next time (see QRG 2.1).

Even once the decision has been made, various pressures, such as human error, moral weakness, self-interest or pressure from others can affect the actual action that is taken. However, it is important to try to follow through on reasoned decisions, as repeatedly acting in ways that are not morally justified can lead to moral distress. It can be helpful at this point not to think of actions as being 'good' or 'bad', but as 'justified' and 'unjustified'.

While not seeking to unduly simplify the challenges and complexity of ethical decision-making in shelter environments, it is worth remembering that ethical reasoning is a skill that can be practised and improved, and that repeated exposure to similar scenarios should improve confidence in decision-making. Veterinary professionals often find themselves in situations where they are choosing the 'least bad option', but ethics is about reality, and it is not the decision-maker's fault that the ideal option is not available – one can only choose from the available options. Sometimes challenging situations are mistaken for ethical dilemmas but in fact are difficult in a different way, for example, because of communication difficulties.

Allocating resources

Three good principles for resource allocation are:

* No animal should be made worse by the charity's work
* No animal should be caused to have a life 'worse than death'
* Resources should not be expended on one animal if that *unreasonably* deprives another needy animal(s).

Principle 1: No animal should be made worse by the charity's work

Animals should not be taken into the shelter (or euthanased) when they would be better off left on the street (e.g. in the case of feral cats) or with an owner. This principle means that one animal cannot be harmed *overall* to benefit another. For example, one animal should not be used as a source of kidneys for transplantation into another rescue animal. Similarly, one dog should not be kept in overcrowded conditions in order to admit more dogs into the shelter.

Principle 2: No animal should be caused to have a life 'worse than death'

An animal is better off being euthanased than suffering a life worse than death. This suggests that when an animal cannot be helped to have a life worth living (for legitimate reasons), it should be euthanased. Of course, it would be better to give that animal a life worth living – and this should be provided where this is possible without breaching these principles. However, when providing a life worth living is legitimately not possible, the duty is to ensure that the animal does not suffer. This principle not only mandates euthanasia where appropriate, but might suggest that some shelters would benefit from having an intake policy of only taking in animals that would otherwise have a life worse than death.

Principle 3: Resources should not be expended on one animal if that *unreasonably* deprives another needy animal(s)

While this principle is important, the allocation of resources can – and sometimes must – mean that one animal is helped *less* to benefit another (e.g. if it requires a less expensive treatment). This will prevent excessive expenditure on one animal. What is 'reasonable' depends on the overall resources available and the needs of the other animals. As a general rule, it is unreasonable to deprive one animal such that it is harmed more than the other animal is benefited.

In some cases, this will imply that resources should be allocated in such a way that gives the greatest good for the greatest number (without breaching the other principles); this means spreading resources thinly and giving a small amount of help to a greater number of animals. In other cases, this may mean choosing between animals, for example, in a situation where there is time to help only one or the other. It may also allow that animals need not be treated equally if their circumstances are different. For example, it might be right to help the animal(s) that is suffering the most, or the animal(s) that would be most easily rehomed (this may legitimize some unpleasant choices, but decisions must reflect reality). This principle also promotes wider resource allocation, for example, diverting resources to address the most intense and long-lasting issues affecting the largest numbers of animals.

In some situations, it might be right to give one animal additional treatment if this subsequently allows more animals to be helped or avoids greater deprivation. For example, sometimes treating one animal extensively is necessary to avoid public criticism that would reduce income from donations and, thus, ultimately deprive more animals. Another example might be carrying out preventive work that frees up resources later. Such scenarios can lead to some animals receiving more treatment than others, but this inequality is better than treating all animals by an equal but smaller amount. Effectively, the unfairness is limited to the wider unfairness caused by society – and the organization is simply doing the best in a bad situation.

Euthanasia

The value of an animal's life, to the animal itself, is entirely dictated by the enjoyment or suffering the animal will experience. A life of suffering is worse than death. Therefore, decisions about 'quantity of life' depend entirely on 'quality of life'.

On the one hand, euthanasia is not justified when an animal would be expected to have a good chance of having a 'life worth living' independently of the shelter's activity (e.g. if it is a healthy stray or feral). It is also unjustified when the animal would be expected to have a good chance of a life worth living if it receives treatment that is in accordance with the above principles of shelter resource allocation (e.g. effective veterinary treatment).

On the other hand, euthanasia is justified – and indeed mandated – when the animal is expected to otherwise have a 'life worse than death' independently of the shelter's activity (e.g. due to a painful cancer for which treatment would be ineffective). It is also justified when treatment would unreasonably deprive other animals or be illegal. In these cases, the treatment option is ruled out, so that euthanasia becomes the best option. Four questions that should be considered in turn when making decisions regarding euthanasia are shown in Figure 2.14.

For example, releasing a non-indigenous species or a dangerous animal would be illegal, so that animal would need permanent kennelling. Permanent kennelling would either need very spacious, well-furnished kennels, the provision of which would deprive other animals, or it would cause long-term suffering. Long-term suffering would be a life worse than death. So euthanasia is better for that animal's welfare. It is vital for veterinary surgeons to recognize that shelters cannot, and should not, provide the same level of care one would expect (or at least hope) owners to provide.

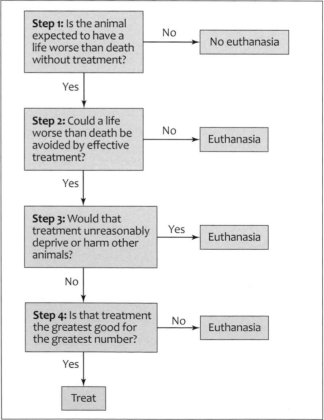

2.14 Flowchart showing the steps that should be considered when making decisions regarding euthanasia.

Transparent decision-making and culture of respect for different ethical positions within the team

Whatever decisions are made in the course of dealing with the ethical and welfare challenges that arise in shelters, it is important that the reasons for making them are clear at the team or even the organizational level (depending on the size of the organization). Individuals with different starting points regarding animal ethics (such as whether animals have a right to life) will react differently to the same decision or outcome. There are many anecdotal reports of significant negative reactions from members of the veterinary team, caregivers and volunteers following controversial decisions (often those involving euthanasia). If such stakeholders feel the decision or outcome is unjustified, this will inevitably affect the morale and effectiveness of the team.

One helpful approach is to make an organizational statement available, outlining the underlying principles used to guide decision-making (perhaps as outlined above for resource allocation or euthanasia). This increases transparency and provides staff with some advance warning of the policies that will be applied in the shelter. Another strategy that can be used to deal with potential discord is to set aside a specific time for ethical discussions around policy-making or regarding particular events. This can be helpful simply because those involved will feel they have had a chance to air their views. Furthermore, knowing that decision-making will be scrutinized by the team may also improve the quality of team members' ethical reasoning.

Variations in the level of knowledge about ethics and ethical reasoning will affect the nature of these discussions (e.g. an outcome may strike someone as being 'just wrong' without their being able to articulate why), and there may be benefit in providing some basic training in ethics for the whole team. Understanding the ethical basis of concerns and making sense of 'spontaneous moral reactions' is likely to facilitate a more objective and less emotionally charged (and potentially personal) discussion about ethically difficult decisions.

In some cases, even the best discussions may not persuade everyone. It is important to allow people opportunities to review decisions and to conscientiously object if they consider that implementing a decision would compromise their moral integrity. However, it is also important to ensure that all colleagues can work together as a cooperative and coordinated team, without constant critiquing or some colleagues not engaging.

A useful compromise is, first, to promote discussion involving everyone until an 'authoritative' decision is made, after which that decision is not to be reviewed unless significant new information comes to light (e.g. an owner is located), and second, to allow conscientious objection except in relation to activities that are 'mission critical', that are compliant with a shelter protocol (see below) or that relate to a fundamental ethical belief (e.g. that euthanasia is better than a life worse than death, or that cats and dogs should be neutered). Colleagues can conscientiously object to these activities by working for another shelter.

Formulating protocols

The formulation of protocols and policies is vitally important for:

- Preventing specific welfare compromises
- Improving biosecurity
- Improving welfare assessment, especially health checks and behavioural evaluations
- Ensuring consistency to optimize resource allocation
- Contingency planning for speedy responses
- Prioritizing work
- Informing others about the principles and objectives of the organization.

Some of these protocols and policies will come from the shelter's trustees or management, hopefully informed by convincing veterinary advice, and veterinary surgeons should aim to provide convincing medical arguments in line with the shelter's mission. This veterinary involvement is especially important for formulating day-to-day and contingency protocols (see Chapter 20 for further details).

References and further reading

FAWC (1993) *Report on Priorities for Animal Welfare Research and Development*. FAWC, London

Parker RA and Yeates J (2011) Assessment of quality of life in equine patients. *Equine Veterinary Journal* **44**, 244–249

Rollin BE (2006) *An Introduction to Veterinary Medical Ethics: Theory and Cases, 2nd edn*. Blackwell Publishing, Oxford

Sandøe P and Christiansen SB (2008) *Ethics of Animal Use*. Wiley-Blackwell, Oxford

Sandøe P, Corr S and Palmer C (2015) *Companion Animal Ethics*. Wiley-Blackwell, Oxford

Yeates J (2013) *Animal Welfare in Veterinary Practice*. Wiley-Blackwell/UFAW, Oxford

Yeates J and Main D (2009) Assessment of companion animal quality of life in veterinary practice and research. *Journal of Small Animal Practice* **50**, 274–281

Yeates J (ed in production) *Companion Animal Care and Welfare*. Wiley-Blackwell, Oxford

Useful websites

The Animal Welfare Act 2006:
http://www.legislation.gov.uk/ukpga/2006/45/pdfs/ukpga_20060045_en.pdf

QRG 2.1: Using ethical reasoning to make decisions

by Dorothy McKeegan and James Yeates

Practical guidance for ethical decision-making

Those working with companion animals often face complex situations that can lead to daunting dilemmas. Ethical reasoning is part of our thinking in many areas of everyday life – we apply rules to our conduct or attempt to balance different interests to produce the best outcomes in a range of contexts. However, the reasoning process behind decisions and actions is not always explicit, and we may not even be aware of it. We may also sometimes make decisions without reasoning (e.g. on the basis of a need to conform to expectations or a 'gut feeling').

For many veterinary surgeons (veterinarians), a more structured approach to ethical reasoning may be helpful. For those without specific ethics training, it may be easier to think about 'influences on my decision' rather than attempt to generate specific ethical arguments. A step-by-step approach to ethical reasoning is outlined below.

1 Prepare

Preparation, at unpressured times, can reduce stress, avoid some difficult situations and allow better and quicker decisions than when you are 'in the thick of it'. This preparation may involve:

- Identifying potential dilemmas you might face
- Identifying the overarching principles you endorse/wish to follow
- Communicating your position to others
- Identifying other stakeholders' ethical views
- Acknowledging any biases you may experience.

2 Describe the options genuinely available

- **Consider all possible options**, including doing nothing.
- **Discount impossible options**, and do not feel guilty for not being able to achieve the impossible.

3 Identify influences on the decision (factual and ethical)

- Ethics is about the real world – every decision is made in a particular context.
- Find out **all the relevant information**, including both clinical data and all pressures on the decision-maker (e.g. laws, owners'/keepers' wishes, charity policies and practice protocols).
- Ethical influences might be **rules or principles** that apply to everyone, such as 'one should avoid killing healthy animals', or might relate to your role, such as 'an owner's refusals should be respected'.
- Dissect the problem to its basic facts and influences to help **grasp the elements of a complex situation** and **reduce the risk of feeling overwhelmed** by large numbers of considerations.

4 Identify interests and weight the influence of each

- Since many dilemmas arise from a conflict of interest, **consider to whom each influence relates** (e.g. the animal, veterinary surgeon, owner, organization or society).
- Evaluate **how important** each of the influences should be in this case. These can be scored (e.g. out of 10).
- Influences should be scored as zero, if they are unimportant in the case, are negations of other pressures (e.g. 'the cat will not suffer') or should be ignored (e.g. selfish motivations or inappropriate pressures from managers or clients).
- Influences should be scored as 10 if they should absolutely never be breached (e.g. 'I should never deliberately harm an animal').
- Other principles should be scored in between, depending on the severity of the effects (e.g. the painfulness of a procedure), the importance of the rule (e.g. not lying is a major ethical tenet) or the stakeholder (e.g. that animals should always have priority). Weightings can also be used to identify how much consideration is being given to different stakeholders.

5 Identify the best option

- If the weighting of any influence or principle is absolute (i.e. scores 10/10) then rule that option out completely.
- In some cases, ruling out multiple options may leave only one option.
- In other cases, identify the overall score for each option by combining the scores for each influence. Compare the scores of each option to determine which one is best.
- If your scores seem wrong, then rethink your 'working' as outlined above.
- If multiple options appear equally acceptable, use an additional decision-making process (e.g. allowing the owner or carer to choose).

6 Act

- **The actual act is often the hardest part**, and we may fail to carry through our decisions because of human error, moral weakness, self-interest or pressure from others.
- Ensuring that decisions are reached and acted upon can be helped by good communication and reminding yourself of your good reasoning.
- It can be helpful to think of outcomes not as 'right' or 'wrong' but as 'justified' or 'unjustified'.

7 Reflect (and prepare for next time)

- **Think back over your decision.** When decisions go well, reflection is enjoyable and motivating, and can identify why things went well. When decisions go badly, reflection can leave us feeling guilty, but it can help to analyse this guilt and ensure that it provides learning for future decisions.
- Reflection can also allow you to consider the 'big' animal ethics issues, such as whether you consider painless death to be an ethical harm.

→

QRG 2.1 *continued*

- **Analyse the decision-making process and not the outcome.** Do not ask 'did it turn out right?' because a decision may have been the right one at the time, even if things turned out badly through, for example, bad luck.
- Useful questions for reflection are:
  - Did I engage in enough discussion?
  - Did I consider all relevant influences and stakeholders?
  - Was my animal welfare assessment accurate?
  - Did I stand by my principles?
  - Did I give myself enough time?

Ethical reasoning is a skill that can be learned and improved with practise. Employing an explicit reasoning process may make discussion of controversial decisions easier, which can promote a culture of respect for the ethical perspectives and actions of others working in veterinary teams. Finally, remember that some ethically problematic outcomes are beyond your control – you can only choose from the available options, and sad or disappointing outcomes are not your fault.

Case example

Jasper, a 4-year-old Staffordshire Bull Terrier, has been in a shelter for 7 months. Jasper is friendly to adults but very aggressive towards other dogs. After many appeals for a home, a man puts in a request of interest to rehome Jasper. Due to Jasper's history of aggression, the shelter is being very careful about potential adopters, but the interested party seems ideal: he is a single man in his thirties, who has previous experience

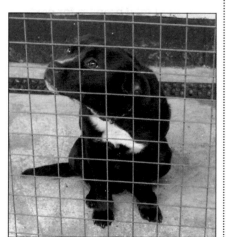

Jasper: a 4-year-old Staffordshire Bull Terrier.

with Staffordshire Bull Terriers. However, the man has a 6-year-old daughter who does not live with him but often stays at his home. A meeting is arranged between Jasper and the daughter, and it does not go well. Jasper shows very obvious signs of aggression and it is clear the adoption cannot go ahead. Should Jasper be euthanased?

1 Prepare

This is a dilemma likely to occur regularly in shelter environments, so discussion of this eventuality can be done in advance. At this time, individual principles or policies regarding the euthanasia of such animals can be considered and discussed to guide future decision-making.

2 Describe the options genuinely available

The options available are:

1. Euthanase Jasper
2. Continue to attempt to rehome Jasper without informing potential adopters of the history
3. Continue to attempt to rehome Jasper while informing potential adopters of the history
4. Keep Jasper at the shelter permanently.

3 Identify and weight influences on the decision, and identify interests

The example ranking shows the influences that might be identified, whose interests are involved in each, and the weighting score assigned.

4 Identify the best option

Based on the example ranking, being dishonest to potential adopters and keeping Jasper permanently in kennels are both scored as having absolute importance, which rules out options 2 and 4. Of the remaining options, there are 51 points in favour of euthanasia and nine against, suggesting that euthanasia appears to be the best option (other cases may not be so simple as this illustrative example).

However, the influences and rankings produced by individuals will differ based on:

- The ethical significance one places on death. In this example, Jasper's right to life is scored 0, as if the veterinary surgeon does not think the dog has such a 'right'. However, if this was scored as an absolute right (i.e. 10), then a euthanasia decision would not be indicated

Influence on the decision	Whose interests?	Example of weighting
Arguments for euthanasia		
• Jasper represents a danger to children • Jasper represents a danger to other dogs	Society Other animals	9 7
• Jasper will not suffer from a painless death	Animal	0
• Jasper's quality of life in kennels is suboptimal in the short term • Jasper's quality of life will involve suffering if he is housed in kennels permanently	Animal Animal	3 10
• The shelter has limited resources and Jasper's place could be taken by another dog more likely to be rehomed	Animal	3
• The shelter's reputation needs to be protected from the risk posed by a rehomed dog causing injury • The shelter should not be dishonest to potential adopters	Organization Adopters	9 10
Arguments against euthanasia		
• Jasper has a right to life	Animal	0
• Jasper is young and healthy, and could have a good life	Animal	5
• Euthanasia is unpleasant to do	Veterinary surgeon	1
• The kennel carers are very attached to Jasper	Organization	2
• Euthanasia of a healthy animal risks reputational harm to the organization	Organization	1

A summary of possible influences on the decision, to whom each influence relates and examples of weighting (0–10, where 10 is the most important). The weighting is based on ethical views and underlying principles, which will vary between individuals. Thus, weighting values may vary considerably within and between organizations.

QRG 2.1 *continued*

- Whether it is acceptable for the needs of many animals to outweigh the interests of one. For example, it could be argued that one should focus on each animal in isolation
- What quality of life is expected. For example, this may affect the weighting in favour of continuing Jasper's life

- What resources are available. For example, better kennels could make option 4 acceptable (if Jasper's quality of life would not be unacceptable), but at the cost of increasing the score for the pressure on the shelter's resources.

5 Act
Minimizing the impact of the euthanasia decision in this case could involve:

- Careful communication with the kennel care staff to explain the basis of the decision
- Finding a veterinary surgeon who is content to carry out the euthanasia.

6 Reflect (and prepare for next time)
Reflection could focus on whether the decision in this case could inform policy-making, and whether there were unexpected outcomes of the euthanasia decision.

Pragmatic decision-making in the charity situation

Sally Everitt, Rachel Dean and Tim Browning

This chapter will introduce some basic concepts of clinical decision-making and evidence-based veterinary medicine, and will suggest how the principles can be applied in a pragmatic way in a shelter or charity environment. Further details of the ethical and animal welfare aspects of clinical decision-making are given in Chapter 2.

To make a decision is to choose a course of action, and clinical decisions will be defined here as those decisions that are taken in the course of caring for patients. In the literature, the terms clinical decision-making, clinical reasoning, clinical judgement, clinical inference and diagnostic reasoning are often used interchangeably (Hardy and Smith, 2008), although it is possible and sometimes important to make a distinction between the process of decision-making and the outcome in terms of the decision made.

It has been shown that the context in which decisions are made, including the expectations and standards of an organization or veterinary practice, have a significant influence on decision-making (Orasanu and Connolly, 1993). Stark differences in the context of shelters and charitable organizations, as compared with private clinical practice, often require correspondingly different decisions to be made. While resources may be limited in both situations, in private practice the primary focus is usually the individual animal. However, in the charity/shelter environment it is important not only to consider the welfare of the animal in a broader context – for example, the likelihood of being able to rehome the animal – but also to consider how best to distribute resources for the benefit of the wider population of animals within the organization.

Introduction to decision-making

Decision-making is part of everyday life, both private and professional, and how decisions are made has been the subject of study in many different disciplines. Decisions imply making a choice between options; consequently, the study of decision-making becomes the study of how and why certain choices are made and perhaps how they could be made better.

Much of the initial study of decision-making took place in the field of economics and proposed a 'rational actor', who selects between options on the basis of stable preferences in the pursuit of explicit goals. This requires knowledge of all the available choices and their consequences. In situations where there is some uncertainty, decision analysis can be used to assign numerical values indicating the probability and utility (value) of each option. Within this theory, a 'good decision' is the one indicated by the highest numerical value based on the likelihood of the outcomes and the values and preferences of the decision-maker, and a 'good outcome' is one that is profitable or otherwise highly valued by the decision-maker (von Neumann and Morgenstern, 1944). However, as the decision-making process may involve elements of uncertainty, a good decision does not guarantee a good outcome.

Studies of decision-making have shown that in the real world people make decisions with less than perfect information, because collecting information has a cost in terms of time and effort but also because the human brain is able to deal consciously with only a limited amount of information. Therefore, people often use shortcuts (rules of thumb or heuristics) in making decisions (see Heuristics and biases box). These enable people to make decisions more rapidly with incomplete information, but can introduce bias into the decision-making process. In many areas of veterinary medicine, clinicians lack information (see Evidence-based Veterinary Medicine) but still have to make decisions; this is particularly true for many aspects of shelter medicine. Understanding the origins and influences of their own personal biases may help facilitate clinicians in coming to collective decisions, even when they have very different perspectives.

In contrast to economic theories that consider how people should make decisions, psychological research has concentrated on how they actually do make decisions. Dual processing theory draws on research in psychology to suggest that humans have access to two different methods of reasoning (Evans, 2003). These have been variously referred to as intuitive–analytic, implicit–explicit, fast–slow and System 1–System 2 reasoning; the last of these is becoming most common as it does not make assumptions about the cognitive processes being used (Evans, 2003; Croskerry, 2009b; Maskrey et al., 2009; Kahneman, 2011; see Figure 3.2).

System 1 processes are considered to be rapid, automatic and involve parallel processing of information. This is considered to be 'fast and frugal', requires little effort and frequently gets the right answer, but is subject to error and bias (Croskerry, 2009a). Clinicians are able to draw on their experience of previous cases to recognize patterns (Heneghan et al., 2009) or deviations from expectations (Klein et al., 1989). However, even experienced practitioners will revert to analytical reasoning in areas with which they are unfamiliar or when presented with novel or complex cases.

System 2 processes, in contrast, are slow, systematic, linear and fully conscious, but because they are reliant on working memory they are limited in the amount of information they can process (Evans, 2003). In clinical decision-making they are associated with systematic review and appraisal of evidence (Maskrey et al., 2009). They are slow and resource-intensive but more likely to reach a correct diagnosis than System 1 processes, at least in those cases that deviate from the classic presentation (Croskerry, 2009b) (Figure 3.1).

Whereas both economic and psychological approaches concentrate on the role of the decision-maker, sociological approaches look at the influence of the context in which decisions are made. Clinical decision-making in veterinary

System 1	System 2
• Quick	• Slow
• Can occur in parallel with other activities	• Serial
• Not fully conscious	• Voluntary/conscious
• Intuitive	• Rational
• Based on past experience	• Based on explicit evidence
• Subject to bias	• Less subject to bias, but subject to error where evidence is poor

3.1 Comparison of System 1 and System 2 decision-making.

Heuristics and biases: veterinary examples

System 1 decision-making is subject to a wide range of heuristics and biases. The technical definition of a heuristic is a simple procedure that helps to find adequate, although often imperfect, answers to difficult questions (Kahneman, 2011). A few examples are given below; further examples from the medical field can be found in Croskerry (2003) and https://first10em.com/cognitive-errors/.

The representativeness heuristic: In this case the decision-maker makes assumptions about the likelihood of an occurrence on the basis of apparent similarities without taking underlying base rates into consideration. A veterinary example would be when considering breed predispositions over prevalence in formulating a differential diagnosis.

The availability heuristic: This describes the phenomenon where predictions of the incidence of an event are based on how easily they are brought to mind rather than how frequently they actually occur. For example, events with a major emotional impact, such as plane crashes, tend to be more readily recalled even though they are very rare. A veterinary example would be the tendency to recall rare or particularly memorable cases over more mundane cases, leading to a distortion in their perceived frequency of occurrence.

The anchoring and adjustment heuristic: This is the tendency of people to assess probabilities by starting from an implicitly suggested reference point (the anchor) and adjusting their estimates from that point until they reach a plausible answer. The anchoring heuristic predicts that a veterinary surgeon who is asked whether they considered the prevalence of a disease to be greater than 65% would arrive at a final estimate higher than if asked whether they thought the prevalence was greater than 45%.

practice is affected by a range of factors, including the resources of the owner, the value placed on the individual animal and the circumstances in which the decision-making takes place. In a shelter or other charity environment, other factors may need to be considered, such as the resources available, considerations of herd health and the ethos of the organization as well as specific organizational protocols (see Chapter 1).

Clinical decision-making

Clinical decision-making is the process of making decisions about the care of patients, and is an integral part of the work of many health professionals (Higgs et al., 2008). Medical decision-making is taken to be a specific example of clinical decision-making by doctors, and has been described as a process involving deciding what information to gather, which diagnostic tests to perform, how to interpret and integrate this information to draw diagnostic conclusions, and deciding which treatments to give (McGee, 2010). Research into medical decision-making has been broadly divided into two approaches. Problem-solving research is primarily aimed at describing reasoning by expert physicians, with the aim of being able to increase the expertise of less experienced clinicians. Psychological decision research aims to identify departures from the statistical models of reasoning under conditions of uncertainty (Elstein and Schwartz, 2002; Norman, 2005).

The major clinical decisions in veterinary medicine relate to making an assessment of the animal's condition (diagnosis), the appropriate management of the problem (treatment) and the likely outcome (prognosis). Information that enables the clinician to establish the condition of the animal may come from the clinical history, the veterinary surgeon's (veterinarian's) own assessment of the animal through physical examination and the results of tests performed either directly on the animal or on samples taken from the animal. This information about the individual (or group/'herd') will need to be integrated with more general evidence about diseases and treatments that the veterinary surgeon has gained from their professional knowledge base, which may be made up of personal experience, accepted practice, expert opinion and published literature.

In contrast to diagnostic decisions, which involve the clinician in a process of clinical judgement based on evidence collected from the clinical history, physical examination and diagnostic tests, treatment decisions are often considered to follow logically from the diagnosis. The paradigm of evidence-based medicine recommends decisions be based on empirical evidence. This should be tempered with shared decision-making, where the patient's (or, in veterinary medicine, the client's) preferences and values are integral. Therefore, the clinician is required to take into account a range of factors into the final decision (see Decision analysis example and Figure 3.3).

Some veterinary professionals would argue that all clinical decisions should be made using explicit, rational, evidence-based (System 2) decision-making processes. However, many veterinary surgeons in fact use similar strategies to their medical colleagues in reaching a diagnosis, with experienced clinicians in primary care frequently using rapid (System 1) techniques, such as spot diagnosis and pattern recognition, reserving hypothetico-deductive reasoning (System 2) for complex cases or those where System 1 reasoning has failed (Evans, 2003; Croskerry, 2009b).

Where there is an appropriate match between the experience of the clinician and the decision to be made, a System 1 approach can be very efficient in enabling diagnoses to be made quickly and cost-effectively. However, it is also important for the clinician to be aware of the types of bias that may be introduced through the use of System 1 reasoning. This requires taking the time to check the results of their 'intuitive' decisions through the brief consideration of differential diagnoses or the use of appropriate diagnostic tests to guard against errors. This combination of System 1 and System 2 decision-making enables the best features of both systems (speed and accuracy, respectively) to be harnessed (Figure 3.2).

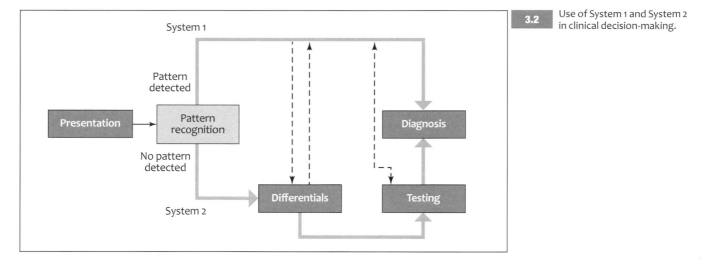

3.2 Use of System 1 and System 2 in clinical decision-making.

Decision analysis example

One way of structuring decisions is to use some form of decision analysis. This involves assigning a numerical value to each outcome, which is made up of the probability that it will occur and the utility (value) to the owner.

For example, consider a dog with a spinal problem that is causing pain and hind limb lameness for which there are two methods of treatment, one medical and one surgical. In a small number of cases (10%), the medical treatment achieves a cure after 1 month, but in the majority of cases (90%) the condition requires ongoing treatment costing around £50 per month.

The alternative is surgical treatment, which has a much greater chance of cure (75%) but also carries a risk of increased disability (20%) or death (5%). This procedure costs £2,000.

For simplicity, we can assign cure a utility value of 1 and death a utility value of 0. Then, we need to assign the other options intermediate utilities. For example, ongoing treatment 0.7, as this will achieve the outcome of a mobile dog at a cost of £50 per month, and disability 0.2, as we will have a dog that is still alive but with restricted function, such as some degree of paresis.

The different options can be arranged in a decision tree (Figure 3.3).

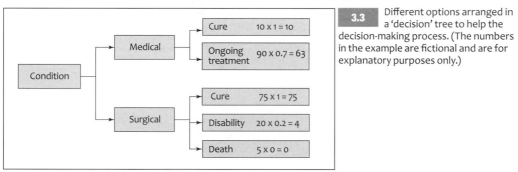

3.3 Different options arranged in a 'decision' tree to help the decision-making process. (The numbers in the example are fictional and are for explanatory purposes only.)

It is important to remember that different people may put a different value on different outcomes. The owner of a young dog may work out that surgery is likely to be the less expensive option, as it costs the same as only 3 years of medical treatment, but they may also consider the risk of disability to be much worse. However, a shelter may not be able to finance the surgery and may opt to try medical treatment for a month or euthanasia.

We also need to consider the impact of any disability on animal welfare whatever the clinical setting (see Chapter 2 and QRG 2.1). When the disability is likely to have significant impact on the animal's quality of life, it may be assigned a negative value and euthanasia may be considered a better and acceptable treatment option.

It is also important to remember that we may not have objective data on all the probabilities, and even if there are published figures in the literature, they may not give the same results that we can obtain in our own practice. In this situation, clinical audit can be useful to provide local (practice-specific) data that is more appropriate.

Even if it is not possible to use the decision tree explicitly, we can use the idea to talk through the options with the client.

Uncertainty

In the medical field, uncertainty has been identified as a key factor affecting both doctors' decisions and their ability to discuss their decision-making process with their patients (Fox, 1989). Types of uncertainty include:

* Uncertainty arising from incomplete mastery of current and expanding medical knowledge
* Uncertainty arising from gaps, limitations and inadequacies in medical knowledge
* Uncertainty due to difficulty in distinguishing between the limitations of medical knowledge and personal ignorance.

Evidence-based medicine may be presented, in some decisions, as a way of reducing the clinician's uncertainty by grading evidence and providing an increasingly numerical approach to discussing risks. However, it may also introduce a further level of uncertainty to the clinician, who may feel inadequately prepared to interpret the published evidence, or it may highlight that evidence is lacking (Timmermans and Angell, 2001).

Where medical knowledge is absent, practitioners make use of their personal experience, opinion and judgement to fill the gaps.

It has been suggested that uncertainty may be even greater in veterinary practice, both because of a lack of scientific evidence to support decision-making (Cockcroft and Holmes, 2003) and because of 'the constraints that may be applied to a diagnostic work up as a result of financial limitations' (Mellanby *et al.*, 2007, p. 26). Embracing the existence of uncertainty in veterinary clinical decision-making and acknowledging that this uncertainty has been identified are key aspects of being able to practice in an evidence-based way (Dean *et al.*, 2017). Identifying aspects of veterinary healthcare that we are uncertain about enables us to question what we do, find or produce evidence that provides more clarity and where appropriate change care.

Shared decision-making

The concept of shared decision-making has been widely advocated in the medical world, where it is contrasted with both paternalistic decision-making, in which the health professional takes decisions in the best interests of the patient, and informed decision-making, in which the role of the professional is seen as that of providing information to enable the patient to make their own decisions through the process of informed consent (Charles *et al.*, 1997). In the most frequently quoted description, shared decision-making is described as a process in which both the clinician and patient:

* Are involved in the treatment decision-making process
* Share information with each other
* Take steps to participate in the decision-making process by expressing treatment preferences
* Agree on the treatment to implement (Charles *et al.*, 1999).

Although shared decision-making has been described as the ideal for the veterinary consultation, it has also been acknowledged that 'there are occasions when some owners do not always act in the best interests of their animal' (BVA, 2009). This situation requires the veterinary surgeon to take a role in educating the client, and requires that clinical decision-making takes account of the ethical concerns regarding the welfare of the animal (Tannenbaum, 1995; Rollin, 2006).

In shelter and charity settings there may not be an individual owner, and there can often be relatively large teams with varying clinical experience working together in a high-volume setting with limited resources. It is important that the team is involved in the development of practice protocols for managing cases (see Chapter 20 for more information). This will ensure appropriate and rational care of the patient that ensures the best possible outcome for that individual as well as for the population and the organization.

Evidence-based veterinary medicine

Evidence-based Veterinary Medicine (EBVM) has been defined as 'the use of best relevant evidence in conjunction with clinical expertise to make the best possible decision about a veterinary patient. The circumstances of each patient, and the circumstances and values of the owner/carer, must also be considered when making an evidence-based decision' (Centre for Evidence-Based Veterinary Medicine, 2018).

The circumstances of veterinary patients and the values and circumstances of their owners/carers can vary massively from one situation to another. The situation of a chronically atopic 6-year-old dog in a rescue shelter is very different from that of a chronically atopic 6-year-old insured show dog with a devoted owner. Although the disease and the scientific evidence are the same in both cases, the respective circumstances may lead to the evidence being applied differently and therefore lead to a different clinical decision (Figure 3.4). The decision-makers are key to implementing EBVM, as they decide how the evidence can be applied to each unique clinical situation.

Implementing EBVM has its challenges. One of the main challenges is often finding and then applying the best available evidence. The evidence base for decision-making in shelters and other charitable settings is increasing, which is important as it can be very hard to apply the findings of research undertaken in first-opinion or referral private practice to the shelter context. It is important for veterinary professionals to promote and become involved with clinically applied research that encompasses the challenges of population medicine as well as individual patients, to ensure there is a scientific basis to shelter medicine.

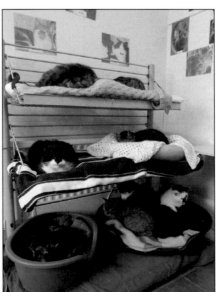
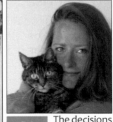

3.4 The decisions made for cats in a shelter environment may be very different compared to decisions made for a privately owned cat with a dedicated owner – the evidence will be the same.
(© Rachel Dean)

The five steps of EBVM

There are five basic steps of EBVM.

1. Ask

Many clinical decisions are made every day and some of those decisions will be more evidence-based than others. The first step of EBVM is to clearly articulate the question to which you need to know the answer. It is important to consider: what am I uncertain about? One way of doing this is to structure clinical queries in three parts; this is often described as a PICO question, as a mnemonic for the three parts:

1. **P:** Specify the **patient** group, problem or population you are interested in
2. **I/C:** This is the **intervention** or action you are interested in and a **comparator** if appropriate. This may be, for example, two treatments, a diagnostic test or a risk factor
3. **O:** This is the clinical **outcome** of interest for the patient group.

For example, you want to know whether giving antibiotics to shelter dogs with kennel cough that are otherwise healthy would speed up the time required to clear the clinical signs, enabling the dogs to be rehomed. This could be structured as:

P: Systemically well dogs with kennel cough
I: Antibiotics
C: No antibiotics
O: Reduced length of clinical signs.

The PICO question is thus: In (systemically well dogs with kennel cough), do (antibiotics compared with no antibiotics) (reduce time to clinical recovery)?

It is very important to establish what the clinical question is and define it well before looking for the evidence or asking for help with a case, as this will ensure that the evidence you find is relevant and useful.

2. Acquire

Before looking for evidence, it is important to think about what type of evidence you are looking for. This can vary from expert opinion, to textbooks and websites, to peer-reviewed primary research. All these types of evidence can be useful for decision-making but it is important to recognize that they will all have sources of bias (see step 3).

As well as the traditional forms of evidence, there are more and more EBVM resources available to clinicians to aid their decision-making. These include secondary sources of evidence, which are summaries of the knowledge on certain topics that have been collated around specific clinical questions. It is worth investigating some of these resources before undertaking a literature search, as they are quick to search and may already contain the evidence you are looking for. Such resources include:

* BestBETs for Vets: https://bestbetsforvets.org/
* BSAVA Library: https://www.bsavalibrary.com/
* Veterinary Evidence (RCVS Knowledge Summaries): https://www.veterinaryevidence.org/index.php/ve
* VetSRev database of veterinary systematic reviews: http://webapps.nottingham.ac.uk/refbase/

If there is nothing relevant in these resources, it may be necessary to undertake a primary search of scientific databases. There is no database or search engine that is exclusively dedicated to veterinary medicine. However, CAB Abstracts has been reported to be the most useful database for the veterinary clinical literature (Grindlay *et al.*, 2012); it can be accessed free of charge by BSAVA members.

3. Appraise

As mentioned above, all types of evidence can be affected by bias, which is anything that may mean you make an erroneous decision that could harm your patient. The systematic critical appraisal of evidence is one of the cornerstones of EBVM and enables you to identify the good and the bad (and potentially biased) parts of any type of evidence. Clinicians require some basic skills to differentiate good science from bad – just because something is published, it does not mean the science is sound. The reader needs to grasp some basic principles when reading veterinary literature, which can make the process very quick. There are various texts that are good guides for clinicians wanting to improve their reading skills (Crombie, 2009; Dean, 2013; Greenhalgh, 2014). The most important parts of a paper to read are the methods and the results; these sections explain what the researchers did and what they found. If there are flaws in the methodology that may lead to bias in the results, the results must be interpreted with caution.

In deciding whether a particular piece of published evidence is relevant to making a particular decision, it can be helpful to ask the following questions:

* What is the question that is being asked/answered? Is it the same as or closely related to the question I want to answer?
* What is the type of study and is it appropriate to answer the question? (Dean, 2013)
* Is the population of animals used in the study sufficiently similar to the animal(s) that I am treating for the evidence to be relevant?
* How have the data been analysed? Do they relate to the original question that was asked, and are all the animals accounted for?
* What are the findings? What are the implications of these findings for the decision I am making? ▶

The five steps of EBVM *continued*

Often, the best way to appraise a paper is by using a structured critical appraisal tool. Some examples can be found at:

* Centre for Evidence-Based Veterinary Medicine: https://www.nottingham.ac.uk/cevm/evidence-synthesis/resources.aspx
* RCVS Knowledge EBVM Learning: http://www.ebvmlearning.org/

Remember it is also possible to critically appraise expert opinion and consider how the information provided may be biased based on their experience, beliefs and the information they have read (no one can read it all).

4. Apply

The first three steps of EBVM are redundant unless the evidence that has been found and appraised is applied to practice where appropriate. The extent to which veterinary clinicians integrate evidence with their expertise is unknown, but if science is not implemented in practice we cannot tell whether it will improve care or not. Applying evidence to a clinical situation can be very difficult, but by using what is found to create or alter protocols and working as a team to implement changes it is possible. It is important to ensure that the whole team wants to make the change and feels it is possible. Hence, small incremental changes often are more successful than bigger ones.

As an example, consider the PICO question outlined above, 'In (systemically well dogs with kennel cough), do (antibiotics compared with no antibiotics) (reduce time to clinical recovery)?' An evidence synthesis may suggest that antibiotics may not make a difference to clinical recovery if a dog is otherwise well (BestBETs for Vets, 2016). However, in a particular shelter it may have been 'routine' for a number of years to dispense antibiotics to dogs with a cough. To apply the evidence into this shelter it would be necessary to ensure that everyone looking after the dogs understands why the practice of dispensing antibiotics is going to change. It is important to include not just the clinical team but also the workers who care for the dogs on a day-to-day basis, any volunteers and also the management team. It is important to make it clear that there is no clinical reason to prescribe antibiotics for most coughing dogs but some dogs may still receive them (e.g. if they are unwell or have a comorbidity). The benefits of not using antibiotics in some dogs include reduced cost and time requirements that will benefit the charity – and, of course, avoiding inappropriate antibiotic use is also important for responsible antibiotic stewardship. Having explained the benefits of the change, actually getting people to change their habits will take time and effort. Enabling shelter workers (and clinicians!) to understand that antibiotics have no benefits in some cases, and that they may even do harm, can be challenging. This is where assessing the effect of change is important – and this is the next step of the EBVM process.

5. Assess

If evidence is applied to or changes clinical practice, it is vital that is it possible to assess the effects of implementing the evidence in terms of clinical and business outcomes. To be able to monitor the effects of a change of practice, an audit is required. The clinical audit process involves:

1. Assessing how a procedure is done
2. Looking at a certain outcome, which can be positive or negative
3. Implementing a change
4. Reassessing the effect of the change on the outcome of interest.

If the application of evidence has improved practice, then this is a step forward. If nothing has changed in terms of outcome, then the cycle of EBVM needs to be reassessed. If the change implemented has had a negative consequence on the outcome of interest, then the change needs to be reverted. Often, the process of applying EBVM to practice generates more clinical questions, and the cycle of EBVM starts once more (Figure 3.5).

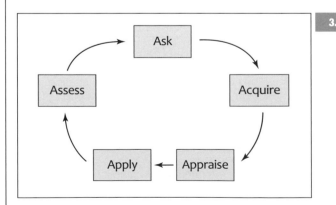

3.5 The cycle of the five steps of Evidence-based Veterinary Medicine.

Further resources about clinical audit include:

* BSAVA: https://www.bsava.com/MyBSAVA/Knowledge-bank/Practice/Practice-Pack/Module-2
* The *BSAVA Manual of Small Animal Practice Management and Development*
* RCVS Knowledge: https://knowledge.rcvs.org.uk/quality-improvement/

Chapter 3 · Pragmatic decision-making in the charity situation

Pragmatic decision-making in a shelter or charity environment

While the principles of clinical decision-making and EBVM are appropriate to all types of clinical setting, there are a number of specific issues that may arise in a shelter or charity hospital environment.

- **Lack of clinical history:** Many animals enter a shelter with a very limited health history, although many have clinical signs of disease or develop them soon after admission to the multi-animal environment. Once an animal has been admitted, it is vital that the resource of experienced staff or staff who can be directed to observe and collect specific information should be utilized immediately. There will often be a lack of information on factors such as previous vaccination or exposure to disease and mating or parity. This is also relevant to behavioural assessments: making decisions around behaviour within the shelter is often limited by a lack of knowledge about the animal's previous behaviour and experience, and accurate assessment can be very challenging as the animal is now in an unfamiliar environment.
- **Prevalence data:** In a shelter or charity population, disease prevalence may be quite different from that in the general population and referral population on which the majority of clinical veterinary publications may be based. Animals may also be presented at a different stage of disease when compared with a typical practice population and/or immediately exposed to a disease that is not normally encountered in a private pet-owning household.
- **Limited resources:** The charitable sector often has limited resources in terms of money and workforce. This may engender a need to be very selective in the choice of diagnostic tests and treatment options. However, the opportunity to reassess animals in a shelter may be greater than in private practice, which may facilitate a 'wait and see'/'test of time' approach as the animals can be re-examined and monitored to assess how their condition progresses.
- **Time:** Time for decision-making may be very limited for clinicians in an overpopulated, under-resourced shelter or busy charity hospital, which may lead them to rely on a System 1 approach to decision-making. However, particularly when making overall population-level or strategic decisions, finding enough time for a considered, transparent and evidence-based approach to decision-making is important. This is where existing well thought out protocols whose importance has been discussed with all clinical and non-clinical staff can be very useful.
- **Protocols and standard operating procedures (SOPs):** The ethos and values of the charity funding the care of the animals may dictate what can and cannot be done and may influence clinical protocols and SOPs. For example, some organizations will not permit ovariohysterectomy of pregnant queens and bitches, which can significantly affect decisions made about the individuals and the population under a clinician's care.
- **Need to consider the group/herd as well as the individual:** Often, individuals presenting with health problems in a charity setting are part of a bigger population that needs to be considered at the same time; this is the crux of shelter medicine (see Chapter 1). It is

essential to be clear about who the patient is – is it just the individual or the population as well? – and the priorities and resources of the owner or carer. For example, a 'good decision' in a shelter with a serious outbreak of cat 'flu may be to euthanase all the vulnerable kittens under 6 weeks of age. This is a difficult decision to make, but the 'good outcome' in terms of animal welfare and of reducing viral load and the spread of disease in the shelter may be achieved more swiftly.

All of the above factors need to be taken into account as the specific context of the decision that is ultimately made. These aspects of common clinical decision-making in shelter and charity environments are covered in Chapters 12–18 and QRGs 3.1, 3.2, 3.3, 14.1 and 15.3.

In order to provide appropriate care to the individual animal in any clinical setting, but particularly within the shelter/charity environment, it may be necessary to take a pragmatic approach to decision-making. This will often require taking a sensible and realistic approach based on practical experience and a good working knowledge of the clinical setting and the values of the organization. It is important to consider if what you are about to do will contribute to the management of a case. For example, in an entire bitch with a purulent vulval discharge and other clinical signs suggestive of pyometra, paying for an abdominal ultrasound examination or extensive diagnostic blood work may not be appropriate, as it will not change the decision on whether to operate or not. Instead, a pragmatic approach may include supportive treatment and fluid therapy prior to neutering or the decision to euthanase the bitch may be made if the resources can be better spent elsewhere within the population.

There are four principal areas in which clinical decisions are made, and the following sections will explore examples of how the concepts discussed above can fit into these areas. They are information gathering; diagnostic testing; drawing together information to form conclusions; and treatment decisions.

Information gathering

Access to information is key to making good decisions. Information gathering may be in terms of accessing the best available evidence for a treatment or policy, using an EBVM approach. Alternatively, it may describe the gathering of other types of evidence relevant to a specific clinical decision.

The main source of information will be the clinical examination of the animal. Where it is not possible to collect a clinical history from the relinquishing owner of the animal or there is no prior owner, it may be necessary to take time to observe the animal's condition over a period of time, to provide some basic information. For example, in a cat with signs of mild upper respiratory tract infection on admission, it may be worth isolating the cat and observing the clinical signs over time to establish whether the signs are progressing or resolving before making further treatment or diagnostic plans. In many situations, these cats may not need any interventions at all.

Keeping good clinical records of a population's health over time provides a benchmark for any intervention. For example, collecting data about outbreaks of diarrhoea in dogs within a shelter population over a period of time, including diagnostic test results, the prevalence of pathogens and the response to treatment, enables 'patterns' of disease to be recognized. This information can be used in future outbreaks to instigate the correct interventions sooner and reduce the number of diagnostic tests needed, and helps to avoid the use of unnecessary treatments, particularly antibiotics. Good clinical records can also be used to enable clinical audit; for example, when seeking to answer a question such as 'What evidence is there to assess the success or failure of previous interventions?'.

Diagnostic testing

Diagnostic tests can be a valuable part of the information-gathering process to support clinical decision-making. However, there is a risk that the deployment of diagnostic tests can be driven by thoroughness or sometimes defensiveness, or that they are used as screening tests rather than truly diagnostic tests. Where resources are limited, it is important to make a cost-benefit analysis of performing a test. The question that should always be asked is 'Is this test going to change the treatment or management of this case/population?'. If the answer is no, then it is not usually appropriate to perform the test in question, but rather to monitor the clinical signs and response to treatment.

For example, rather than undertaking a battery of diagnostic tests on a recently admitted old and underweight cat, it would be beneficial to wait for a few days and observe the cat's appetite and behaviour and look for signs of gastrointestinal disease. In a shelter setting it can be too expensive to 'screen' for hyperthyroidism or chronic kidney disease, and it is better to use specific diagnostic tests only in those cats with a high index of suspicion for the disease (see QRG 3.1).

It is also important to remember that tests must not be interpreted in isolation but must always be referenced to the predictive value of the tests (see Chapter 17), the clinical context and the overall quality of life of the animal. For example, if a charity is able to manage a diabetic dog it may not be possible to follow the usual protocols used with a privately owned pet. Observing the dog's appetite, bodyweight and polyuria/polydipsia daily in their own environment may be an acceptable approach for stabilizing the patient, rather than performing daily blood glucose testing, transporting the dog to a practice for blood glucose curves or paying for regular assessment of blood fructosamine levels. In scenarios such as this a balance must be struck between an 'ideal' protocol and the course of action that is likely to be of greatest benefit to the animal. This may be different for an animal in a charitable setting compared with a privately owned pet.

It is very important to recognize that the most expensive diagnostic or treatment decisions are not necessarily the 'best' for every patient or setting.

Assimilating information to form conclusions

Once information is gathered, it must be appropriately weighted with reference to the overall picture. Often, the information gathered can be incomplete, and a decision may be required as to whether to gather more information (i.e. perform more diagnostic tests) or proceed with a course of action. In a pragmatic situation, this may require strategies such as observing a response to treatment rather than seeking to obtain a definitive diagnosis.

Using the 'test of time' (sometimes called 'watchful waiting') may in some instances be a preferred option (while taking into account factors such as the responsible use of antibacterial agents) to undertaking a time-consuming and expensive series of diagnostic tests, and be more likely to lead to a 'good outcome' for the patient and organization.

For example, in a dog presented at a shelter or charity hospital with acute paraplegia with no history of trauma, the cause may be unclear after initial assessment. However, an absolute diagnosis is not necessary before treatment with analgesia and anti-inflammatory agents, and in the absence of opportunities and financial resources for advanced imaging, this may represent a good, pragmatic option that is 'best' for this particular patient.

Treatment decisions

Where treatments are selected, they should have a clear risk-benefit profile and be appropriate to the patient in question. For example, any treatment plan that involves hospitalization of a feral cat is unlikely to benefit that animal's welfare overall, due to the stress involved. Especially, when formulating protocols that will be applied to a large number of animals, the overall financial cost must be balanced against the benefit. For example, current evidence only supports the use of angiotensin-converting enzyme (ACE) inhibitors in cats with chronic kidney disease (CKD) that are proteinuric; there is a suggestion that this treatment may also improve quality of life. A private client may wish to fund the use of ACE inhibitors in their cat with non-proteinuric CKD. However, if this were to be used as the standard treatment within a shelter for every cat with CKD, it would represent a significant cost without a corresponding known benefit. This financial outlay could deprive other cats of care by the same organization.

A pragmatic approach to clinical decision-making that considers the circumstances in which the animal will be treated is important in all situations and particularly pertinent in shelter medicine (Figure 3.6). For example, the 'best' treatment for a given condition may be a medication that is to be administered three times a day but achieving this in a multi-animal environment with a limited workforce is impossible, so this option becomes the 'worst' treatment and alternatives would constitute a 'better outcome'.

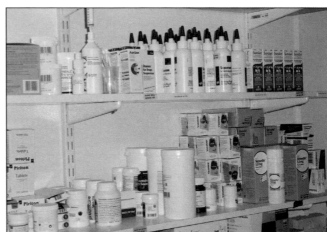

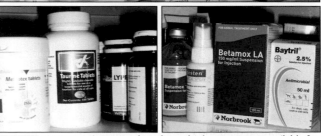

3.6 A pragmatic approach to the multiple treatments available for many conditions involves careful consideration of which drug will make the most difference.
(© Rachel Dean)

Summary of the principles of pragmatic decision-making

1. It is a 'big picture' approach that avoids the over-focusing on a single defined cause but takes into account overarching, complex, social and animal welfare/quality of life issues.
2. It is a step-by-step approach, pragmatically considering the different choices, without second-guessing the outcome. At any one point in time it is important that the way forward is deliverable, and that the owner/carer is involved with the decision-making as much as possible. Ensuring adequate timescales following any actions means the 'test of time' can be used and the natural processes of the diseased can be seen to progress one way or the other.
3. Act as the animal's advocate. If clinical decisions are based on an objective assessment of an animal's welfare (see Chapter 2 and QRG 2.1), they are easier to explain to the carer of the animal when opinions about the course of action differ.
4. Good communication with the right members of staff at the clinic or the shelter is essential.
5. Focus on the most critical treatable conditions that will give a major return on 'investment' in terms of improving animal welfare, by using discriminatory clinical judgement to prioritize the treatment of different comorbidities.
6. Be aware of the law of diminishing returns, both in treatment and in diagnosis. In veterinary medicine there is almost always another step, another drug that can be prescribed or a procedure that can be done. Often, the first test or drug contributes the most, with a marked clinical effect. Subsequent tests or drugs may be added over time, but frequently have progressively less effect. This is why choosing the right first course of action promotes the best care.
7. Be realistic, flexible and honest about the skill levels and resources available. Just because something can be done in theory, it may not be possible in a particular circumstance, and the right thing can still be done so long as the patient's health and welfare remains at the centre of any decision made.
8. Develop clinical judgement. Every diagnostic test should aid the development of clinical assessment rather than seeking to replace it. Each test should have a consequence; if the test will not change your clinical approach to an individual or a population then it should not be used.
9. Do no harm, and 'if in doubt, leave it out'. 'Harm' can be caused to an individual through over-diagnosis and over-treatment. 'Harm' can be done to an organization by using up too much of its resource in terms of money, workforce and time, as well as compromising its ethos and values. 'Harm' can be done to a population if too much resource is spent on a single animal, which then compromises the treatment or management of the rest of the population.
10. Do not panic! When the situation is difficult and complicated and a definitive diagnosis or course of action seems impossible to work out, shelter medicine is at its most challenging. It raises the complications of herd health as well as the health and wellbeing of the individual patient. There is always a valid and pragmatic next step, which may involve difficult decisions, but by working as a team with all stakeholders in the organization involved it is usually possible to reach a sensible decision.

Using a team approach to pragmatic decision-making

Pragmatic decision-making in the shelter environment often involves the need to make decisions with incomplete information, and may involve difficult choices in the allocation of resources and consideration of factors beyond the treatment options for the individual animal. In order to avoid conflict and guilt, the members of the team need to discuss the creation of protocols and SOPs and consider together where the decision points might be questioned.

The following points can help in the development of a culture in which all team members are able to contribute to the decision-making process and understand the reasoning when decisions are made.

1. An initial discussion of the challenges of decision-making in a charity/shelter environment. The whole team (including the non-clinical team at the shelter where appropriate) should discuss the priorities and agree the need for and advantages of an approach. It is important to include nursing staff, who also understand the importance of of doing no harm and ensuring that the minimum, but necessary, treatments are employed. Understanding the reasoning behind having to withhold treatment or euthanase animals in certain circumstances can reduce the stress to staff when individual decisions have to be taken.

2. A systematic development of diagnostic and treatment protocols for the most common conditions can provide decision-making aids. Experienced team members can bring their varying past experience to this process, and the less experienced members may be able to contribute knowledge about the current best available external evidence. It is important to ensure that protocols and SOPs are always open to discussion and renegotiated as evidence and practice move forward. Standard approaches to care can be particularly important in charitable settings, and they enable continuity of care between individuals in busy clinical environments where a number of different carers have contact with patients. Protocols and SOPs can be specifically designed with the whole population as well as individuals in mind as the specifics of the population demographics and dynamics are understood.

3. The decision points, such as entry and exclusion criteria, for each protocol should be addressed. The level of blood testing and other diagnostic tests should receive special attention in order to avoid unnecessary discussion about individual cases. The staging of initial 'work-ups' and longer-term monitoring can also be agreed.

4. Once protocols have been agreed, clinical audit can be introduced to measure the deployment of agreed processes (against targets) and subsequently the outcomes of those processes once they are in place (against expectations). Assessing clinical effectiveness

is vital for safeguarding patient care and giving the team clinical confidence in the processes in place. In addition, auditing clinical activity to ensure the needs of the charity are met and the demands of veterinary care do not compromise the financial and workforce aspects of running the charity is key to knowing whether a good service is being provided. Clinical audit is a cornerstone of good decision-making and should be performed periodically to assess decisions made and lessons learned.

5. Less formal case conferences and ward rounds enable discussion of the application of protocols to individual cases. This process enables the sharing of experience within the team and will enable less experienced staff to learn from the experience of others and develop confidence in pattern recognition. Questions like 'Have you seen this before?', 'Can you make a decision, however tentative the diagnosis?' are useful. Discussing working diagnoses backed up by following cases and the outcomes of pragmatic choices can build confidence and encourage reflective learning.

6. The management of common but important breed-related problems and preventable 'lifestyle' problems such as obesity should be discussed by the team. This will give perspective to animal wellbeing and preventive care messages, and encourages a holistic approach rather than focusing narrowly on single 'technical' fixes.

7. Discussion of the concept of acting as the animal's advocate, and of the need to see the animal existing in its own right and not just as a projection of the needs of the owner/carer and perhaps the clinician (see Chapter 2). The ethical reasoning tool described in QRG 2.1 can be useful for this aspect of decision-making.

8. Clinical team members will need to undertake continuing professional development (CPD). The new knowledge gained from these activities should be brought back and actively reflected upon against the pragmatic protocols that are in place. The cost-benefit of new techniques should be considered against the wider welfare implications, and the evidence base of any individual expert opinion should be considered. CPD may stimulate clinical audit points and the development or refinement of protocols.

9. Recruitment into the team should involve a discussion of the challenges of decision-making, including euthanasia in a charity/shelter environment. If the team member can understand the approach, the team will be strengthened. The use of the term 'pragmatism' in itself may facilitate discussion about case management.

10. It should be made clear to members of the team that a no-blame culture exists and they should feel able to raise any concerns that they may have. Audits, review of critical incidents and encouraging open, less formal, discussions will help support pragmatic case management.

Summary

Pragmatic case management is an important tool for vets in charity and shelter work, and is commonly utilized, even in private practice. It does not mean substandard care; it means making careful and transparent choices that balance the needs of the individual animal with the available resources within each unique clinical and charitable setting.

References and further reading

BestBETs for Vets (2016) Antibiotics in dogs with kennel cough. https://bestbetsforvets.org/bet/166. Accessed June 14, 2018

BVA (2009) The role of the vet in treatment choice decision-making. Available from https://www.bva.co.uk/Workplace-guidance/Ethical-guidance/Role-of-the-vet-in-treatment-choice/. Accessed June 11, 2018

Centre for Evidence-Based Veterinary Medicine (2018) Evidence-based veterinary medicine. https://www.nottingham.ac.uk/cevm/about-the-cevm/evidence-based-veterinary-medicine-(evm).aspx. Accessed June 14, 2018

Charles C, Gafni A and Whelan T (1997) Shared decision-making in the medical encounter: what does it mean? (or it takes at least two to tango). *Social Science & Medicine* **44**, 681–692

Charles C, Gafni A and Whelan T (1999) Decision-making in the physician-patient encounter: revisiting the shared treatment decision-making model. *Social Science & Medicine* **49**, 651–661

Clarke C and Chapman M (2012) *BSAVA Manual of Small Animal Practice Management and Development*. BSAVA Publications, Gloucester

Cockcroft P and Holmes M (2003) *Handbook of Evidence-Based Veterinary Medicine*. Blackwell Publishing, Oxford

Crombie IK (2009) *The Pocket Guide To Critical Appraisal, 2nd edn*. Wiley-Blackwell, Oxford

Croskerry P (2003) The importance of cognitive errors in diagnosis and strategies to minimize them. *Academic Medicine* **78**, 775–780

Croskerry P (2009a) Clinical cognition and diagnostic error: applications of a dual process model of reasoning. *Advances in Health Sciences Education: Theory and Practice* **14(Suppl 1)**, 27–35

Croskerry P (2009b) A universal model of diagnostic reasoning. *Academic Medicine* **84**, 1022–1028

Dean R (2013) How to read a paper and appraise the evidence. *In Practice* **35**, 282–285

Dean R, Brennan M, Ewers R *et al.* (2017) The challenge of teaching undergraduates evidence-based veterinary medicine. *Veterinary Record* **181**, 298–299

Elstein AS and Schwartz A (2002) Clinical problem solving and diagnostic decision making: selective review of the cognitive literature. *British Medical Journal* **324**, 729–732

Evans JSBT (2003) In two minds: dual-process accounts of reasoning. *Trends in Cognitive Sciences* **7**, 454–459

Fox R (1989) *The Sociology of Medicine: A Participant Observer's View*. Prentice-Hall, Englewood Cliffs

Glasziou P, Rose P, Heneghan C and Balla J (2009) Diagnosis using 'test of treatment'. *British Medical Journal* **338**, b1312

Greenhalgh T (2014) *How to Read a Paper: The Basics of Evidence-Based Medicine*. Wiley-Blackwell, Oxford

Grindlay DJ, Brennan ML and Dean RS (2012) Searching the veterinary literature: a comparison of the coverage of veterinary journals by nine bibliographic databases. *Journal of Veterinary Medical Education* **39**, 404–412

Hardy D and Smith B (2008) Decision making in clinical practice. *British Journal of Anaesthetic and Recovery Nursing* **9**, 19–21

Heneghan C, Glasziou P, Thompson M *et al.* (2009) Diagnostic strategies used in primary care. *British Medical Journal* **338**, b946

Higgs J, Jones MA, Loftus S and Christensen N (2008) *Clinical Reasoning in the Health Professions, 3rd edn*. Elsevier/Butterworth Heinemann, Amsterdam

Kahneman D (2011) *Thinking, Fast and Slow*. Allen Lane, London

Klein G (2008) Naturalistic decision making. *Human factors: The Journal of the Human Factors and Ergonomics Society* **50(3)**, 456–460

Maskrey N, Hutchinson A and Underhill J (2009) Getting a better grip on research: the comfort of opinion. *InnovAiT* **2**, 679–686

McGee DL (2010) Clinical decision-making strategies. In: *Merck Manual*. Merck Sharp & Dohme, Whitehouse Station

Mellanby RJ, Crisp J, De Palma G *et al.* (2007) Perceptions of veterinarians and clients to expressions of clinical uncertainty. *Journal of Small Animal Practice* **48**, 26–31

Norman G (2005) Research in clinical reasoning: past history and current trends. *Medical Education* **39**, 418–427

Orasanu J and Connolly T (1993) The reinvention of decision making. In: *Decision Making in Action: Models and Methods*, ed G Klein, J Orasanu, R Calderwood and CE Zsambok, pp 3–20. Ablex, Norwood

Rollin BE (2006) *An Introduction to Veterinary Medical Ethics: Theory and Cases*. Blackwell Publishing, Ames

Tannenbaum J (1995) *Veterinary Ethics: Animal Welfare, Client Relations, Competition and Collegiality, 2nd edn*. Mosby, St Louis

Timmermans S and Angell A (2001) Evidence-based medicine, clinical uncertainty, and learning to doctor. *Journal of Health and Social Behavior* **42**, 342–359

von Neumann J and Morgenstern O (1944) *Theory of Games and Economic Behavior*. Princeton University Press, Princeton

QRG 3.1: Dealing with the elderly thin cat

by Sarah Caney and Rachel Dean

Many cats entering a shelter may be considered elderly (aged 11 years or older). Elderly cats are vulnerable to a number of age-related diseases, and comorbidities are common. Establishing a diagnosis can be time-consuming and costly, so a pragmatic approach is recommended. A stay in a rehoming centre can be stressful for older cats that tend to be more 'set in their ways' and especially traumatic for those cats suffering from cognitive dysfunction, a common condition of elderly cats. Owners considering relinquishment of their thin older cat should be encouraged to have their cat examined by a veterinary surgeon (veterinarian) and a targeted mini-profile performed (e.g. free-catch urine specific gravity and dipstick tests; blood sampling for packed cell volume and serum proteins, urea, creatinine, alanine aminotransferase and alkaline phosphatase) to rule out significant illness, which could be a barrier to rehoming. When significant health issues are identified it may be better from a welfare perspective to consider euthanasia rather than subjecting the cat to the stress of a move to a rehoming centre with little prospect of finding a new home.

History

A thorough history is an essential starting point. The value of the history may be limited if the carer has known the cat for only a short period, if several carers are involved or if the cat is housed in a group or a busy shelter.

Particular focus should be placed upon the following:

- Bodyweight – Was the cat weighed on admission? Has there been any change in weight? What is the cat's body condition score? Is the cat underweight?
- Appetite – How much is the cat eating? Resting energy requirements are approximately 50 kcal (210 kJ)/kg bodyweight per day. Is the cat polyphagic? Is the cat showing any signs of inappetence or dysphagia? Is halitosis apparent?
- Diet and feeding regime – How much is being eaten and what diet is being fed? Is the diet adequate to meet the cat's requirements? Physiological weight loss can be encountered in elderly cats due to their reduced ability to digest proteins and fats, combined with a reduced sense of smell and taste, which can decrease appetite. Group-housed cats may need extra care to ensure that they are not prevented from accessing sufficient food – for example, by ensuring that adequate food bowls are present for the number of cats in the group
- Thirst – How much is the cat drinking? Does the carer consider the cat's thirst to be excessive?
- Faeces – Colour? Any evidence of blood? Diarrhoea? Frequency of defecation?
- Urine – Most healthy cats urinate once or twice daily. Does the cat's litter tray contain more urine clumps or seem heavier than expected (indicating polyuria)?
- Vomiting or regurgitation – Vomiting may be associated with metabolic, endocrine and primary gastrointestinal disease
- Mobility – Osteoarthritis is very common in elderly cats. Clinical signs most commonly reported include stiffness, reduced jumping, reduced grooming and behavioural changes consistent with chronic pain (e.g. aggression, more withdrawn)
- Behaviour – Examples of abnormal behaviour commonly seen in elderly cats include excessive vocalization (especially at night), hyperactivity, altered relationships with other animals or people in the home, anxiety, withdrawal and aggression
- Grooming and coat condition – Coat condition can deteriorate in association with endocrine conditions such as hyperthyroidism; pain associated with osteoarthritis may lead to reduced grooming.

Clinical examination

The history may point to a certain body system or possible disease; however, it is essential to perform a complete clinical examination so that comorbidities are not missed.

Particular focus should be placed upon the following:

- Behaviour and demeanour – Behavioural changes are not specific and can be seen with a range of causes. Cognitive dysfunction is common in elderly cats. Behavioural changes can also accompany common illnesses such as hyperthyroidism, osteo-arthritis and systemic hypertension
- Mouth (including submandibular lymph nodes) – Look for signs of dental disease and oral masses

Illness	Comments
Bacterial urinary tract infection	Reported to affect approximately 12% of hyperthyroid and diabetic cats and 22% of cats with chronic kidney disease
Chronic kidney disease	Estimated to affect approximately 30% of elderly cats
Cognitive dysfunction	Age-related deterioration in brain function, which results in behavioural changes such as toileting accidents, increased vocalization, confusion, forgetfulness and altered sleep patterns. This is estimated to affect more than 50% of cats over the age of 15 years
Dental disease	Estimated to affect more than 50% of elderly cats
Diabetes mellitus	Estimated to affect up to 1% of cats
Hyperthyroidism	Estimated to affect approximately 12% of cats over the age of 9 years
Neoplasia (cancer)	The most common sites for cancer are the skin, mouth, gastrointestinal tract, mammary glands and bone marrow
Osteoarthritis	One study estimated this to affect more than 90% of cats over the age of 12 years
Systemic hypertension	Estimated to affect more than 20% of cats with chronic kidney disease and 10–15% of cats with hyperthyroidism

Common health problems in older cats that may be associated with weight loss.

QRG 3.1 *continued*

- Mucous membranes – Pallor may be seen in association with anaemia due to chronic kidney disease (CKD)
- Eyes – Ocular examination is helpful for identifying changes consistent with systemic hypertension and those associated with infectious diseases such as feline immunodeficiency virus (FIV) infection and feline infectious peritonitis (FIP)
- Ears – Deafness is common in elderly cats and can sometimes be associated with excessive earwax
- Cervical region – Careful palpation for an enlarged thyroid (goitre) is important because hyperthyroidism affects approximately 12% of cats over the age of 9 years. The presence of a goitre is not diagnostic of hyperthyroidism because non-functional goitres can also occur. Diagnosis of hyperthyroidism requires confirmatory blood tests
- Thorax – The presence of a systolic heart murmur may be associated with hyperthyroidism, systemic hypertension, primary cardiac disease or anaemia
- Abdomen – Careful palpation may reveal common conditions such as constipation, or possible neoplasia. Thickened bowel loops may be identified in patients with diffuse infiltrative conditions such as inflammatory bowel disease or intestinal lymphoma
- Joints and mobility assessment – Although joint thickening and reduced range of movement may be identifiable in osteoarthritic joints, clinical examination may be challenging and is often not specifically helpful; a thorough clinical history may be more useful in such cases
- Weight and body condition score – Weight loss of 5% or more is clinically significant and should not be ignored (see below)
- Blood pressure assessment – Systolic blood pressure readings, ideally using Doppler methodology, should be obtained for all elderly cats in addition to an ocular examination for evidence of target organ damage. Systemic hypertension is commonly associated with CKD and hyperthyroidism.

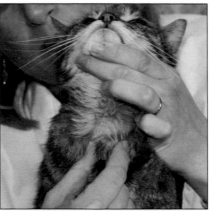

Palpation for a thyroid nodule (goitre) is an essential component of physical examination of the elderly cat. Approximately 80% of cats with hyperthyroidism have a palpable goitre.
(© Sarah Caney)

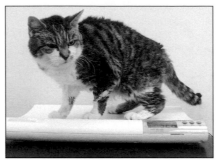

Assessing the bodyweight of a cat.
(© Sarah Caney)

Accurate bodyweight assessment and calculation of percentage changes in weight are helpful in assessing the significance of weight loss. Percentage weight changes are calculated using the following equation:

Percentage change =

$$\frac{\text{Old weight} - \text{New weight}}{\text{Old weight}} \times 100\%$$

Changes <2.5% (either gain or loss) are probably not significant, although trends in previous weights should be reviewed. A 2.5–5% change is likely to be significant; a change >5% is definitely significant

PRACTICAL TIP

If there are no significant abnormalities on clinical examination, the history is limited and the cat is not compromised, it may be acceptable to ask for the cat to be observed for a short period of time and the history and clinical examination repeated 7–10 days later before initiating diagnostic investigations

Further investigations

If physical examination of a thin elderly cat finds no significant abnormalities, the major differential diagnoses are hyperthyroidism, CKD, diabetes mellitus, diffuse inflammatory or neoplastic bowel disease, or a combination of two or more of these diagnoses. Other causes of weight loss that are generally more straightforward to diagnose on physical examination would include oral and dental disease or neoplasia. Sometimes the clinical history and examination will point to one of these diagnoses, and therefore targeted investigations and/or treatment can be undertaken. However, sometimes nothing remarkable is found, and failure to gain weight with good nutrition over a period of time, or continued weight loss, needs to be investigated. A pragmatic approach is needed to ensure that a sensible progression of diagnostic testing is undertaken to reach a diagnosis without using excessive time or financial resources. Euthanasia should be considered if a single case will take up significant funds that could be used more effectively elsewhere.

Diagnostic tests that may be considered in thin elderly cats include initial laboratory tests. An extremely cost-effective initial test would be a simple urinalysis (specific gravity and dipstick) of a free-catch sample; this is a helpful starting point in identifying cats with diabetes mellitus, CKD and hyperthyroidism. If initial blood and urine panels are inconclusive, further laboratory tests that may be helpful include faecal parasitology and bacteriology, feline pancreatic lipase immunoreactivity, and screening for feline leukaemia virus and FIV. Survey radiography, ultrasonography and endoscopy are of value in looking for neoplasia and diffuse alimentary pathology, although an exploratory laparotomy is likely to be a more cost-effective option.

QRG 3.1 *continued*

Test	Result	Interpretation and further action
Urine specific gravity (USG; measured using a refractometer)	<1.035–1.040	Generally abnormal but rule out physiological/iatrogenic causes such as being fed a liquid diet and/or furosemide therapy. Common pathological causes include CKD, hyperthyroidism, diabetes mellitus. Dipstick evaluation, haematology, biochemistry and T4 tests may be indicated depending on the history and clinical findings
	>1.035–1.040	Normal renal concentrating ability. Dipstick evaluation, haematology, biochemistry and T4 tests are still recommended in thin elderly cats
Serum biochemistry (blood collected after an 8-hour fast)	Elevated liver enzymes	Rule out hyperthyroidism before considering primary hepatopathies
	Elevated urea ± creatinine	Azotaemia can be seen with pre-renal disease (e.g. dehydration, poor cardiac function), primary renal disease and post-renal disease (e.g. urethral obstruction, bladder rupture). If USG <1.035 this indicates primary renal disease
	Hyperphosphataemia	Commonly associated with hyperthyroidism, CKD
	Hypokalaemia	May be associated with poor appetite, iatrogenic causes (e.g. furosemide, overzealous administration of i.v. fluids, insulin), hyperthyroidism, hyperaldosteronism, CKD
Haematology	Non-regenerative anaemia	Consider any chronic disease, CKD
Total thyroxine (T4)	Above reference range	Hyperthyroidism highly likely as most diagnostic tests have a low false-positive rate
	Upper half of reference range	Hyperthyroidism possible – if compatible clinical signs are present, consider repeating the total T4 test ± adding free T4 and thyroid-stimulating hormone (TSH) to confirm the diagnosis. Cats with hyperthyroidism usually have elevated total and free T4 with low or undetectable levels of TSH
	Low or lower half of reference range	Hyperthyroidism unlikely
Glucose	Elevated	Diabetes mellitus is possible; beware stress hyperglycaemia
FIV testing	Positive antibody result	Unless cat is from a country where vaccination is possible, likely to indicate persistent infection

Initial laboratory tests that may be helpful in feline patients with undiagnosed weight loss.

Supportive care for unexplained weight loss

The following strategies may be helpful while awaiting the results of diagnostic tests, or when following a more conservative approach to the old thin cat:

- Providing a high-calorie diet (e.g. convalescent food)
- Trial therapeutics – for example:
  - Appetite stimulants, e.g. mirtazapine at 1.9 mg/kg q24–48h
  - Anti-nausea treatments, e.g. maropitant at 1 mg/kg q24h
  - Analgesia, e.g. buprenorphine at 10–30 μg/kg sublingually q8–12h
- Close monitoring including repeat history, physical examination, weight and body condition scoring.

Treatment of common causes of weight loss in elderly cats

Chronic kidney disease

Many cats with International Renal Interest Society (IRIS) Stage 1 and 2 CKD have an excellent quality of life for several years following diagnosis. Cats in IRIS Stage 3 and 4 (creatinine >250 μmol/l) are likely to have greater medication requirements and a worse prognosis, which may make them difficult to rehome. The most proven treatment for cats with CKD is feeding a specially formulated diet for renal patients (Roudebush *et al.*, 2009). On average, a cat with CKD that eats one of these diets will live for two to three times longer after diagnosis than a cat with CKD that is fed a standard commercial cat food. Although 'renal diets' have multiple modifications, the one felt to be most beneficial in terms of survival and quality of life is phosphate restriction. Therefore, for cats that refuse a 'renal diet', or where it is not possible to feed such a diet for other reasons, mixing oral phosphate binders with the food offered is recommended. Blood phosphate levels should be kept below 1.5 mmol/l if possible. A wide variety of additional treatments may be beneficial for cats with CKD, depending on clinical findings. These could include, as appropriate, treatment for proteinuria, appetite stimulants, anti-emetics and antihypertensive medications. It is important to target treatment to clinical findings; for example, only cats with CKD and accompanying proteinuria (which is a relatively small subset), require ACE inhibitors or angiotensin receptor blockers.

Diabetes mellitus

The majority of cats diagnosed with diabetes are suffering from type II diabetes mellitus, in which there is peripheral insulin resistance in addition to an absolute or relative deficiency of insulin. Aggressive early treatment with insulin and a specially formulated low-carbohydrate ('diabetic') diet can result in diabetic remission, and this is always the primary goal of treatment. For those cats that do not go into diabetic remission, the goals are to resolve the clinical signs associated with the diabetes (e.g. polydipsia, weight loss) and to reduce blood glucose such that for most of the day levels are below the renal threshold (12–14 mmol/l) while not risking clinical hypoglycaemia (<5 mmol/l). Cats with long-standing diabetes (particularly those showing signs of insulin resistance or having variable insulin requirements) are difficult to stabilize and hence less easy to rehome. Diabetic cats are also expensive to care for in the shelter, and a pragmatic decision to euthanase may be appropriate in some cases.

Hyperthyroidism

Treatment options for hyperthyroidism include oral or transdermal antithyroid medications, feeding an iodine-restricted food, surgical thyroidectomy →

QRG 3.1 *continued*

(following medical stabilization) and radioactive iodine treatment. In a shelter setting, surgical thyroidectomy may be the most cost-effective option for long-term management. If concerns exist about the patient's suitability for anaesthesia and/or surgery (e.g. no palpable goitre, raising the suspicion of an ectopic thyroid mass), then oral medical management is likely to be the most cost-effective option. Additional complications of hyperthyroidism, such as systemic hypertension and cardiac failure, should be treated as needed.

Rehoming cats with ongoing conditions

Clinical disease is common in elderly cats and often makes them harder to rehome. Although many illnesses of older cats are manageable, not all prospective owners wish to take on a cat requiring daily medication or a special diet. Prolonged residence in a rehoming centre is not ideal from a welfare perspective and may prevent the shelter from accepting other cats that would be easier to rehome. While some conditions may be straightforward to stabilize, in other cases the prognosis may be more guarded. In situations where significant long-term clinical disease is present, euthanasia may be more appropriate.

References and further reading

Roudebush P, Polzin DJ, Ross SJ *et al.* (2009) An evidence-based review of therapies for feline chronic kidney disease. *Journal of Feline Medicine and Surgery* **11**, 195–210

http://bestbetsforvets.org/bet/174

QRG 3.2: Dealing with the elderly dog
by Gemma Bourne and Zoe Belshaw

Initial assessment of the older dog

Older dogs arriving at a rehoming organization have a considerable life history. If the dog is from a home environment, it may be possible to obtain relevant medical information from the owner. However, some owners may withhold information for fear of prejudicing the dog's chances of being offered a place or being subsequently rehomed. Other dogs will arrive as strays; for these dogs, an assessment of health and wellbeing will be necessary given the absence of any background information. In all cases it is pertinent not to assume anything, and a full clinical examination is always a good starting point.

Older dogs may be at increased risk of succumbing to ill health in a kennel environment due to comorbidities. It is unwise to assume that older animals will have strong immunity to infectious diseases, as this will depend on their previous exposure and vaccination history. Proactive preventive healthcare, including worming and full vaccination, is therefore warranted unless a history of appropriate preventive healthcare is provided (see Chapter 11).

Some conditions are more prevalent in older animals, but not all of these are obvious within the confines of a consulting room. As well as assessing for evidence of lameness, dental disease, mass lesions, visual or auditory deficits, it is advisable to ask care staff to observe older dogs as they go about daily life within the shelter. Simple monitoring sheets can be designed to facilitate this task. As a minimum, monitoring should include assessment of appetite, thirst, mobility and exercise tolerance. This can also prove very useful if a dog's condition deteriorates, as it is impossible to quantify any changes without first understanding what is 'normal' for an individual animal. For instance, a Yorkshire Terrier that has always lived with one doting owner may flatly refuse to eat dry dog food on day 1 after arrival, because it is used to sharing a roast chicken. This dog's appetite could be expected to improve over time. However, a stray dog that eats well at first, but subsequently becomes inappetent, may be showing early signs of illness. Where abnormalities are detected, consideration must be given to how far investigation and treatment are feasible. The value of in-house testing should not be underestimated, with cheap and simple tests such as urinalysis being extremely valuable.

Caring for the older dog in a shelter

Older dogs often prove challenging to rehome and may be resident within an organization for extended periods. Communication is essential in monitoring their health and wellbeing, and regular checks of parameters such as weight and general body condition are advisable. Few organizations work with a single designated veterinary surgeon (veterinarian), and the more likely scenario is that the animals within a shelter are looked after by a number of different veterinary surgeons. It is essential that animals are clearly identified both by shelter staff and in veterinary records, and that comprehensive clinical notes are maintained so that information can be transferred between professionals. This is particularly important in the absence of an owner to provide updates.

A clear system for medication administration should be established. Questions to ask include whether a specific member of staff takes responsibility for administering drugs, and what happens if the responsible person is absent. It is advisable to keep written records at the shelter of what medication has been given, when and by whom. This will improve compliance and reduce the incidence of accidental overdose. Medications should be labelled very clearly to ensure that they are administered to the correct dog, and the importance of timely and accurate dosing should be emphasized. If medication is usually given in food, a clear plan should be provided as to →

QRG 3.2 *continued*

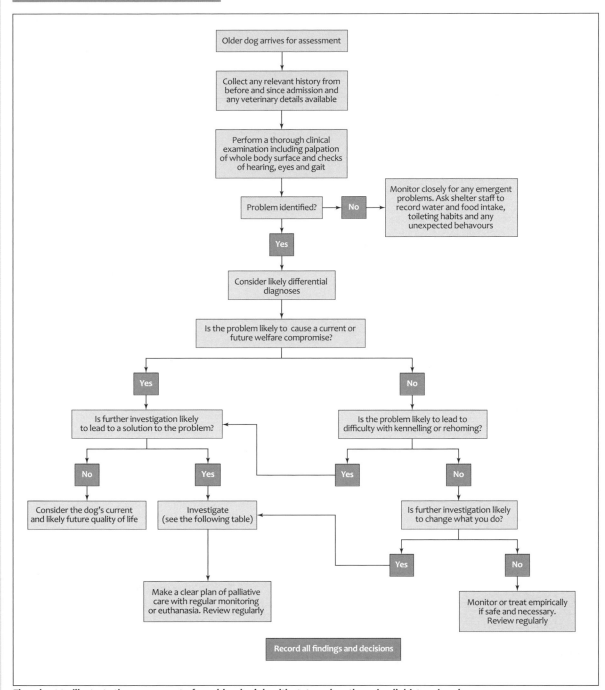

Flowchart to illustrate the assessment of an older dog's health status when the animal's history is unknown.

whether and how to administer it if the dog does not eat its meal, as the significance of this can easily be missed by lay staff. Clear information on common side effects of each medication and what to do in case of overdose or missed doses should be provided by the veterinary surgeon, and a record left on site for consultation.

Even in the absence of any specific disease processes, older dogs need special consideration.

Dogs from a home environment may benefit from familiarity and maintaining a routine; providing their usual diet or maintaining the training that they have been taught can help to manage stress. Older dogs may be at more risk of sleep deprivation in a busy kennel environment, and providing a quiet resting place with a soft, warm bed away from damp or draughts will help. However, it is equally important to ensure that older dogs have enough stimulation to

keep them interested and alert, to prevent boredom and minimize weight gain. Walks should be tailored to each dog's ability and the use of interactive toys can help prevent boredom while placing less emphasis on physical exercise. Arranging social contact with appropriate people or other dogs can also help older animals to keep stimulated during their time in the shelter.

QRG 3.2 *continued*

Clinical sign	Information to be collected by the shelter	Initial investigations if finances are limited
Heart murmur	Exercise tolerance, evidence and nature of coughing, recording resting respiratory rate over 1 minute	Auscultate thorax and assess pulses – sinus arrhythmia makes clinically significant cardiac disease unlikely
Lameness	The number of limbs involved, whether the lameness improves on exercise or is exacerbated on different floor surfaces, severity of lameness	Thorough orthopaedic examination. Radiography only if it is likely to change the outcome
Mass lesions	Examine all dogs for masses regularly; monitor size changes in any recognized masses	Fine-needle aspiration of mass lesions, palpation ± aspiration of draining lymph node
Cough	Frequency and nature of cough, any change over time, anything that exacerbates it (e.g. pulling on the lead, excitement). Any change in bark that may suggest laryngeal paralysis	Full clinical examination, neck palpation, thorough thoracic and cardiac auscultation in a quiet room. If multiple dogs are affected, check worming and vaccination history, and possibly the kennel environment to assess ventilation and ease of direct and fomite transmission of infection
Excessive thirst, urination or urinary incontinence	Record exact water intake over 24 hours. Collect free-catch urine sample in a sterile container. Monitor whether the dog is unconsciously leaking urine (e.g. wet bedding) to differentiate incontinence and polyuria (both may be present simultaneously)	Urine specific gravity, dipstick and sediment examination. Free-catch urine sample culture – negative result makes urinary tract infection very unlikely. If the result is positive, consider catheterized or cystocentesis repeat sample to rule out environmental contaminants, confirm infection and optimize antibiotic choice
Decreased appetite	Monitor food intake, try different food types, various bowls and different food environments. Record behaviour around food	Thorough feeding history and full clinical examination to differentiate behavioural and medical causes
Weight loss	Observe feeding behaviour from the time the food is given to when it is removed. Record appetite, ideally the exact amount of food consumed in a 24-hour period – may necessitate weighing food. Record nature of faeces (i.e. any evidence of diarrhoea) and any vomiting or regurgitation	Collect relevant feeding behaviour history. Assess whether weight loss is muscle, fat or both. Calculate the amount of food the dog should be eating and ascertain whether it is receiving it. Ascertain whether there are kennel-related factors that may be inhibiting eating or leading to excessive energy expenditure (e.g. cold weather, compulsive pacing). If there is weight loss in the face of adequate food intake, consider blood biochemistry and urinalysis
Abnormal faecal nature	Ascertain the frequency and consistency of faeces passed plus any change in faecal weight (both can be used to differentiate small *versus* large intestinal diarrhoea, which have different differential diagnoses). Assess appetite, any relevant dietary history, worming status (including drugs active against *Giardia*) and, where relevant, identify any potential stressors. Note any other abnormal clinical signs or behaviours that may point to a more systemic problem	Many dogs will have diarrhoea on first admission that resolves with no treatment. If it persists and kennel-related factors appear an unlikely cause, switch to a different protein and carbohydrate diet for at least 3 weeks and repeat comprehensive worming. If obvious stressors are identified, minimize these. If a cohort of dogs has diarrhoea, consider faecal culture and parasite assessment from a proportion of dogs, but consider how much additional investigations will change the course of action. Assessment of blood vitamin B12 levels (or empirical supplementation) in chronic cases of small intestinal diarrhoea may be worthwhile

Common presenting problems and potential pragmatic courses of initial investigation for older dogs.

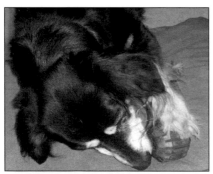

Providing some of the daily feed in suitable toys can help prevent boredom in older dogs with reduced exercise tolerance.
(© Gemma Bourne)

Rehoming the older dog: veterinary considerations

Veterinary surgeons typically do not have much of a role in the rehoming of dogs from rescue centres, but it is useful to understand some of the difficulties faced by shelters in rehoming older dogs. Additionally, shelter staff may be unaware of the veterinary-related implications of adopting an older dog, for example, potential insurance exclusions, the prevalence of certain age-related diseases and the cost of their management, so they may appreciate guidance.

Dog age is known to play a significant role in adoption (Siettou et al., 2014). Older dogs may not be able to cope with a busy, active lifestyle, so may not be suitable pets for prospective owners who are looking for company on long walks. There is some evidence that older owners may be well suited to provide a good quality of life for senior dogs (Pitteri et al., 2014), but this must be balanced with the burden of care described by owners of chronically ill dogs (Christiansen et al., 2013). Other practicalities are worth consideration. For example, smaller old dogs may be easier to rehome; a 50 kg dog with osteoarthritis may pose significantly more practical and financial challenges than one weighing 5 kg.

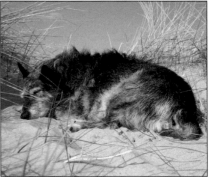

Older dogs may appreciate a more sedentary lifestyle.
(© Zoe Belshaw)

QRG 3.2 continued

Taking the example of a large dog with osteoarthritis, rehoming staff should be aware that steep steps, hills and stairs may be a problem for this dog, that the dog may need to be lifted into a car and that the ongoing treatment costs may be significant. It is therefore useful to discuss with prospective owners whether their house would be easy for the dog to access, and whether they would be able to lift the dog if needed.

Potential adopters should be made aware of the needs of any dog in which they are interested, including its past and present health problems, potential insurance exclusions, and the importance (and ideally an estimate of the cost) of any ongoing medications. It would be useful for adopters to be able to take any relevant veterinary history with them when they collect the dog. This is particularly important for animals on any prescription medication. The shelter may appreciate the provision of information sheets written by a veterinary surgeon in simple language, explaining conditions such as osteoarthritis, renal and cardiac disease, which can be given to both staff and potential owners.

A generic fact sheet on caring for the older dog may be useful for new owners, covering aspects such as managing deafness, recognizing behavioural changes, spotting early signs of arthritis, checking for mass lesions and monitoring water intake. It is important that adopters of an older dog are made aware of these conditions and know that they are manageable, to encourage them to present the animal to a veterinary surgeon early if any abnormalities arise; however, this must be balanced with the risks of dissuading owners from adopting an older dog.

Not all dogs will be suitable for rehoming and some elderly dogs will not adapt to life in a shelter. Fostering may be an option for some, but euthanasia may be better in welfare terms than a long stay in a shelter for dogs that are unlikely candidates for rehoming. However, there is no doubt that older dogs can make rewarding companions, and age should be only part of the assessment for their rehoming potential.

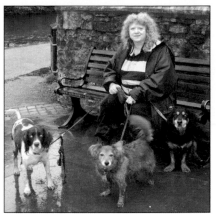

Rehoming an older dog can be very fulfilling for dog and owner alike.
(© Zoe Belshaw)

References and further reading

Christiansen SB, Kristensen AT, Sandoe P *et al.* (2013) Looking after chronically ill dogs: impacts on the caregiver's life. *Anthrozoos* **26**, 519–533

Pitteri E, Mongillo P, Adamelli S *et al.* (2014) The quality of life of pet dogs owned by elderly people depends on the living context, not on the owner's age. *Journal of Veterinary Behavior: Clinical Applications and Research* **9**, 72–77

Siettou C, Fraser IM and Fraser RW (2014) Investigating some of the factors that influence "consumer" choice when adopting a shelter dog in the United Kingdom. *Journal of Applied Animal Welfare Science* **17**, 136–147

QRG 3.3: Dealing with heart murmurs in dogs and cats

by Virginia Luis Fuentes and Jessie Rose Payne

Heart murmurs are common in dogs and cats, but the prognostic significance of a murmur can vary enormously depending on the underlying cause. This poses a particular problem in shelter settings, where a realistic estimate of prognosis is essential for successful rehoming of an animal but resources for further investigations may be limited. The most accurate prognosis will be obtained with referral to a veterinary cardiologist for echocardiography but, unless a sympathetic local cardiologist can be found who will offer a discount for investigation and treatment, other options may be necessary. The value of auscultation should not be underestimated. In dogs, characterization of the murmur is the best way to narrow the list of differential diagnoses and incurs no additional costs. In cats, auscultation of murmur characteristics is less useful, but the detection of other auscultation abnormalities (gallop sounds or arrhythmias) may be useful indicators of serious disease.

In both species, an 'in-house' echocardiogram can provide very useful information on prognosis, but the value is highly user-dependent. Recognition of left atrial enlargement is a key skill, as this finding indicates a worse prognosis in dogs with myxomatous mitral valve disease and dilated cardiomyopathy, as well as in cats with cardiomyopathies. A combination of skilled auscultation and even a basic level of echocardiographic skill is likely to be the most cost-effective approach to determining prognosis in shelter animals.

Dogs

Physical examination (particularly auscultation) and any history that is available is vitally important in establishing the most likely differential diagnoses prior to carrying out any investigative tests. Accurate characterization of murmurs can help to eliminate differentials, and signalment profiling can help to organize the differentials according to likelihood.

Characterization of murmurs
Timing

'Long' systolic murmurs: These murmurs (holosystolic or pansystolic) last throughout systole. Examples include mitral or tricuspid regurgitation and ventricular septal defect. ➡

QRG 3.3 *continued*

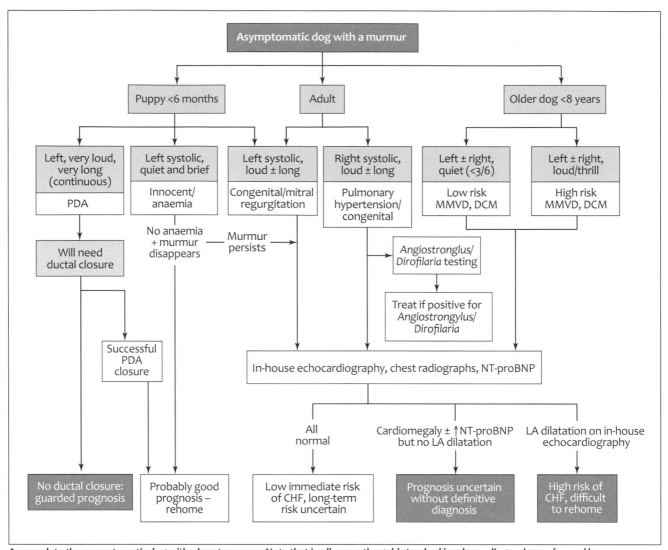

Approach to the asymptomatic dog with a heart murmur. Note that in all cases, the gold standard is echocardiography performed by a cardiologist. If not available, see suggestions above. CHF = congestive heart failure; DCM = dilated cardiomyopathy; LA = left atrium; MMVD = myxomatous mitral valve disease; NT-proBNP = N-terminal pro B-type natriuretic peptide; PCV = packed cell volume; PDA = patent ductus arteriosus; PH = pulmonary hypertension.

'Brief' systolic murmurs: These murmurs are of short duration, typically lasting only for the first 30–50% of systole. Most brief murmurs are ejection murmurs. Ejection murmurs are heard best over the aortic and pulmonic valves at the heart base, and can be associated with anything that increases stroke volume (e.g. increased sympathetic tone, bradycardia, anaemia); in such cases they are called functional or physiological murmurs. They may be called innocent murmurs if there is no underlying disease process. Ejection murmurs can also be associated with mild aortic or pulmonic stenosis (note that more severe stenosis results in longer murmur duration).

Very long murmurs: Murmurs that are continuous – systolic extending well into diastole – are likely to indicate patent ductus arteriosus (PDA).

Diastolic murmurs: These murmurs are most commonly associated with aortic insufficiency due to aortic endocarditis.

Intensity

Murmur intensity is generally graded from 1 to 6: grade 6/6 murmurs being the loudest, grade ≥4/6 murmurs being considered loud and grade 1–2/6 murmurs being considered quiet. Grade 5/6 and 6/6 murmurs are

associated with palpable precordial thrills. Murmur intensity may correlate with severity in some conditions (e.g. mitral valve disease, aortic and pulmonic stenosis) but not at all in others (e.g. dilated cardiomyopathy, ventricular septal defect). A murmur that is both quiet and brief is very likely to be a functional murmur.

Point of maximum intensity

Most murmurs are left-sided, but the whole thorax should be auscultated thoroughly. Ejection murmurs are typically heard best at the left base (i.e. under the triceps muscle), whereas longer holosystolic murmurs are often louder at the

QRG 3.3 *continued*

left apex (i.e. the murmur becomes quieter as the stethoscope chest-piece is moved cranially into the left axilla). Right-sided murmurs include murmurs of tricuspid regurgitation and ventricular septal defects. Tricuspid regurgitation is often present with mitral valve disease and dilated cardiomyopathy, but may also be an indication of pulmonary hypertension. Where geographically appropriate, *Angiostrongylus vasorum* or *Dirofilaria immitis* should be ruled out, as these are treatable causes of pulmonary hypertension.

Cardiac enlargement on thoracic radiographs can indicate clinically significant cardiac disease, but there is substantial breed variation that

Top tip

Always auscultate the whole thorax. PDA murmurs are often missed because a quiet murmur of mitral regurgitation is found and further auscultation is abandoned

makes interpretation of heart size challenging. Measurement of plasma concentrations of the biomarker N-terminal pro B-type natriuretic peptide (NT-proBNP) can play a role in helping to identify dogs with clinically significant cardiac disease, but biomarkers are less useful than in cats.

Cats

Overall, innocent murmurs are more common in cats than pathological murmurs, so the approach in cats is

different from that in dogs. Murmur characterization is very difficult in cats, as is obtaining a definitive diagnosis without expert echocardiography, so the emphasis should instead be on identifying cats at high risk of cardiac complications (such as congestive heart failure (CHF) or aortic thromboembolism). This is easier to achieve and more useful than differentiating cats with functional murmurs from those with mild hypertrophic cardiomyopathy; fortunately, a good prognosis can be expected in cats with both of these conditions.

Top tip

Most murmurs in cats are loudest over the sternum

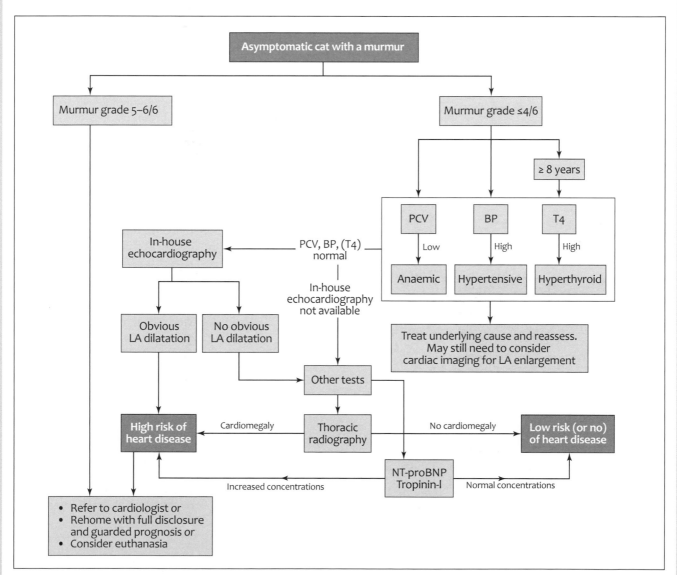

Approach to the asymptomatic cat with a heart murmur. BP = blood pressure; LA = left atrium; NT-proBNP = N-terminal pro B-type natriuretic peptide; PCV = packed cell volume; T4 = thyroxine.

QRG 3.3 *continued*

The general approach to a cat with a murmur should be:

- Palpate the chest to identify precordial thrills – their presence indicates congenital disease
- Rule out systemic disease that can result in a heart murmur – measure packed cell volume for anaemia, blood pressure for hypertension and serum thyroxine in older cats for hyperthyroidism
- If possible, consider 'in-house' echocardiography to assess the size of the left atrium. Cats with an obviously enlarged left atrium are at risk of CHF or aortic thromboembolism, and this requires a more basic level of echocardiographic skills than diagnosing the type of heart disease
- If in-house echocardiography is not feasible, consider thoracic radiography to assess cardiac size – cardiomegaly is more likely in 'high-risk' cats
- Cardiac biomarkers may also be usefully measured if finances allow – plasma N-terminal pro B-type natriuretic peptide (NT-proBNP) concentrations increase as heart disease severity worsens, and elevated concentrations of serum troponin-I indicate a poorer prognosis.

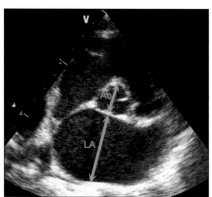

Right parasternal short-axis echocardiographic view showing the aortic valve (Ao) and left atrium (LA) in a cat with left atrial enlargement. A normal LA:Ao ratio is <1.5; values >1.8 are likely to indicate left atrial enlargement.

Homing animals with a heart murmur

Not all animals with a heart murmur have a poor prognosis; many will have a normal life expectancy and can be successfully rehomed. Obtaining a definitive diagnosis can be difficult without access to high-quality echocardiography, but it may be possible to differentiate animals at high risk *versus* low risk of cardiac complications with the use of thoracic radiography, measurement of cardiac biomarkers and, in some instances, echocardiographic assessment of the size of the left atrium. Dogs or cats already showing signs of CHF are at very high risk of future episodes and will require lifelong therapy. Euthanasia should be considered for these high-risk cases. It is also important to bear in mind that insurance cover is likely to exclude cardiac conditions for animals with a history of a murmur.

Asymptomatic dogs considered low risk

Quiet, brief or disappearing murmurs are often functional and considered low risk. Prospective owners should be made aware of the heart murmur and informed that the likelihood is that the prognosis will be good, but that this cannot be guaranteed without a definitive diagnosis. Specialist imaging will be necessary for an accurate diagnosis, but prospective owners can treat such dogs as normal with no lifestyle restrictions.

Asymptomatic cats considered low risk

Many low-risk cats have dynamic murmurs that come and go, and the murmur itself is not necessarily a good indicator of disease, as these cats may have mild myocardial disease or no cardiac disease at all. Prospective owners should be warned that although the cat is currently considered 'low risk', this could change over time. Disappearance of the murmur is not necessarily a good prognostic sign and annual re-evaluation should be recommended (e.g. by measurement of NT-proBNP and troponin-I or assessment of left atrial size).

Asymptomatic dogs considered high risk

It is important to identify a continuous murmur, as the prognosis for dogs with a PDA is very poor without treatment. However, PDA is potentially curable with surgical ligation or a catheter intervention for device closure of the ductus if funds allow. For older dogs with cardiomegaly and elevated cardiac biomarker concentrations, there is a high risk of CHF and prospective owners should be warned of this. Monitoring for early signs of heart failure can be achieved very cheaply by teaching new owners how to measure resting or sleeping respiratory rate. A resting respiratory rate above 40 breaths/min may indicate CHF in a high-risk dog, and this should prompt the owner to seek veterinary attention. There may be substantial costs associated with the treatment of heart failure once there is clinical deterioration. For younger dogs, the prognosis is even less certain, and prospective owners should be warned that it is not possible to predict a prognosis. With high-risk dogs, owners should be warned that they should avoid deliberately encouraging the dog to sprint (i.e. do not throw balls for the dog to chase), but regular exercise can still be encouraged.

Asymptomatic cats considered high risk

Cats with dilatation of the left atrium are at risk of aortic thromboembolism, which is a devastating complication. Euthanasia may need to be considered, but if not, these cats should receive lifelong treatment with clopidogrel, which is not always easy to administer. If rehoming is considered, prospective owners should be taught how to measure resting or sleeping respiratory rate, as these cats are also at high risk of CHF. As with dogs, a respiratory rate above 40 breaths/min may indicate CHF.

Chapter 4

Concepts in free-roaming population control

Ian MacFarlaine and Andy Gibson

Domestication of the two most common companion animal species is believed to have taken place over a period of thousands of years – around 10,000 for the cat and around 20,000 to 30,000 for dogs. Although the mode and purpose of domestication of the cat and the dog differed, the ability of both species to spread globally via human-mediated movement has been significant.

One of the earliest-dated finds of feline remains, buried in association with human remains on an island where there are no naturally occurring felids, indicates that humans were transporting cats with them on colonization and settlement expeditions at least 9500 years ago. The feline overpopulation that now exists in many areas is in part linked to the original path of domestication in the cat, which was initially passive, driven by the actions of cats to seek out a good food supply (rodents attracted to human settlement). This process is repeated regularly when free-living cats approach human habitations as a good source of food.

Humans have selectively bred dogs for desired physical and behavioural traits to meet our needs. As a result, domesticated dogs provide value to society through security, rescue, detection and assisting those with disabilities, but by far their broadest contribution is their unwavering companionship. In most settings domestic dogs cannot survive and reproduce without resources provided either intentionally or unintentionally by humans. Although cats are seen as less directly dependent on humans, the breeding success of feline populations is also strongly driven by human behaviours such as feeding the cats and dumping rubbish. Therefore, modifying human behaviour is the most powerful tool in managing dog and cat populations.

This chapter aims to provide an overview of the key aspects of population management from a practical standpoint and some of the emerging techniques and technologies that are likely to be instrumental in how cat and dog populations are managed in the future.

Population structures

In most Western countries it is deemed unacceptable for dogs to roam unsupervised on the streets and such animals are actively removed by local authorities for holding, rehoming or euthanasia. In this context, definition of ownership by confinement is usually straightforward. However, in countries where there is a culture of allowing dogs to roam freely, an individual dog's degree of ownership and confinement can fluctuate. In contrast, cats have remained a generally free-roaming species and, with the exception of some parts of the USA and Australasia, indoor–outdoor or wholly outdoor models of ownership are the norm. The situation is therefore complex, with cats and dogs falling on a spectrum of ownership/dependency, and there is huge variation in local attitudes, tolerance and welfare expectations for both species. However, a degree of simplification can be helpful. Therefore, here ownership and confinement are considered independently, with owned animals being categorized as responsibly owned or irresponsibly/quasi-owned. The overlap between owned and free-roaming animals, which exists in many cat and dog populations, is illustrated in Figure 4.1.

Categorization by confinement

Free-roaming

A 'free-roaming' dog or cat refers to any animal that is not physically restricted to private property or under the direct control of an owner at the time of sighting. These are sometimes referred to as 'street', 'stray' or 'free-ranging', but in many cases a high proportion of these animals are owned in some capacity. These animals may be intermittently confined to private property and allowed to roam for some of the day, or never confined and therefore free to roam at all times. As a result, their dependency on humans can vary from having all of their resources provided by a person, to being fully independent of resources intentionally provided by people, or somewhere between these two extremes.

Fully confined

Fully confined dogs and cats are generally considered as 'pets'. They are supervised by an owner whenever they leave the owner's property and therefore never have the opportunity to roam freely. These animals are entirely dependent on the owner for provision of food, water, shelter, exercise, socialization, preventive veterinary care and veterinary attention when sick or injured. They are more likely than free-roaming animals to be responsibly owned, but this is not necessarily the case, with irresponsible breeding and failure to provide for basic welfare needs and veterinary care still being a major problem in many parts of the world.

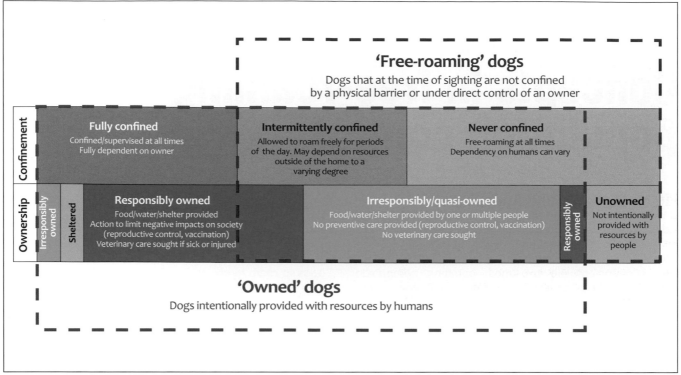

4.1 Diagram illustrating the overlap between owned and free-roaming populations of dogs. The size of each compartment relates to the size of the respective populations, which varies greatly depending on the local situation. Note that some fully confined animals are not responsibly owned, and some unconfined animals may be responsibly owned. Shelter animals are, by definition, confined and may be responsibly or irresponsibly owned.

Intermittently confined

Depending on the location and culture, many dogs and, especially, cats may be intermittently confined by their owner or carer, either with access to the outside at the owner or animal's time of choosing (e.g. via a cat flap) or allowed to be free-roaming at specific periods. These populations may form an important link between fully confined and fully free-roaming populations.

Categorization by ownership
Owned

The definition of ownership is often blurred in situations where animals are allowed to roam freely and have variable dependency on one or several people. Ownership, and therefore accountability for an animal, is classically defined by someone claiming possession of the animal; however, this is likely to be influenced by the context. For example, if claiming ownership is likely to result in a financial or legal burden, an individual might deny ownership of an animal, while that same person may demand the right to give consent in the event of the animal needing treatment or euthanasia. This fluctuating definition of ownership can present many difficulties both in describing populations and when implementing practical population management strategies.

If a person is regularly and intentionally providing resources to an animal, they are facilitating its survival and influencing its ongoing wellbeing and ability to reproduce. One could therefore argue that they have some degree of responsibility for or ownership of that animal. Although this definition is perhaps unconventional, it is far more ecologically and socially relevant than the classical definition. Therefore, for the purpose of this chapter, an 'owned' animal is one that is intentionally being provided with resources by one or more people – for example, if the

answer to the question 'Do you feed this animal?' is 'Yes', the animal could be said to be owned by that person. This definition of ownership can be subdivided into *responsibly owned* and *irresponsibly* or *quasi-owned* animals.

Responsibly owned: Responsibly owned animals are provided with an appropriate diet, exercise, social interaction and healthcare; in addition, the owner prevents detrimental impacts on society through aggression, the spread of zoonotic diseases and the breeding of unwanted litters. These animals generally have low reproductive capacity as, although litter survival rates would be high in animals whose welfare needs are met, reproduction is controlled by neutering or restricted access to mates. Therefore, responsibly owned animals will be bred only in a planned manner to supply a known need. This is especially relevant in terms of dogs in the UK, where the canine overpopulation problem is dominated by the preponderance of certain types of dog. For example, in the UK currently bull breeds and their crosses disproportionately present as stray or unwanted, however, fashionable trends for other breeds that prove to be inappropriate for many owners are a cyclical problem. The distinction is less clear for cats, where an absolute overpopulation currently exists in the UK, and therefore almost any breeding of cats contributes to the overpopulation problem.

Irresponsibly owned/quasi-owned: Irresponsibly owned or quasi-owned animals are those that are provided with resources such as food or shelter to enable their survival, but no action is taken to maintain their wellbeing or prevent negative impacts on society. In some situations an owner may want to provide preventive care for an animal, but is unable to do so owing to a lack of accessible services. In such instances one could argue that this degree of care is not irresponsible, but may be insufficient to meet the animal's needs fully, and therefore the animal could be said to be 'quasi-owned' (it is provided with some of its needs by human caregivers). On the other hand, if that person is aware of accessible services but fails to make use of them for an animal they feed, then they could be said to be irresponsible. From a population management perspective both of these cases have the same potential for poor animal welfare and spread of zoonotic disease. These animals have the highest reproductive capacity, especially if allowed to roam; they have high fertility and litter survival rates as well as unrestricted access to breeding partners.

Unowned

Unowned animals are those that are not intentionally provided with resources by humans. These animals may be lost or abandoned, or may have never been owned and survive by scavenging. For unowned dogs, their reproductive capacity is usually low because, although they have high access to potential mates, they are generally less fertile due to poor nourishment and have high litter mortality rates. The death of large numbers of puppies in these litters may warrant targeting reproductive control efforts at this population on welfare grounds.

In contrast, cats are able to breed successfully with very little intentional input by humans, meaning that unowned cats can contribute very significantly to overall overpopulation problems. In societies with highly developed feline ownership norms, and with a welfare and shelter infrastructure, stray cats still form a significant proportion of the pet population.

There is often a flux of animals between the owned and unowned populations. Shelters may facilitate the movement of animals from being unowned to owned. As such, when an animal is in the care of a shelter, this may be regarded as a form of ownership, which implies a duty of care. Shelters fulfil animals' basic needs to a variable extent, and this can be considered as analogous to responsible (or sometimes irresponsible) ownership.

Coexistence of roaming cat and dog overpopulations in the same zone

Experience suggests that where a roaming canine population is large, the roaming cat population in the same area may be smaller. Although predation of younger kittens by roaming dogs may play a small part in this, it is more likely that competition for food or discomfort felt by the cats in relation to the proximity of a larger potential predator may be the cause. Figure 4.2 shows cats and dogs scavenging together at a passive feeding point; however, this is not a typical finding in many places. It must be remembered that, for example, a neutering programme to control the dog population may lead indirectly to a rebound increase in the cat population.

What is overpopulation?

'Overpopulation' is dependent on the concerns of the individual(s) describing it as such. For the animal welfare sector, the relentless demand for foster and shelter space for cats may indicate that there is overpopulation. However, overpopulation may be relative; for example, many shelters in the UK have large numbers of adult and elderly cats needing homes, while demand for kittens is comparatively high. A similar scenario is seen with a demand for puppies contrasting the large numbers of inadequately socialized adolescent dogs of bull breeds in shelters.

Inputs into overpopulation

There are several possible inputs into overpopulation of animals (Figure 4.3):

* Inadequately controlled or accidental breeding – reproduction is either not controlled at all, or is controlled only after puberty and after the production of a litter, meaning that the animals have not only replaced themselves in the potential breeding population but have also increased their number before control is commenced
* Deliberate breeding where the offspring produced outnumber the demand for them – the individuals in the litter that is bred do not all find homes (or, it could be argued, usurp the placement of others in homes in a 'domino' effect)
* Abandonment and relinquishment either into the shelter population or directly into the environment (see below)
* Straying of animals without subsequent reunion with the owner.

Relinquishment (which is referred to within the shelter sector variously as 'signing over', 'gifting', 'surrendering', 'intake' and 'handover') is the transfer of legal ownership of an animal from an owner to a rescue or rehoming organization, with the animal being taken into shelter care or fostering. In most shelter situations the potential for intake is greatly exceeded by the demand, and

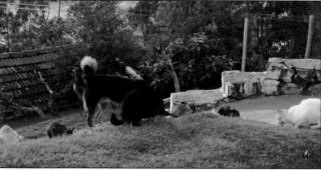

4.2 Free-roaming dogs and cats feeding side by side at a roadside fish-gutting point in Ootacamund, India.
(© Mission Rabies)

Inputs into overpopulation
• Owned roaming animals
• Inappropriate overbreeding of owned animals
• Abandoned animals
• Lost animals
• 'Community' animals
• Feral/street animals

Common control measures in overpopulation
• Trap-neuter-return (TNR) of animals
• Caught animals:
• Rehomed
• Housed in shelters
• Euthanasia
• Animals adopted from the street
• Death of animals (e.g. from injury or disease)
• Animals killed (e.g. poisoned or shot)

4.3 Inputs into and impacts of overpopulation.

consequently shelters run at or exceed capacity much of the time. Where there is little or no shelter infrastructure it is common for animals to be abandoned at other locations. This may be casually, by being turned out into the street, or at critical points such as veterinary practices, pet shops, markets or at existing colonies of feral or stray animals.

The point at which there are too many animals is relative, and only where the population reaches a level or local permeation that gives rise to risk of harm does welfare compromise ensue. However, while many organizations begin population management because the welfare of animals is already compromised, others begin to intervene because they recognize that the population may soon reach a point where welfare will be compromised. Historically, in the UK it has been the animal welfare sector that has led the drive to control cat populations, rather than conservation or statutory bodies. In contrast, the government has a much more active role in controlling stray dog populations, and this is perhaps reflected in the differing legal status of these two species (see Chapter 21).

The potential for compromised welfare is inherent when there are large numbers of animals that lack access to basic requirements such as a regular food supply and veterinary attention, or are confined to shelters such that their behavioural needs cannot be fulfilled. However, there are a number of other factors that also drive attempts to control pet overpopulation (Figure 4.4).

Problems experienced by dogs
• Suffering resulting from untreated disease and injury • Malnutrition • High mortality, especially in puppies
Problems experienced by humans
• Public health risk due to the spread of zoonotic diseases (e.g. rabies) • Fear and injury resulting from biting and aggressive behaviour • Nuisance caused by noise and fouling • Road traffic accidents caused by animals straying on to roads
Impact on the economy and wildlife
• Cost of treating people with dog bite wounds • Economic burden of rabies: post-exposure treatment, dog vaccination, livestock losses, travel costs, lost income and premature death • Increased cost of managing poorly controlled populations – dog pounds, large-scale interventions • Negative impact on tourism due to fear, nuisance and animal welfare concerns • Impact on wildlife species (e.g. vultures and wild dogs) through competition and the spread of disease (e.g. distemper)

4.4 Problems resulting from poorly managed populations of dogs. (Adapted from ICAM Coalition, 2008)

Factors motivating population control
Public health

In rabies-endemic countries, the risk of human infection via dog bites is an important motivator for population control. Other zoonotic pathogens, such as *Toxocara canis* and *Toxoplasma gondii*, can be spread by animal populations via contamination of public areas. Additionally, public health and nuisance concerns include a risk of dog bites, spreading of refuse, urine and faeces, and the noise of dogs and cats fighting and mating. Alternatively, feeding activities may constitute a nuisance or eyesore more than the individual animals themselves (Figure 4.5).

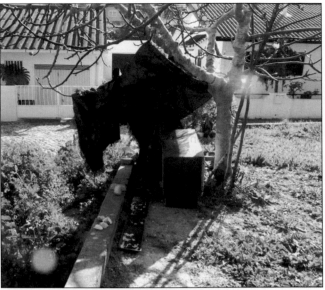

4.5 Unsightly feral cat feeding station in Portugal. (© Ian MacFarlaine)

Civic image

Concern may exist about citizens' or visitors' perceptions of the local environment, especially in tourist areas or capital cities, and stray animals may be one factor implicated in these concerns. A population of animals that appears sick or underweight, or shows signs of fight injuries or constant pregnancy, will be perceived negatively, both by those who dislike the animals (because they convey a poor image of the area or city) and also by those who are animal lovers but who are distressed to see animals that are in a poor state.

Concern for wildlife

There are differing assessments of the threats that free-living dogs and, especially, cats pose to small mammal and bird species. Although cats are clearly important predators in some situations, the extent of the threat they pose to wildlife is controversial. Some cat eradication programmes have found that rats fill the niche left by the cats, and have a similarly deleterious effect on eggs and chicks. Conflict frequently arises when wildlife organizations oppose the return to site of cats that have been through a trap-neuter-return (TNR) programme and propose that the cats should be euthanased rather than returned. An alternative concern may be over species dilution when domestic or feral cats interbreed with an indigenous wild species, such as the Scottish wildcat (*Felis silvestris silvestris*). This is equally significant in places with populations of other small felids that are genetically similar enough to *Felis catus* to be able to hybridize with them.

Concern for conspecifics

There may be concern over the potential for unowned and free-roaming owned animals to transmit diseases to pets. Although in some populations there is evidence that the prevalence of significant contagious diseases in unowned cats mirrors that in the local pet population, some risk of transmission may occur, particularly from entire animals or where the stray/free-roaming population has a high prevalence of disease.

Features of free-roaming populations

Carrying capacity and human tolerance

The carrying capacity of a species is the largest stable population that an environment can support with the available resources (food, water and shelter), at which point the birth rate equals the death rate. Human tolerance also has a significant impact on carrying capacity. If human tolerance is low, there may be fewer animals than the available resources would support, due to culling or neglect. Conversely, if human tolerance is high, a larger population may be maintained through active feeding of free-roaming animals. Human attitude is likely to be the most influential factor in the survival and proliferation of a particular species within a society, and this will be influenced by a vast number of cultural, historical and religious factors unique to each location. For example, male dogs are frequently over-represented in countries with free-roaming dog populations, especially within owned dog populations (Davlin and VonVille, 2012). This preferential ownership of male dogs may be due to perceived advantageous behavioural traits, such as guarding behaviour, or because of the greater burden of ownership of (unneutered) bitches associated with managing litters and unwanted male attention during oestrus. As a result, people in these societies may be more inclined to abandon, neglect or kill female puppies at a young age (Matter and Daniels, 2000).

A pragmatic view is that many environments have the capacity to sustain the presence of stray and feral animals. Although in ideal circumstances this capacity would be eliminated via education, waste management and other changes to human behaviour, in some circumstances a more viable goal, at least initially, may be to limit the free-roaming animal population size and improve its welfare.

Location and interaction with humans

The dynamic of ownership and carrying capacity varies greatly between rural and urban settings. As human population density increases, the potential for animals to have access to unintentionally provided resources increases. For example, poor waste management creates the opportunity for scavenging food, and abandoned buildings and building sites provide shelter where females can rear young. These resources increase the carrying capacity of the environment independently of ownership and mean that animals are potentially more likely to survive without an owner. There are some differences in the ways in which human populations tend to interact with free-roaming dogs and cats.

Dogs

Many studies have documented estimations of dog:human ratios, which can vary greatly with settlement density (city, town or rural area) both within and between countries. Generally, there will be a larger ratio of dogs to humans in rural areas compared with urban settlements, which is most likely a result of higher rates of ownership and suggests that there is a greater demand for dogs in many rural settings. Studies from many urban settings around the world place the urban owned dog:human ratio at between 1:4.3 and 1:8 (Brooks, 1990; Matter and Daniels, 2000; Kitala *et al.*, 2001; Kato *et al.*, 2003; Flores-Ibarra and Estrella-Valenzuela, 2004; Kongkaew *et al.*, 2004; Ratsitorahina *et al.*, 2009; Acosta-Jamett *et al.*, 2010); however, studies from urban locations in India and Tanzania showed lower dog:human

ratios of 1:14 and 1:35, respectively (Sudarshan *et al.*, 2006; Gsell *et al.*, 2012). Care should be taken in applying these data to unstudied locations, as the dog population is highly influenced by local factors and human tolerance, as mentioned above (Leney and Ramfry, 2000).

Cats

In any city or society, cat populations will present as a spectrum, with true wild-living feral examples of the domestic cat species (rare) at one pole, and domestic indoor or indoor–outdoor pets at the other (Sparkes *et al.*, 2013). Cats will sit at varying points along this spectrum, according to their level of interaction and sociability with humans, and their willingness to tolerate and engage in close contact with people, as well as their reliance on them. The levels of handling tolerated, comfort with confinement and self-defending aggression are often erroneously seen as indicators of the level of a cat's 'feral' nature. However, given that a cat's level of sociability with humans and fear of, or lack of, close contact with them is strongly determined by experiences in the first 7 weeks of life (see QRG 19.4), it is not uncommon to find feral cats that are comfortable in proximity to humans, and sometimes even with close handling (albeit sometimes only by specific people). A small proportion of these cats may be regarded as adoptable, although this is the exception rather than the rule. For cats involved in a TNR programme, adoption may be more successful if the cat is adopted some time subsequent to its return to its territory, rather than attempting to do so at the time of initial TNR. In many cases a cat-centric programme of adoption can be a functional adjunct to TNR, provided it is focused on socialized animals and young kittens, and does not compromise the welfare of these animals or add to an already overburdened shelter population.

Notwithstanding the above, considerable energy remains invested on the fringes of feline rescue and welfare operations in trying to 'tame' or 'bring round' feral cats, sometimes tied into strong 'no-kill' beliefs. However, it should be borne in mind that life on the street may not in itself always be a bad thing for these cats. 'Rescue' should be for a purpose, not just because one can carry it out, and the perception of risk to the cat may irrationally place some risks (e.g. lack of food or water), which are tangible, as being of higher significance than the more intangible and more hidden risks of stress or fear.

To try to manage any one part of the overpopulation problem without managing the whole, or to do so solely by surgical neutering, is at best a temporary local fix and at worst futile, as it does not take account of the extreme fluidity of the different segments of the population and the frequency with which they interface. If the reasons why a population exists are not tackled in conjunction with neutering, any programme will be in a constant state of 'fire-fighting'. Therefore, a balance must be found between dealing with the population that exists and constructing a feasible long-term plan to avoid recurrence of the problem in the future.

Components of population management strategies

There are a number of component parts to a successful population management strategy. While every component may not be equally useful or necessary in any given situation, all should be considered. Utilizing a single component alone (for example, neutering without education or community engagement) is unlikely to give rise to meaningful sustained benefits.

Legislation

Legislation to require all owners to neuter their animals unless required for breeding has been proposed on a number of occasions in different countries and municipalities, including Los Angeles and the island of Bermuda. Opponents of such legislation point to the potential for it to incite huge public resentment, the cost of implementation and enforcement if there is not already an animal policing infrastructure in place, and the impracticality of enforcement.

To date, it is relatively uncommon for population management programmes to focus on legislation of this type. However, other relevant laws must be explored and, if necessary, clarified or changed for some aspects of a programme to be viable. Examples include the ear-tipping of feral cats (see Chapter 5), which may be prohibited as a mutilation in some jurisdictions, and the release of feral or stray animals as part of a TNR programme, which is legally classified as animal abandonment in some locations. Professional regulations concerning veterinary practice, including recognition of foreign qualifications and access to controlled drugs, must also be recognized and adhered to, as they vary significantly from country to country (see Chapter 21).

Education to catalyse behaviour change

Education is likely to be the most important factor in shaping how people perceive dogs and cats and in stimulating sustained change in societies. Changing people's attitudes and behaviour towards animals not only has a direct impact on the welfare of individual animals in the short term, but also has a profound effect on population dynamics and the propagation of unwanted pets in the future. Local animal welfare organizations have a powerful role to play in educating the community and other groups about animal welfare and public health issues surrounding animals. However, inducing behavioural changes in humans is inherently challenging. Encouraging changes in behaviour by using innovative methods that engage the local culture has been effective in some settings (Panter-Brick et al., 2006). The approach to education will vary depending on the local culture and the target audience; it is important to address the various groups whose behaviour will impact on the free-roaming animal population.

Pet owners

Irresponsible pet owners that allow unneutered, unvaccinated animals to roam unsupervised are more likely to be the source of unwanted litters and problems relating to dogs and cats in the community. This group of people are often passionate about their animals; however, may not be aware of the impact of their actions or may not have access to basic preventive healthcare such as neutering and vaccination. Accessing these pet owners can be challenging, as they may not be in regular contact with existing animal healthcare services where pet care information is easily disseminated. Improving access to basic veterinary services and affordable/subsidised preventive healthcare, while concurrently educating owners about the benefits of vaccination and neutering, can help a shift towards a culture of responsible pet ownership.

The public

Educating the wider public about responsible acquisition of pets, the benefits pets bring to society, the services available to address problems with pets and, where appropriate, signs that animals have been neutered or vaccinated (e.g. collar, ear tip) and what this means will help to reduce fear and encourage responsible pet ownership. In addition, education of the general public regarding the impact of feeding free-living animals (whether deliberately or inadvertently via poor waste management) may be an important part of a population control programme.

Children

Children are highly susceptible to new ideas and learning. Instilling a culture of empathy towards animals, and teaching children that animals also feel pain, cold and hunger, can be lacking in poor communities. Basic lessons can address feeding, shelter, exercise and people's responsibilities towards animals, including vaccination and reproductive control (Figure 4.6). Children are at greatest risk of dog bites in rabies-endemic countries, and so combining lessons on how to avoid dog bites and what to do if bitten (washing the wound, telling an adult and finding a doctor) could save lives.

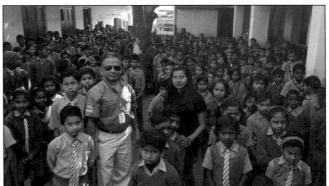

4.6 A team of animal welfare educators visiting a school in India as part of a rabies vaccination and population control programme.
(© Mission Rabies)

Reproductive control

The approach to canine and feline population management is likely to change dramatically over the coming decades with significant progress being made in the development of new non-surgical methods of neutering. However, at present, surgical removal of the reproductive organs remains the most effective permanent method of reproductive control for both pet and mass population control settings. The risks and benefits of neutering animals, whether surgically or non-surgically, need to be weighed against the consequences of no intervention, uncontrolled breeding or euthanasia.

Surgical neutering

The facilities, expertise and financial resources available in private veterinary clinics and mass population control settings are often very different, and working in a resource-limited setting can present a number of challenges to the clinician (Figure 4.7).

Mass neutering programmes aim to optimize patient throughput in order to have maximal impact on population control for a given investment of finance, manpower and time. A number of techniques have been described to increase throughput for neutering in the clinic (see Chapters 5 and 6). However, this must be balanced with maintaining high core clinical standards and patient care. It is important to appreciate that any intervention that interrupts an animal's normal activities will result in some degree of compromise to its welfare in the short term. Every effort should be made to limit this negative impact at each stage of the process, where possible. Figure 4.8 summarizes the steps at which an animal's welfare may be compromised during a TNR initiative.

Parameter	Private veterinary clinic	Mass population control
Enforcement of minimum veterinary standards	Minimum standards of practice are clearly outlined and the threat of disciplinary action from the governing veterinary body usually ensures basic minimum standards are upheld	Standards may not be defined and policed, and so there is a greater risk of substandard practices going unchecked
Surgical competence of veterinary surgeons	Higher undergraduate exposure to aseptic technique and surgical principles, rigid undergraduate examination to ensure at least minimum standards before unsupervised surgery is permitted	Variable exposure/examination in aseptic technique and basic surgical principles before graduation, meaning that a veterinary surgeon may be able to operate unsupervised with a lower degree of surgical competence
Support staff expertise	Support staff will generally be qualified or training veterinary nurses with an interest in caring for animals, innate minimum standards of animal welfare and higher levels of clinical competence	Working with animals may be seen as 'dirty' or 'low-class' work and is often poorly paid. As a result, support staff may not have an inherent understanding of animal welfare, and it can be difficult to source staff who already have clinical experience
Animal handling	Animals are used to being handled by their owners and can be brought to the clinic	Animals may need to be transported from the place of capture to the clinic. Animals may not be used to being handled. Additional precautions should be taken in rabies-endemic countries
Previous health status	Usually an owner will report any previous medical problems the animal has had, and the practice may have a full history of previous treatment	Medical history usually unknown
Anaesthesia	Inhalation anaesthesia enables minute-by-minute adjustment of anaesthetic depth and rapid anaesthetic recovery	Total injectable anaesthesia often means that anaesthetic complications are harder to correct and recovery is generally slower
Anaesthetic monitoring	Generally there is one-to-one monitoring of anaesthesia, regular assessment of basic clinical parameters such as heart rate, breathing rate, oxygen saturation and pulse quality	Usually one-to-one anaesthetic monitoring is not feasible, and there is less capability for monitoring such as pulse oximetry or indirect blood pressure measurement
Analgesia	Pre-, intra- and postoperative analgesia is provided, usually involving multimodal analgesia tailored to the individual animal's clinical signs. Analgesia can be continued for the postoperative period	Analgesia protocols will vary greatly with local availability of medication; however, as a minimum they should include a non-steroidal anti-inflammatory drug (NSAID) and an opiate at the time of surgery. Ability to provide postoperative analgesia will depend on the retention time
Postoperative care	The animal's activity can be restricted in the postoperative period. Usually an owner will be able to check the wound daily and return the animal for veterinary attention immediately should complications occur	Following release, detection of postoperative complications is dependent on reporting by the local community. There is potentially a higher risk of complications not being detected or reported

4.7 Comparison of conditions typically encountered in the private veterinary clinic and in mass population control settings.

Stage of TNR protocol	Factors impacting on an animal's stress level/welfare
Capture	Method of capture – catch pole, sack/loop, net, free hand, manual or automated trap
Transportation	Individual cages, multiple animals per cage[a], unconfined in a covered trailer, individual nets
Waiting period	Individual nets, individual cages, multiple animals per cage/kennel[a]
Surgery	Perioperative analgesia, surgical technique, aseptic technique, tissue handling
Anaesthetic recovery	Level of monitoring, ability to monitor basic clinical parameters such as mucous membrane colour, heart rate, pulse rate and pulse quality
Monitoring period	Housing facilities, ability to keep clean, ensure water and food availability, risk of contracting infectious diseases from animals in close contact
Transfer from holding cage to transport	Depending on the temperament of the animal, type of housing and experience of the handler, the use of a restraint aid may be needed to assist in moving the dog to the vehicle in some cases – the care and skill of the handler(s) will have a significant impact on the animal's level of stress during this transition. Transfer of cats should be managed calmly, using a small closed room to avoid escape, and covering the destination cage
Transportation	As before
Release	How the animal is handled to remove it from the vehicle to its release point will also be a potential period of stress. Possibilities include by hand or with the assistance of a net or catch pole for dogs
Return to home territory	If the animal is not returned to the precise location of capture it will have to find its way back to its home territory. This may involve a period of increased stress
Recovery	The remaining postoperative recovery period will be approximately 14 days, during which time there is the potential for discomfort and postoperative complications

4.8 The stages of a TNR protocol and the potential factors that could impact on animal welfare to consider at each stage. Every effort should be made to reduce stress at every step of the procedure. [a]Note that cats caught in a trap together will typically cope without fighting, if kept calm and covered until being separated for anaesthesia.

It is important that animals that have undergone surgical neutering are observed during the postoperative period by a local guardian or community after being released, and that avenues to seek veterinary attention are made easily accessible to caretakers by providing an emergency contact telephone number.

Non-surgical contraceptive methods

Chemical contraception broadens access to reproductive control to a much wider population of animals, with potential welfare and cost benefits over surgical neutering due to the lack of surgical risks and lack of requirement for anaesthesia, specialist staff or facilities. Since the announcement of the Michelson Prize and Grants programme in 2008, pledging $75 million towards research and development of non-surgical methods of contraception in dogs and cats, there has been a dramatic rise in interest and progress in this field. Mechanisms of action currently showing the most promise include gonadal ablation, immunocontraception using gonadotropin-releasing hormone (GnRH)-targeted vaccines and interrupting the hypothalamic–pituitary–gonadal axis. It is important to note that with any form of non-surgical contraception in males, fertility may persist for up to 30 days after cessation of sperm production due to the presence of motile sperm in the vas deferens and epididymis.

Gonadal ablation: Chemical 'castration' has many benefits over surgical neutering; however these benefits must be balanced against the possible limitations. Chemical castration can be applied on a large scale in locations where the clinical facilities or surgical expertise required for neutering are not available. It is inexpensive, can be administered under sedation and so has a shorter recovery time than surgery, and it is not technically challenging.

The only product currently authorized for use in dogs is zinc gluconate neutralized by arginine for intratesticular injection. Permanent infertility is achieved following a single treatment. Although injection has been demonstrated to be well tolerated in conscious animals, light sedation is recommended for administration. The importance of training in the correct administration protocol is emphasized by the manufacturer to limit the risk of complications, most commonly injection site reactions (reported in 1.2% of cases). The impact of ongoing testosterone production is variable, with the majority of dogs continuing to maintain testosterone levels similar to pre-administration baseline levels; however, in a proportion of dogs the decrease in testosterone was comparable to that associated with surgical neutering (Alliance for Contraception in Cats and Dogs (ACC&D), 2015). Other products for chemical castration, such as a formulation of calcium chloride, are likely to become more widely available in the future.

Population control relies predominantly on female reproduction; however, neutering of male animals also carries benefits (as described later in this chapter). Many of the welfare and social benefits of surgical castration relate to reduction in testosterone-mediated behaviours such as roaming, mounting and fighting. Further research is needed to investigate whether such benefits are also achieved by chemical castration; if they are not, its value as a component of population management strategies may be questionable.

Immunocontraception: Vaccines targeted at inducing an immune response against GnRH have the benefit of producing infertility in both males and females, as well as suppressing the release of hormones responsible for sexual behaviours. GnRH-targeted vaccines work by coupling the small GnRH decapeptide to a large foreign protein, in order to elicit an immune response against GnRH produced by the body. An adjuvant is generally added to further stimulate the immune system and strengthen the response. A GnRH–haemocyanin conjugate vaccine formulation, which is authorized for use in deer and wild horses, generated multi-year infertility from a single injection. Initial trials in dogs with the same product resulted in unacceptable injection site reactions and an inconsistent immune response. However, recent research with alternative adjuvant formulations and combined with rabies vaccines have indicated an adequate immune response to both components, with less severe local side effects (Bender *et al.*, 2009). Initial trials in cats have been more promising, with female cats developing a stronger and more sustained immune response than males. Development of late-onset injection site reactions in a proportion of cats raised the concern that vaccine-induced granulomatous reactions could increase the risk of malignant injection site sarcoma (Levy *et al.*, 2011).

The fact that reproductive capacity returns after approximately 2–3 years is a limitation to population control compared with permanent methods of neutering. However, shorter average lifespans in free-roaming dog populations could mean that a multi-year contraceptive will produce infertility in an animal for a substantial proportion of its life, which could still have a significant impact on population stabilization. The effects of booster vaccination and potential side effects in dogs and cats have not yet been reported. Further research is required before a safe, effective immunocontraceptive will be available for use in dogs and cats.

GnRH agonist implants: GnRH agonists have been used as non-surgical contraceptives in wildlife species for over 15 years. They cause infertility by inducing down-regulation of the GnRH receptors on the pituitary gland, so that the pituitary gland becomes 'desensitized' to endogenous GnRH. They are usually administered as slow-release subcutaneous implants. There is one authorized product, deslorelin acetate, currently available as a subcutaneous implant. GnRH agonists have the disadvantage that they can induce oestrus in bitches and increase sexual behaviour when first administered. As with GnRH-targeted vaccines, fertility returns once the GnRH agonist is exhausted. The use of these implants for population control of free-roaming dogs and cats is currently limited due to the need for repeated administration and the potential side effects of persistent oestrus and initial increase in sexual behaviour. However, research into lengthening their duration of action is ongoing and may make these agents a useful component of strategies to manage free-roaming populations in the future.

General principles of any population control programme

In order to be successful, any population control programme needs to:

* Have a successful, well-planned veterinary intervention (see Chapter 5 for further information)
* Engage with stakeholders to provide clear, common objectives
* Assess the target population
* Evaluate the success of the project.

Engage stakeholders and clarify objectives and actions

In any population control programme, there will be numerous stakeholders. These are individuals, groups and organizations, or vocal representatives of organizations, whose presence or absence from the programme in executive, planning or simply moral terms will mean success or failure (World Organisation for Animal Health (OIE), 2015). Establishing a multi-stakeholder committee that encompasses all the groups involved in population management will ensure that the opinions and experience of all relevant stakeholders are benefited from (International Companion Animal Management (ICAM) Coalition, 2008; OIE, 2015).

Early consultation with the stakeholders involved in all aspects of animal overpopulation is essential to ensuring that solutions are acceptable and feasible. Problems and concerns raised by a multi-stakeholder committee can be prioritized, and priority points of intervention can be identified. Most often, identified problems relate to irresponsible/quasi-ownership of animals that are allowed to reproduce unchecked. Out of this consultation, core objectives of the programme can be formulated (Figure 4.9). The actions required to achieve these objectives can then be defined and planned.

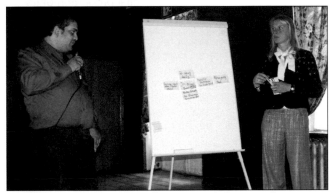

4.9 Prioritization exercise for a cat population control programme in Lithuania.
(© Jenny Stavisky)

Government – local and central

The responsibility for free-roaming stray and feral animals will often sit with the lowest or second lowest tier of government. In some countries, cats are simply not covered by local laws or bylaws. The UK, for example, has well defined municipal programmes for the handling of stray and lost dogs, but there is no equivalent programme, governed by law, for cats. This vacuum is filled by the ungoverned actions of charities (non-governmental organizations (NGOs) and non-profit organizations) and individuals. However, central governments may sometimes take an interest in feline populations from the viewpoint of rabies and other notifiable diseases, and from the perspective of being the custodians of new national legislation (e.g. relating to animal welfare). Local or municipal governments may also have an interest in cats from public health or civic image perspectives (as described earlier; see also Chapter 21).

Many legislatures recognize cats as 'non-biddable' – that is, as animals that cannot be directly and continuously controlled by their human carers, which are able to freely enter and leave and move around their home environment and the surrounding land. Some legislatures (including the UK) have the control of roaming and stray dogs built into local municipal functions, but do not include cats (either in statute or in enforcement/practice) as a species deemed to be controllable. Other legislatures (including many countries in Europe) control both cats and dogs in a similar way, which can lead to negative consequences for both species when control schemes do not take full account of the different needs of each.

The animal husbandry/veterinary authority is usually the main point of contact in relation to population management. However, other departments, including public health, environment (refuse collection), education and tourism, are also likely to be crucial to certain aspects of the population management programme. Population management is a continuous activity that will be required in some capacity as long as there are pets within a society. The responsibility for population management should lie with local and central government, with local NGOs or private organizations being enlisted where necessary to provide specific services.

Veterinary staff

Veterinary surgeons (veterinarians) and veterinary nurses are key players in the management of stray, feral and shelter populations. This role may be as private practitioners providing services for a fee (which may be reduced or discounted), working free of charge, or as state or municipal veterinary officers. It is essential for veterinary staff working in population control programmes to understand the differences in animal management that may be required compared with work for private clients. For example, allowing trapped feral cats to be transported directly to a quiet area of the practice, rather than coming in via a noisy waiting room full of dogs, can be very helpful.

Reducing the age considered to be routine for neutering, particularly for cats, is viewed as being of high priority by many animal welfare charities, in light of the high proportion of unplanned litters (Murray *et al.*, 2009; see also Chapter 6). Some veterinary surgeons may have practical or ethical concerns regarding neutering of paediatric or pregnant animals and euthanasia policies. Involving veterinary surgeons as stakeholders in the project and ensuring that they clearly understand the organizational requirements (and the reasons behind these requirements) can aid successful treatment and surgery.

Veterinary surgeons also play a crucial role in disease surveillance and public education, and can bring much needed local expertise to the project. They are also important ambassadors for responsible pet ownership through their contact with owners.

Non-governmental organizations, charities and non-profit organizations

These organizations take all forms and will be stakeholders in overpopulation issues in numerous ways – as existing providers of TNR schemes, shelters (open-admission and no-kill) and as providers of advocacy and education. It is important to have as many sympathetic and informed animal welfare groups on board as possible. Statistics on shelter intake, rehoming and euthanasia rates will provide information on the current situation, and partnering with established organizations can make use of existing infrastructure and experience. Discussing a plan and policy for managing challenging cases, particularly with regard to euthanasia, can help to maintain a positive partnership from the planning stages onwards. National and international organizations working together in animal welfare and public health can help to raise awareness and provide experience, expertise and funding (see Chapter 23).

Animal owners, feeders and carers

Pet owners commonly have misconceptions or are confused about the ideal timing of neutering, the age of puberty, the perceived need for the animal to have a season or litter before being neutered, the side effects of neutering (and potential change in the 'personality' of the animal) and the exact nature of what they need to do for their animals. Having a common and consistent message expressed by all the veterinary and animal welfare staff and volunteers involved in the programme, and providing evidence where appropriate to back up practices, can help considerably in clarifying these misconceptions.

Such attitudes may also transfer with emigration, when people move to live in a different country, so it is important to consider the cultural norms of clients from diverse communities and be sympathetic to their fears and ready to explain the process of neutering. It is important to remember that owners from all backgrounds may not understand the process and have misplaced fears surrounding its complexity, logistical process or cost.

Common owner apprehensions and bars to neutering are:

* Fear of their animal dying
* Anthropomorphic considerations about the animal deserving a sex life
* Perception that the animal would be a good parent or needs to breed to 'replicate' itself
* Money, transport or time factors, or lack of access to veterinary services
* Gender-specific pride issues (especially in males)
* Cultural or religious attitudes
* Perception of neutering as harmful to the animal's natural behaviour
* Ignorance of the efficiency of reproduction, including precocious puberty, high fecundity and frequency of oestrus (especially in cats).

Cultural attitudes towards pets and perceptions of the positivity or negativity of 'altering' an animal by neutering are often confused with religious doctrine. Doctrine and practice can differ, and there may be variability in the way in which religious teachings are interpreted. Cultural views or concerns are often inaccurately attributed to religious beliefs because the demographic happens to be of a particular religion. It is therefore important when tackling what may be perceived as apprehension over neutering in a particular community, to be especially sure of the true nature of the concerns.

Different stakeholder groups will attempt to appeal in various ways to owners' sense of duty to the animal or to the wider society, or to raise awareness of the number of excess animals being euthanased. More successful approaches often focus on the owner's role in protecting their animal and how the benefit of taking such actions can make for a safer pet. Use of language is important in communication with owners: for example, an event named 'Protect Your Pet Roadshow' will appeal more than 'Neutering Campaign', and making reference to 'preventing your boy cat from becoming an unexpected father' may appeal more than 'castrating your tom cat'.

Social media can be used in campaigns to make neutering of animals more socially acceptable. Often, the message can be attached or linked to an image or video that is quirky or funny – providing that the link to the message is not too subtle for viewers to make quickly! However, the use of images of kittens and puppies in promotional or campaign material can often be counter-productive, as people focus on the image but do not link it to the message of trying to produce fewer of these animals.

Local community

An understanding of the local context of pet ownership and the problems caused by stray, free-roaming and irresponsibly owned dogs and cats will enable a management strategy to be tailored to the specific setting and more effectively address the problems at their source. Gaining support from the public and key stakeholders will provide sustainability in the longer term, and so it is important that interventions are socially and culturally acceptable and are perceived by the local community to have value. Investing in a period of assessment will enable perceived problems to be identified and interventions to be targeted at the root of these problems.

Community engagement has become a linchpin of work in local communities where an animal welfare project is proposed. Trying to manage companion animal populations in a community is a complex process. The actions of individual citizens and vocal opponents and proponents of the project can have a huge impact.

Not every community can provide the specialists needed to kick-start a welfare programme. However, during the development of any initiative, local people can be recruited to support the work in numerous ways, whether as collectors of newspapers or blankets, as population counters or as drivers. Sometimes these tasks can be undertaken by a committed group of local volunteers, and sometimes it will be necessary to pay people to provide services. Bringing local people into the project is a good way of starting a 'ripple effect' as they may tell their families, friends and neighbours about the project or even recruit them to help out.

Other stakeholders may include the media, public health sector, law enforcement, educational bodies, veterinary orders and regulators (e.g. the RCVS), veterinary schools, and many others. Sometimes unconventional stakeholders will turn out to be the most effective tool for implementation – several cat neutering schemes on local council estates in the UK have been driven forward by local dog wardens, housing wardens or police officers.

Catch/trap-neuter-vaccinate-return

In catch-neuter-vaccinate-return (CNVR) (also known as trap-neuter-vaccinate-return, TNVR) programmes, cats and dogs are collected from the street (or brought to the clinic by their owners), neutered, vaccinated, marked for identification purposes and then returned to their point of capture. If performed correctly, this is a cost-effective method of population control, although a reduction in the population is not seen immediately. Policy-makers must be educated in the aims of moving towards a stable, healthy and vaccinated free-roaming population with lower disease prevalence. The effectiveness of this approach has been demonstrated in studies of cities in Rajasthan, northern India, where CNVR programmes have been in place for a number of years. Neutering of 62–87% of dogs in Jodhpur resulted in a reduction in the dog population and improvement in the health of both dogs that had been and dogs that had not been neutered ▶

Catch/trap-neuter-vaccinate-return *continued*

compared with areas without population management programmes (Totton *et al.*, 2010, 2011; Yoak *et al.*, 2014).

A cost-effective CNVR project in Italy described the concept of 'block dogs'. These were free-roaming dogs that had been caught, health checked, neutered, microchipped and vaccinated before being returned to the point of capture, where they were fed and cared for by the community, but were the responsibility of the local authority. A proportion of dogs were not returned to the street after neutering and identification, but were either euthanased if sick, kennelled or adopted by new owners (Høgåsen *et al.*, 2013). This model places a duty of care on members of the community and may help to bridge the gap towards responsible ownership. The community does not pay for neutering, vaccination or identification of the dogs, but must permit the local authority to do this and take responsibility for the animals thereafter. Providing some support to help people manage their dogs is likely to be needed in poorer areas, while encouraging steps towards responsible ownership.

In settings where they are responsibly owned and well tolerated by the community, dogs and cats that are allowed to roam freely could arguably have a better quality of life and more freedom to express normal behaviour than some of their counterparts that are confined indoors or kept in some shelters. These benefits must be balanced against the potential for disease and injury; however, if these risks are reduced through vaccination, neutering and veterinary care, then it may be possible for the culture of free-roaming animals to continue in a more controlled fashion.

Public relations

Local press are key allies in providing cheap publicity to a broad audience. Inviting members of the press to an event and sending press releases giving updates on the progress of work or reporting on interesting cases and events within the project are inexpensive ways of capturing media attention. If support for the project has been provided by the local municipal authority or sponsors, enlist their help to promote their involvement through the production of posters and banners. These should be distributed in advance of work beginning in an area, informing the local community of the nature of the work and when it will be happening. Emphasis should be placed on what owners can gain, for example, 'free dog vaccination'. Radio interviews and investigating avenues for free advertising airtime can also be very effective, especially when a simple message is used.

A telephone number should be distributed to the public for use in the event of any concerns regarding animals that have been neutered and then returned to the community. It is useful to provide this information on business cards which can be distributed via local shops and community gathering points; cards are more likely to be retained than leaflets. Records of complaints and complications should be maintained so that trends can be monitored over time and early action can be taken to correct potential problems.

Assessing the population

A period of assessment to gather information about the target population of animals is beneficial in a number of ways:

- Assessing the size of the population enables estimation of the amount of resources and time frame required to achieve specific goals
- It allows identification of subgroups or geographical areas that are particularly contributing to the problem, enabling targeting of resources
- Assessing the health status of the population identifies additional intervention that may be required, such as preventive treatment
- Factors that could impact on how the project is managed can be identified, e.g. accessibility of animals, proportion of owned/stray/free-living/shelter animals
- Gathering baseline data allows comparisons to be made by carrying out repeat surveys, therefore measuring the impact of the intervention.

For the most part, assessing free-roaming and owned populations requires separate methods, which are outlined in Chapter 5.

How many animals need to be neutered?

With any population management initiative there will be finite budget and resources, often to address a large population. When competing against a constantly replenishing population, targeting the resources enables a far greater impact to be achieved than if work is carried out haphazardly across the whole population.

Females control population growth, depending on the success with which they produce offspring; every fertile female that is neutered will reduce the production of future litters, whereas a single male cat or dog left intact can father litters with all females in a given area. There is an argument that female dogs and cats only should be neutered, while vaccinating and releasing males; however, castration of males can benefit the population in more ways than simply by reproduction control, mostly through reduction in hormonally driven sexual behaviours such as fighting, mounting, spraying and extensive roaming (Hopkins *et al.*, 1976; Neilson *et al.*, 1997). This contributes to reduced spread of disease and nuisance behaviour, as well as improved welfare and lifespan. Neutering of both males and females sends also sends a clearer message to the community. These benefits need to be weighed against the impact of the procedure itself on animal welfare and the use of resources that could otherwise be focused on neutering females only. There is currently no research directly comparing the outcomes of female only neutering *versus* male/female neutering programmes; however, the benefits of combined male/female neutering strategies are well documented.

The proportion of animals that needs to be neutered in order to stabilize the population can be difficult to estimate, as the factors that control population growth, such as female survival rate, fertile lifespan and average litter size/frequency, are often unknown and vary greatly between locations. A more practical approach is to target neutering to the population with the greatest likelihood of producing unwanted litters. This requires periodic evaluation of the impact achieved, to ensure that the selected strategy is appropriate and allow it to be modified if necessary.

Targeting reproductive control to specific populations: status dogs in the UK

One of the emerging problems resulting from dogs, predominantly bull breeds, in the UK is their use as 'status' animals and the link to antisocial behaviour, violence and animal abuse (Hughes *et al.*, 2011). Breeds typically used as status animals (bull breeds, Rottweilers and Akitas or their crossbreeds) now make up a considerable proportion of the animals presented to shelters and charity veterinary services, accounting for 22% of the 110,000 stray dogs handled by local council authorities between April 2013 and March 2014 (Dogs Trust, 2014) and 30% of dogs relinquished to RSPCA rehoming centres nationally in 2013 (unpublished data). At the Mayhew Animal Home, a charitable animal welfare organization in London, 46% of relinquished dogs in 2013 were Staffordshire Bull Terriers. In response to this, and in an effort to reduce the number of unwanted dogs, the charity launched a free bull breed neutering scheme in 2006, focusing investment in neutering efforts on the population that most commonly contributes to the unwanted dog population.

Geographical strategy

Scattered approaches will have a minimal impact on population size, particularly in areas with a high population turnover, where neutered animals are rapidly 'diluted' by the birth of new puppies and kittens. It is more effective to concentrate efforts in a region-wise manner to ensure the desired level of intervention has been achieved in each location before moving on to focus on another area.

For example, if there are sufficient resources (manpower, finance and infrastructure) to neuter 2000 dogs over the course of a year, a greater impact on population turnover can be achieved if these dogs are taken from a problem population of 3000 dogs than a larger area containing 6000 dogs. Particular regions of a city or socioeconomic groups may have been identified in the initial assessment as being greater contributors to the unwanted animal population, and so these can be mapped and targeted in a similar fashion. The availability of accurate maps is limited in many places; the use of free online tools (such as Google My Maps) enables the creation of custom working boundaries or importation of local government administrative boundaries as KML files by which to conduct work in a strategic manner (Figure 4.10).

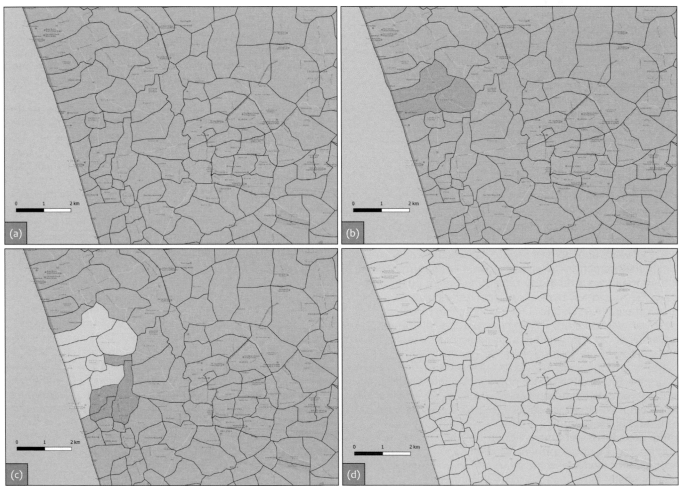

4.10 Geographical strategy for work. Map data: Google, Google Maps 2015; boundaries created using Google My Maps. (a) Divide the area of work into workable regions using maps (2–3 km²). (b) Concentrate neutering/vaccination of dogs in a single or limited number of regions. Once staff suspect that the desired proportion of dogs has been neutered/vaccinated, or no more dogs can be caught, conduct a dog sight survey of the region counting the number of neutered/unneutered dogs. Calculate the percentage of neutered dogs by region and repeat capture of dogs from that area if below the desired threshold. (c) Repeat this process of capture–survey until the desired percentage of dogs has been neutered/vaccinated, then move to the next region. (d) Continue in this manner until all regions are complete to the desired percentage. Grey = incomplete; Pink = active; Green = complete.
(© Mission Rabies)

Evaluating the success of population control interventions

Whatever the population control programme and methodology used, monitoring and evaluation are essential to demonstrate the output achieved from a given investment and to assess ways of improving efficiency and impact. NGOs are often born out of a desire to address a problem, such as suffering within an animal population, and as a result the prime focus of resources and effort is placed on the 'doing'. This focus on doing as much good as possible with the available resources sometimes means that little attention is directed towards the process of evaluating the change being achieved. Although the social and ecological systems involved in population management may be complex, identifying simple measurable indicators and assessing them over time can make the difference between a project that evolves towards being more efficient and beneficial, and one that endlessly swallows money with unknown effect. Funders of animal welfare and population management initiatives are increasingly (and rightfully) demanding reporting of evidence to demonstrate the impact of the work and lessons that have been learned before further funding can be applied for (see Chapter 7).

The process of monitoring and evaluation does not need to be expensive or time consuming, but should be at the forefront of the work for a project. It is important to carefully consider what information is most relevant to gather and to invest time in data analysis and interpretation. Different stakeholders will measure 'success' by different markers. For example, a government body may define success by the size of the dog population, but an NGO grant giver may be more interested in markers of animal welfare, such as the incidence of disease. Three universal questions need to be answered by the monitoring and evaluation activities (Garbutt, 2013):

1. Are we doing what we said we would do?
   - This feeds back to the managers on the intervention to ensure that the agreed work has been completed (internal validation)
2. Are we making a difference?
   - This is relevant to all stakeholders, but especially donors who are interested in the change achieved from the funds given (impact assessment)
3. Are these the right things to do?
   - This is aimed at those involved in planning the intervention, to ensure that activities are effective and relevant, or to determine whether there is a better alternative (strategic relevance).

As far as possible, it is best to use tools and methods that gather data passively and add to the dataset without increasing workload, as these methods are most likely to be used accurately and sustainably. For example, surveys conducted following a vaccination drive in which animals are marked not only provide information about the percentage of coverage achieved, but can also be used to assess the size of the population (see Chapter 5). For shelters, this may include measures such as the proportion of days they were full to capacity, the length of their waiting list and infectious disease rates, which can be increased by overcrowding (ICAM Coalition, 2015).

Other measures of success for shelter-based organizations could include:

- Reduction in the number of requests for intake of animals, assuming that the organization remains equally contactable over the period in question. A like-for-like measure across a 12-month period (resampling at similar times of year) is useful, but can be influenced by other factors (such as an economic recession or downturn). To measure this, organizations should log all requests for intake in a consistent way
- An increase in the mean or modal age of animals being relinquished, indicating a decrease in the number of unwanted litters being born
- Whether the location (e.g. by postcode) of animals that are the subject of intake requests increases in distance (e.g. geographical radius) from the shelter, assuming the organization does not change its catchment area
- The number of pregnant animals admitted
- Telephone or face-to-face interviews assessing community members' attitudes to, and experiences of, cats and dogs locally.

The purpose of monitoring and evaluation should be to identify both activities that have succeeded in achieving the desired change and those that have failed. There is no 'one size fits all' model for successful dog and cat population management, as each local area will have its own cultural, ecological, political and geographical challenges. Therefore, it is only by evaluating the effect of previous and ongoing efforts, and by sharing successes and shortcomings of these programmes, that shelters and other animal welfare organizations can learn and adapt future interventions to be more effective.

In any intervention it is important to re-evaluate the effectiveness of the equipment used during capture. This can often become a poor subsidiary to the 'veterinary' part; something that often gets left to the 'catchers'. Methods including manual trapping and acclimatizing animals to traps prior to the exercise are extremely important. The availability of catchers to capture as many animals as possible before operated-on animals are returned will determine success. The Oak Tree Animals' Charity, UK, has a 99.5% neuter rate in feline colonies (n = 300 cats across 25 colonies) by combining the use of acclimatization, manual trapping, and a relentless effort to catch during the first 24–36 hours of an operation. Adequate and functional, well designed TNR equipment is also essential for this kind of work (Oak Tree Animals' Charity, 2017)

Adverse results of effectiveness

There have been instances of neutering programmes being 'too successful' and creating a short-term shortage of kittens or puppies in an area. A certain percentage of potential owners will desire to take on only a young animal, and will in no circumstances be willing to accept an adult. When rescue facilities do not have kittens or puppies readily available, some potential owners may be persuaded to adopt an adult animal, but others will seek their pets from a commercial source. To avoid this problem, shelters should make a concerted effort to examine their rehoming practices alongside neutering campaigns. For some organizations it may be necessary to relax some traditional bars and barriers to rehoming – while not placing animals at risk – to avoid driving a large number of responsible owners to obtain animals from a commercial source at the expense of adoption.

Conclusion

Management of these populations of dogs and cats is a complex issue for which there is no quick fix. Sometimes compassion inadvertently results in suffering. People who feed an unowned free-roaming animal out of kindness also need to accept responsibility for controlling the reproduction of that animal and its ability to spread disease and feel pain. More than ever, we have the tools and knowledge to be able to control dog and cat populations humanely. However, the problem is vast, and many of the animals – and people – most at risk of suffering the backlash of human kindness are in the poorest communities, who are least able to solve the problem themselves. Helping communities to stabilize their animal populations by sharing knowledge and demonstrating practices that are effective, sustainable and locally appropriate, will help to move towards a situation where all animals are cared for responsibly, whether on the street or in a home.

References and further reading

Acosta-Jamett G, Cleaveland S, Cunningham AA and Bronsvoort BMD (2010) Demography of domestic dogs in rural and urban areas of the Coquimbo region of Chile and implications for disease transmission. *Preventive Veterinary Medicine* **94**, 272–281

Alliance for Contraception in Cats and Dogs (ACC&D) (2015) Zeuterin™/Esterilsol™ product profile and position paper. Available from: www.acc-d.org/docs/default-source/Research-and-Innovation/pppp-zeuterinesterilsol-revised-june2015-for-web.pdf?sfvrsn=2

Bender SC, Bergmann DL, Wenning KM *et al.* (2009) No adverse effects of simultaneous vaccination with the immunocontraceptive GanoCon and a commercial rabies vaccine on rabies virus neutralizing antibody production in dogs. *Vaccine* **27(51)**, 7210–7213

Brooks R (1990) Survey of the dog population of Zimbabwe and its level of rabies vaccination. *Veterinary Microbiology* **127**, 592–596

Davlin SL and VonVille HM (2012) Canine rabies vaccination and domestic dog population characteristics in the developing world: a systematic review. *Vaccine* **30**, 3492–3502

Dogs Trust (2014) *Stray Dogs Survey 2014*. Prepared by GfK NOP Social Research for Dogs Trust. Available from: www.dogstrust.org.uk/news-events/news/stray%20dogs%202014%20report.pdf

Flores-Ibarra M and Estrella-Valenzuela G (2004) Canine ecology and socio-economic factors associated with dogs unvaccinated against rabies in a Mexican city across the US-Mexico border. *Preventive Veterinary Medicine* **62**, 79–87

Garbutt A (2013) Monitoring and evaluation: a guide for small and diaspora NGOs. Available from: http://www.intrac.org/wpcms/wp-content/uploads/2013/10/ME_A-Guide-for-Small-and-Diaspora-Organisations.pdf

Gsell AS, Knobel DL, Cleaveland S *et al.* (2012) Domestic dog demographic structure and dynamics relevant to rabies control planning in urban areas in Africa: the case of Iringa, Tanzania. *BMC Veterinary Research* **8**, 236

Hiby E, Atema KN, Brimley R *et al.* (2017) Scoping review of indicators and methods of measurement used to evaluate the impact of dog population management interventions. *BMC Veterinary Research* **13**, 143

Høgåsen HR, Er C, Di Nardo A and Dalla Villa P (2013) Free-roaming dog populations: a cost-benefit model for different management options, applied to Abruzzo, Italy. *Preventive Veterinary Medicine* **112**, 401–413

Hopkins S, Schubert T and Hart B (1976) Castration of adult male dogs: effects on roaming, aggression, urine marking, and mounting. *Journal of the American Veterinary Medical Association* **168**, 1108–1110

Hughes AG, Maher J and Lawson C (2011) Status dogs, young people and criminalisation: towards a preventative strategy. Available from: http://www.cardiff.ac.uk/socsi/resources/wp139.pdf

International Companion Animal Management (ICAM) Coalition (2008) Humane dog population management guidance. Available from: http://www.ifaw.org/sites/default/files/Dog%20POP%20Management.pdf

International Companion Animal Management (ICAM) Coalition (2015) Are we making a difference? A guide to monitoring and evaluating dog population management interventions. Available from: http://www.icam-coalition.org/downloads/ICAM_Are_we_making_a_difference_updated_Nov2015.pdf

Kato M, Inukai Y, Yamamoto H and Kira S (2003) Survey of the stray dog population and the health education program on the prevention of dog bites and dog-acquired infections: a comparative study in Nepal and Okayama Prefecture, Japan. *Acta Medica Okayama* **57**, 261–266

Kitala P, McDermott J, Kyule M *et al.* (2001) Dog ecology and demography information to support the planning of rabies control in Machakos District, Kenya. *Acta Tropica* **78**, 217–230

Kongkaew W, Coleman P, Pfeiffer DU *et al.* (2004) Vaccination coverage and epidemiological parameters of the owned-dog population in Thungsong District, Thailand. *Preventive Veterinary Medicine* **65**, 105–115

Leney J and Ramfry J (2000) Dog population management. In: *Dogs, Zoonoses and Public Health*, ed. CNL Macpherson *et al.*, pp. 299–331. CABI, Wallingford

Levy JK, Friary JA, Miller LA, Tucker SJ and Fagerstone KA (2011) Long-term fertility control in female cats with GonaCon™, a GnRH immunocontraceptive. *Theriogenology* **76**, 1517–1525

Matter HC and Daniels TJ (2000) Dog ecology and population biology. In: *Dogs, Zoonoses and Public Health*, ed. CNL Macpherson *et al.*, pp. 17–62. CABI, Wallingford

Murray JK, Roberts MA, Whitmarsh A and Gruffydd-Jones TJ (2009) Survey of the characteristics of cats owned by households in the UK and factors affecting their neutered status. *Veterinary Record* **164(5)**, 137–141

Neilson J, Eckstein R and Hart B (1997) Effects of castration on problem behaviors in male dogs with reference to age and duration of behavior. *Journal of the American Veterinary Medical Association* **211**, 180–182

Oak Tree Animals' Charity (2017) Feral cats and hoarding. Available online: www.oaktreeanimals.org.uk/community/feral-cats-hoarding.html

OIE (2015) Chapter 7.7. Stray dog population control. In *Terrestrial Animal Health Code*. Available from: http://www.oie.int/index.php?id=169&L=0&htmfile=chapitre_aw_stray_dog.htm

Panter-Brick C, Clarke SE, Lomas H, Pinder M and Lindsay SW (2006) Culturally compelling strategies for behaviour change: a social ecology model and case study in malaria prevention. *Social Science and Medicine* **62**, 2810–2825

Ratsitorahina M, Rasambainarivo JH, Raharimanana S *et al.* (2009). Dog ecology and demography in Antananarivo, 2007. *BMC Veterinary Research* **5**, 21

Sparkes AH, Bessant C, Cope K *et al.* (2013) ISFM guidelines on population management and welfare of unowned domestic cats (*Felis Catus*). *Journal of Feline Medicine and Surgery* **15(9)**, 811–817

Sudarshan MK, Mahendra BJ, Madhusudana SN *et al.* (2006) An epidemiological study of animal bites in India: results of a WHO sponsored national multi-centric rabies survey. *Journal of Communicable Diseases* **38**, 32–39

Totton SC, Wandeler AI, Ribble CS, Rosatte RC and McEwen SA (2011) Stray dog population health in Jodhpur, India in the wake of an animal birth control (ABC) program. *Preventive Veterinary Medicine* **98**, 215–220

Totton SC, Wandeler AI, Zinsstag J *et al.* (2010). Stray dog population demographics in Jodhpur, India following a population control/rabies vaccination program. *Preventive Veterinary Medicine* **97**, 51–57

Yoak AJ, Reece JF, Gehrt SD and Hamilton IM (2014) Disease control through fertility control: secondary benefits of animal birth control in Indian street dogs. *Preventive Veterinary Medicine* **113**, 152–156

World Society for the Protection of Animals (WSPA) (2007) Methods for the euthanasia of dogs and cats: comparison and recommendations. Available from: http://www.icam-coalition.org/downloads/Methods for the euthanasia of dogs and cats- English.pdf

Useful websites

Google My Maps:
http://www.google.com/mymaps

ICAM guidance:
http://www.icam-coalition.org/downloads/ICAM_Guidance_Document.pdf

Chapter 5

Practical management of free-roaming populations

Ian MacFarlaine and Andy Gibson

Trap-neuter-return (TNR) is the name given to the capture, neutering and returning to home of groups of feral and free-roaming cats and dogs. The objective is to humanely stabilize and then reduce the population in a manner that incorporates euthanasia only for reasons of welfare, and is only acceptable to caregivers, the authorities and all other stakeholders. It is alternatively known as catch-neuter-return (CNR) or CNR combined with vaccination (CNVR). Typically, TNR is the term used for cats, and CNR for dogs. In the UK, TNR of cats is relatively common, while CNR of dogs is not practised; however, this chapter describes a set of procedures and practices that are common to control of free-roaming dog and cat populations worldwide.

TNR of cats gained momentum in the 1960s in a number of countries, especially the UK. An early attribution (Remfry, 2001) of the method to the animal rescue worker and welfare charity founder Celia Hammond noted that, while cats were initially returned to the site of trapping because of a lack of rescue holding capacity, the cats enjoyed higher psychological welfare if they were neutered and left on site than if they were moved through the 'shelter' system (Berkeley, 2004).

Other alternatives to TNR, such as 'catch and kill' and 'catch and relocate', may already be in place at the start of a project. These methods are often perceived to be cheaper and quicker than more humane interventions; however, they are ineffective and inevitably more expensive in the long term. The humane euthanasia of animals is costly and labour intensive, and so mass killing by inhumane methods is often reported, including indiscriminate poisoning with strychnine or shooting (Dalla Villa *et al.*, 2010). Other inhumane methods of culling, including beating, strangulation, gassing and electrocution, have also been reported in some countries. Although culls are often carried out in response to complaints from members of the public about free-roaming animals, the campaigns are not supported by all citizens owing to the suffering caused to the animals and, in some regions, a high proportion of free-roaming dogs and cats being owned. In order for culling strategies to have a long-term impact on population growth, a significant proportion of free-roaming animals must be culled and sources of new animals must be stopped. Otherwise, culling produces a short-term reduction in the population, followed by a return to carrying capacity through increased reproductive rate and repopulation from the surrounding area as animals take advantage of uncontested resources. Consequently, regular culls must continue indefinitely to have a sustained impact on population size. Furthermore, influx of new animals is likely to increase the spread of diseases (including rabies in endemic regions) from surrounding areas. The same principles apply to 'catch and relocate' practices where animals are caught from one area and moved either to a different area or to mass housing facilities; both of these options have serious welfare ramifications and the same long-term outcomes as 'catch and kill'. These practices are expensive to carry out and do not address the core problems of overpopulation.

While TNR/CNR is not universally appropriate or practical in every circumstance, it has been repeatedly observed to be more effective than large-scale culling or relocation, albeit only when applied correctly. It is important to evaluate the effectiveness of TNR over a given area and target colonies or districts on an 'assess-sweep-evaluate-move on' basis. All TNR/CNR projects require clearly defined aims and strategy, along with well defined and measurable outcomes. In this way, errors and failures can be learned from, and successes and cumulative change can be identified and used both as tools for planning and as a catalyst for acceptance and funding of future projects.

Stakeholder engagement

Before beginning any project, it is important to engage the relevant stakeholders, including government, local non-governmental organizations (NGOs), the local and regional veterinary practices, and interested members of the community. Each stakeholder has a different role to play in helping to ensure that a project's aims are appropriate and achievable. This topic is covered in more detail in Chapter 4; however, some practical suggestions are provided below.

Veterinary professionals

Encouraging local private sector and government veterinary surgeons (veterinarians) to regularly take part in the population management initiative and training can help stimulate interest in humane methods of population management, improve standards of surgery and introduce progressive ideas about euthanasia. These veterinary surgeons are often in direct contact with the animal-owning public and should be encouraged to educate the public in the principles of responsible pet ownership in the course of their everyday work. Veterinary surgeons recruited to the project should be carefully assessed for competence, as standards can vary hugely even within a region. Some veterinary surgeons will have specialized in surgical neutering techniques, maintaining excellent standards of patient care, asepsis and tissue handling, while achieving a high throughput of animals undergoing neutering. Equally, however, enforcement of minimum standards can be very poor in some regions and the need to provide basic or refresher training in asepsis, anaesthetic monitoring, analgesia, surgical technique, and appropriate use and methods of euthanasia should be anticipated.

Local community

Engaging with the local community to identify perceived problems caused by free-roaming animals helps to ensure that the proposed interventions are relevant and sustainable to that setting. Focus group discussions, semi-structured interviews and household questionnaires are tools that can be used to assess public opinion. Focus groups provide a forum in which a particular subject can be discussed openly, with the aim of gathering a cross-section of opinions across all geographical, demographic and cultural variations in the society. Semi-structured interviews allow exploration of related topics with individual members of the community and key stakeholders, whereas household questionnaires are useful for gathering quantitative data about a specific topic or opinion. Detailed information on conducting these kinds of activities has been provided by the International Companion Animal Management (ICAM) Coalition (http://www.icam-coalition.org; ICAM Coalition, 2015).

A useful method is to work as a group to select a zone and establish whether the group has a good picture of the free-roaming animals in the area by assigning a percentage to each subset of the population (percentage owned, percentage lost/abandoned, etc.). Although this can be very effective, there can be an inbuilt bias if the exercise is carried out by a single stakeholder (e.g. a TNR volunteer will have a very different perception from a private veterinary surgeon, who in turn will have a different perception from a local community member), so it may be more effective to target and bring together several stakeholders to try to map the issue they are facing.

Animal owners, carers and feeders

In any TNR/CNR programme, the collaboration and support of those who care for and/or feed free-roaming animals is essential to ensure success. However, it is important to remember that, at least initially, some apprehension may be encountered. Modern veterinary practice in developed countries has offered safe and ethical neutering by surgical means for over 50 years, with mortality and complication rates in countries with advanced veterinary professions being negligible. In countries where infrastructure is poor and veterinary capacity is limited, neutering may not be normal practice and may not be readily available. Owners in such countries will not seek neutering because of ignorance of its existence, lack of knowledge of its benefits or fear of its complication rate. The failure of owners to request neutering of their animals perpetuates the lack of availability of this service, as veterinary surgeons see no commercial gain in investing in the training, equipment or procedural changes to provide such a service. By engaging animal owners, and dealing with the myths and apprehensions surrounding neutering in advance, it is possible to avoid disruption to catching/trapping activities and attempts to hide animals.

Planning

Staff recruitment and training

In the weeks before work begins, it is often necessary to budget and accommodate for a period of recruitment and training of lay staff, who may not have previous experience of or initial interest in animal welfare. It may be necessary to use experienced staff from outside the region initially, to help train and establish a permanent local team. It is important to invest in practical training in humane handling techniques, and also in building a sense of expertise, compassion and pride in the work. Providing a uniform and identity badges will help to solidify the team ethos and sense of worth in a job that deserves to be viewed as a skilled vocation. It is imperative that all staff in contact with animals in rabies-endemic countries are fully vaccinated against rabies and that staff vaccination records are maintained.

Volunteers

Both local and international volunteers can bring a great deal to a project. Local volunteers are likely to be well known to the community, to have detailed knowledge of the local setting, and are motivated to serve their community. They can therefore have a positive impact on community opinion and understanding of the project through public relations and education activities. Volunteer veterinary surgeons and veterinary nurses can provide valuable help in delivering quality training on a wide range of topics to both lay and veterinary staff, as well as bringing new ideas and experience.

Volunteers from outside the local community, or from other countries, bring an additional dynamic to the project and may enhance the perceived value of the work to local staff and members of the public. However, it is essential that animal welfare is seen as an organic and integral part of life and that good veterinary care and resources are (or become) intrinsic to the local society. Allowing the provision of animal control to be delivered primarily by external personnel and totally reliant on foreign aid can create a sense of helplessness among the community, with the risk of suspicion and perceived insult, and can therefore disengage a community that does not feel empowered or listened to.

Surgical training and the learning curve

Ovariohysterectomy is a technical surgery that carries the potential for life-threatening complications. Veterinary undergraduates in the UK report significant anxiety relating to attaining competence in this technique, and a degree of support from an experienced supervisor is inevitably required during the learning curve to competence (Bowlt et al., 2011). In addition, a higher rate of complications, in particular rectus sheath dehiscence and intraoperative haemorrhage, has been documented with inexperienced surgeons, and presents a particular concern in the mass neutering setting.

There is a trend for UK students to seek early surgical experience with charities overseas, where there may be greater opportunity for hands-on surgical exposure. However, the facilities and support available in such projects should be carefully researched, to ensure that the volunteer has an appropriate level of competence before they attend. The benefits and risks to both the surgeon and animal welfare should be carefully considered in such a situation. There are now a number of facilities established to provide training in all aspects of surgical neutering in a carefully supported environment. These programmes match the abundant caseload provided through population control initiatives with high demand from both local and international candidates for further surgical experience and training.

Data recording

Accurate data about a population of animals before the start of an intervention are often limited and carrying out basic surveys can provide valuable baseline information. However, data gathered during the intervention can provide a great deal of much-needed information about the population at little extra cost if accurate records are kept throughout. The basic dataset for each animal should include:

- Location the animal came from (e.g. village or municipality ward for dogs; colony location for cats)
- Name of the veterinary surgeon
- Sex (male/female)
- Age based on dentition
- Skin condition (i.e. no skin disease, mild skin disease (0–20% hair loss), moderate skin disease (20–80% hair loss) or severe skin disease (80–100% hair loss))
- Body condition score (Figures 5.1 and 5.2)
- Surgical complications

- In females, evidence of lactation (so that the animal's return to the site of capture can be expedited if appropriate).

If every animal is also visibly marked and its location of capture/release is recorded, the number of marked animals released in a specific location can be known. If a survey of that region is subsequently conducted, the proportion of marked animals sighted can be used to estimate the size of the population (see Mark–resight surveys below; Hiby *et al.*, 2011).

Mobile technology in population management

Mobile technology is becoming an increasingly important and powerful tool in data collection and improving disease surveillance and the response to outbreaks of disease in remote and resource-limited settings. Free smartphone applications ('apps') have been developed that allow users to enter data on to customized questionnaires, which are then synchronized to a cloud-based server for collation and analysis. Functionality to capture GPS (geographical location), photographic, video and even microchip data are increasing the versatility and application of these tools. Mapping of populations and disease outbreaks in real time helps with strategic direction of animal capture efforts, and also enables better visualization of field work for presentation to policy-makers and project funders.

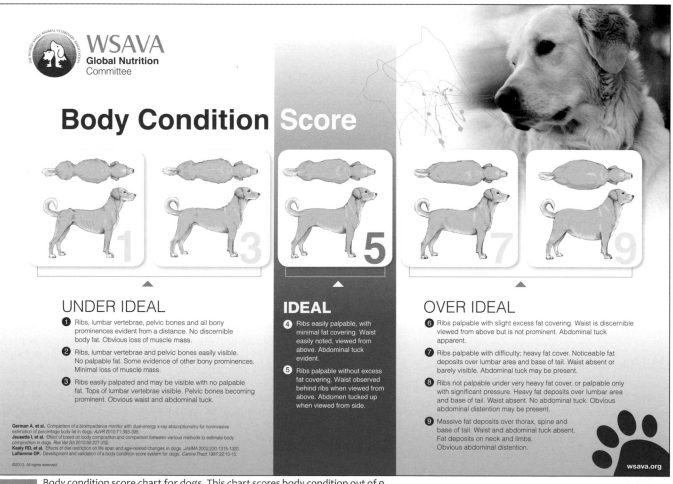

5.1 Body condition score chart for dogs. This chart scores body condition out of 9.
(Courtesy of WSAVA Global Nutrition Committee)

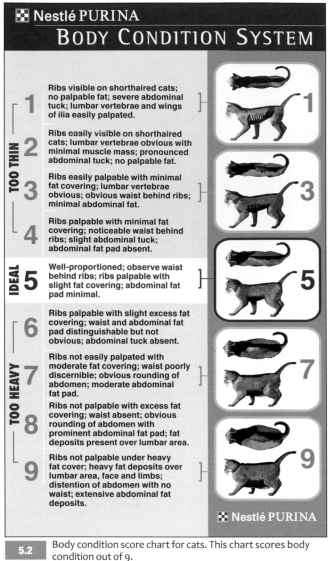

5.2 Body condition score chart for cats. This chart scores body condition out of 9.

(© Nestlé Purina PetCare and reproduced with their permission)

TNR/CNR in free-roaming dog populations

Assessing the free-roaming dog population

A free-roaming dog population can be assessed by direct sight surveys. These involve a survey team travelling through the streets of a designated region or along a pre-defined path, counting dogs and recording information about each dog seen. Surveys can be used to estimate the size of the population, assess the proportion of vaccinated/neutered dogs or monitor trends in the dog population.

Counting method

Every effort should be made to standardize the methods used and the routes travelled for all surveys conducted for a particular project. This enables data gathered from different surveys to be compared more reliably. Before the surveys begin, the methods for data collection should be set out as clearly as possible and all staff trained to use the same protocol.

Factors that should be decided in advance of undertaking a survey include:

- Time of day – the number of dogs roaming varies with the time of day, with dogs often being most active at night and in the hours following dawn, before the volume of road traffic and the temperature increase. Intermittently confined dogs may be allowed to roam only during certain periods of the day, so defining a survey period (such as 6–10 am) helps to avoid differences in counts due to diurnal variation in roaming dog activity
- Method of travel – this should enable the surveyor to cover the region of study within a manageable time, but also allow thorough detection of roaming dogs. Walking, cycling, or travel by motorcycle or rickshaw are all feasible, and each method will have its own merits and drawbacks in different settings
- Counting protocol – for surveys of free-roaming dogs, dogs that are confined or tied up on private property should not be included. It should be agreed how dogs at boundaries are counted, as it is important that survey regions do not overlap. For example, the centre line of boundary roads could be defined as the boundary; dogs sighted outside the boundary should not be counted (World Society for the Protection of Animals (WSPA), 2007)
- Details recorded – a simple system to record the type of dog sighted allows assessment of sex, age and, in bitches, lactation. The survey record sheet should include the date, time, name of surveyor and region being surveyed. One method for recording dogs that are sighted is a simple letter code to denote adult male (M), adult non-lactating female (F), adult lactating female (LF) and puppy (P). The proportion of actively lactating females is generally a more useful indicator of the reproductive capacity of a population than the sighting of puppies (ICAM Coalition, 2015). As the dog population management intervention progresses, the proportion of lactating females should reduce. For mark–resight surveys, the record sheet can include columns for the presence/absence of a mark (indicating that the dog has been trapped and neutered; see later), under which the type of dog is recorded. This enables the proportion of marked dogs to be calculated for estimating the population size or neutering/vaccination coverage (see Mark–resight surveys).

Estimating the size of the population

Estimating the size of a dog population before commencing neutering/vaccination will facilitate appropriate allocation of resources and planning of a TNR/CNR strategy. It is often not logistically feasible to survey the entire area, and so a representative sample of locations within the area of interest is selected and used to estimate the population in the area as a whole. A random sample may be representative in small areas where the dog population density is consistent; however, the population is likely to vary across larger areas, with variation in human population size and activities. To help overcome this problem, regions can be grouped (stratified) according to known factors, such as land use or human population density, and sampling sites randomly selected from within each group (stratum). The population is then extrapolated for each stratum and combined to estimate the total population (Boone and Slater, 2013).

It is possible to get an idea of the number of free-roaming dogs in a defined survey region by counting dogs sighted in all the streets in the area; however, it is important to appreciate that not all free-roaming dogs will be seen. The proportion of the total population that is sighted in a single survey is called 'detectability' and will be affected by the survey methods and movements of dogs during the survey. Simple dog sighting surveys can be termed 'rapid surveys', as they are relatively quick to conduct, but other survey methods are needed to estimate the proportion of dogs not seen (see below) (Boone and Slater, 2013).

Mark–resight surveys

Mark–resight surveys are one method of trying to account for animals that are not sighted during rapid surveys. First, a group of animals in a defined region is marked and then allowed to mix within the general population. A survey is then conducted in the same area to count the numbers of marked and unmarked animals. The proportion of marked animals seen in this survey is assumed to be the same as the proportion of marked dogs in the total population, and so, because the number of animals that were originally marked is known, the size of the total population can be estimated (Figure 5.3).

If dogs are marked during a neutering/vaccination campaign, these surveys not only enable the size of the population to be estimated, but also provide an estimate of the neutering/vaccination coverage achieved by the intervention; to facilitate this, it is important to record the number of marked animals that have been released in the area being surveyed. The time between releasing the marked dogs and surveying the population must be sufficient to allow the dogs to mix evenly, but not so long that there is an increased risk of movement of animals in and out of the population, or loss of marks, deaths or births. In situations where temporary marks are used, such as in vaccination campaigns, 1–3 days is sufficient.

This method makes several assumptions about the population, such as marks not being lost and all dogs in the population being equally likely to be caught or seen during the survey. In reality, these assumptions may not hold true, resulting in an inaccurate estimate. For example, if marks are lost or overlooked, the calculated estimate will be higher than the true population size. Further research is needed to understand the errors involved in dog surveys and to develop and refine predictable methods for studying free-roaming dog populations.

Monitoring dog populations

It is not necessary to estimate the total dog population in order to monitor the effect of a population management intervention. Indicator counts provide a snapshot of the number of dogs sighted along a particular route at a given time. If these counts are repeated along the same routes annually, using standardized methodology and in the same weather conditions, it is possible to plot trends of increase or decrease in the number of free-roaming dogs over time. Indicator counts do not enable estimation of the total dog population, but can be a powerful tool in providing evidence of the impact of dog population management activities and can therefore be used to, for example, demonstrate the need for further support. A defined survey path is plotted across the city or region of interest, including a proportion of minor and main roads roughly equal to the proportion in the overall area. This path should be able to be covered in a period of approximately 2–3 hours by motorcycle (around 15–20 km) at the time when roaming dog activity is greatest (Hiby and Hiby, 2014). The route is then surveyed on at least 2 days at the

Stage	Comments	
1	The number of dogs that are marked in a defined area is recorded	
2	The marked dogs are allowed to mix into the unknown total population	
3	The same defined area is surveyed 1–3 days later and a proportion of dogs are sighted. Each sighted dog is recorded as marked or unmarked	
4	The total population is estimated	

Total population estimation

The total population size is estimated using the following equation:

Total population size =

$$\frac{\text{Total number of dogs sighted on survey} \times \text{Total number of dogs initially marked}}{\text{Number of marked dogs sighted on survey}}$$

Advanced calculation

To gain an idea as to how precise the population estimation is, 95% confidence limits should be calculated. This gives an upper and lower value. There is a 95% chance that the true population size is within this range.

Total population size (N) is estimated as:

$$N = n_1 \times n_2/m_2$$

Where:

n_1 = number of dogs marked and released on the first occasion
n_2 = total number of dogs sighted on the second occasion
m_2 = number of marked dogs sighted on the second occasion

Calculation of confidence limits

First calculate P

$$P = m_2/n_2$$

Then calculate the two values:

$$W_1, W_2 = P \pm \left[1/(2n_2) + 1.96\sqrt{p(1-p)(1-m_2/n_2)/(n_2-1)}\right]$$

Finally, divide W_1 and W_2 into n_1 to calculate the upper and lower confidence limits for the estimated population size:

Lower confidence limit = n_1/W_1
Upper confidence limit = n_1/W_2

5.3 Calculating an estimate of the total population size using mark–resight methodology.

(Adapted from Sutherland, 2006)

same time of year, avoiding days with adverse weather. The mean number of dogs counted each year is plotted on a graph so that change can be monitored over time (WSPA, 2007). The additional benefit of this type of survey is that it provides the average number of dogs per kilometre of street surveyed. This can provide a number that is more meaningful to residents and other stakeholders than an estimate of the total dog population of the city would be (Hiby and Hiby, 2014).

Assessing the owned dog population

Information about the owned dog population is better gained through household questionnaires. These should include questions relating to the number and breed of dogs owned, as well as whether the dogs are allowed to roam outside the property and, if so, at what times of day. The questionnaires can also include questions exploring owners' attitudes towards dogs, reasons for dog ownership, the litter size, survival and any disease in their dogs, use of/access to veterinary services, sources of new dogs and attitudes towards neutering and vaccination. A detailed guide to planning and conducting questionnaire surveys has been produced by the ICAM Coalition (2015).

Trapping and handling free-roaming dogs

During population management interventions, dogs will need to be handled periodically, whether for vaccination, treatment or transportation to a clinic for surgical neutering. These are times at which the animal is likely to experience greatest stress, particularly if it is not used to being handled by people, and this stress may make an animal harder to catch and handle in the future. Furthermore, support from the local community is essential for the ongoing success of any project, and inhumane handling methods are unlikely to be tolerated by the public. Therefore, good handling techniques not only ensure the safety of the animal and the handler, but are also important for the future success of the project. In rabies endemic countries, animal bites and scratches carry additional risk and require post exposure rabies vaccination. Therefore it is essential that staff are trained in humane handling methods before they start unsupervised work.

The extent to which dogs are comfortable being handled by people will depend largely on local ownership practices. In African countries, the majority of dogs (up to 98%) are owned and are therefore accessible through presentation by their owner and manual restraint (Jibat et al., 2015). However, this type of approach has only limited success in many Asian countries, with many free-roaming dogs being less amenable to handling, and so catching dogs using nets is more often required in order to access a significant proportion of the population (Pal, 2001; Morters et al., 2014). The temperament of the individual dog, the immediate environment and the skill and experience of the handler will all have an effect on which method of restraint is most appropriate. The chosen method should aim to ensure the safety of the handler while minimizing stress to the animal and the risk of it escaping.

Methods of capture

Manual catch and restraint: Manual catch and restraint is often the most desirable form of capture for dogs that are comfortable being handled; however, this is highly dependent on the temperament of the dog and the skill of the handler. Food can be used to tempt free-roaming dogs and

a testing object can be useful in assessing the dog's response to touch in cases where the dog appears unpredictable. The skill and time required to catch dogs manually often mean that manual capture cannot be used as the primary method in situations where free-roaming dogs are not readily amenable to handling.

Pole nets and butterfly nets: Pole nets are lightweight if made from aluminium and effective for catching free-roaming dogs that are not amenable to manual restraint in urban areas. Once caught, dogs will often calm quickly; however, they may become stressed by handling and can bite through the net. Dogs can be transferred into ring nets that do not have a pole attached for transportation. Care should be taken in hot climates to avoid heat stroke, particularly in larger dogs, and handlers must be trained to recognize the early signs of, and to treat, heat stress. A catching net with example dimensions is shown in Figure 5.4.

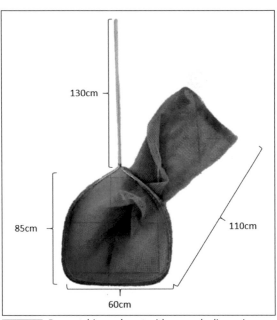

5.4 Dog catching pole net with example dimensions.
(© Mission Rabies)

Catch pole: Catch poles should be used with caution, as they can result in serious welfare issues if used inappropriately or by an inadequately trained operator. As with any form of neck restraint, animals can become distressed and there is a risk of airway obstruction if the catch pole is used incorrectly. They may be necessary for restraining unpredictable dogs in confined or semi-confined areas, but fearful dogs may react violently and can injure their teeth by biting on the pole. Care must be taken to avoid over-tightening and causing obstruction of the airway, and it is essential that the tightening and release mechanism is checked for faults before use. Dogs should never be lifted by the catch pole alone; the weight of the animal must always be supported by an assistant during lifting (Figure 5.5).

Sack and loop: Some organizations have developed a successful and economical method of catching dogs using hessian sacks. This is likely to be a more humane method of catching than using lassoes or catch poles and may have advantages over pole nets in narrow streets and markets (Figure 5.6).

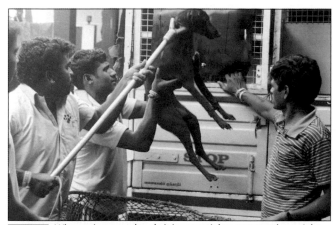

5.5 When using a catch pole it is essential to support the weight of the dog during lifting.
(Courtesy of WVS India)

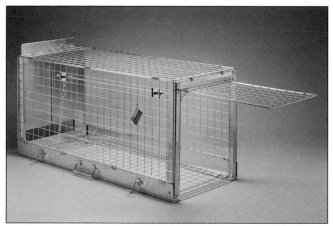

5.7 An example of a cage trap for dogs.
(© MDC Exports)

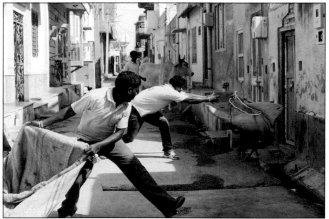

5.6 Catching dogs with hessian sacks is an alternative method that can be used in some locations, but it requires highly skilled operators.
(© Mission Rabies)

Chemical means of capture: Dart guns and blow pipes can be used in less densely populated areas to catch animals that cannot be approached. These methods require skilled staff who have been trained in safe injection technique, drug dose calculation, assessing the depth of anaesthesia and management of anaesthetic emergencies. There is a risk of dogs escaping immediately after darting and subsequently becoming anaesthetized, as well as the risk to staff and public safety associated with the use of anaesthetic darts in public areas.

Cage traps: Manually activated or pressure-activated cage traps can be useful for capturing dogs in open spaces where other methods have failed. Patience is often required, and it is essential that the trap is checked regularly, contains water and is sheltered from the weather. Repeat capture of the same dogs can be a problem. It may be necessary to secure traps if they are left unattended, as they are an expensive asset to lose to theft. The use of local volunteers to check traps can save on manpower, but the required financial and time investment, combined with low capture rates, usually prohibit the use of traps on a large scale (Figure 5.7).

Restraint tools

Basket muzzles: These are easy to apply and effectively reduce the risk of the handler being bitten; however, some dogs poorly tolerate application of the muzzle.

Tape muzzles: Using tape to create a temporary muzzle is an economical and easily accessible method. Tape muzzles enable the dog's mouth to be immobilized while the animal is handled, examined and treated, but must be applied correctly. Tape muzzles should not be used in unenclosed areas as dogs that escape while muzzled could die from dehydration.

Slip leads: Slip leads can be used to restrain friendly dogs that are used to being handled on a lead, and can also provide a temporary muzzle for animals receiving a potentially painful stimulus such as an injection. Dogs that are not used to being handled on a lead may become panicked, and alternative methods of restraint may be more appropriate for these animals.

Veterinary treatment
Surgical technique

Excellent surgical technique is essential in the mass neutering setting, both from an animal welfare perspective and in the context of achieving the wider aims of population control and optimizing the cost–benefit of the programme. The limitations in anaesthetic monitoring, maintaining an aseptic environment, perioperative analgesia and postoperative follow-up in this setting all emphasize the importance of a short anaesthetic and surgical time with minimal tissue handling and trauma, and the need for low intraoperative and postoperative complication rates. In addition, efficient use of suture material and a short anaesthetic time will increase throughput and reduce the cost of surgery per dog, which, when scaled up to potentially thousands of dogs, can significantly increase the financial feasibility of a CNR programme and its impact on population control.

There is some evidence for ovariectomy being recommended over ovariohysterectomy as the technique of choice for surgical neutering of healthy bitches. Ovariectomy is arguably less technically challenging, time-consuming and traumatic than ovariohysterectomy and has been shown to be equivalent in terms of long-term problems such as endometritis, pyometra and urinary incontinence (van Goethem et al., 2006). In bitches that have visible uterine pathology or older bitches that may have cystic endometrial hyperplasia, it is advisable to perform ovariohysterectomy to avoid the risk of future uterine disease.

Analgesia

All surgical patients should be provided with appropriate analgesia. As a bare minimum, this should consist of a potent analgesic (preferably an opioid) and a non-steroidal anti-inflammatory drug (NSAID) at the time of surgery, with additional analgesia being provided as appropriate after individual case assessment. A more detailed discussion of analgesic and anaesthetic protocols for surgical neutering is provided in Chapter 6.

Preventive care and treatment

One of the core aims of many population management interventions is to improve and maintain the health of the population, and a high incidence of disease may have been one of the primary reasons for taking action to begin with. Skin disease, wounds, emaciation and tick infestations are commonly reported welfare issues in free-roaming dog populations, and may be a result of overpopulation, lack of accessible veterinary services, irresponsible ownership or lack of enforcement of animal welfare legislation, or a combination of these factors. Sick or injured animals in the population will need to be treated in the short term while activities are implemented to address the cause of the problem in the future.

Preventive care: Preventive care focuses on keeping the population healthy, as opposed to just treating individuals that are sick. Combining reproductive control with preventive care maximizes the benefit achieved each time an animal is handled, thus making the greatest use of the resources invested in catching the animal and minimizing repeated disruption to its welfare. The specific preventive treatments used will be highly dependent on the diseases seen in the local population and the cost *versus* the welfare benefit of treatment. It may be necessary to prioritize what is considered treatable and appreciate what is outside the capacity of the available resources.

Rabies not only has clear animal and human health and welfare consequences, but also represents a significant economic burden to rabies-endemic countries through loss of life and treatment of humans (Hampson *et al.*, 2015). Free-roaming dog populations act as a reservoir within which the virus circulates, intermittently spilling over into the human population. Annual vaccination of 70% of the dog population has been demonstrated to be effective in eliminating rabies (Cleaveland *et al.*, 2003; World Health Organization, 2013). Slowing dog population turnover through reproductive control helps to ensure that vaccination coverage is maintained for longer, and so neutering and vaccination are often combined. It is important to realize, however, that rabies elimination can be achieved with vaccination alone, and mass vaccination of large populations of dogs with strategic neutering targeted at subpopulations that contribute most to the unowned dog population is likely to be more effective than untargeted combined neutering and vaccination.

During neutering initiatives there is increased potential for the transmission of disease between animals kept in close confinement; for example, dogs in a neutering and vaccination programme in Jodhpur, India, were found to be at increased risk of skin disease and tick infestations after being released (Yoak *et al.*, 2014). Attempts to improve kennelling protocols and cleaning, or providing prophylactic treatment against ticks and mange at the time of neutering, may limit the detrimental impacts of keeping dogs in close quarters (see Chapter 11).

Sick dogs: At the outset of an initiative there may be a high proportion of sick or injured animals among those captured. The decision-making around these individuals in the face of limited resources can be challenging and upsetting for animal care staff, as well as having serious welfare implications for each animal. The level of care provided will depend largely on the clinic's capacity and caseload. Factors such as the number and expertise of staff, the infrastructure and the diagnostic and treatment options available will affect the decision-making process regarding individual animals.

When presented with a sick or injured free-roaming dog with no identifiable owner, the options are to:

* Do nothing (appropriate only for minor self-healing injuries)
* Leave the dog where it is and give treatment (on a single occasion or repeatedly through visits to the site)
* Take the dog to a treatment facility, treat and return it
* Take the dog to a treatment facility, treat and rehome it
* Euthanase the animal.

Alternatives to hospitalizing free-roaming dogs should be used by preference, if possible. Clinical facilities are expensive to run while maintaining adequate standards of hygiene and care. Additionally, animals that are unfamiliar with being confined may experience greater levels of stress and therefore have an increased risk of infection and delayed recovery times, as well as being exposed to the risk of infectious disease transmission. For chronic disease or minor injuries it may be possible to manage the animal as an 'outpatient' if a local person can be designated as a guardian to monitor the animal and give treatment. In cases where hospitalization is required, minimizing the period of hospitalization will help to maintain a high throughput of treated animals and limits detrimental impacts on the animals' welfare.

It is beneficial to develop and follow clear standard protocols for the management of specific conditions, especially for contagious diseases such as distemper and parvovirus, where variations in practice could put other animals at risk. Where the demand for treatment outweighs the capacity to provide it, triage and euthanasia are essential components of population control and maintaining minimum welfare standards.

Visual confirmation of neuter status

Simple methods of visually identifying whether an animal has been neutered can be of great benefit, especially in dogs that have the potential to become free-roaming at any time. For animals undergoing surgery, a visible notch can be cut from the tip of the pinna (Figure 5.8), followed by haemostasis using cautery, during anaesthesia. Staff must be trained in proper cautery technique to prevent unnecessary trauma to the pinna, which could increase the risk of fly strike.

Dogs not undergoing an anaesthetic can be marked using non-toxic paint or dye that marks the fur for a period of days, long enough to carry out a repeat survey of the region (see above). These simple markings benefit the animal as they mean it will not be repeatedly caught in subsequent catching efforts. For bitches that are not permanently marked, there is a risk of repeat laparotomy, which carries significant welfare ramifications associated with the repeat anaesthetic and surgical risks. Therefore, permanent marking of unowned bitches undergoing surgery should be considered compulsory, although it is

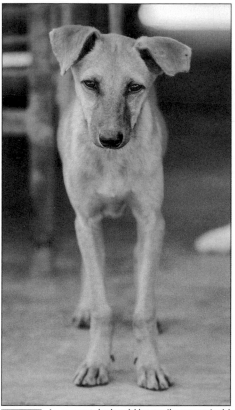

5.8 An ear notch should be easily recognizable at a distance.
(© Richard Murgatroyd Photography)

also important to secure approval from the local government authorities to do so.

Marking treated dogs is also of benefit to the project, as surveys can be performed to estimate the proportion of dogs treated and monitor the population size. Methods that allow identification of individual animals, such as a tattooed code on the inside of the ear or microchipping, can allow tracing of when and where the animal was first caught and, in the case of microchips, will enable owner contact details to be obtained. If individually marked animals are subsequently caught again, information can be gathered about their roaming patterns and lifespan. A comprehensive description of marking methods is available on the ICAM Coalition website (http://www.icam-coalition.org).

Timing of release

There is no standardized recommendation for the length of time that an animal should be hospitalized following surgical neutering, and appropriate time of release has often been debated among animal welfare communities. A period of hospitalization allows for perioperative pain management and early detection of postoperative complications. However, these benefits must be balanced against the difficulty in maintaining hygiene, risk of transmission of diseases such as rabies, parvovirus, mange and distemper and the welfare concerns of confining free-roaming dogs in a kennel environment for protracted periods. Stress can impair the immune response and delay healing and, therefore, kennelling may actually contribute to a delayed recovery and a decreased immune response to vaccines. Thorough clinical examination before release is essential for the detection of potentially life-threatening anaesthetic or surgical complications. It is important that the local community is made aware of potential postoperative complications and that direct avenues of communication

are available for reporting these to the programme should they occur. Capacity to respond to public concerns and complaints should be considered when planning the intervention.

For same- or next-day release to be ethically acceptable, it is essential that a thorough pre-release examination is performed and that high standards of asepsis and surgery are maintained to minimize the risk of postoperative complications.

Pregnant bitches, or any animal that experiences surgical or anaesthetic complications, should be hospitalized for observation, analgesia and treatment as necessary until they can be safely returned to the place of capture. Sufficient cages and staff to accommodate and care for a proportion of the daily patient throughput for a lengthened hospitalization period should be factored into the surgical neutering plan, as a contingency. For example, to retain 5% of the daily caseload for a period of 5 days in a clinic operating on 40 dogs per day would require the capacity to hospitalize an additional 10 dogs at any one time.

TNR/CNR in free-roaming cat populations

Assessing the free-roaming cat population

Unlike with dogs, there is no accepted available technique for estimating population size in cats, although at the time of writing studies are ongoing to develop suitable methods. In assessing individual colonies of cats, it is important to carry out a visual count both at a regular feeding time and also at an 'opposite' time. Some factors that must be taken into account when counting dog populations also have relevance for cats, especially:

- Time of day – cats are crepuscular by choice, unless environmental factors cause this to change
- Environmental factors – the presence of humans, other cats or roaming dogs (either free-roaming or those that are allowed out at certain times) will affect cat activity
- Feeders – cats are food-oriented and will attend at the times feeders are present, or at a time when a passive food source is available (e.g. restaurant opening or closing times)
- Weather – cats will hide at their usual feeding time if the weather is inclement, especially if they are not hungry
- Unusual events – similarly to weather, an event such as a football match may disrupt their routine.

There may be an absence of itinerant peripheral adult males from a count site at a time of year when cats are not reproducing, or queens may be absent from the count site if they have very recently kittened; this effect will be made more pronounced by queens being in synchronous reproductive cycles. It is worth enquiring into particular anomalous trends that are noticed – a lack of young cats may indicate that kittens are being culled, while a higher than expected percentage of males may indicate the culling of female kittens.

Three useful reliable commonalities are:

- The number of cats counted can be extrapolated reliably by adding 40% or 50% to give a closer estimate of the true number present (useful when allocating funding or determining surgical capacity)

- Females will comprise around 60–70% of the core cluster of cats
- Manual trapping and acclimatizing techniques are essential, especially when targeting females, which are anecdotally more likely to be suspicious and 'trap-shy'.

Methods of capture

A common failure of TNR programmes for cats is that trapping fails to yield a sufficient neuter rate in each location to achieve stasis and then reduction in population size. A slowdown in the rate of population increase is in itself a positive outcome and contributes towards stalling an increasing population (as well as benefiting each individual cat), but does not achieve the aim of population control of any programme.

Trapping should be planned to:

- Achieve a high neuter rate and outpace breeding
- Never result in a cat being released from, or escaping from, a trap unneutered
- Catch the cats in a logical order of priority (pregnant queens first, other female cats next, male cats last), as well as focusing on more wary cats first
- Be of sufficient reliability to justify clinics reserving blocks of time for neutering procedures
- Demonstrate visibly that the programme is reliable and effective even in the short term.

There are a number of problems that may present themselves during TNR operations, ranging from difficulty finding parking spaces in urban areas to disruption by members of the local community, but these can be mitigated if the cats' feeders, landowners and residents are cooperative and supportive and if there is good publicity in advance of the programme beginning. TNR operations may also be impaired by the weather – for example, bad weather can disrupt a trapping intervention on a particular day when the movement and transit patterns of cats change in response to the conditions, or their appetite may be reduced during long spells of hot weather meaning it is harder to trap the cats. The climate can also affect TNR by making it difficult to execute trapping operations during certain times of the year.

Acclimatization

Acclimatization is the process of getting animals accustomed to safely entering and leaving a trap before trapping begins, to build up a 'credit' of positive experiences for the cats. Food is added to the deactivated trap for 2–7 days before trapping, and no food is provided anywhere outside the trap. If there is concern that the caregiver may start trapping the cats prematurely, then it may be worth removing and taking away the transfer door (if the trap has one), to prevent overzealous catching by carers. Acclimatization will dramatically improve the catch rate and reduce the problem of trap-shyness. Trapping is difficult, time-consuming and can be emotionally draining for TNR operators, who are often volunteers. Rarely can a cat be caught a second time, so once cats are trapped, they should never be released without being neutered, regardless of their age or pregnancy status. Failure to do so will undermine attempts to control the population.

Trapping equipment

Manual traps: With a manual trap, closure of the door is controlled by the trapping operator rather than being activated by the cat standing on a treadle plate (Figure 5.9). This allows more than one cat to be caught with each closure of the trap, as well as selectivity by the operator targeting the cats in order of priority and not catching those that have already been neutered. Given that the sound of a cat being trapped is likely to be a noxious and aversive stimulus to the other cats that have not yet been caught and observe or hear the trapping, then increasing the number of cats per catch means that one noxious stimulus gives rise to more cats being neutered. Careful selection of the subject(s) to be trapped is important to prevent unnecessary or wasted trappings. For example, some cats (typically males) make repeat visits to a trap; repeatedly trapping such cats not only wastes effort, but may also lead to trap-shy females avoiding the location due to the noise of the trap being activated.

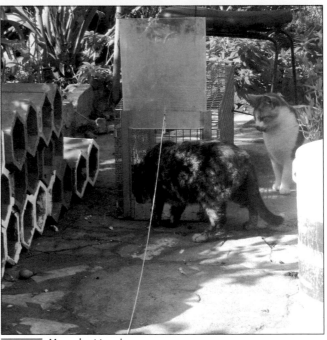

5.9 Manual cat trap in use.
(© Ian MacFarlaine)

Automatic traps: The cage trap includes a mechanism (e.g. a treadle plate) which activates the door closure when triggered by a cat entering the trap. These traps need to be well maintained. It is important to bear in mind that, unlike manual trapping, automatic traps are totally indiscriminate in terms of which cats are trapped. If used as the sole option, automatic traps frequently contribute to trap-shyness.

Drop traps: A drop trap is a large bottomless cage-type device that can be dropped over a group of feeding cats (Figure 5.10), which may be less reluctant to go under a drop trap to reach food than into another type of trap. Drop traps can catch up to five or six cats at once. The cats must be transferred into transport cages at the capture point, as the drop trap has no floor and so cannot be moved with the cats contained within it.

Trap transfer (squeeze/crush) cage: This type of cage incorporates a sliding end door to allow hands-free transfer of a cat from a trap with a similar sliding end door, and also includes a moveable 'squeeze' panel to push the cat to one side of the cage (e.g. for intramuscular injection of anaesthetic agents).

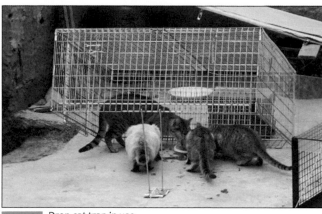

5.10 Drop cat trap in use.
(© Ian MacFarlaine)

Handling, transporting and temporary holding of cats

Key elements to minimizing stress and trauma when handling feral cats are:

- Keeping to a minimum the duration of confinement, captivity, exposure to unfamiliar stimuli and proximity to people
- Safe handling begins before and continues after the arrival of cats at the veterinary clinic for surgery
- Good trapping methodology
- Personal time management on the part of the field team, so that they are able to respond quickly, monitor frequently and thus reduce the amount of time that trapped cats are left unattended
- Good communication between the field operators and the veterinary service provider.

Baskets or traps containing cats should be kept covered during transportation and throughout the time at the veterinary clinic or mass neutering facility. This reduces the risk of cats panicking and attempting to escape. A determined feral cat can get out of most plastic cat carriers and is capable of wedging open the sliding door at the end of a trap or restrainer cage if this is not secured or tied closed, so plastic cable ties, plastic/wire bag ties or strong cord should be used to secure all cages and traps to prevent escape (Figure 5.11).

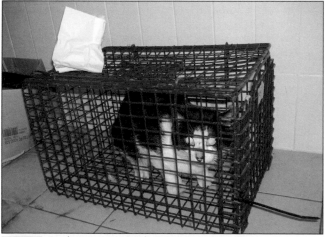

5.11 Feral tom cat in a crush cage prior to anaesthesia. Note the identification label, which remains with the cat at all times and cable ties securing the cage to prevent escape.
(© Jenny Stavisky)

Within a veterinary practice, housing feral cats in noisy dog wards, high throughput and busy cat wards, busy preparation rooms or anywhere with a radio or telephone should be avoided.

Veterinary treatment
Restraint for anaesthesia

Feral cats should never be manually handled unless anaesthetized, because they are effectively wild animals. Squeeze baskets/crush cages allow handling without direct physical contact. They should incorporate a sliding door at one end that matches the door on most traps, to allow easy transfer of cats from the trap to the cage. The moving panel should be in good working order and bolts and nuts checked and tightened regularly. The most common design of basket has protruding frames which, when squeezed together, hold the partition firm; this obviates the need to push the cat against the side of the cage when injecting anaesthetic, which can result in discomfort and injury (including reported rib fractures) to the animal. An alternative method is to use an 'isolator' or 'trap divider' (Figure 5.12), a strong blunt-ended pitchfork-type device that fits through the bars of the trap or cage and pushes the cat to one end, so that the cat can be maintained in its own trap or cage rather than needing to be transferred. Whether a squeeze basket or divider is used, it must be cleaned and disinfected between each use, to reduce the risk of transmission of infectious disease.

Transfer of a cat from a trap into a squeeze basket/ crush cage requires the cage and trap to be steadied (using either a wall or an assistant's foot). The destination cage is covered (e.g. with a blanket) and the trap is uncovered, encouraging the cat to seek shelter in the cage (Figure 5.13). Blowing on the cat will also encourage it to move across into the cage. Where a drop trap is used, the process is reversed so that the trap remains covered while the cage is left uncovered, encouraging the cat to move from the drop trap into the cage. Transfer must take place in a secure room with all doors and windows locked (with the exception of drops which, having no floor, have to be transferred from at the site of capture as they cannot be moved). A bathroom can be an ideal transfer room in field situations.

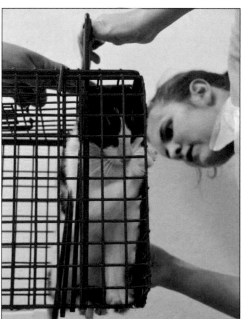

5.12 Use of an isolator to restrain a cat for injection.
(© Ian MacFarlaine)

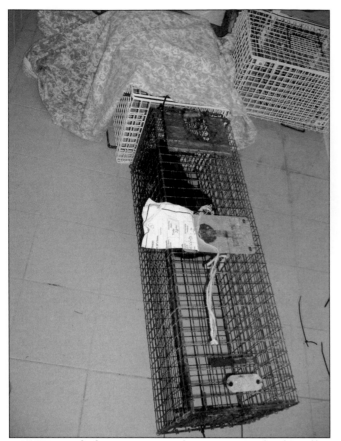

5.13 Transfer from a trap to a crush cage is most easily achieved by placing them end to end and covering the crush cage. Most cats will naturally prefer to be covered and will move into the cage. This should be carried out in a secure closed room.
(© Jenny Stavisky)

Anaesthesia and analgesia

Cats in general, but especially adult feral cats, will generally require at least 10 minutes to reach a suitable depth of anaesthesia after injection with intramuscular induction agents (for additional information regarding specific protocols, see Chapter 6). During this time it is essential that the cat is removed from the busy preparation area and allowed to achieve induction in a quiet area without external stimuli, with time allowed for the drugs to reach effect. Cages should be covered, lights switched off and noise kept to a minimum.

Occasionally, cats do not achieve a sufficient depth of anaesthesia as a result of excessive stimulation due to a noisy environment or repeated checking after injection, and a 'top-up' of the anaesthetic agent is required. If the cat appears to be sufficiently immobile to remove it from the basket and place it on a table, sometimes covering the head will reduce stimulation and give the opportunity for agents that have already been injected to achieve a better effect. This can avoid the need to top up the anaesthetic further.

Even with feral cats, calmer and slower, gentle restraint can result in a more effective induction. When bringing cats from the ward or holding area into the preparation or induction room, placing the cat in its basket/cage on to the table and then waiting 2–3 minutes before injecting the anaesthetic will have a beneficial effect, as will slow but deliberate use of the squeeze cage or restraining devices.

Perioperative treatment

Intraoperative analgesia should always be administered early (ideally using an opioid within the initial induction combination) and NSAIDs should also be given promptly, especially if surgery and then reversal are soon to follow. Good analgesia will help feral cats to return to their normal routine as soon as possible after surgery, as a cat that is in pain will be reluctant to forage, return to its base zone and sometimes even to eat. Therefore, an opioid and a NSAID should be considered a minimum requirement, especially for females.

Opinion ranges widely regarding the routine use of perioperative antibacterials during TNR. The necessity to use antimicrobials responsibly must be evaluated and weighed against the fact that cats that are neutered in a TNR programme return to challenging environments after release, and are not subject to postoperative confinement, wound hygiene or monitoring/checking. Antimicrobials should never be seen as a substitute for high standards of hygiene and appropriate surgical asepsis within a facility.

Emptying the urinary bladder of the cat once it is anaesthetized will make for a more comfortable recovery. This may also benefit the surgeon, especially given that diuresis secondary to the administration of alpha-2 agonists may make the bladder very prominent. Every cat should be checked for tattoos and microchips before clipping, ear tipping (see later) or any procedure that leaves a mark. In queens, it may be of benefit to clip a small area of the midline to check for a scar from a previous ovariohysterectomy, even if the plan is to approach by a flank incision, and *vice versa*.

Although the intravenous administration of fluids is difficult in a TNR setting, there may be some value in routinely administering subcutaneous fluids to every cat going through TNR, or at least to debilitated, pregnant, lactating and early-neutered cats. For adults, a standard 500 ml bag of 0.9% saline with a giving set can be used to provide fluids to a number of cats at low cost. A suitable gauge hypodermic needle (which must be changed between cats) is used to give 30–40 ml per cat across several injection sites; this will be of benefit in adults. In younger kittens, it may be easier to manually inject fluids with 2 ml syringes. During TNR of feral cats, providing access to oral fluids can be problematic and cats' fluid intake can be compromised during the 24–36 hours confinement, so any fluid input is helpful. Placing an empty water bowl in the basket while the cat is unconscious (to be filled from outside the cage with a squeeze bottle when the cat has recovered) is extremely useful in aiding cats' hydration postoperatively.

Lactating cats

Feeding of kittens is a shared activity among queens within cat colonies, so kittens left without their mother will not starve in a large colony situation. However, a robust and rehearsed system should be in place to ensure the swift post-surgery return to site of cats that are either known to be lactating when trapped or found to be lactating once anaesthetized. Monitored TNR programmes demonstrate that the removal of nursing queens for a brief period for TNR does not increase kitten mortality, and kittens of the correct age and colour corresponding to the mother are often seen soon after the intervention.

Pregnant cats

The issue of neutering pregnant cats is often controversial. The operators of some TNR programmes refuse to neuter pregnant feral queens as they consider it to be against the best interest of the cat or they feel the process is unsafe; in this situation, the cat is released and then must be caught again (which will be more difficult due to the cat's previous aversive experience of trapping).

A pregnant feral queen released or left until its kittens are born and weaned, and then trapped, could potentially be pregnant again or in oestrus when next caught. Thus, it can be almost impossible to find an ideal window in the reproductive cycle. As well re-trapping the queen, there would also be the kittens to trap and neuter. Alternatives such as keeping a pregnant feral cat in a cattery until parturition and weaning of the kittens will result in enormous stress for the queen and possible problems with returning the animal to the colony after a delay. Therefore, despite many veterinary surgeons and volunteers finding it distasteful, neutering queens at any stage of pregnancy once they have been trapped may well represent overall the least worst option.

Sick cats

With adequate resources, testing sick feral cats for feline immunodeficiency virus (FIV) and feline leukaemia virus (FeLV) may be recommended, but routine screening provides little benefit from either a financial or an effectiveness point of view. Mathematical models suggest that, in a trade-off between testing and neutering, neutering is a more efficient means of containing disease in the whole population, through reduction of transmission due to sexual or sex-linked behaviours. If testing is undertaken, a clear policy must be in place and agreement needs to be reached between clinicians and other stakeholders regarding procedures for individual cats that test positive. It is not possible to release a feral cat and then re-catch and re-test it later in an attempt to guard against euthanasia of animals that give a false-positive result on patient-side screening tests; nor is it humane to confine a cat for the time necessary for either re-testing or awaiting the results of confirmatory tests.

Major surgeries are unjustifiable in a cat that must survive in the wild, including limb amputation or surgical fracture repair. However, minor procedures, such as pinnectomy to treat early carcinoma or enucleation, can be successful. Enucleation should be confined to recent injuries where the cat is still in pain, rather than to remove an eye remnant from a historic injury purely for aesthetic reasons.

When deciding what to treat, it is important to bear in mind that the cat should be able to be returned to site, fully recovered and functional, within 5 days of capture, as well as needing no further treatment. Cats kept beyond this time, especially if they are sick, may find it difficult to reintegrate with their colony when released.

Additional health interventions

Antiparasitic spot-on treatments may be of value, provided that an understanding of the mechanism of effect of the product is in place, given the inability to treat the environment. Vaccination, even by only the single dose that can be given during TNR, is also of value and delivers some considerable immunity despite being administered during the TNR process (and appears not be especially compromised by stress and anaesthesia) (Fischer *et al.*, 2007). In countries where rabies is present, it is responsible (and often a legal requirement) to include rabies vaccination as part of the core TNR process.

Visual confirmation of neuter status

Ear tipping of neutered feral cats is now standard across the UK and much of the world. The method of choice (and in common use) is a straight-across cut, as opposed to tattoos, v-notches or curved cuts, all of which can either be missed or mistaken for fight-related injuries. The left ear is always used, and the cut line should be straight, running parallel to the base of the ear (Figure 5.14). This should not bleed profusely if a straight haemostat is applied and used to guide a cut with a scalpel blade, and the haemostat left in place for 5 minutes afterwards. It is important that the cut is obviously a man-made mark that can be seen from a distance when manually trapping cats. The amount of ear tip removed will vary between 3 mm and 8 mm (occasionally up to 10 mm) in each cat; it should not be too large as feeders, while normally tolerant of a standard ear tip, may be upset by something closer to ear cropping, and may withdraw future consent for neutering. Education of feeders who decline ear tipping is more important than compromise; simply warning them in advance that it is to happen and is integral to the process will reduce problems. It is also important to ensure that free-roaming unowned cats that are not going to enter adoption programmes are ear tipped when neutered, even if brought in as an individual cat by a private feeder.

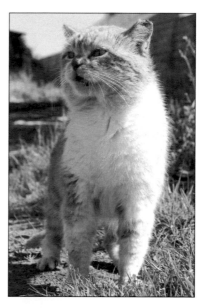

5.14 An ear tip should provide a clear mark that is distinguishable from fight wounds in even the most battle-scarred tom cat.
(© Ian MacFarlaine)

Timing of release

In most cases where a good surgical process has been used, release to the site the day after surgery is appropriate for most cats, with an additional day perhaps indicated for larger midline surgeries (i.e. heavily pregnant queens). Same-day release has been trialled for canine CNR in some countries with considerable success and, while there is no supportive evidence for same-day release of cats in the UK, further investigation may be of value.

References and further reading

Berkeley EP (2004) *TNR Past, Present and Future: a history of the trap-neuter-return movement*. Alley Cat Allies, Bethesda, Maryland

Boone JD and Slater, M (2013) A generalized population monitoring program to inform the management of free-roaming cats. Report for ACC&D. Available from: http://www.acc-d.org/docs/default-source/think-tanks/frc-monitoring-revised-nov-2014.pdf?sfvrsn=2

Bowlt KL, Murray JK, Herbert GL *et al.* (2011) Evaluation of the expectations, learning and competencies of surgical skills by undergraduate veterinary students performing canine ovariohysterectomies. *Journal of Small Animal Practice* **52**, 587–594

Cleaveland S, Kaare M, Tiringa P *et al.* (2003) A dog rabies vaccination campaign in rural Africa: impact on the incidence of dog rabies and human dog-bite injuries. *Vaccine* **21**, 1965–1973

Dalla Villa P, Kahn S, Stuardo L *et al.* (2010) Free-roaming dog control among OIE-member countries. *Preventive Veterinary Medicine* **97**, 58–63

Feline Advisory Bureau (2006) *Feral Cat Manual*. International Cat Care, Tisbury

Fischer SM, Quest CM, Dubovi EJ *et al.* (2007) Response of feral cats to vaccination at the time of neutering. *Journal of the American Veterinary Medical Association* **230**, 52–58

Hampson K, Coudeville L, Lembo T *et al.* (2015) Estimating the global burden of endemic canine rabies. *PLOS Neglected Tropical Diseases* **9**, e0003709

Hiby LR and Hiby EF (2014) "Dogs seen per km" monitoring of a dog population management intervention. Available from: http://www.wa2s.org/uploads/5/8/8/9/5889479/american_strays_canine_survey_methods.pdf

Hiby LR, Reece JF, Wright R *et al.* (2011) A mark-resight survey method to estimate the roaming dog population in three cities in Rajasthan, India. *BMC Veterinary Research* **7**, 46

ICAM Coalition (2011) Humane cat population management guidance. Available from: http://www.ifaw.org/sites/default/files/ICAM-Humane%20cat%20population.pdf

ICAM Coalition (2015) Are we making a difference? A guide to monitoring and evaluating dog population management interventions. Available from: http://www.icam-coalition.org/downloads/ICAM_Guidance_Document.pdf

Jibat T, Hogeveen H and Mourits MCM (2015) Review on dog rabies vaccination coverage in Africa: a question of dog accessibility or cost recovery? *PLOS Neglected Tropical Diseases* **9**, e0003447

Lapiz SMD, Miranda MEG, Garcia RG *et al.* (2012) Implementation of an intersectoral program to eliminate human and canine rabies: the Bohol Rabies Prevention and Elimination Project. *PLOS Neglected Tropical Diseases* **6**, e1891

Levy JK and Crawford PC (2004) Humane strategies for controlling feral cat populations. *Journal of the American Veterinary Medical Association* **225(9)**, 1354–1360

Morters MK, McKinley TJ, Horton DL *et al.* (2014). Achieving population-level immunity to rabies in free-roaming dogs in Africa and Asia. *PLOS Neglected Tropical Diseases* **8**, e3160

Pal SK (2001) Population ecology of free-ranging urban dogs in West Bengal, India. *Acta Theriologica* **46**, 69–78

Remfry J (2001) *Ruth Plant, a Pioneer in Animal Welfare*. Jenny Remfry, Barnet

Sutherland WJ (2006) *Ecological Census Techniques, 2th edn: a handbook*. Cambridge University Press, Cambridge

van Goethem B, Schaefers-Okkens A and Kirpensteijn J (2006) Making a rational choice between ovariectomy and ovariohysterectomy in the dog: a discussion of the benefits of either technique. *Veterinary Surgery* **35**, 136–143

World Health Organization (2013) WHO expert consultation on rabies. Available from: http://apps.who.int/iris/bitstream/10665/85346/1/9789240690943_eng.pdf

WSPA (2007) Surveying roaming dog populations: guidelines on methodology. Available from: http://www.icam-coalition.org/downloads/Surveying%20roaming%20dog%20populations%20-%20guidelines%20on%20methodology.pdf

Yoak AJ, Reece JF, Gehrt SD and Hamilton IM (2014) Disease control through fertility control: secondary benefits of animal birth control in Indian street dogs. *Preventive Veterinary Medicine* **113**, 152–156

Useful websites

ICAM Coalition:
http://www.icam-coalition.org

Mission Rabies:
http://www.missionrabies.com

QRG 5.1: Trap/catch-neuter-return (TNR/CNR) checklist

by Andy Gibson and Jenny Stavisky

Preparing the ground

- Is there a need for a TNR/CNR programme? Is there an animal overpopulation? Is someone else doing the job already? Are the programme's aims sensible and in keeping with the local culture?
- Are there community organizations and/or non-governmental organizations (NGOs) to partner with? Have they been contacted, listened to and allowed to provide input and engage?
- Are the animal feeders or carers engaged, informed and willing to cooperate? For example, if feeders withhold food for 12–24 hours before trapping is carried out, the animals will be hungry and easier to trap.
- Is there a long-term plan? Single or occasional bouts of neutering will achieve little in the long term.

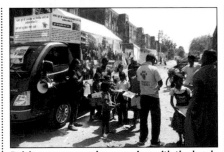

Raising awareness by engaging with the local community, as well as other local animal welfare workers, is essential to the success of a project, as seen here in a rabies control project in Ranchi, India.
(© Mission Rabies)

Training and empowering a local community and upskilling volunteers should be part of any project.

- Consider laws around trapping/releasing – is it legal to release animals following treatment? Do ordinances (by-laws) about mutilation need to be amended to allow ear-tipping?

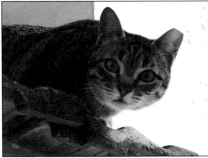

A method for identifying treated animals, such as ear-tipping for cats, is essential.
(Courtesy of H Eckman)

- What are the local laws about controlled or prescription drugs? What drugs are available locally?
- If veterinary staff from overseas are helping, are their qualifications and professional indemnity valid in this context?
- Has a population survey been carried out and a logical, targeted and achievable plan been made?

$\rightarrow$

QRG 5.1 *continued*

Staffing requirements

- Good, experienced trappers, able to plan, trap and also monitor animals post release.

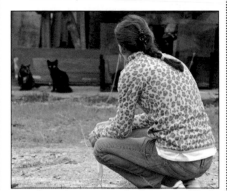

Experienced trappers and volunteers will help not only with collecting animals, but also with monitoring post release.
(Courtesy of H Eckman)

- Confident, experienced veterinary surgeons.
- Confident, experienced veterinary nurses or technicians.
- If students are involved (whether veterinary students or qualified veterinary surgeons seeking to expand their surgical experience), there must be a suitable staff:student ratio to ensure they are closely supervised and that the welfare of the patients is never jeopardized.
- Extra staff/volunteers are helpful to aid cleaning and disinfection of traps and kennels and to do many other small jobs.

Clinic location and equipment

- The location should be easy to access. Ideally, separate quiet areas should be available for preoperative preparation and recovery.
- If hospitalization of patients is anticipated, an isolation area with its own entrance, water supply and drainage is recommended.
- Appropriate record keeping – catching sheets (including a description of each animal and its location of capture) and a surgical register (including details of animals undergoing surgery).
- Means of identifying each patient (e.g. disposable collars or numbered plastic tags on thin breakable string – NB bits of paper tend to go astray so there

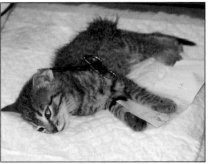

Each patient must be identifiable at all times. This male kitten is prepared for castration. Note the use of eye lubricant, haemostat on the ear, and identification card.
(© Jenny Stavisky)

should always be a way of cross-referencing paperwork to an animal).
- Autoclave (or other means of generating asepsis).
- Waste disposal (including appropriate methods for sharps and clinical waste).
- Lighting, heating and water supply.

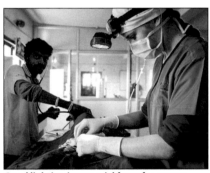

Good lighting is essential for safe surgery. Creative solutions, such as this head torch, can be found.
(Courtesy of Worldwide Veterinary Service)

- Appropriate parvocidal disinfectant.
- Mops and buckets.
- Towels, sheets and newspaper – for covering cages (to reduce stress), lining kennels and mopping up spills.
- A means of weighing animals – scales are preferred, but a spring balance can be used for caged cats.

- Surgery kits – these can be quite minimal in content but must be sterilized between each patient.
- Sterile surgical gloves.
- Sterile drapes.
- Scrub sink and scrub solution.
- Clippers or other means of shaving the surgical site.

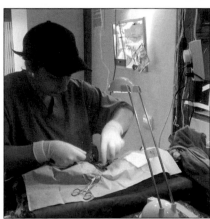

Even in field clinic conditions, basic necessities for sterility, such as gloving and draping, should not be neglected.
(© Jenny Stavisky)

- Means of keeping animals warm if necessary. Perioperative warming methods can be improvised using gloves or soft drink bottles filled with warm water.
- Anaesthesia – appropriate options.
- Analgesia – a non-steroidal anti-inflammatory drug (NSAID) and an opioid as the minimum.
- An appropriate antibiotic.
- Endo- and ectoparasiticides and/ or vaccines if these treatments are part of the scope of the project. If vaccines are to be used, refrigeration facilities are essential.
- Sterile suture material.
- Basic pharmaceutical supplies – needles, syringes, scalpels, swabs.
- Euthanasia option, preferably pentobarbital.
- Suitable equipment for marking neutered animals (e.g. by ear-tipping).

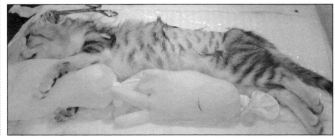

Feral female kitten prepared for neutering. Note the bubble wrap and gloves filled with warm water to help maintain body temperature.
(© Jenny Stavisky)

QRG 5.1 *continued*

Cats

- Crush cages, transfer baskets.
- A room that can have all the doors and windows secured is essential for transferring cats to crush cages.
- Cable ties to secure wire baskets (see Figure 5.11).

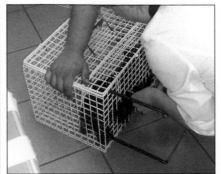

Administration of an injectable intramuscular anaesthetic combination to a feral cat in a crush cage. A blanket can be used to cover the cage to minimize stimulation after injection.
(© Jenny Stavisky)

Dogs

- An appropriate number of secure recovery kennels with some extra capacity.
- Appropriate handling and restraint equipment (e.g. muzzles, catch pole, gauntlets).

QRG 5.2: Euthanasia
by Andy Gibson

The aim of animal population control programmes is to create a situation in which the supply of animals matches demand. Ideally, all unwanted animals are rehomed to suitable owners, where they can go on to experience a good quality of life. In poorly managed populations, however, it is likely that the number of unwanted animals outweighs the number of suitable homes available. In these settings, the euthanasia of some animals may be the only alternative to lifelong housing in suboptimal conditions.

Moral and ethical considerations

The term euthanasia, meaning 'good death', should be used only to describe humane methods that do not cause pain and result in a rapid loss of consciousness followed by death. Here, euthanasia is discussed only in the context of animals.

Euthanasia is a strongly emotive topic with deep personal, cultural and religious significance, which varies with geographical location and personal experience. Euthanasia of animals can be seen as a powerful tool in maintaining animal welfare and alleviating suffering in animals that are unlikely to experience an acceptable quality of life long term or permanently. In some countries, however, the concept of euthanasia is commonly rejected. The teachings of many religions, including Hinduism and Buddhism, place paramount importance upon the preservation of life and non-injury of sentient beings, and this doctrine can present significant moral conflict relating to the practice of euthanasia. It is important to be sensitive to the views and beliefs of anyone involved in the process, while at the same time striving to uphold the welfare of animals in our care and prevent unnecessary suffering.

An additional challenge can arise in deciding what quality of life is acceptable for an animal and at what level of impairment euthanasia is appropriate. What constitutes 'a life worth living' will vary from one person to the next, let alone between regions or countries. Prior to starting any new programme/intervention, and at periodic reflection points, it can be useful to discuss the subject of euthanasia in an open and unimposing forum in which team members can raise their views and share their thoughts on the situations in which euthanasia would be indicated. In this way the team can pre-emptively agree on criteria for euthanasia in a non-stressful and non-emotional setting based on the best interests of the animal in each scenario.

Euthanasia and alternatives

The argument for euthanasia will be clearer in some situations than in others. For instance, where an animal is suffering from an untreatable disease and facing a prolonged, painful death, the benefit of euthanasia in relieving suffering is clear. There are, however, situations where relatively healthy animals may need to be euthanased because it is not safe for them to be returned to where they came from and there are no suitable rehoming or kennelling options.

In situations where demand for resources exceeds supply, as is often the case when working with large populations of animals, triage is an essential tool for benefiting the greatest number of animals possible with the finite resources available. In such situations, euthanasia becomes crucial for maintaining minimum welfare standards, by preventing suffering in those animals that cannot be helped in another way.

In the majority of cases, increasing the effectiveness and capacity of rehoming centres directly reduces the number of animals euthanased, and so innovative and novel ways to promote the rehoming of dogs and cats should always be explored. The use of fostering systems can overcome many of the problems of permanent →

QRG 5.2 *continued*

infrastructure, such as staffing levels, maintenance of welfare and hygiene standards, disease transmission and behavioural problems related to kennelling, and may ultimately provide a better quality of life for those animals that are fostered. Fostering systems have even proven successful in avoiding the need for a permanent shelter, and should be considered wherever possible.

As veterinary surgeons it is our obligation to consider the alternatives to euthanasia on a case-by-case basis. Coming to a reasoned and thought-through conclusion will help to ensure that euthanasia is used for reasons of compassion and that people involved in the process feel confident in their actions and ethics. It is important to be aware of local animal welfare laws relating to euthanasia which may define specific situations where euthanasia is and is not lawful.

In some veterinary colleges around the world, euthanasia continues to be viewed as unacceptable and appropriate methods of euthanasia are still not taught. The table below summarizes acceptable methods of euthanasia and how they can be administered.

References and further reading

American Veterinary Medical Association (2013) *AVMA Guidelines for the Euthanasia of Animals: 2013 Edition*. Available from www.avma.org

WSPA (2007) *Methods for the euthanasia of dogs and cats: comparison and recommendations*. Available from www.icam-coalition.org

Method	Preference	Important additional requirements	Remarks
Intravenous injection of 20% pentobarbital (pentobarbitone) solution	Recommended	Experienced handlers trained in restraining animals correctly and carrying out intravenous injections quickly and competently	• Rapid acting • May be used in conjunction with a sedative drug if the animal is fearful, fractious or aggressive. Note that some sedatives will slow the action of the pentobarbital, leading to a delay in cessation of the heartbeat
Intraperitoneal injection of 20% pentobarbital solution	Acceptable	Larger dose required than for intravenous administration, therefore may not be suitable for euthanasia of large animals	• Slow acting • May be a practical alternative in small animals (fractious cats, neonatal kittens and puppies) where intravenous access is limited • Use of pre-anaesthetic drugs may prolong the time to death
Intravenous injection of overdose of anaesthetic agents (e.g. thiopental (thiopentone) or propofol)	Acceptable	Underdose may lead to recovery	• Large volumes or high concentrations are required to euthanase animals, potentially making this method impractical for routine use • Cost may preclude routine use
Intracardiac injection of 20% pentobarbital solution after general anaesthesia	Conditionally acceptable	Only acceptable in unconscious animals	• Unacceptable in conscious animals – administration of anaesthetic agents is essential if the animal is conscious • Requires training and understanding of anatomy
Intravenous or intracardiac injection of potassium chloride (KCl) after general anaesthesia	Conditionally acceptable	Only acceptable in unconscious animals	• Should never be used in conscious animals due to severe cardiac pain caused prior to death • Conscious animals must be anaesthetized prior to administration • Operator must be trained in assessing adequate anaesthetic depth prior to administration
Intravenous or intracardiac injection of magnesium sulphate (MgSO₄) after general anaesthesia	Conditionally acceptable	Only acceptable in unconscious animals Large volumes are required for euthanasia	• Should never be used in conscious animals due to severe cardiac pain caused prior to death • Conscious animals must be anaesthetized prior to administration • Operator must be trained in assessing adequate anaesthetic depth prior to administration • A saturated solution is required – this is a very viscous liquid, which can make administration difficult
Shooting a free bullet to the head	Conditionally acceptable	Only acceptable in emergency situations where no other acceptable method is possible because the animal cannot be handled or given pre-anaesthetic drugs	• Requires training, skill and precision • Firearm use is likely to be subject to national and local regulations; operator may require a licence • Dangerous and unpleasant for operator and any other people present

Acceptable methods of euthanasia. (Adapted from WSPA[a] (2007)) [a]WSPA is the former name of World Animal Protection.

Chapter 6

Optimizing neutering programmes

David Yates and Kate White

Why neuter shelter animals?

When considering neutering pet animals, there are two issues to take into account. The first is the balance of risks and benefits for the individual animal, and the second is the potential impact on the welfare of the overall population (Palmer *et al.*, 2012). When practising shelter or charity medicine, often the population concerns are of prime importance; however, it is essential to bear in mind the individual factors too, so that appropriate policies can be developed, assessed and revised over time.

Population risks and benefits

There is a large overpopulation of pet animals in the UK, as in many other countries. The reasons for this are complex and differ between cats and dogs. Many pet owners lack understanding about dog and cat reproduction (New *et al.*, 2004). Not being able to tell when a bitch is 'in heat' or knowing that puberty in queens may occur as early as 4 months of age may contribute to mistimed, unplanned or unwanted breeding. In the UK, 80% of cat litters are unplanned (Welsh *et al.*, 2014), probably as a result of cats being polyoestrous, along with owners' generally poor understanding and management of breeding. As a consequence, there is an absolute overpopulation of cats in shelters and charity practice due to sheer numbers of animals. The number of unwanted dogs is slightly smaller. It has been suggested that owners' lack of understanding of dog care, behaviour and husbandry contribute heavily to dog relinquishment, with perceived behavioural problems consistently being the primary reason given. A study in the UK in 2010 showed that over 80% of dogs and cats in shelters are either surrendered by their owner or are found as strays. The remainder may originate from other rescue organizations, veterinary practices or confiscations for welfare reasons (Stavisky *et al.*, 2012) (Figure 6.1).

Source	Dogs (%)	Cats (%)
Surrendered by owner	56.3	45.2
Stray	25.8	42.3
Another welfare organization	12.3	1.3
Veterinary surgery	0.3	1.8
Confiscation for welfare reasons	3.6	8.4
Other	1.6	1.0

6.1 Sources of dogs and cats entering UK shelters in 2010. (Stavisky *et al.*, 2012)

In another study, over one-third of the shelter animal intake resulted from unplanned litters (Alexander and Shane, 1994). Clearly, the problem is complex, and the solution is unlikely to be simple. Owner education and public engagement programmes will be necessary to improve people's understanding of pet ownership. However, neutering provides a permanent solution to unwanted breeding of each neutered individual, and is therefore a key weapon in the battle to improve welfare and reduce the number of unwanted animals.

Individual risks and benefits

Neutering may confer certain benefits upon the individual animal. The relative balance between the risks and benefits associated with the procedure depends on a number of factors. For example, the breed or species of animal, its age and its sex all affect the surgical risk and the potential changes that may occur after neutering (Kustritz, 2007). As well as physiological changes, another benefit that could be considered is whether behavioural changes following neutering will increase an animal's acceptability as a pet. The successful formation of a bond with a human caregiver is likely to be associated with reduced risk of future relinquishment or abandonment. Whatever the risks and benefits may be on an individual basis, all shelter animals should be routinely neutered, if possible, prior to rehoming.

Cats

An entire male cat is likely to exhibit behaviour that increases the likelihood of trauma, as a result of fighting with other cats and road traffic accidents. An unneutered male cat with outdoor access is therefore likely to have a reduced lifespan, and during that time is more likely to suffer from diseases linked to these behaviours, such as infection with feline immunodeficiency virus (Muirden, 2002). Castration greatly reduces this sexually dimorphic behaviour. Few veterinary surgeons (veterinarians) would suggest that an entire male cat should not be castrated on health grounds. Additionally, the behaviour of entire male cats (mounting, aggression and urine spraying) would make them generally unpleasant pets. The surgical procedure of castration of male cats is brief and complications are uncommon. In some studies, gonadectomy has been identified as a risk factor for feline lower urinary tract disease in both male and female cats. However, other studies have reported that prepubertal gonadectomy does not decrease urethral diameter in male cats, nor does it increase the incidence of the disease. Weight gain, stress and lifestyle are considered important factors in the development of this multifactorial disease (Buffington *et al.*, 2014).

The issues to consider in the female cat are more complicated. The surgery (ovariohysterectomy or ovariectomy) is slightly more invasive than castration, and therefore potentially carries a higher risk to the individual, although reported complications are most commonly limited to swelling or discharge from the surgical site (Coe *et al.*, 2006). Conditions such as mammary neoplasia, uterine and ovarian neoplasia and pyometra are either reduced or the risk of disease is eliminated with neutering. The behaviour of an entire queen may be difficult to accept in many households. This assertion may be supported by the fact that most owners eventually neuter their queen. Entire, sexually receptive females may be more likely to stray, become involved in road traffic collisions or produce unwanted litters.

It is understood that neutered pets have a reduced energy requirement and may be more likely to gain weight after neutering if their food intake does not decrease. Neutered cats have therefore been found to be at increased risk of obesity and type 2 diabetes mellitus.

Dogs

Castration of dogs will also reduce straying behaviours and unwanted litters, but the reproductive issues associated with dogs are different from those in cats. Unwanted litters are less common in dogs as the reproduction of dogs is more closely controlled by humans and is possible during only one or two periods of oestrus (seasons) per year.

Neutering bitches will prevent reproduction and has additional benefits such as preventing pyometra and reducing the likelihood of mammary tumours (Beauvais *et al.*, 2012a) (Figure 6.2).

Concerns about neutering dogs and bitches because of the increased risk of some types of neoplasia, urinary incontinence (Beauvais *et al.*, 2012b), orthopaedic disease and diabetes are common among many owners, especially owners of purebred dogs (Figure 6.3). In the bitch, post-surgical complications are more likely with increasing bodyweight and anaesthetic time. A reduced morbidity in

Benefits	Comments
Preventing pseudopregnancy	Pseudopregnancy is common in bitches and can occur after each oestrus, resulting in behavioural problems, anorexia and distress to the bitch and owner
Preventing oestrus and associated problems, and unwanted litters	Oestrus occurs approximately twice a year and can cause unwanted behaviours, and requires close supervision of the bitch
Reduction in the prevalence of mammary tumours	This is often cited as a benefit, but the evidence is weak (Beauvais *et al.*, 2012a)
Reduction in incidence of pyometra	Neutering a bitch will prevent pyometra and other uterine diseases. This reduces the risk of having to neuter an older bitch with potentially toxic pyometra as an emergency
Risks	**Comments**
Increased risk of certain neoplasms	Neutering is associated with a small increased risk of developing transitional cell carcinomas, mast cell tumours, haemangiosarcomas and osteosarcomas, although cause and effect have not been defined. Neutering is also associated with a longer lifespan and this may be a factor
Increased risk of orthopaedic disease such as cranial cruciate ligament rupture	This may be associated with the obesity that can occur after neutering. Dietary control is important
Increased risk of urinary incontinence	Evidence for this association is weak
Changes in the working ability of the bitch	There is currently no evidence of any negative effects with respect to training

6.2 Benefits and risks of neutering bitches.

Benefits	Comments
Preventing excessive sexual behaviours towards bitches (and humans)	These behaviours can be a nuisance to the owner and the neighbourhood. Dogs can show behavioural changes and anorexia when in the vicinity of bitches in oestrus
Preventing roaming and associated problems, and unwanted litters	These behaviours can be a nuisance to the owner of the bitch, the owner of the dog and the neighbourhood
Reduction in the prevalence of testicular tumours, perianal adenomas and prostatic hypertrophy	The absence of testicles and a small prostate confer these advantages
Reduction in aggression	Aggression is multifactorial and can be breed-specific and behavioural too
Risks	**Comments**
Increased risk of certain neoplasms	Castration is associated with a small increased risk of developing prostatic carcinomas, lymphosarcomas, osteosarcomas and haemangiosarcomas, although cause and effect have not been defined. Castration is also associated with a longer lifespan and this may be a factor
Increased risk of orthopaedic disease such as cranial cruciate ligament rupture and hip dysplasia	This may be associated with the obesity that can develop after neutering. Dietary control is important
Changes in the working ability of the dog	Neutering and the age of neutering are not associated with any negative effects with respect to training

6.3 Benefits and risks of neutering male dogs.

the prepubertal patient can be predicted because of a slender abdomen, smaller quantity of abdominal fat and reduced vascularity to the 'immature' reproductive tract (Muraro and White, 2014). There is no evidence to support the claim that bitches should be allowed to have one oestrous period before being neutered.

Why do owners choose not to neuter?

Owners may choose not to neuter their pets for a variety of reasons. For some, the choice is a conscious one, either because they plan to breed, show or otherwise work the animal. Others may have cultural, moral or religious objections to neutering. Many owners, however, do not make active choices regarding their animal's reproductive status, and these owners and animals are often implicated in unplanned irresponsible breeding.

Recent research shows that over 92% of cats are eventually neutered (Murray *et al.*, 2009), but only 66% of cats between 6 and 12 months of age are neutered. This leaves a window of opportunity (from 4 months) for unplanned breeding. Without closing this window, efforts to control the cat overpopulation crisis by neutering large numbers of public-owned cats will be futile. Lowering the recommended neutering age for cats to below the age of puberty is essential.

Why do shelters neuter?

Most shelters will aim to neuter the animals they rehome in order to reduce the constant influx of new unwanted animals. Post-adoption neutering contracts, by which new owners undertake to have their new pet neutered if they adopt an unneutered animal, may suffer from poor compliance rates and so increase the risk of unplanned breeding (Alexander and Shane, 1994). Ensuring compliance can be time-consuming, and even low rates of non-compliance can significantly hamper a population control programme.

Within a shelter, a neutered animal may have a greater chance of being adopted. The shelter's neutering strategy should aim to reduce the likelihood of return of individual animals and also eliminate the possibility that an adopted animal may contribute to pet overpopulation. If all shelter animals were neutered before adoption, this would clearly satisfy the requirement that individual animals would not contribute to overpopulation. In charity veterinary practice, owners' compliance and knowledge of pet reproduction may be suboptimal. In such circumstances, unplanned pregnancies occur in both dogs and cats. Many owners are unaware of the possibility of pregnancy when they present their cats for surgery. The frequency of unplanned pregnancies discovered at surgery in cats is influenced by the photoperiod. In the UK summer, up to 30% of public-owned queens presented for elective neutering may be pregnant (Jennett *et al.*, 2016).

The bitch is not as prolific a breeder as the queen. Accidental matings can be more readily avoided by careful planning around the time of the two oestrous periods each year. Fewer bitches are likely to live an outdoor lifestyle and encounter wandering fertile males. Less than 1% of public-owned bitches presented for elective neutering are discovered to be pregnant (RSPCA, unpublished data), and these cases are spread throughout the year.

Neutering before puberty

Assuming that most owners want to neuter their cat or dog, the issue becomes one of timing. Prepubertal neutering is a valuable tool for shelter veterinary surgeons. It excludes the possibility of owners failing to adhere to post-adoption neutering contracts, and eliminates the manpower requirement involved in chasing up these owners. It also makes the timing of the neutering procedure simpler; a bitch that is in oestrus after being adopted may need to be scheduled for surgery at time that is both convenient for the owner and that reduces the likelihood of morbidity (surgical haemorrhage, mammary development, etc.).

There are a number of circumstances in which prepubertal neutering offers distinct practical advantages (Figure 6.4). For example, in the charity veterinary sector, many pet owners have low and fixed levels of income. They may struggle to attend routine appointments and their compliance with pre-booked surgical appointments may be suboptimal. Therefore, to reduce the need for repeat visits to the practice, neutering before puberty may be combined with the routine vaccination schedule.

Scenario	Advantage of prepubertal neutering
Feral kittens	Avoids the difficulties associated with recapture
Shelter puppies and kittens	Avoids the difficulties associated with poor compliance seen in post-adoption contracts or voucher schemes
Owned puppies and kittens (charity client)	Reduces the number of visits to the practice
Owned puppies and kittens (private client)	Eliminates the risk of accidental breeding
Breeders	Breeders can sell an animal that cannot be used for breeding and protect their genetic material

6.4 Opportunities to exploit some of the advantages associated with prepubertal gonadectomy (early neutering) in cats and dogs.

Similarly, feral cat neutering schemes require a high capture rate to achieve population control (McCarthy *et al.*, 2013). It would be both unwise and practically demanding to release kittens and attempt to recapture and neuter them at a later date. Instead, feral kittens should be neutered at the earliest opportunity. The (small) physical size of a kitten is unlikely to hinder the performance of a competent surgeon (Joyce and Yates, 2011) (see QRG 6.1).

Surgical time, anaesthetic recovery time and pain scores are likely to be reduced in younger animals (Polson *et al.*, 2014). Indeed, complicating factors such as mammary hyperplasia, ovarian cysts, and the increased friability and vascularity of the uterus of a queen at oestrus are avoided if surgery is carried out before puberty. Earlier neutering is likely to have a significant protective effect against mammary neoplasia when compared with neutering after puberty (Overley *et al.*, 2005).

Uterine and ovarian neoplasia are both treated and prevented by ovariohysterectomy at any age. The low incidence of these diseases makes consideration of age at neutering relatively unimportant. Similarly, pyometra is treated by ovariohysterectomy. The risk of pyometra increases with age and may be a significant cause of morbidity and mortality in older queens and bitches. However, it is unlikely to be a sole reason for a shelter to adopt a prepubertal neutering policy.

Early neutering undoubtedly alters male cats. The penis of a sexually mature cat has a different visual appearance to that of a cat castrated before puberty. For example, dissolution of the balanopreputial fold and the formation of penile spines are androgen dependent (Figure 6.5). The

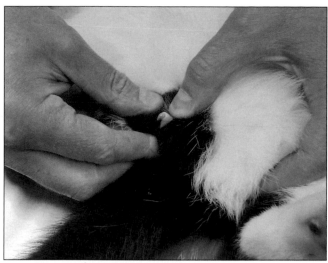

6.5 Penis of an early-neutered cat. Note the absence of spines and persistence of the balanopreputial fold.

(© David Yates)

facial shape of a male kitten neutered before puberty is more slender than that of a cat castrated after puberty. However, the conventional age for neutering of 6 months for cats has been rather arbitrary; there are likely to be few differences seen when this timeframe is shifted to 4 months or earlier (Porters *et al.*, 2014).

The remaining conditions of common concern when making decisions about the timing of neutering (obesity, lower urinary tract disease and diabetes mellitus) are multifactorial in origin. Although gonadectomy is a risk factor for obesity, no correlation has been found between age at neutering and bodyweight. Similarly, in female cats, neutering is a risk factor for the development of both diabetes mellitus and lower urinary tract disease when compared with sexually intact queens. However, studies have not evaluated the effect of age at neutering on the likelihood of disease (Spain *et al.*, 2004).

Fewer dogs than cats are presented for early neutering, but when litters of young puppies are presented to a shelter, neutering before rehoming should also be considered. However, the remit of a shelter is very different from, for example, a charity veterinary hospital, and the aim in the context of a shelter is to neuter these dogs before rehoming, primarily for population control. These concerns are valid, but with owned animals it is more likely to be necessary to discuss the risks and benefits of early neutering on an individual basis. Many shelter dogs are mature animals that have been abandoned or relinquished owing to behaviour problems or changes of circumstances, and the opportunity to neuter these animals before puberty is at best limited.

Neutering at any age will predispose a dog to becoming overweight, but early neutering of dogs does not invariably lead to fat dogs. Owners must be educated about the need to reduce food intake after neutering in both dogs and cats (Wei *et al.*, 2014). Obese animals may be predisposed to other conditions, such as cranial cruciate ligament disease (Duval *et al.*, 1999), cancers and diabetes (German, 2006). Again, however, many of these conditions that develop later in life are likely to be multifactorial in origin.

Neutering as an elective procedure

Prepubertal neutering is invariably an elective procedure. For example, testicular torsion is a rare event in young animals and surgical emergencies relating to the reproductive system (e.g. pyometra, ovarian neoplasia) are far more likely after puberty.

Consequently, this allows a degree of flexibility in scheduling the procedure before the animal leaves the shelter. For example, a kitten with a heavy flea burden on arrival at the shelter will require veterinary treatment and corrective nutrition to address a potential anaemia. It may also receive vaccinations before surgery is carried out. It would be counterproductive to rush surgery for such an animal just to speed up the adoption process. The low surgical morbidity associated with early neutering is dependent upon careful patient selection (Howe 1997).

The shelter environment

Assuming that all of the animals in a shelter are to be neutered before adoption, neutering may be carried out on site (if facilities are available) or by transporting the animals to a veterinary practice located elsewhere. There are some key differences between these options that may be worth consideration (Figure 6.6).

Considerations	Neutering onsite	Neutering offsite
Impact on animal	• Familiar environment • Current disease risk	• Stress of transportation • Exposure to new disease risk
Shelter considerations	• Requires financial investment • Staff may need training • Responsibility improves staff morale	• External fees are payable • Trained support staff are available • Gives the practice an awareness of shelter medicine
Veterinary considerations	• Local knowledge if carried out by shelter veterinary surgeon • What if things go wrong?	• Veterinary surgeon may be unaware of local issues • Back-up available if carried out at a veterinary practice • Risk of disease spreading from shelter animals to private clients

6.6 Some key differences between neutering at the shelter and at an off-site veterinary facility.

Neutering shelter animals should not be seen as an opportunity to 'cut corners' and provide suboptimal veterinary care. The patients may not have a permanent owner, but they require the same high level of care as any privately owned animal to ensure that neutering is a procedure of low morbidity. The surgery is predictable and of short duration, and the throughput of animals is likely to be high. For example, an abandoned litter of kittens will all be due for surgery at around the same time. Furthermore, there is a high degree of seasonality to both breeding and shelter occupancy. Cat breeding is influenced by the photoperiod (Faya *et al.*, 2011); summer in shelters in the UK can be a hectic time, meaning that more young animals are likely to be presented for neutering. This 'production line' work suggests the need for a rigid protocol.

Animal care staff should ensure that shelter animals have received the appropriate range of preventive treatments (vaccinations, worming and flea medication). Animals scheduled to be neutered should be free from signs of disease and should be in good body condition. The staff should be familiar with standard growth charts for puppies and kittens, and regular weighing and body condition scoring systems should be in place.

Healthy male patients should be screened for cryptorchidism. Bitches with conditions that are likely to improve by allowing a first oestrus, for example, juvenile vaginitis, should be excluded from the surgical list. Postponing the procedure is less likely to influence pet overpopulation in the dog (as outlined earlier); the cat is a far more successful and prolific breeder (Figure 6.7).

Cat	Dog
Most cats in the UK are mixed breeds, i.e. the result of unplanned matings	Even in charity practice or shelters, many dogs are purebred
A sexually mature female given outdoor access will conceive, as entire males are readily available	Accidental breeding requires significant timing of the mating event and irresponsible ownership
Puberty may be as early as 4 months	Puberty relates to breed size. Larger breeds may not be fertile for up to 2 years
Many veterinary surgeons neuter female cats at around 6 months – this is too late	Many veterinary surgeons neuter bitches at around 6 months – this may be prepubertal in some breeds

6.7 Key differences between dog and cat breeding and the bearing that these differences have on shelter neutering strategies.

Physiology of kittens and puppies

The terminology describing young animals can be quite confusing. *Paediatric* can describe animals up to 12 weeks of age, although some texts extend this definition until 24 weeks (Mathews, 2008). The paediatric period can be further subdivided into *neonatal* (0–2 weeks), *infant* (2–6 weeks), *weanling* (6–12 weeks) and *juvenile* (3–6 months). In this chapter, the term paediatric is used and refers to animals of approximately 6–16 weeks of age.

In general, kittens and puppies cope well with the anaesthesia and surgery for neutering. Studies have shown that one of the advantages of performing the surgery in juvenile patients is a reduction in surgical time, thereby reducing the likelihood of hypothermia. It is unnecessary to insist on a prolonged starvation period before anaesthesia in these paediatric patients. A maximum of 2–3 hours is recommended, to prevent hypoglycaemia, and there is no need to withhold water. Young animals have less glycogen stored in the tissues than adults, and their ability to increase their blood glucose concentrations via gluconeogenesis or glycogenolysis will be hampered by their immature liver. It is important to feed paediatric patients immediately on recovery. Hypoglycaemia can predispose kittens and puppies to prolonged recovery and hypothermia. Group housing of litters can minimize stress before anaesthesia and reduce heat loss in the perioperative period (Figure 6.8). Hypothermia can occur rapidly in paediatric patients because of their low muscle mass and body fat, reduced ability to shiver and maintain normothermia, and their high body surface area to volume ratio (relative to adult animals), which predisposes them to greater heat loss.

The tissue oxygen demand of a paediatric patient is 2–3 times greater than that of an adult. Paediatric patients have a more rapid respiratory rate and no end-expiratory pause. Additionally, the work of breathing is higher due to

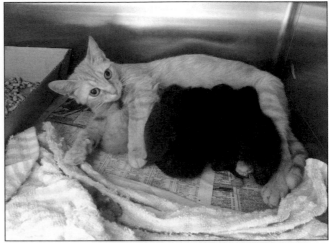

6.8 An abandoned cat with a litter of kittens. The kittens will be neutered in several weeks' time. When they are housed for neutering, they can remain together in one cage. Group housing of litters reduces the burden on cage space at the shelter and reduces stress to the animals. Furthermore, the kittens and dam can recover from anaesthesia for neutering together, which will reduce heat loss.
(© David Yates)

a narrow upper airway and increased resistance. The result of these differences is that the fresh gas flow used in non-rebreathing circuits needs to be high enough to avoid rebreathing and hypoxaemia. Occasionally, some very young patients may require careful ventilation. In addition, these animals are at risk of airway complications because of a combination of a relatively large fleshy tongue, a narrow upper airway and a low functional residual capacity. Intubating the kitten/puppy will secure and protect the airway and allow oxygen to be administered.

In cats less than 8 weeks old, the hepatic microsomal enzymes are not fully mature, resulting in prolonged metabolism of drugs that are dependent on extensive hepatic metabolism. Notably, in humans, there is more rapid metabolism of some drugs in children of certain ages compared to the rates in adults, necessitating higher dosing. Whether this occurs in domestic species is unknown, but it is certainly true that paediatric cats and dogs tolerate and appear very comfortable with relatively high doses of certain drugs, for example opioids.

Total body water and extracellular fluid volumes are relatively greater in the paediatric patient, and plasma albumin concentrations do not reach adult values until approximately 8 weeks of age. Consequently, these patients are at greater risk of dehydration and have a larger volume of distribution for the water-soluble drugs. Theoretically, this may mean that some drugs require a higher initial dose to achieve an adequate plasma concentration, due to the increased volume of distribution. In veterinary clinical practice, however, this dose adjustment is uncommon, in comparison to the situation in human medicine. The renal function of paediatric patients is not fully developed, and these patients' inability to concentrate urine can manifest in an inability to cope with a fluid load. Although theoretically the relative lack of albumin in neonatal animals may predispose these very young patients to a risk of overdose in the period when and immediately after the drugs are administered, due to the greater proportion of free drug in the circulation, in practice this is not clinically obvious.

The cardiac output in a paediatric patient is primarily rate dependent. These patients have a relatively fixed stroke volume and do not cope well with changes in preload and afterload. There is parasympathetic dominance, and in the face of bradycardia the heart is unable to increase cardiac output; this can result in a serious hypotension. Consequently, the clinician must understand that drugs such as alpha-2 agonists can have a profound effect in some of these patients. Using a combination of drugs can potentially reduce the side effects of each individual agent, as lower doses of each can be used. Furthermore, a mild degree of blood loss can result in severe hypotension, and this, coupled with the fact that effective haemopoiesis does not start until 2–3 months of age, means that a moderately small volume of blood loss will result in a significant reduction in oxygen delivery.

Currently, there are limited published sets of haematological and serum biochemistry values for kittens and puppies. These values need to be interpreted with care in view of the lack of standardization of reference ranges between laboratories.

Awareness of these differences in physiology will contribute to safer anaesthesia of the younger patients that are presented for neutering.

Anaesthesia

Preoperative preparation

All puppies and kittens should undergo a full clinical examination before anaesthesia. However, in some feral feline patients this is impractical, and a clinical examination is possible only when the animal is anaesthetized. The risk of this approach is that animals suffering from unidentified severe disease and lacking the reserves to cope with anaesthesia may undergo anaesthesia, risking complications. However, there are conditions where examination under anaesthesia is preferred (e.g. where radiography is required, fractious patients, examination of a painful ear). Animals should undergo a minimal period of fasting. Routine administration of antibiotics is contraindicated. Antibiotics should be reserved for animals with pre-existing infection or where there is a break in surgical asepsis. With some female patients there may be uncertainty as to whether the animal has been neutered previously. The animal's flank and midline should be examined for surgical scars before surgery. Abdominal and rectal palpation of the uterine body can also be attempted, but it must be borne in mind that the animal may have undergone a previous ovariectomy with the uterus left *in situ*. In some female cats, an exploratory laparotomy may be necessary to determine their status. In male cats, penile spines start to develop at 12 weeks of age and are usually fully present by 5–6 months of age. The spines regress after neutering and will have fully disappeared within two months of the surgery. The absence of spines may falsely indicate neutered status in a very young entire male. The presence of penile spines may also falsely indicate entire status in a recently neutered male in which the penile spines have not yet disappeared. It is therefore important to check the patient for signs of surgery. Hormonal assays are also available, but are not totally reliable.

Anaesthetic agents

There is no single ideal anaesthetic agent. The small size of many feline patients and the significant number of feral cats needing neutering favours the use of a combination of intramuscular agents. Puppies can be anaesthetized using an intramuscular combination or treated in the same way as an older dog, with premedication administered by the intramuscular or subcutaneous route followed by an intravenous induction agent. The protocol used should offer analgesia, good surgical conditions, muscle relaxation and ideally be reversible.

Phenothiazines

Acepromazine is frequently used for premedication of adult cats and dogs, but its use in paediatric patients can be associated with hypothermia and a prolonged recovery, so it is best avoided.

Benzodiazepines

These drugs have a wide therapeutic index and cause minimal cardiopulmonary depression. Both diazepam and midazolam provide muscle relaxation and marked sedation in younger patients and act synergistically with the opioids, ketamine and alpha-2 agonists.

Alpha-2 agonists

Xylazine has been largely superseded by medetomidine and dexmedetomidine, and these sedatives are routinely used. One of the advantages of the alpha-2 agonists is that they can be reversed with the antagonist atipamezole. These drugs can cause profound bradycardia. The risk of this side effect can be reduced by using low doses of an alpha-2 agonist in combination with other anaesthetic and analgesic agents. Alpha-2 agonists also provide a degree of moderate analgesia that is relatively short lived (up to 1 hour). Reversing the alpha-2 agonist at the end of a procedure will also reverse the analgesia. The timing of administration of the reversal agent should be considered carefully, as with some protocols early reversal of an alpha-2 agonist can result in a stormy recovery due to the remaining ketamine (see Reversal, below).

Opioids

The opioids provide very good analgesia, and are best used in combination with other anaesthetic agents as they can reduce the subsequent dose of induction or maintenance agent. Pre-emptive use will ensure that the patient is more comfortable postoperatively.

Intravenous induction agents

Both propofol and alfaxalone are used in adult cats for induction of anaesthesia, usually after a premedicant combination of drugs. However, the lack of venous access in small patients makes these drugs less useful for the paediatric patient.

Ketamine

Ketamine is a dissociative anaesthetic that causes minimal cardiopulmonary depression. It can be used alone, although muscle relaxation is improved when it is combined with other sedative agents. Ketamine provides mild visceral analgesia and good somatic analgesia. It can be administered intravenously or intramuscularly.

Inhalant agents

Anaesthesia can be induced with a volatile anaesthetic agent delivered via mask or induction chamber, or these

Basic monitoring

Plane of anaesthesia

The same reflexes and parameters can be used for assessment of anaesthetic depth in paediatric and adult animals. The patient should be continually monitored and parameters recorded at regular intervals on an anaesthetic record. The main clinical parameters that should be continually assessed include eye position, palpebral reflex, jaw tone, muscle relaxation, mucous membrane colour, capillary refill time, pulse rate and chest movement/respiratory rate/movement of the reservoir bag. In protocols where a dissociative agent (ketamine or tiletamine) has been used, the eye may remain central with no rotation. It is advisable to apply artificial tears or ocular lubricant to the eyes to prevent corneal drying.

Heart rate

An oesophageal stethoscope can be pre-measured (from the nares to the point of the olecranon), lubricated and gently introduced over the endotracheal tube into the oesophagus. Small-diameter oesophageal stethoscopes are available for use in paediatric patients. The tube is advanced until both the cardiac and respiratory sounds can be heard optimally. These stethoscopes can be worn by the veterinary surgeon or nurse to facilitate continuous assessment of heart and respiratory sounds and rates.

Otherwise, the heart rate can be regularly evaluated using a precordial stethoscope. Peripheral pulses should be palpated concurrently.

Pulse oximetry

A pulse oximeter can also be useful in monitoring. These devices give an audible signal and display a heart rate and percentage saturation of haemoglobin with oxygen. The tone of the audible signal (beep) also corresponds to the level of saturation. In very small cats, it can be difficult to get a reading if a probe designed for use in adult humans is being applied to the tongue, ear or paw. These probes are held in place by a strong spring that, with time, can exert sufficient pressure to occlude blood flow to the area; this necessitates regular re-placement of the probe at a different area as the quality of the signal declines. Rectal and oesophageal probes may offer a useful alternative. In animals that have received alpha-2 agonists, the signal can sometimes be difficult to detect because of the vasoconstriction that these drugs cause.

Respiratory rate

Respiratory rate and function are assessed by observing the chest and the reservoir bag for the rate and nature of excursions, and listening to the respiratory sounds via an oesophageal stethoscope.

Additional monitoring equipment

A variety of equipment and procedures are available to aid anaesthetic monitoring. While their use is not always practicable in field or charity situations, where finances and logistics permit, their use should be considered.

Ideally, every anaesthetized patient should have its blood pressure assessed, but in practice this is often not the case, especially in short, routine procedures in a healthy population of animals. Non-invasive blood pressure monitors are often inaccurate and fail to work on small patients such as puppies and kittens; however,

Doppler devices can be more useful and provide a reassuring audible signal indicating the pulse rate. For longer procedures, it is advisable to monitor blood pressure, as this will aid in tailoring the depth of anaesthesia and fluid therapy to the individual patient. An electrocardiogram can be monitored during anaesthesia but this is uncommon in high-throughput neutering programmes.

Respiratory monitors with apnoea alerts are available, but a capnograph will offer additional monitoring and security. A capnograph is invaluable for monitoring the adequacy of ventilation and for alerting the veterinary surgeon to the development of complications such as apnoea, airway obstruction and disconnection from the breathing circuit, as well as cardiovascular complications such as low cardiac output. A limiting factor can be the small tidal volume of paediatric animals, which can result in artificially low end-tidal carbon dioxide concentrations due to dilution of the tidal volume by the relatively high gas flow rates and high sampling rates. Mainstream (non-aspirating) capnographs offer benefits over side-stream sampling models. Irrespective of the type of capnograph employed, neonatal adaptors should be used between the patient and the breathing circuit to reduce the dead space volume and prevent rebreathing. Sidestream capnographs can also be set to sample a smaller volume per minute to reduce the volume of gas diverted for sampling. However, with a lower sampling rate a greater degree of error is possible, and the end-tidal carbon dioxide concentration may be underestimated.

Analgesia and pain

In healthy cats and dogs, the use of a single subcutaneous perioperative dose of a non-steroidal anti-inflammatory drug (NSAID) such as meloxicam or carprofen is commonly used. However, these drugs do not have marketing authorization in patients less than 6 weeks old or cats less than 2 kg bodyweight, and therefore care must be taken to ensure that paediatric patients are accurately weighed, they are healthy and have a good hydration status. This will reduce the likelihood of renal insult.

Providing analgesia as a priority cannot be stressed strongly enough. Painful early experiences have been shown to alter subsequent responses to pain in human infants (Taddio et al., 1997), and the assumption that this also occurs in other species should be borne in mind. The alpha-2 agonists, opioids and ketamine all offer valuable analgesia. Combining these agents with a NSAID provides an excellent example of a multimodal pre-emptive approach to analgesia.

The use of local anaesthetics should also be considered. Although used infrequently in dogs and cats, local anaesthetics can be used in castrations and ovariohysterectomies. For example, lidocaine can be administered subcutaneously and intratesticularly before castration to obtund and blunt the nociceptive impulses associated with surgery (Moldal et al., 2013).

It is important to calculate the dose of local anaesthetic carefully and not to exceed 2 mg/kg lidocaine. For example, in male cats, using a 2% (20 mg/ml) solution of lidocaine (with or without adrenaline), 0.1 ml/kg can be used per cat. The dose should be divided between the testes and infiltrated subcutaneously on withdrawal of the needle (Figure 6.11). In female cats, lidocaine infiltrated subcutaneously, into the wound, and irrigated on to the mesovarium and ovaries has been shown to decrease anaesthetic requirements during ovariectomy (see later for discussion of the use of lidocaine in ovariohysterectomy of bitches).

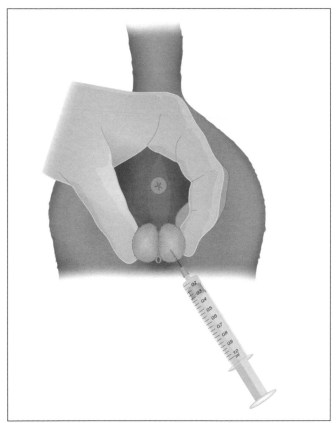

6.11 Local analgesia can be provided by intratesticular injection before castration in the dog and cat. The dose of lidocaine should not exceed 2 mg/kg. For example, in cats 0.1 ml/kg of a 2% lidocaine solution can be divided between the testes and then infiltrated subcutaneously on withdrawal of the needle.

Reversal

If a protocol including an alpha-2 agonist is used, the alpha-2 agonist can be reversed using an antagonist such as atipamezole. The dose and timing of administration of the antagonist is dependent on the procedure. For example, if the procedure is short (e.g. 10–15 minutes), it is advisable to reverse the alpha-2 agonist at approximately 30–40 minutes after administration of the alpha-2 agonist. In protocols that include ketamine, earlier reversal of the alpha-2 agonist can result in a stormy recovery due to residual ketamine. The dose of atipamezole can be tailored to the patient, but it is rarely necessary to administer a full dose of antagonist. It is important to remember that administering an antagonist will reverse the sedative and analgesic effects provided by the alpha-2 agonist, potentially resulting in a faster recovery. In cases where the patient has received ketamine, an opioid and a NSAID, reversal of the residual analgesia afforded by the alpha-2 agonist is rarely detectable and probably of little clinical significance (Hasiuk *et al.*, 2015). For longer procedures it may not be necessary to administer a reversal agent.

Surgical approach

Cats

Male kittens

The testes of prepubertal kittens are small and mobile. Careful and gentle palpation is required to determine whether a kitten has normal or cryptorchid testes. If there remains doubt after this examination, the kitten can be re-examined at a later date or by a more experienced member of staff. An exploratory laparotomy (which will have a prolonged surgical time) to locate abdominal testes may constitute an unnecessary risk to a paediatric patient, and it may be safer to postpone surgery until closer to puberty, when the testes are larger and become 'fixed' in the scrotum.

When the patient is anaesthetized, any doubt surrounding whether the testes have descended can be removed by palpation of the inguinal region: digital pressure will return the testis to the scrotum (Figures 6.12 and 6.13).

A number of surgical techniques can be used to castrate kittens. The tunic may be incised (open castration) and then:

- The blood vessel and vas deferens can be tied to each other (Figure 6.14)
- The blood vessel and vas deferens can be secured with an absorbable ligature (Figure 6.15)
- A pair of mosquito forceps can be used to form a knot combining both structures.

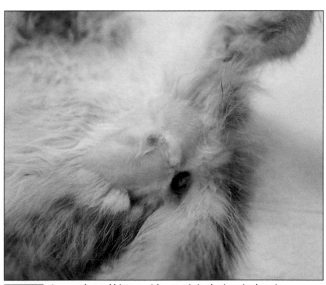

6.12 A prepubertal kitten with a testis in the inguinal region.
(© David Yates)

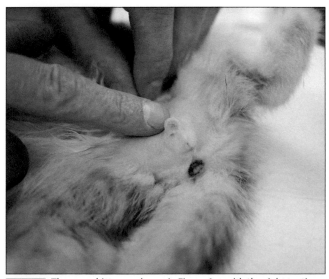

6.13 The same kitten as shown in Figure 6.12 with the right testis pushed into the scrotum by applying digital pressure.
(© David Yates)

Similarly, the tunic may be kept closed and a ligature or the forceps technique (Figure 6.16) applied to achieve haemostasis.

The testes are smaller in kittens than in sexually mature cats. The vessels are also smaller, and care should be taken to avoid excess traction, which may cause damage, when manipulating them. Otherwise, the surgery is quick and simple, and kittens rapidly return to normal behaviour after this intervention.

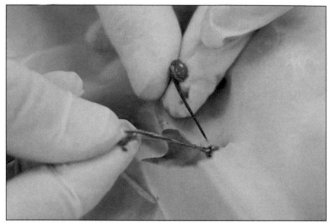

6.14 Haemostasis in an open cat castration can be achieved by tying together the testicular blood vessel and vas deferens.
(© David Yates)

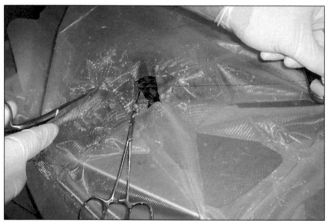

6.15 An absorbable ligature may be also be used to achieve haemostasis. This image shows an open castration.
(© David Yates)

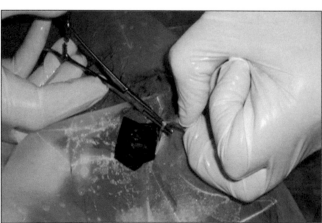

6.16 Some veterinary surgeons may prefer to perform an instrument tie using mosquito forceps, as in this closed castration.
(© David Yates)

Female kittens

Any healthy female kitten can be neutered. In very small patients (approximately 0.5 kg bodyweight) the surgery should be performed delicately. However, the reduced subcutaneous and abdominal fat in small patients makes location of the reproductive tract straightforward. One significant difference in kittens compared with adult cats may be the presence of a small volume of clear abdominal fluid. This is of low specific gravity and can be removed using gentle swabbing.

Using a midline approach, the following tips may help an inexperienced surgeon gain confidence in the procedure.

- The bladder of the anaesthetized patient should be expressed before surgery (Figure 6.17).
- The incision should be two-thirds the distance from the umbilicus to the pubic brim in a kitten less than 12 weeks of age (Figure 6.18).
- A full colon may be a useful landmark for finding the uterus.
- After opening the abdomen, the author uses forceps to push the intestines and omentum cranially. The search for the uterus then begins in an area between the bladder and colon. The author retrieves the left uterine horn, which sits on top of the descending colon (Figure 6.19).

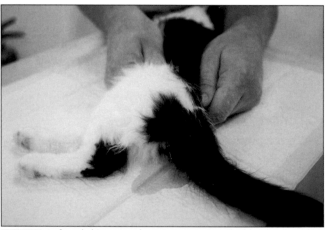

6.17 In female kittens undergoing neutering, the bladder should be expressed before surgery to prevent accidental perforation and to aid visualization of the uterus.
(© David Yates)

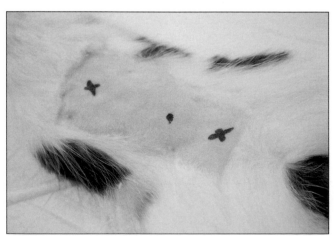

6.18 Landmarks for making the surgical incision in kittens less than 12 weeks of age are shifted slightly caudally for a midline ovariohysterectomy compared with their positions in older patients.
(© David Yates)

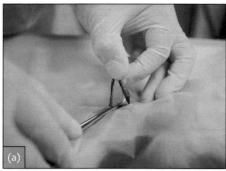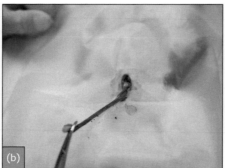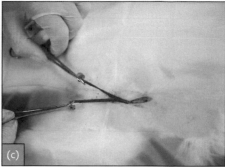

6.19 (a) The first ovary is located and a window made in the broad ligament to enable placement of a ligature. (b) Using gentle traction, the second uterine horn is exteriorized. (c) Once both ovarian pedicles have been ligated and transected, the cervix can be clamped and ligated.
(© David Yates)

There are few differences between conventional neutering and prepubertal neutering once the uterus is identified. The surgery is predictable, and there are no complicating factors such as mammary development, pregnancy or a friable uterus, which may be seen in sexually mature queens that are in oestrus.

The left flank approach may be preferred by some surgeons. There is sufficient elasticity in the right ovarian pedicle to achieve adequate exposure when this approach is used. However, in some cases the surgeon may be unable to remove all of the uterine body via a left flank approach. This is a minor technical point, as ovariectomy and ovariohysterectomy will achieve similar results. In the context of shelter medicine, the key is to neuter lots of cats, as early as possible, by whichever method suits the individual surgeon (see Figure 6.20 for the advantages and disadvantages of the flank and midline approaches to feline ovariohysterectomy).

Pregnant queens

Considering the origin of many shelter animals, it is likely that a significant proportion of queens, in particular, may be pregnant on arrival. Unwanted pets are less likely to have been neutered, and entire animals are more likely to stray when in oestrus.

There are a number of considerations regarding the decision whether to perform ovariohysterectomy in pregnant queens:

- Shelters exist (at least in part) because of a pet overpopulation problem. The shelter veterinary team have a responsibility to manage this problem
- Allowing a cat to give birth in a shelter may expose the neonates to a greater risk of infectious disease

- Staff may spend a disproportionate amount of time caring for young animals that are perceived to be 'more appealing'. This may indirectly compromise the care afforded to other animals housed in the shelter
- Vaccination schedules within a shelter may need to be refined for pregnant animals
- Ovariohysterectomy of the pregnant queen is uncomplicated if done early. (In contrast, morbidity is likely to be higher in pregnant bitches; see later)
- The length of stay for 'less desirable' shelter animals may be extended if they are 'competing' with kittens and puppies for a new owner.

The surgical results achieved with ovariohysterectomy in early pregnancy are more likely to resemble those of conventional surgery in a non-pregnant cat. Using a midline approach (the authors' preference), an experienced veterinary surgeon is likely to complete the procedure in less than 30 minutes. Postoperative pain and healing are similar for non-pregnant postpubertal and pregnant cat ovariohysterectomies.

A flank incision for ovariohysterectomy of a late-stage pregnant queen (>5 or 6 weeks) is likely to cause significant damage to several muscle layers. This means that postoperative pain would be more difficult to control. A midline approach is therefore preferred. Meticulous dissection is required to avoid significant mammary blood vessels and mammary tissue; milk may leak from damaged tissues and obscure the surgical field.

The ovarian vessels, although engorged in the pregnant queen, are easy to exteriorize (Figure 6.21). The ovarian suspensory ligament is long and relatively elastic – it will have stretched while supporting the gravid uterus. Blood vessels running in the broad and round ligaments may need to be ligated. The thickened vaginal stump requires transfixing

Surgical approach	Advantages	Disadvantages
Flank	• Less wound tension from abdominal contents • Less likelihood of catastrophic wound breakdown • Easier to check wound postoperatively (e.g. in feral cats when monitoring from a distance) • Quicker	• More traumatic and technically demanding in pregnant queens • May be more difficult to expose the bifurcation of the uterus • Possibly more wound complications • Need to convert to midline in cases of uncontrolled haemorrhage or in heavily pregnant queens that were not identified before surgery
Midline	• Fewer complications • Easier to teach to students • Approach of choice for queens in season and pregnant queens • Less painful/tender compared to flank approach	• Slightly longer to perform • Identification of the uterus can take longer • Bladder emptying is advisable before surgery – requires gentle expression • Catastrophic wound breakdown is more likely, especially when using only catgut suture

6.20 Advantages and disadvantages of the flank *versus* midline approach to ovariohysterectomy in the cat.

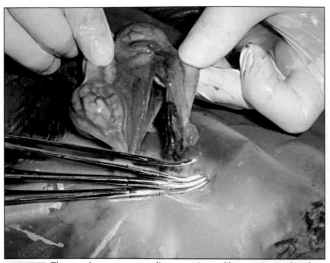

6.21 The ovarian suspensory ligament is readily exteriorized in the pregnant queen. Although the blood vessels are engorged, multiple haemostats can be applied to facilitate haemostasis.
(© David Yates)

ligatures. Non-transfixing ligatures are likely to slip as the reproductive tract involutes. The flaccid abdominal muscles are easily sutured with a synthetic absorbable material such as polydioxanone. Care must be taken to close the dead space to prevent seroma formation.

The duration of anaesthesia and surgery for ovario-hysterectomy of a pregnant queen is likely to be longer than for a non-pregnant animal. The combinations of intra-muscular anaesthetic drugs can be supplemented with a low concentration of inhalant agent (0.5–1% isoflurane) after 35–40 minutes, to prolong the anaesthesia. Provision of analgesia is important and so a NSAID should also be administered.

There is no evidence to suggest that queens suffer from behavioural problems after ovariohysterectomy while pregnant. However, the resolution of mammary hyper-plasia may need to be monitored. Occasionally, milk reten-tion cysts may develop and require aspiration (Figure 6.22).

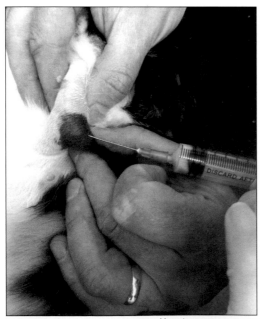

6.22 This queen was neutered late in pregnancy, at approximately 8 weeks of gestation. Several weeks after surgery, a mammary cyst required aspiration.
(© David Yates)

Identification of neutered cats

Ear tipping is a well recognized method of identifying feral or free-roaming cats that have been neutered. Tattoo ink can also be applied to the ear or midline (see Chapter 5 and QRG 5.1).

Dogs

Anaesthesia considerations

There is less reliance on intramuscular combinations to provide anaesthesia in puppies than in kittens. The time to sexual maturity is very variable across the wide range of breeds of dog that exist, but the vast majority of animals presented for 'early' neutering are likely to be prepubertal. Most juvenile dogs can undergo an anaesthetic protocol similar to those used in adult dogs. It is important to be able to secure intravenous access in order to administer intravenous agents, and premedication will facilitate this. Intravenous access will also facilitate the administration of fluid therapy if necessary, for example, during a prolonged surgery to neuter a bitch, or in an animal that under-goes significant haemorrhage during surgery. Attention to thermoregulation is vitally important in young dogs and of equal importance in adults.

Premedication protocols and anaesthetic induction protocols suitable for use in healthy dogs are listed in Figures 6.23 and 6.24, respectively.

Male puppies

There is a greater likelihood of cryptorchidism in the dog compared with the cat (Yates *et al.*, 2003). However, cryptorchidism can be screened for relatively easily by raising the forelimbs of a conscious puppy and palpating the inguinal region. Abdominal cryptorchidism may be a valid reason to delay surgery until closer to puberty. In a sexually mature dog, the testes are larger and can be more easily located.

Prepubertal castration of puppies can be carried out using either a scrotal or midline prescrotal approach. The scrotal approach is suitable for puppies up to about 5 kg (about the size of a large male cat) and is similar to the technique used in cats. One additional step used in dogs is the need to apply tissue glue to the scrotal wounds. Puppies housed in groups in a shelter may be more likely to lick and soil their castration wounds.

The prescrotal approach is simple in the puppy. There is less obvious skin bleeding than in the sexually mature dog. However, the testes are more mobile and difficult to hold firmly during surgical dissection. The testicular vessels are easy to ligate with absorbable suture material or can be ligated to the vas deferens in smaller puppies (Figures 6.25).

Female puppies

During their training, veterinary surgeons usually learn to neuter male animals before females. A logical progression would be castration of cats and then dogs, followed by ovariohysterectomy of queens and then bitches. Having gained confidence in neutering bitches, a novice surgeon would then add ovariohysterectomy of pregnant animals, Caesarean sections and pyometra cases to their reper-toire. Ovariohysterectomy of prepubertal bitches sits somewhere on the spectrum of difficulty between ovario-hysterectomy of a cat and of a lean, anoestrous bitch weighing 10–15 kg. It should be regarded as the ideal time to operate with regard to surgical morbidity.

Drug(s)	Dose and route	Comments
Acepromazine (A) + Opioid (one of the following): Butorphanol (B) or Buprenorphine (Bu) or Methadone (Me)	0.03–0.05 mg/kg i.m. (A) + 0.2–0.4 mg/kg i.m. (B) or 20 µg/kg i.m. (Bu) or 0.2–0.5 mg/kg i.m. (Me)	Commonly used combination in adult dogs In puppies, the acepromazine may predispose to prolonged recovery and hypothermia Morphine does not have marketing authorization
Medetomidine (M) + Opioid (one of the following): Butorphanol (B) or Buprenorphine (Bu) or Methadone (Me)	10–20 µg/kg i.m. (M) + 0.2–0.4 mg/kg i.m. (B) or 20 µg/kg i.m. (Bu) or 0.1–0.2 mg/kg i.m. (Me)	Provides profound sedation Medetomidine can be reversed with atipamezole The medetomidine + methadone combination will necessitate reduced doses of induction agent^a, such as: • Propofol at 1 mg/kg i.v. or • Alfaxalone at 0.5 mg/kg i.v. or • Ketamine at 2 mg/kg i.m. or • Mask induction with isoflurane
Midazolam (Mi) + Methadone (Me)	0.3–0.4 mg/kg i.m. (Mi) + 0.2–0.5 mg/kg i.m. (Me)	Midazolam does not have marketing authorization
Dexmedetomidine (D) + Opioid (one of the following): Butorphanol (B) + Buprenorphine (Bu) + Methadone (Me)	125–375 µg/m² i.m. (D) + 0.1–0.4 mg/kg i.m. (B) or 10–20 µg/kg i.m. (Bu) or 0.1–0.2 mg/kg i.m. (Me)	Provides profound sedation Body surface area formula ensures accuracy of dosing across a range of sizes of dog Dexmedetomidine can be reversed with atipamezole The dexmedetomidine + methadone combination will necessitate reduced doses of induction agent^a, such as: • Propofol at 1 mg/kg i.v. or • Alfaxalone at 0.5 mg/kg i.v. or • Ketamine at 2 mg/kg i.m. or • Mask induction with isoflurane
Midazolam/diazepam (Mi/D) + Ketamine (K)	0.25–0.5 mg/kg i.m., i.v. (Mi/D) + 5–10 mg/kg i.m., i.v. (K)	Expect profound sedation/light general anaesthesia Use lower doses i.v.

6.23 A selection of premedication protocols for use in healthy dogs undergoing neutering. ªAll intravenous induction agents should be given slowly and to effect. Doses are provided as a guide only, and the total dose will depend on the effect of the premedication. i.m. = intramuscular; i.v. = intravenous.

Drug(s)	Dose and route	Comments
Isoflurane	Mask induction or for maintenance of anaesthesia following an i.v. or i.m. induction	Unpleasant odour No analgesia Environmental pollution and health and safety considerations for staff Marketing authorization
Sevoflurane	Mask induction or for maintenance of anaesthesia following an i.v. or i.m. induction	No analgesia Environmental pollution and health and safety considerations for staff Marketing authorization
Propofol	4–6 mg/kg i.v. Lower dosages may be required after profound sedation caused by premedication	Intravenous access required, which may be difficult in small puppies No analgesia Marketing authorization Requires maintenance with inhalant anaesthesia or TIVA Premedication advisable
Alfaxalone	2–3 mg/kg i.v. Lower dosages may be required after profound sedation caused by premedication	Intravenous access required, which may be difficult in small puppies Marketing authorization No analgesia Premedication advisable Requires maintenance with inhalant anaesthesia or TIVA
Xylazine (X) + Ketamine (K)	1–2 mg/kg i.m. (X) + 10 mg/kg i.m. (K)	Marketing authorization Unsuitable for ovariohysterectomy Anaesthesia can be prolonged with an inhalant agent
Midazolam/diazepam (Mi/D) + Ketamine (K)	0.25–0.5 mg/kg i.v., i.m. (Mi/D) + 5–10 mg/kg i.v., i.m. (K)	Premedication improves the plane of anaesthesia The benzodiazepines do not have marketing authorization Poor analgesia, can be improved with addition of an opioid Anaesthesia can be prolonged with an inhalant agent or TIVA Painful i.m. injection
Medetomidine (M) + Ketamine (K)	40 µg/kg i.m. (M) + 5–7.5 mg/kg i.m. (K)	Marketing authorization Provides analgesia Superior to xylazine + ketamine Reversal with atipamezole at 20–40 µg/kg Anaesthesia can be prolonged with an inhalant agent Addition of an opioid will improve analgesia

6.24 A selection of anaesthetic protocols for use in healthy dogs undergoing neutering. Induction agents should be given slowly and to effect. Doses are provided as a guide only, and the total dose will depend on the effect of the premedication. Veterinary surgeons should consult individual product data sheets for further details. Additional analgesia can be provided by instillation of a local anaesthetic agent and a perioperative non-steroidal anti-inflammatory drug (see text for details). Oxygen provision should be available at all times. i.m. = intramuscular; i.v. = intravenous; TIVA = total intravenous anaesthesia.

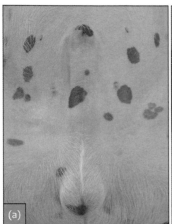 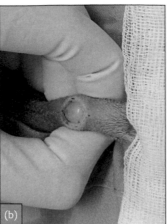 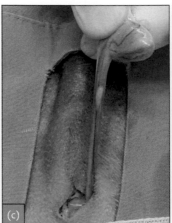 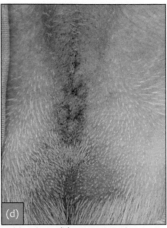

6.25 (a) Castration of prepubertal puppies generally requires a smaller incision and less vascular surgery than in older dogs. (b) A prescrotal approach is generally used in prepubertal puppies, as for adult castrations. (c) Prepubertal puppies lack the vascularity and fibrous tissue present in older dogs. (d) Intradermal sutures will improve postoperative comfort and promote healing.
(Courtesy of R Elmore)

The prepubertal bitch is generally lean (indeed, it would be unwise to perform an elective ovariohysterectomy on an overweight animal). There is very little subcutaneous or abdominal fat. The uterus is thin and relatively avascular. There may be an increased volume of clear abdominal fluid, as compared with an adult. The approach is similar to the midline approach in a cat. In a puppy less than 12 weeks of age, the incision should be made approximately halfway between the umbilicus and the pubic brim. The left flank approach is unlikely to achieve sufficient exposure of the right ovary in the prepubertal bitch, and is therefore not recommended.

There is some debate about whether ovariohysterectomy or ovariectomy is preferable in the bitch. Ovariectomy is associated with a shorter procedure and may be less invasive compared with ovariohysterectomy. In addition, there is no evidence to associate ovariectomy with a higher incidence of pyometra. In older bitches, particularly where there is evidence of cystic change, ovariohysterectomy is generally recommended. The choice of which surgery to perform rests with the surgeon, but certainly in the UK ovariohysterectomy is more common.

Pregnant bitches

A heavily pregnant middle-aged bitch with significant mammary engorgement is unlikely to be neutered in a shelter environment. Many shelters would allow such a bitch to give birth, perhaps in experienced foster care away from the busy shelter environment.

The anaesthesia and surgical time for neutering a pregnant bitch will be significantly longer than for a non-pregnant bitch because of the extra time needed to achieve haemostasis, exteriorize the gravid uterus and close a longer incision. If possible, it is recommended to measure the patient's blood pressure and consider the administration of an isotonic crystalloid solution during anaesthesia to maintain normovolaemia. Postoperative analgesia is necessary for the somatic and visceral pain, and the administration of a NSAID is recommended. Local anaesthetic can be injected in a 'fan-like' manner in the muscle and fascial planes either side of the incision to provide local anaesthesia. Careful calculation of the volume of local anaesthetic is necessary to prevent overdose. The total dose of lidocaine should not exceed 2 mg/kg.

Evaluating the impact of pre-adoption neutering in shelters

When any procedure is changed, it is essential to monitor the impact of the change. This applies as much to changing the age of neutering as to any other procedural change.

The impact of pre-adoption neutering can be measured from two perspectives. The first relates to the individual animal in the programme. Has the animal benefitted from the intervention? Did the puppy or kitten find a new home more quickly because it was healthy, neutered, vaccinated and microchipped? Did the animal stay with the new owner and live a long and healthy life? A neutered, vaccinated dog is less likely to be relinquished, as it is unlikely to display the behaviours associated with being sexually mature (roaming, aggression, oestrus) that most owners find unacceptable.

The second evaluation is the impact of neutering on the whole population – that is, on animal overpopulation. Has the shelter reduced the likelihood of animals contributing to future breeding? Does a shelter that rehomes high-quality neutered animals displace those obtained from disreputable sources such as puppy farms and online sales? Over many years, do successful shelters educate a cohort of animal adopters to return to the shelters for all of their future pets?

In an ideal world, all pets would be responsibly owned. Decisions on treatment would be made following an informed discussion between a veterinary healthcare professional and the individual pet owner. The best available evidence for and against an intervention would be put forward and evaluated during that discussion. However, evidence from a recent report suggests that less than 5% of pet owners consider veterinary advice before choosing their pet (PDSA, 2013). Until such time as all pet owners make educated, informed choices regarding their pet's reproduction, it is likely that prepubertal neutering will remain an important measure in reducing the abuse, neglect and euthanasia of unwanted pets.

Conclusion

There are a number of advantages to lowering the age for neutering dogs and cats. There is a reduction in the risk to staff associated with handling smaller animals – they are less likely to sustain lifting injuries, and younger patients are less likely to inflict serious injuries during handling and restraint. Additional procedures, such as microchipping and blood sampling, can be conveniently carried out along with the neutering procedure. The anaesthetized patient is also easier to examine more comprehensively. For example, heart murmurs (in kittens) may be easier to hear and luxating patellae (in small breeds of dog) easier to screen for in the unconscious patient. In addition, problems such as transmissible venereal disease (which is a problem in some countries outside the UK) can be evaluated.

Littermates can be group housed to reduce stress before surgery; this will also improve kennel occupancy levels. Both surgical time and anaesthetic recovery time are reduced in younger patients – this, too, improves the turnaround time on the surgical list. Even in a high-throughput shelter, providing animals are screened before surgery and monitored during recovery, perioperative morbidity should be appreciably lower than that seen in animals neutered at over 2 years of age (Pollari et al., 1996).

References and further reading

Alexander SA and Shane SM (1994) Characteristics of animals adopted from an animal control center whose owners complied with a spaying/neutering program. Journal of the American Veterinary Medical Association 205, 472–476

Beauvais W, Cardwell JM and Brodbelt DC (2012a) The effect of neutering on the risk of mammary tumours in dogs – a systematic review. Journal of Small Animal Practice 53, 314–322

Beauvais W, Cardwell JM and Brodbelt DC (2012b) The effect of neutering on the risk of urinary incontinence in bitches – a systematic review. Journal of Small Animal Practice 53, 198–204

Buffington CAT, Westropp JL and Chew DJ (2014) From FUS to Pandora syndrome: where are we, how did we get here, and where to now? Journal of Feline Medicine and Surgery 16, 385–394

Coe RJ, Grint NJ, Tivers MS et al. (2006) Comparison of flank and midline approaches to the ovariohysterectomy of cats. Veterinary Record 159, 309–313

Duval JM, Budsberg SC, Flo GL et al. (1999) Breed, sex, and body weight as risk factors for rupture of the cranial cruciate ligament in young dogs. Journal of the American Veterinary Medical Association 215, 811–814

Faya M, Carranza A, Priotto M et al. (2011) Domestic queens under natural temperate photoperiod do not manifest seasonal anestrus. Animal Reproduction Science 129, 78–81

German AJ (2006) The growing problem of obesity in dogs and cats. Journal of Nutrition 136, 1940S–1946S

Grint NJ, Murison PJ, Coe RJ et al. (2006) Assessment of the influence of surgical technique on postoperative pain and wound tenderness in cats following ovariohysterectomy. Journal of Feline Medicine and Surgery 8, 15–21

Hasiuk MM, Brown D, Cooney C et al. (2015) Application of fast-track surgery principles to evaluate effects of atipamezole on recovery and analgesia following ovariohysterectomy in cats anesthetized with dexmedetomidine-ketamine-hydromorphone. Journal of the American Veterinary Medical Association 246, 645–653

Jennet AL, Jennet NM, Hopping J and Yates D (2016) Evidence for seasonal reproduction in UK domestic cats. Journal of Feline Medicine and Surgery 18, 804–808

Joyce A and Yates D (2011) Help stop teenage pregnancy! Early-age neutering in cats. Journal of Feline Medicine and Surgery 13, 3–10

Kustritz MV (2007) Determining the optimal age for gonadectomy of dogs and cats. Journal of the American Veterinary Medical Association 231, 1665–1675

Mathews KA (2008) Pain management for the pregnant, lactating, and neonatal to pediatric cat and dog. Veterinary Clinics of North America: Small Animal Practice 38, 1291–1308

McCarthy RJ, Levine SH and Reed JM (2013) Estimation of effectiveness of three methods of feral cat population control by use of a simulation model. Journal of the American Veterinary Medical Association 243, 502–511

Moldal ER, Eriksen T, Kirpensteijn J et al. (2013) Intratesticular and subcutaneous lidocaine alters the intraoperative haemodynamic responses and heart rate variability in male cats undergoing castration. Veterinary Anaesthesia and Analgesia 40, 63–73

Muirden A (2002) Prevalence of feline leukaemia virus and antibodies to feline immunodeficiency virus and feline coronavirus in stray cats sent to an RSPCA hospital. Veterinary Record 150, 621–625

Muraro L and White RS (2014) Complications of ovariohysterectomy procedures performed in 1880 dogs. Tierärztliche Praxis. Ausgabe K, Kleintiere/Heimtiere 42, 297–302

Murray JK, Roberts MA, Whitmarsh A et al. (2009) Survey of the characteristics of cats owned by households in the UK and factors affecting their neutered status. Veterinary Record 164, 137–141

New JC Jr, Kelch WJ, Hutchison JM et al. (2004) Birth and death rate estimates of cats and dogs in U.S. households and related factors. Journal of Applied Animal Welfare Science 7, 229–241

Overley B, Shofer FS, Goldschmidt MH et al. (2005) Association between ovarihysterectomy and feline mammary carcinoma. Journal of Veterinary Internal Medicine 19, 560–563

Palmer C, Corr S and Sandøe P (2012) Inconvenient desires: should we routinely neuter companion animals? Anthrozoös 25, 153–172

PDSA (2013) PDSA Animal Wellbeing (PAW) Report. Available from www.pdsa.org.uk

Pollari FL, Bonnett BN, Bamsey SC et al. (1996) Postoperative complications of elective surgeries in dogs and cats determined by examining electronic and paper medical records. Journal of the American Veterinary Medical Association 208, 1882–1886

Polson S, Taylor PM and Yates D (2014) Effects of age and reproductive status on postoperative pain after routine ovariohysterectomy in cats. Journal of Feline Medicine and Surgery 16, 170–176

Porters N, Polis I, Moons C et al. (2014) Prepubertal gonadectomy in cats: different surgical techniques and comparison with gonadectomy at traditional age. Veterinary Record 175, 223

Posner LP, Pavuk AA, Rokshar JL et al. (2010) Effects of opioids and anesthetic drugs on body temperature in cats. Veterinary Anaesthesia and Analgesia 37, 35–43

Spain CV, Scarlett JM and Houpt KA (2004) Long-term risks and benefits of early-age gonadectomy in cats. Journal of the American Veterinary Medical Association 224, 372–379

Stavisky J, Brennan ML, Downes M et al. (2012) Demographics and economic burden of un-owned cats and dogs in the UK: results of a 2010 census. BMC Veterinary Research 8, 163

Taddio A, Katz J, Ilersich AL et al. (1997) Effect of neonatal circumcision on pain response during subsequent routine vaccination. Lancet 349, 599–603

van Oostrom H, Krauss MW and Sap R (2013) A comparison between the v-gel supraglottic airway device and the cuffed endotracheal tube for airway management in spontaneously breathing cats during isoflurane anaesthesia. Veterinary Anaesthesia and Analgesia 40, 265–271

Wei A, Fascetti AJ, Kim K et al. (2014) Early effects of neutering on energy expenditure in adult male cats. PLOS ONE 9, e89557

Welsh CP, Gruffydd-Jones TJ, Roberts MA and Murray JK (2014) Poor owner knowledge of feline reproduction contributes to the high proportion of accidental litters born to UK pet cats. Veterinary Record 174, 118

Yates D, Hayes G, Heffernan M et al. (2003) Incidence of cryptorchidism in dogs and cats. Veterinary Record 152, 502–504

QRG 6.1: General anaesthetic protocols for early neutering
by David Yates

Kittens

Kittens entering a rescue centre may have come from a poor environment and may require corrective nutrition and treatment for fleas and endoparasites before surgery. It is vital that each kitten is compared to a standard growth chart to estimate its age and physical development. The body condition score should be determined and the patient accurately weighed.

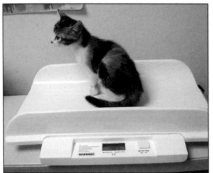

Accurate digital scales are essential for safe prepubertal neutering. The volumes of injectable agents may be calculated from charts that convert patient bodyweight to body surface area (see below).
(© David Yates)

The patient should be weighed to an accuracy of at least 100 g (preferably 10 g). The result should lie between the minimum female and maximum male mass points (shown on the chart below) for a particular age in weeks.

Male kittens are likely to weigh more than their female siblings. Kittens that are significantly underweight compared with their littermates should be re-examined on a weekly basis. If concerns exist, the procedure can be rescheduled for a time when these smaller kittens have caught up with their siblings.

Dosing anaesthetic drugs on the basis of bodyweight may result in an inadequate plane of anaesthesia for prepubertal patients. Due to the dosing precision required for kitten anaesthesia, calculations are best based on body surface area rather than bodyweight, similar to the calculation of doses of potent chemotherapy agents.

The 'kitten quad' combination is an effective, safe and convenient total injectable protocol based on body surface area:

- Medetomidine 600 µg/m² +
- Ketamine 60 mg/m² +
- Midazolam 3 mg/m² +
- Buprenorphine 180 µg/m².

This combination gives an identical volume for injection of each

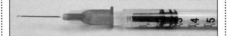

This syringe has an additional projection on the plunger, which is useful for reducing dead space in the hub.
(© David Yates)

agent. The use of fine-gauge needles and syringes that reduce 'dead space' will improve reliability.

The body surface area of the cat can be estimated from the equation:

$$\text{Body surface area} = \frac{10.4 \times \text{bodyweight}^{0.67}}{100 \text{ m}^2}$$

The volume of each agent in the anaesthetic combination can be calculated from the table below. This non-linear dosing is also shown in graphical form. The volume in millilitres of each agent in the quad is 0.6 x cat body surface area (m²).

Bodyweight (kg)	Volume of each agent in quad protocol (ml)
0.25	0.02
0.5	0.04
0.75	0.05
1.0	0.06
1.25	0.07
1.5	0.08
1.75	0.09
2.0	0.10
2.25	0.11
2.5	0.12

Dosage chart for routine neutering of prepubertal kittens.

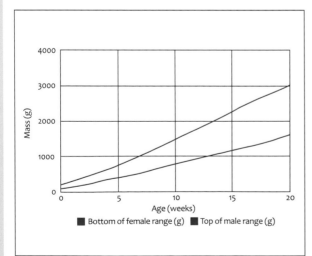

Kitten growth chart developed at the RSPCA Greater Manchester Animal Hospital. Ideally, the bodyweight of all the kittens in a litter should lie between the two extremes.

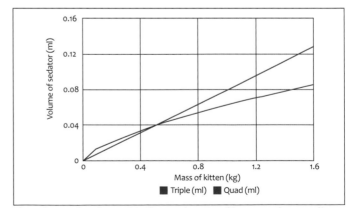

The volume of each agent in the quad protocol increases in a non-linear relationship with bodyweight. This improves the reliability of the combination in smaller animals (<1.5 kg) and reduces the amount of anaesthetic required in postpubertal patients (likely to be >3 kg). The graph shows the volume of medetomidine (600 µg/m²) used in the quad protocol compared with the linear dosing (80 µg/kg) used in the 'cat triple' protocol.

QRG 6.1 *continued*

As an example, the quad combination for a 1.2 kg kitten would be 0.07 ml of each constituent, giving a total volume of 0.28 ml. This should be given by deep intramuscular injection. The author routinely uses the quadriceps muscle group.

After a few minutes, the patient can be intubated with a non-cuffed endotracheal tube. Application of ocular lubricants will prevent corneal desiccation.

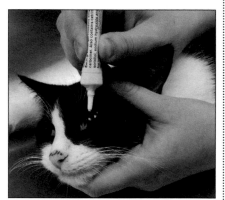

Protection of the globe using an ocular lubricant. Anaesthetic combinations containing ketamine may increase the likelihood of corneal desiccation during surgery.
(© David Yates)

Although non-steroidal anti-inflammatory drugs (NSAIDs) are not currently licensed for cats of body-weight less than 2 kg or under 6 weeks of age, in the UK they are routinely used under the prescribing cascade to provide postoperative analgesia. Anecdotally, despite their frequent use, side effects are uncom-mon provided kittens are adequately hydrated and provided with food and water as soon as possible postopera-tively (as soon as sternal recumbency can be maintained).

Atipamezole at half of the original volume of medetomidine can be given by intramuscular injection at least 45 minutes after induction in order to reverse the effects of the medetomidine.

The littermates can be reintroduced to each other once they are able to stand and eat.

Puppies

A number of considerations may influence anaesthetic planning for neutering of puppies. The physical size of the puppy may make intravenous access difficult. Lengthy premedication periods should be avoided as these are possible contributors to hypothermia. Body surface area dosing, as described above, may improve both the reliability of the anaesthetic combination and the quality of analgesia provided.

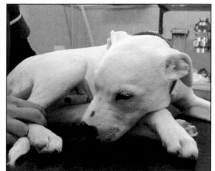

Puppy premedicated before induction for castration.
(© David Yates)

Several different intramuscular medetomidine–ketamine combinations have been used in puppies. Some of these are shown in the table below. These may be more applicable to smaller puppies (<5 kg) where intravenous access is difficult.

The safest anaesthetic protocol is likely to be the one that is most familiar to the anaesthetist. Indeed, there is no reason to significantly deviate from protocols for adult dogs, except in particularly small puppies. Hypothermia and hypoglycaemia should be avoided – they may significantly extend the recovery time. Avoid withholding food for long periods of time prior to anaesthesia – for kittens, a 3-hour fast is sufficient. Patients should be fed as soon as is safely possible postoperatively.

Analgesia should be carefully tailored to the individual. It should be noted that higher doses of analgesic agents than those used in adults may be required; this is likely to be due to increased metabolic clearance rather than an increased requirement in young animals.

Combination	Dose rate	Comments
Medetomidine (M) + Butorphanol (B) + Ketamine (K)	25 µg/kg i.m. (M) + 0.1 mg/kg i.m. (B) + Wait 15 minutes 5 mg/kg i.m. (K)	Licensed 'triple' combination Analgesia may be insufficient for bitch spays
Medetomidine (M) + Buprenorphine (Bu) + Ketamine (K)	25 µg/kg i.m. (M) + 20 µg/kg i.m. (Bu) + Wait 20 minutes 5 mg/kg i.m. (K)	Improved analgesia compared with licensed 'triple'
Medetomidine (M) + Ketamine (K)	1000 µg/m² i.m (M) + 5 mg/kg i.m. (K)	Body surface area dosing improves reliability in dogs <5 kg compared to linear bodyweight dosing seen in 'triple'. Will require additional opioid analgesia for bitch spays
Medetomidine (M) + Methadone (Me) + Propofol (P) or Alfaxalone (A) or Ketamine (K) or Isoflurane	20 µg/kg i.m. (M) + 0.2 mg/kg i.m. (Me) + Wait 10–15 minutes 1 mg/kg i.v. (P) or 0.5 mg/kg i.v. (A) or 2 mg/kg i.m. (K) or Mask induction with isoflurane	Profound analgesia Risk of respiratory depression (methadone) Readily reversible especially if using mask induction

Examples of intramuscular combinations suitable for neutering of prepubertal puppies. i.m. = intramuscular; i.v. = intravenous.

Chapter 7

Shelter metrics

Janet M. Scarlett and Jenny Stavisky

This chapter will consider what can be achieved through the use of metrics and provide real-world examples and guidance around how to begin using them. Readers should think of metrics as numbers that enable shelters to measure and track important information over time to assess their progress towards achieving specific health-related goals. This is a similar process to clinical audit, with the ultimate aim of identifying where improvements can be made and tracking the success or failure of initiatives to boost performance.

Metrics is defined as a 'method of measuring something, or the results obtained from this' (Oxford Dictionaries, 2014a). The term 'metric' is also defined as 'a system or standard of measurement' (Oxford Dictionaries, 2014b). Both definitions apply in the context of animal shelters. The use of 'metrics' in this chapter will refer sometimes to data as a measure of what a shelter is doing (e.g. the shelter's intake of cats last year was 745), and at other times as a measure of how a shelter is progressing (e.g. benchmarking its progress over time towards meeting its goals). Overall, though, practising shelter metrics simply means collecting information regarding how a shelter is functioning. From a veterinary perspective, this clearly means tracking the rate of disease occurrence. However, this is inextricably linked with key indicators of shelter performance such as the number of animals rehomed and their length of stay. Currently, these important pieces of information are often recorded poorly, if at all.

Shelters striving to optimize the physical and mental welfare of the animals in their care cannot do so without a sound, comprehensive population health programme that actively promotes both individual and population-level health. Collection, maintenance, periodic analysis and dissemination of health-related data are essential components of a comprehensive population health programme (Newbury et al., 2010). Without data, population health can at best be described with imprecise words (e.g. excellent, good, fair) based on subjective impressions that are difficult to define or to compare across and within populations or over time. The components of population health (or herd health) programmes are described elsewhere (Hurley, 2004; Cannas da Silva et al., 2006; Newbury and Hurley, 2013).

Knowledge of the relative frequency of various diseases is essential to formulating and prioritizing health management goals and tracking progress towards minimizing disease occurrence. Establishing the baseline rates of disease is the foundation of a disease surveillance programme.

Disease surveillance

Disease surveillance is defined as the ongoing systematic collection, orderly consolidation, analysis and interpretation of health-related data in populations, and the prompt dissemination of this information to the people who are in a position to act on the data (Dwyer et al., 2014). Surveillance data are used to plan, implement and evaluate preventive and control measures for diseases in populations (Salman, 2003; Scarlett, 2013).

Disease surveillance programmes should include a clear understanding of why monitoring is important, good individual animal identification, clear definitions of the diseases to be included, a medical records system, incentives to report disease and a clear plan for management of affected animals. Timely analysis, interpretation and dissemination of information to pertinent stakeholders are essential.

Surveillance requires the calculation of metrics that summarize the frequency of medical 'events' in populations. These events most often include diseases, conditions, incidents of euthanasia and deaths, but may also include clinical signs, treatments, outcomes (e.g. recovered), medical and surgical procedures, complications (surgical and medical) or the results of diagnostic tests. Computerization of the medical data greatly facilitates this process, but is not essential.

In order to optimize communication and ensure data consistency, shelters must standardize their medical terminology. The terms 'diagnosis', 'condition', 'clinical signs' and 'symptoms' are often used interchangeably by veterinary surgeons (veterinarians) and by software providers. Data entry protocols need clear definitions and directions regarding the input of medical data. Ideally, clinical signs of disease should be distinguished from definitive diagnoses of disease. However, the techniques described in this chapter can be applied to both syndromic surveillance (e.g. for 'cat 'flu' or diarrhoea) and definitive or presumed diagnoses (e.g. positive parvovirus or dermatophytosis tests). Rather than use the words disease, condition or clinical sign interchangeably in this chapter, the word 'disease' is used to encompass all of these terms.

Why metrics are important to veterinary surgeons

It is likely that currently only a few veterinary surgeons rely on metrics to assist them in providing care for animals in shelters. Regular monitoring of medically related metrics can enhance the quality of care that veterinary surgeons offer in a number of ways.

- Metrics summarize the characteristics of our 'population patients' (so called because, in this context, patients are almost invariably populations rather than individuals).
- They are essential for optimal population health management.
- They allow recognition of disease outbreaks.
- They enable assessment of the effectiveness of protocols and recommendations.
- They can identify groups of animals and time periods in which there is a high risk of disease.
- They can enhance communication about the health status of shelter populations.
- They can provide the basis for funding requests to improve animal health.

In the following sections, each of these reasons will be explored in terms of how it applies to the shelter population, using relevant examples.

Summarizing the characteristics of 'population patients'

Shelter veterinary surgeons have both individual animal patients and 'population patients'. They care for populations of cats, dogs and, often, other species. During the physical examination of an animal, a veterinary surgeon needs to be mindful of that animal's species, sex, breed and age, because these characteristics are strongly associated with disease risk and prognosis. Similarly, the species, sex, breed and age distributions of shelter animal populations must be characterized for the same reasons. As discussed in Chapters 1 and 8, a shelter history and physical examination are critical to knowing the patient, and shelter metrics form a key component of this.

Optimal population health management

After noting an individual animal's physical characteristics, a veterinary surgeon looks for signs of disease, such as sneezing, in an individual patient. Measures of disease frequency (e.g. the percentage affected by 'cat 'flu') are the

equivalent of clinical signs when applied to the 'population patient', and can be used to inform decision-making on, for example, where to target resources. A shelter population of puppies with an incidence of canine parvovirus (CPV) of 15% requires much more urgent veterinary intervention to reduce the frequency of this disease compared with a population with an incidence of only 1%. An optimal health management programme begins by characterizing the nature and frequency of disease in shelter populations.

It can be helpful to generate an Annual Medical Profile to help identify and monitor diseases of importance to the wellbeing of the animals and the running of the shelter.

Recognition of disease outbreaks

Without a clear understanding of the frequency of common diseases and causes of death within a shelter population, the veterinary surgeon will be making medical policy decisions and drafting medical protocols based on only impressions and opinions. This is akin to prescribing treatments for an animal without doing a physical examination. This is not acceptable for individual animal care, and veterinary surgeons should strive to incorporate morbidity and mortality metrics into their population health management plans for shelters.

Prompt recognition of disease outbreaks is a component of good population health programmes. A disease outbreak is defined as an occurrence of cases of disease in excess of what would normally be expected in a specified population, geographical area or season (Gordis, 2014). Many outbreaks of infectious disease (e.g. CPV) in shelters are obvious, but it can be more difficult to recognize that an outbreak is occurring if the usual incidence of disease is unknown.

Assessment of the effectiveness of protocols and recommendations

Shelter medicine veterinary surgeons write protocols, manage threats to population health and respond to disease outbreaks. Without a means to measure the impact of these efforts, it is impossible to know whether or how well an intervention has worked. It is just as important to identify a failed intervention as a successful one, as it allows the veterinary surgeon to try something different, if needed, next time.

Example – basic population characteristics

The distributions of basic population characteristics of incoming animals for Somewhere Shelter are summarized in the Annual Intake Profile shown in Figure 7.1. Each shelter can tailor an Intake Profile to meet its needs.

7.1 Annual Intake Profile for dogs and cats for Somewhere Shelter, USA. [a] Total intake for 2017 for dogs and cats. [b] The percentages of returned adoptions were calculated using the total intake as the denominator, as the intent of this table is to show the distribution of animals from all sources (e.g. in this case the percentage of dogs returned is 93 ÷ 3569 = 2.6%). A shelter could also show these percentages as a proportion of all adoptions to emphasize the effectiveness of efforts to successfully 'match' animals to long-term owners. [c] 'Service-in': this includes owner-intended euthanasia (in the USA, owners may request that a shelter performs euthanasia of their owned animal), special cremations, feral cat surgeries, disposal and other miscellaneous reasons (e.g. temporary housing for the animals owned by victims of domestic abuse).

Year: 2017 **Shelter description:** Open admission
Animal control contract: No **Cruelty investigation:** Yes
Overall intake = 12,504

Intake category	Dogs (n = 3569)[a]		Cats (n = 8935)[a]	
	n	%	n	%
Source				
Owner/guardian surrender	2145	60.1	6782	75.9
Stray	114	3.2	732	8.2
Returned adoption[b]	93	2.6	107	1.2
Transfer in	389	10.9	340	3.8
Seized	239	6.7	706	7.9
Service-in[c]	589	16.5	268	3.0
Age group				
0–5 months	478	13.4	3369	37.7
6–11 months	518	14.5	1012	11.3
1–9 years	1756	49.2	2397	26.8
10 years and older	485	13.6	556	6.2
Unknown	136	3.8	769	8.6

Example – annual medical profile

The annual medical profile for Somewhere Shelter (Figure 7.2) summarizes the annual incidence of the most common infectious diseases in the shelter, the prevalence of feline leukaemia virus (FeLV), feline immunodeficiency virus (FIV) and heartworm infections among incoming animals, the overall annual mortality, and the number and proportion of animals euthanased for medical reasons. The decision as to which diseases and other medical information are included in a given shelter's annual medical profile should be made on the basis of the frequency, severity and importance of specific diseases to the shelter.

Disease	Cats		Dogs	
	No.	% affected	No.	% affected
Coccidiosis[a]	43	22.8 (43/189)	22	18.3 (22/120)
Giardiasis[a]	22	11.6 (22/189)	10	8.3 (10/120)
Sarcoptic mange[a]	–	–	8	8.2 (8/98)
Upper respiratory infection ('cat 'flu')/ kennel cough (CIRD)[b]	249	15.8 (249/1575)	11	2.2 (11/501)
Heartworm[b]	–	–	3	0.8 (3/393)
FeLV[c]	15	1.0 (15/1532)	–	
FIV[c]	6	0.4 (6/1532)	–	
Mortality (all causes)	25	1.7 (25/1443)	3	0.7 (3/447)
Euthanasia for medical reasons	97	6.2 (97/1575)	5	(5/501)
Treatable[d]	0	–	0	–
Non treatable	97	6.2 (97/1575)	5	1.0 (5/501)

7.2 Annual medical profile of Somewhere Shelter. [a]Animals positive for this organism among those tested with signs possibly associated with this disease. [b]Disease that developed among the shelter animals while they were resident in the shelter. [c]Animals positive for this organism among those tested during the intake examination. [d]Conditions that could be treated in the future if additional resources were available. CIRD = canine infectious respiratory disease; FeLV = feline leukaemia virus; FIV = feline immunodeficiency virus.

Example – recognition of outbreaks and clinical audit

Somewhere Shelter experienced an outbreak of post-ovariohysterectomy incision infections in cats in 2016. This was documented by comparing the rates of incision infections in 2016 and in 2015 (Figure 7.3). If these data had not been collected and compared over consecutive years, the fact that the rate of wound infections had more than doubled could have been missed. By identifying the problem, the cause (inconsistent preoperative skin preparation) could be identified and addressed.

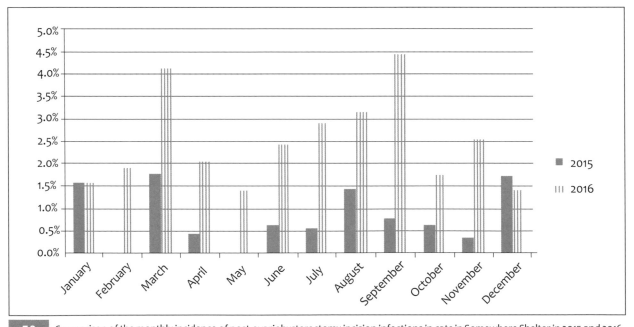

7.3 Comparison of the monthly incidence of post-ovariohysterectomy incision infections in cats in Somewhere Shelter in 2015 and 2016.

Observations such as 'there seems to be less disease' or 'the isolation unit does not seem as full' are imprecise and often inaccurate assessments of the progress that may (or may not) have been made. Assessments of the incidence of disease before and after the implementation of disease prevention or control protocols will enhance population care both at the time and in the future.

Identifying groups of animals and time periods of high disease risk

Knowledge of the behaviour of infectious diseases in a shelter population is important for tailoring preventive and control efforts. Identifying high-risk groups of animals and risky time periods facilitates targeted disease prevention and management strategies.

Example – assessing the impact of management changes

Somewhere Shelter had the goal of reducing the incidence of feline upper respiratory tract disease (FURTD, 'cat 'flu') in its cat population. In early 2012, the shelter instituted changes to minimize FURTD and tracked the monthly incidence of FURTD in the cats, documenting important declines over 2012 and 2013 (Figure 7.4).

Shelters can make comparisons of this type and monitor their progress towards reducing disease without using formal statistical tests. However, it is important to recognize that while large changes are more convincing than small ones, those that are sustained and grow over time are of greatest importance.

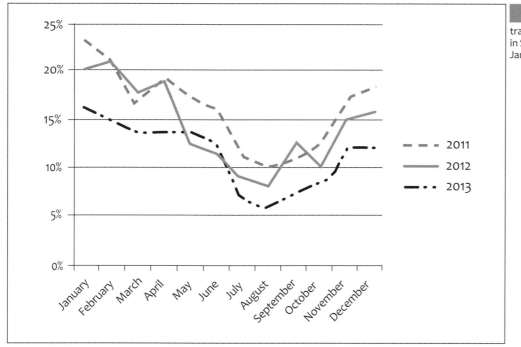

7.4 Monthly incidence of upper respiratory tract infections ('cat 'flu') in cats in Somewhere Shelter from January 2011 to December 2013.

Example – identifying at-risk groups

Somewhere Shelter tracked FURTD rates in its cats by season (Figure 7.5). To the surprise of staff members, the incidence of FURTD was generally highest during the winter months, and adult cats (>6 months of age) were at higher risk than kittens for most of the year. It was true that staff saw more cases of disease in kittens during the summer months. When the numbers were converted to rates, however, the risk of FURTD was actually higher during the winter months and for adult animals. The apparently high rate in kittens over the summer was a misconception – it was simply the case that the summer was when the kitten population was at its highest. Overall FURTD rates actually peaked during the winter months. This recognition prompted the staff to adhere more strictly to the shelter's disease management protocols during the high-risk months and for adult cats.

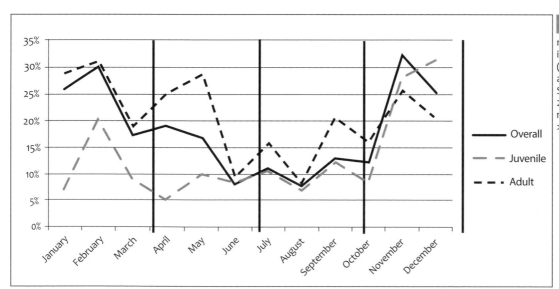

7.5 Incidence of upper respiratory tract infections by month (divided into seasons) and by age group in Somewhere Shelter in 2017. Juvenile = <6 months of age; adult = >6 months of age.

Enhancing communication about the health status of shelter populations

Actual measurements of the nature and frequency of the diseases that occur in shelter populations are the clearest and most precise means to communicate about population health to staff members, members of the shelter's Board of Directors and the wider community. Using a common language with clearly defined terms allows the whole shelter team to work together more effectively towards the same goals. These numbers can be used to highlight progress and continuing medical challenges for the shelter.

Providing the basis for funding requests to improve animal health

When appropriately analysed and presented, metrics data can be a persuasive element in successful requests for funding from the Board of Directors, prospective donors and granting agencies. Demonstrating a need through numbers is a time-tested strategy to attract funding. Funding campaigns centred on a definitive, recognizable goal are often most effective. By accurately assessing a shelter's key needs, it is possible to identify a single significant focus around which to centre a fundraising campaign. For example, a shelter with a high incidence of 'cat 'flu'/feline upper respiratory tract disease (FURTD) could request funding for the construction of a new isolation ward to separate affected cats from healthy cats.

Everyone connected with an animal shelter has a vested interest in the health of the shelter's animal population. Disease causes suffering and is a major threat to animal welfare. Shelters that do not strive to minimize disease will perpetuate suffering. An essential component of an effective health management programme that minimizes disease is the collection, retrieval, analysis and interpretation of population-level metrics.

Getting started with using shelter metrics

Many shelters do not currently collect data in a structured way. Although many record the number of animals rehomed per year, more detailed data, such as length of stay, disease incidence rates and number of 'empty pen' days are rarely recorded. This may seem surprising, as these data are key to optimizing shelter performance. After all, the number of animals successfully rehomed will, for most shelters, be the benchmark of performance, and the factors noted above will clearly affect the number rehomed.

Veterinary surgeons working with or in shelters have a real opportunity to demonstrate to shelters the value of this kind of data collection, and guide them in using it to improve throughput, performance and animal health and welfare.

This is a different kind of practice to the 'fire-brigade' reactive response of treating cases of infectious diseases such as FURTD or CPV as they arise. However, in the same way as a proactive preventive approach is now the cornerstone of cattle herd health, shelter metrics offers the opportunity to create systems for management whereby disease is actually averted.

With shelters for which this approach is novel or feels unfamiliar, the veterinary surgeon may prefer to begin with a small project with a simple measurable outcome. For example, you may decide to measure the incidence of 'cat 'flu'/FURTD and the increase in average length of stay for cats that develop FURTD. From this, it is possible to calculate how a decrease in the incidence of FURTD will decrease the average length of stay of cats in the shelter.

Example – communication around change

In 2013, the veterinary surgeon of Somewhere Shelter became concerned by the relatively low survival (~72%) of unweaned kittens in foster care (Figure 7.6). The veterinary surgeon communicated these concerns to the Executive Director of the shelter and to the foster care providers. Special evening meetings were scheduled with the foster care providers to review newly revised health protocols for unweaned kittens, and progress towards increasing kitten survival was monitored over the next several years.

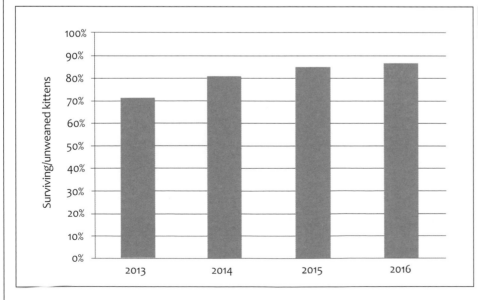

7.6 Survival (%) of unweaned kittens (0–4 weeks of age) in Somewhere Shelter from 2013 to 2016.

Example – disease and length of stay

The relationship between disease and length of stay is bidirectional; animals that stay in the shelter longer are at increased risk of many diseases and, conversely, sick animals will have an extended length of stay. Therefore, reducing length of stay (e.g. by removing barriers to adoption) is likely to reduce the occurrence of disease. Reducing disease levels can, in turn, further reduce length of stay, improving throughput.

Cats'R'Us shelter has the capacity to house 100 cats per day. Overall, 30% of cats will develop FURTD during their stay. The shelter is unwilling to implement extra biosecurity (e.g. using disinfectant hand gel between handling each cat) due to constraints on staff time.

- Currently, the average length of stay for a cat that does not have FURTD is 20 days; for cats that show clinical signs of cat 'flu, the average length of stay is 32 days.
- The average length of stay is therefore:
  (0.3 x 32) + (0.7 x 20) = 23.6 days
- By multiplying the number of cages by the number of days in the year, it is possible to assess the number of cage-days per year – in this case:
  100 x 365 = 36,500 cage-days of space available for housing cats.
- If this number is then divided by the overall average length of stay, the approximate number of cats that the shelter can rehome per year can be calculated:
  (100 x 365) ÷ 23.6 = 1546 cats per year
- If the proposed biosecurity plan means that only 20% of cats get FURTD instead of 30%, the average length of stay drops to:
  (0.2 x 32) + (0.8 x 20) = 22.4 days
  a decrease of just over 1 day per cat.
- Taken at face value, this might not seem like much. However, this decrease means the shelter could rehome approximately:
  (100 x 365) ÷ 22.4 = 1629 cats per year
  which is equivalent to an extra 83 cats or 5% more cats rehomed per year.

Cat 'flu has been used here only as an example – shelter veterinary surgeons can choose the outcome that is most important to the shelter, or perhaps one that is most easily measured – but this example shows the power of this kind of data to demonstrate how relatively small changes can have a powerful impact in the longer term. It can also be used to persuade shelter staff to make a change and show them very clearly how that change is impacting on the things that are most important to them.

Basics of analysing population-level medical metrics

When considering levels of disease in a population, the most intuitive measure is typically the prevalence. Prevalence is simply a spot measure of what proportion of animals have a given disease at a given point in time (this point may be 'today', 'this month' or 'this year').

For example, if we counted 15 out of a total of 50 dogs in a shelter as having CIRD/'kennel cough' today, the point prevalence would be 15/50, or 30%.

As a simple starting point, it is possible to chart the prevalence of the disease in question over a period of time (Figure 7.7), to provide a very approximate measure of changes in health.

Month	Number of dogs in shelter	Number of cases of kennel cough	% of dogs with kennel cough during the month
January	52	10	19.2
February	28	6	21.4
March	66	15	22.7
April	39	6	15.3
May	54	7	13
June	61	7	11.5

7.7 Example of monitoring the percentage of cases of a disease (the disease prevalence) on a monthly basis. CIRD = canine infectious respiratory disease.

The above approach provides a rough estimate of disease levels and can be a useful way to start disease monitoring. However, the usefulness of prevalence as a measure for monitoring disease is limited by the fact that prevalence is affected by how long a disease lasts clinically as well as how infectious it is. For example, if a dog with CIRD typically coughs for 3 weeks post infection, and prevalence is assessed by counting on a weekly basis, the same dogs will end up being counted three times.

For this reason, the most useful medical metrics for evaluating population health are measures of the incidence of disease. Incidence measures the risk of developing a particular disease in a population. Note that 'cumulative

▶

Basics of analysing population-level medical metrics *continued*

incidence' is, strictly speaking, the term used in relation to measuring the risk of developing disease, but in the veterinary literature it is often used interchangeably with 'incidence' or 'incidence rate'. For readers interested in conducting epidemiological research in shelters, references that discuss incidence density are listed at the end of this chapter (Rothman, 2012; Fletcher *et al.*, 2014; Gordis, 2014). To calculate cumulative incidence, a time period of interest is specified (e.g. a year, a season, a month) and the number of **newly diagnosed** cases of a specific disease that occurred in that period is counted. These newly diagnosed cases are called 'incident cases'.

For example, if a shelter sees 33 newly diagnosed cases of CIRD in September, then the shelter had 33 incident cases of kennel cough in that month. By itself, the number of incident cases is potentially misleading, as it is unclear how many dogs were also in the shelter but did not develop CIRD during the same period.

To make the number more meaningful, the number of incident cases is divided by the total number of animals at risk of developing the disease of interest. For example, if 28 new cases of CPV are diagnosed in July and there are 140 dogs at risk of developing the disease during that time, then the cumulative incidence of CPV for the month is 28/140, or 20%. Other ways of expressing the same data are to say that the probability that a dog developed CPV in July is 20%, or one in five dogs became ill with CPV. The total number of new cases during a period of time can be calculated by some shelter software, in a spreadsheet that the veterinary surgeon maintains, or by some other method of the veterinary surgeon's choosing. Regardless of the method chosen, the diagnosis, the date of diagnosis and a unique identifier for each affected animal must be collected for each disease in the shelter's disease surveillance plan.

How is the population at risk defined?

For most diseases, the answer to this question is impossible to know definitively. That said, the 'at risk' population can be estimated using the best available information. Animals in the shelter that already have the disease or have recovered from the disease before the period of interest began are not counted. See Figure 7.8 for sample data for a theoretical shelter and a worked example of calculating cumulative incidence using a formula. Figure 7.9 shows a step-by-step 'recipe' for calculating cumulative incidence, using the same sample data, which some readers may find easier to follow. Note that if the numbers of animals that have recovered or currently have the disease are small, they can be ignored. This makes the calculation simpler without jeopardizing its value.

The cumulative incidence data from a previous year or years can be used to anticipate what might occur in the future if the characteristics of animals entering the shelter

1. Identify the total intake for the period (e.g. August) = 111.
2. Subtract cats that entered the shelter with FURTD from those entering in August (111 – 6 = 105). These are the cats at risk of FURTD that entered in August.
3. Get the cat census (i.e. total number of cats already resident) for August 1 (= 39).
4. Count the number of cats with FURTD on August 1 (do not include cats entering the shelter with FURTD on August 1 (= 11).
5. Count the cats in the shelter on August 1 that have recovered from FURTD (= 3). This is often a small number and, if so, can be ignored.
6. Add the cats with FURTD on August 1 (Q 4) to those that have recovered from FURTD (Q 5) (11 + 3 = 14). These cats are not at risk of FURTD in August.
7. Subtract the sum of those with FURTD on August 1 and recovered from FURTD on August 1, (those in Q 6), from the cat census on August 1 (39 – 14 = 25). These are the cats in the shelter on August 1 that remain at risk of FURTD.
8. Now add the cats entering the shelter at risk to those in the shelter at risk on August 1 (105 + 25 = 130). These are all of the cats at risk in August of developing FURTD.
9. Of these 130 cats at risk, 35 or 26.9% developed FURTD $\left(\frac{35}{130 \times 100\%}\right)$.

7.9 Steps to estimate the population at risk and cumulative incidence of feline upper respiratory tract disease (FURTD) for the shelter in Figure 7.8.

(e.g. age), and conditions within the shelter do not change much from year to year. For example, a shelter could ask the question 'What is the probability that a cat entering the shelter this August will develop FURTD?' Using the data for the number of cats that entered last year in August, their FURTD status at entry and the number of those cats that went on to develop FURTD, one could estimate how many cats entering the shelter this August would be expected to develop the disease. This can also be used to monitor progress year on year, which can be useful for diseases that have a seasonal component which makes month-by-month monitoring more difficult to interpret.

Which diseases should be part of the surveillance programme?

Diseases that are most frequent or severe should be routinely monitored. The diagnoses of interest must be agreed upon, defined and recorded in a standard fashion by the veterinary surgeon, Executive Director of the shelter and other relevant staff members. The list of diseases needs to be practical. Attempting to monitor too many diseases

Description of data	Values
Time frame	*August*
Number of newly diagnosed FURTD cases that developed in the shelter in August	35
Cats that entered in August with FURTD	6
Cats already in the shelter on August 1 with FURTD	11
Cats in the shelter on August 1 that had recovered from FURTD while in the shelter prior to August 1	3
Total intake of cats in August	111
Total cats in shelter on August 1	39
Therefore total number of cats at risk in August = **(Cat intake – those entering with FURTD) + (cats in the shelter on August 1 – cats with FURTD on August 1 – cats recovered from FURTD while in the shelter prior to August 1)**	

Cumulative incidence (C.I.) = $\dfrac{\text{Number of new cases}}{\text{Population at risk}}$

Cumulative incidence = $\dfrac{\text{Number of animals that developed FURTD in August}}{\text{Total number of cats at risk in August}}$

Plugging into the formula:

Cumulative Incidence = $\dfrac{35}{(111-6) + (39-11-3)} = \dfrac{35}{130} = 0.269$ or 26.9%

7.8 Example of the calculation of the cumulative incidence of feline upper respiratory tract disease (FURTD) among cats in a shelter in the month of August.

can overwhelm staff, leading to failure to record findings consistently and, ultimately to inaccurate, incomplete or inconsistent data. The goal is to record quality information that enables the shelter to set and evaluate progress towards goals of minimizing disease.

Once the diseases of interest have been identified, protocols should be developed to help ensure that accurate and complete data are collected. The protocols must describe the criteria by which each disease is identified and what should be entered on the record, when and by whom. If and when the shelter makes changes to disease definitions or diagnosis lists, record when and why the changes were made in a Log of Events and Changes in Protocols. This will enhance the veterinary surgeon's ability to interpret the medical data in the future. The Log of Events and Changes in Protocols should include revisions to protocols, changes in policies and any other events (e.g. flooding) and their dates. This is essential because, for example, changes to disease definitions could affect how disease rates in the shelter are recorded over time and thus hinder accurate comparisons between periods of time.

How often should diseases be formally monitored?

How often particular diseases are monitored (defined as being counted, graphed and reviewed) depends on many factors. Diseases with a high incidence are usually monitored on a monthly basis, whereas the number of cases of a disease such as CPV might be reported only annually if it is rarely diagnosed in the shelter population. Incidences reviewed for periods of less than a month are usually highly variable because of the relatively small number of animals contributing to the data. In the midst of outbreaks, however, the incidence of new cases might be monitored much more frequently (e.g. daily) to track the effectiveness of control measures in bringing the outbreak under control.

Diseases that may recur while an animal is in the shelter

Some diseases (e.g. certain respiratory infections) may occur more than once in the same animal during a particular timeframe. Calculations of cumulative incidence are made on the basis of the first episode only. If a shelter is interested in recurring illnesses in a particular timeframe, however, second occurrences can be counted and the incidence of second occurrences reported separately. When the incidence of second occurrences is calculated, the denominator should include only animals that have had a first occurrence as the animals at risk of a recurrence of disease. Fortunately, most animals do not usually reside in a shelter long enough to experience a second occurrence of most diseases and, therefore, the numbers of recurrences are often ignored.

What if a diagnosis is not made?

It is not uncommon for shelter animals that show clinical signs to never receive a definitive diagnosis. For this reason, some software programs enable shelters to record both 'diagnoses' and 'clinical signs'. If recording software is not available, these data can be recorded in a spreadsheet or in a paper file. From a disease surveillance perspective, recording a definitive diagnosis is preferable, when it can be made. However, when this is not possible, recording and monitoring important clinical signs (e.g. diarrhoea, vomiting) is the next best approach and can also be very useful.

Length of stay

The time animals spend in a shelter is associated with their risk of developing infectious diseases. This has been documented for feline and canine respiratory and gastro-intestinal infections, but is probably true for other infectious diseases as well (Edinboro et al., 2004; Dinnage et al., 2009; Stavisky et al., 2012). This is a function of both the increasing opportunity for exposure to infectious agents as time passes and the stress associated with residence in a shelter (as stress can adversely affect the immune response). Length of stay also affects the efficiency of flow of animals through the shelter, the likelihood of overcrowding and the per-animal costs of care. Therefore, strategies to minimize the average (mean or median) length of stay of animals in the shelter population must be an integral part of the shelter's health management programme. As such, the average length of stay should be monitored routinely.

Capacity

As discussed above, an excessively long mean or median length of stay can significantly affect a shelter's ability to provide good-quality care and its housing capacity. Exceeding the shelter's housing capacity (overcrowding) and the staff's ability to provide adequate care will both have adverse effects on the welfare of shelter animals and their risk of disease.

When collating length of stay data, it can be useful to divide it into two periods of time:

* The time from when the animal enters the shelter to when it is ready for rehoming
* The time from when the animal is ready for rehoming to when it is rehomed.

The first period correlates with how efficient the shelter is in terms of its intake, assessment and clinical procedures, while the second correlates with how 'rehomeable' the animal is and how efficient the rehoming processes are.

If there is an extended length of time between an animal entering a shelter and being declared 'fit for rehoming', protocols for assessment and isolation should be reviewed to ensure there is no unnecessary delay. If, on the other hand, there is typically a long period of time between an animal being 'fit for rehoming' and actually leaving, the rehoming protocols should be examined to identify unnecessary barriers or delays to the rehoming process.

It may seem counterintuitive to increase throughput by decreasing the number of animals housed in a shelter. However, routinely exceeding the shelter's ideal capacity can have severe consequences. Rising stress levels and disease burden associated with overcrowding will lead to an increase in the average length of stay. A lack of reserve capacity limits the shelter's ability to deal with unexpected admissions or disease outbreaks, leading to increased transmission of disease. Therefore, by contributing to an increase in disease rates and consequently extending the average length of stay, adding 'just a few' extra animals in excess of the ideal capacity can actually decrease throughput. By maintaining strict control of the number of animals admitted, the shelter may well be able to care for more animals overall. Projects based on this principle have succeeded in increasing shelter throughput (for more information, see Newbury et al., 2010). Other metrics regarding both housing and staff capacity have been developed (Newbury and Hurley, 2013).

Example – managing length of stay

A shelter established the goal of reducing the median length of stay of animals in early 2016. The strategies instituted to meet this goal were daily rounds (to ensure efficient movement of animals) and scheduling owner surrenders. Daily rounds include determining what happens next for each animal and assigning a member of staff who is responsible for ensuring that the next action happens in a timely manner. Planned relinquishments by owners can be pre-scheduled (perhaps by using a waiting list) and unscheduled walk-in relinquishments discouraged so that housing space in the shelter is used optimally. The effectiveness of these efforts is reflected in the decline in the median length of stay in 2016 and 2017 shown in Figure 7.10.

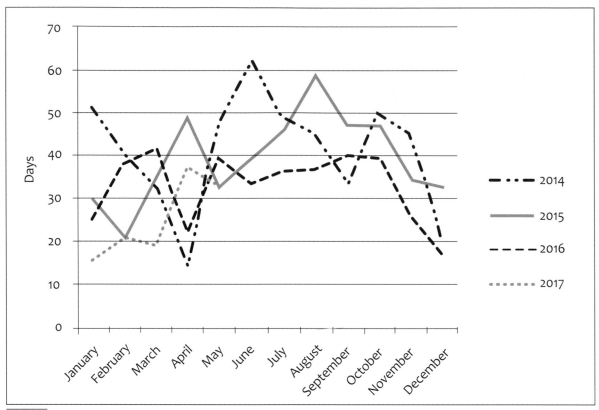

7.10 Median length of stay (in days) by month for cats in Somewhere Shelter from January 2014 to May 2017.

The added benefit of making these changes was reflected in declining rates of FURTD in this shelter's cats (data not shown).

The shelter also documented the impact of FURTD on the cost of care of their cats. They showed that 'cat 'flu' more than tripled the cats' length of stay. These data were presented to the shelter's Board of Directors as a powerful message that changes to the shelter's protocols were needed (Figure 7.11).

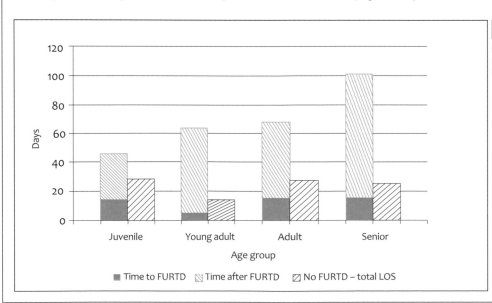

7.11 Effect of feline upper respiratory tract disease (FURTD) on the median length of stay (LOS) of cats by age group in Somewhere Shelter in 2017.

Example – monitoring capacity and overcrowding

A shelter counted the cages in all areas of the shelter to estimate its total housing capacity for dogs (Figure 7.12, dashed line). The shelter then plotted the average monthly census of dogs in the shelter on a graph for several years after initiating changes to reduce the average length of stay and to relieve overcrowding. With time, this shelter was able to reduce its dog population and avoid periodic overcrowding. This led to decreased disease rates and an increase in the number of dogs which the shelter was able to rehome each year.

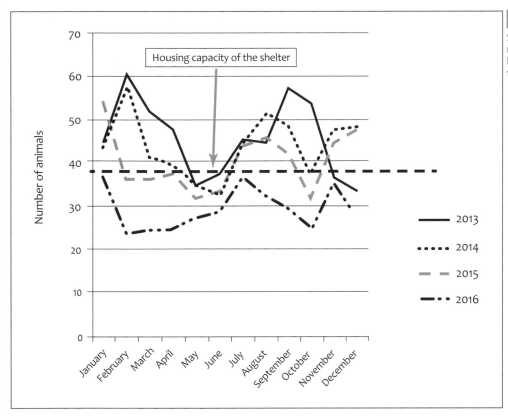

7.12 Graph of the average daily census of dogs in Somewhere Shelter by year in relation to the shelter's dog housing capacity (indicated with the dashed line) from 2013 to 2016.

Example – occupancy and throughput

Relationship between:

- Occupancy (average number of animals at the shelter)
- Throughput (average number of animals entering/ leaving the shelter per day)
- Length of stay (average length of stay in days):

    **Estimated occupancy =
    Throughput × Average length of stay**

So, for example, if three animals leave the shelter on a daily basis and their average length of stay is 15 days, then the shelter will need approximately 45 pens/kennels or animals on site to meet this throughput. Having too many animals leads to stagnation and unnecessarily increased overheads (Figure 7.13). Paradoxically, if the length of stay can be reduced, then for the same throughput, the number of animals on site can also be reduced, leading to cost savings and an improved environment for the animals.

In any shelter organization, a key performance indicator is likely to be the number of animals taken in over a specified period of time (which, over time, must equal the number of animals that leave the shelter). The outcome for these animals may include rehoming, reclaiming or euthanasia, depending on the situation and the type of shelter.

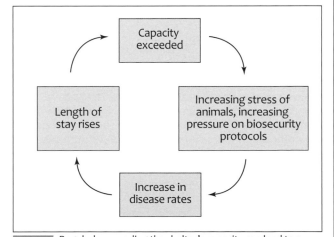

7.13 Regularly exceeding the shelter's capacity can lead to a vicious cycle, causing increased average length of stay, declining animal health and welfare and increases in stress to both the staff and animals. Although it may seem counterintuitive, reducing the number of animals in the shelter can be a powerful tool to promote health and welfare, and actually increase overall rehoming rates.

Why have shelter veterinary surgeons been slow to utilize metrics in population health programmes?

Various metrics have been integral to herd health for livestock species for decades. For example, the calving interval and incidence of mastitis are two of the many metrics routinely used by dairy veterinary surgeons to inform and guide their herd health programmes (Figure 7.14). There are numerous reasons why health-related metrics are not more widely used in animal shelters, including:

- Rudimentary training in and understanding of 'herd health' by veterinary surgeons as it relates to companion animal health
- The time and difficulty involved in recording the data
- Difficulty in retrieving the necessary data if it has been recorded
- Fear of 'stats' and lack of skills to conceive pertinent questions and interpret the numerical answers
- Lack of explicit population-level health goals.

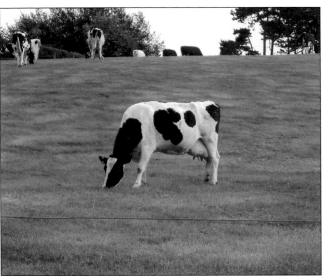

7.14 Metrics are a familiar means of proactively addressing health concerns in dairy cattle.
(© Jenny Stavisky)

Although veterinary students receive training in herd health for livestock species, veterinary surgeons rarely use metrics when practising companion animal medicine. Most companion animal practitioners work primarily with individual animals, and those who work with catteries or kennels often have no access to summary health metrics for these populations. These practitioners are likely to be unfamiliar with setting and monitoring population health goals and, since they do not routinely use summary metrics, they may lack skills to analyse and interpret such data. In addition, shelter-specific software is relatively new and, while constantly improving, the companies producing these programs have not made medical data entry and retrieval a high priority until recently. Many shelter veterinary surgeons, including those in academia, have been frustrated by the time and effort required to enter their medical data and as a consequence have not used (nor taught the extensive use of) medical metrics. The good news is that this situation is changing, and in the next several years, medical data should become more readily available to shelter veterinary surgeons.

Summary

Metrics are a vital component of any population health management programme, including those in shelters. They are the basis for disease surveillance and enable shelter veterinary surgeons to assess the effectiveness of their disease prevention and control recommendations and protocols. Disease management strategies do not always work as predicted in all populations and, even when they are effective, the degree of effectiveness can vary widely. Shelter veterinary surgeons must know whether and how well their population health measures are working, and be prepared to be adaptive and try different strategies – there is no 'one size fits all' approach to varied shelter populations.

Metrics also help to identify new goals for continuously reducing the incidence of disease. They facilitate communication regarding the welfare of a shelter's animals with the shelter's many stakeholders (including staff members, those on the Board of Directors, donors and people within the local community). Since veterinary surgeons rely heavily on shelter staff and volunteers to implement animal health protocols, demonstrating changes in disease rates can be a powerful motivator for these people to adhere to shelter protocols.

Tools for the entry and retrieval of medical information are improving. However, veterinary surgeons must insist that progress continues until such time as they can easily access population metrics that are essential to providing optimal 'herd health' for shelter animals. Optimal population health is synonymous with minimizing disease and the suffering that accompanies it.

References and further reading

Cannas da Silva J, Noordhuizen JP, Vagneur M *et al.* (2006) Veterinary dairy herd health management in Europe: constraints and perspectives. *Veterinary Quarterly* **28**, 23–32

Dinnage J, Scarlett JM and Richards JR (2009) Descriptive epidemiology of feline upper respiratory tract disease in an animal shelter. *Journal of Feline Medicine and Surgery* **11**, 817–825

Dwyer D, Groves C and Blythe D (2014) Surveillance and outbreak detection. In: *Infectious Disease Epidemiology, 3rd edn*, ed. KE Nelson and C Masters Williams, pp. 106–107. Jones & Bartlett Learning, Burlington

Edinboro CH, Ward MP and Glickman LT (2004) A placebo-controlled trial of two intranasal vaccines to prevent tracheobronchitis (kennel cough) in dogs entering a humane shelter. *Preventive Veterinary Medicine* **62**, 89–99

Fletcher RH, Fletcher SW and Fletcher GS (2014) *Clinical Epidemiology. The Essentials*. Wolters Kluwer/Lippincott Williams & Wilkins, Philadelphia

Gordis L (2014) *Epidemiology, 5th edn*. Elsevier Saunders, Philadelphia

Hurley KF (2004) Implementing a population health plan in an animal shelter: goal setting, data collection and monitoring, and policy development. In *Shelter Medicine for Veterinarians and Staff, 1st edn*, ed. L Miller and S Zawistowski, pp. 211–234. Blackwell Publishing, Ames, Iowa

Newbury S, Blinn MK, Bushby PA *et al.* (2010) *Guidelines for Standards of Care in Animal Shelters*. www.sheltervet.org/assets/docs/shelter-standards-oct2011-wforward.pdf

Newbury S and Hurley K (2013) Population management. In: *Shelter Medicine for Veterinarians and Staff, 2nd edn*, ed. L Miller and S Zawistowski, pp. 93–113. Wiley-Blackwell, Ames, Iowa

Oxford Dictionaries (2014a) Metrics. Available from: www.oxforddictionaries.com/us/definition/american_english/metrics

Oxford Dictionaries (2014b) Metric. Available from: www.oxforddictionaries.com/us/definition/english/metric

Rothman KJ (2012) *Epidemiology: An Introduction, 2nd edn*. Oxford University Press, Oxford

Salman M (2003) Surveillance and monitoring systems for animal health programs and disease surveys. In: *Animal Disease Surveillance and Survey Systems: Methods and Applications*, ed. M Salman, pp. 3–13. Iowa State Press and Blackwell Publishing, Ames, Iowa

Scarlett JM (2013) Epidemiology of infectious diseases in shelter populations. In: *Shelter Medicine for Veterinarians and Staff, 2nd edn*, ed. L Miller and S Zawistowski, pp. 287–296. Wiley-Blackwell, Ames, Iowa

Stavisky J, Pinchbeck G, Gaskell RM *et al.* (2012) Cross sectional and longitudinal surveys of canine enteric coronavirus infection in kennelled dogs: a molecular marker for biosecurity. *Infections, Genetics and Evolution* **12(7)**, 1419–1426

Chapter 8

Principles of infectious disease and transmission

Jenny Stavisky and Wendy Adams

Overview of infectious pathogens

Infectious diseases can be a major problem in the shelter environment. This chapter provides a very brief overview of the infectious agents that can cause disease, how the pathogens of importance are transmitted, and how they might be managed and treated. Specific important infectious diseases are dealt with in their own chapters within this section of the manual.

Viruses

A virus is a package of genetic material, along with essential replication equipment. Viruses cannot replicate alone; they need a host cell in order to reproduce.

The genetic material of viruses may exist as single-stranded or double-stranded deoxyribonucleic acid (DNA) or ribonucleic acid (RNA). DNA viruses tend to have stable genomes that mutate relatively rarely. An example would be feline herpesvirus (FHV), which exists as a single strain, FHV-1; as a consequence, all cats infected with FHV have a genetically similar virus, which behaves in a predictable manner.

In contrast, RNA viruses, such as feline calicivirus (FCV), mutate readily. This is due in large part to their replication equipment: in order to reproduce, they require RNA polymerase, which lacks a 'proofreading' function, making it prone to copying error. Therefore, when RNA viruses replicate, an assorted population of similar viruses is produced; these are known as 'quasispecies'. Some of these mutated versions will be poorly adapted to survive and will die out, while others will have adaptations that allow them to thrive or alter their virulence. This means that RNA viruses are more variable and changeable than DNA viruses and, as a consequence, a greater variety of clinical signs can be associated with them. In an outbreak, or sometimes even within an infected individual, this means that an infection can consist of a population of closely related, similar viruses rather than a single strain. This changeable nature can also make development of vaccines and diagnostic tests for RNA viruses more difficult.

Enveloped viruses are surrounded by a fragile layer of phospholipid, often derived from the host cell membrane. They are reliant on the integrity of this structure to survive, so enveloped viruses tend to be relatively easily killed by heat, cold, ultraviolet (UV) light and a wide variety of disinfectants, although there is some variation between different viruses. Examples of enveloped viruses include canine coronavirus (Figure 8.1), FHV and feline leukaemia virus (FeLV). Conversely, non-enveloped viruses are environmentally stable and can survive for months or even years, given the right conditions. Examples of non-enveloped viruses include canine parvovirus (CPV) and FCV.

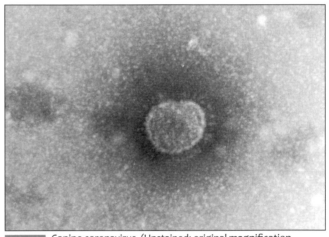

8.1 Canine coronavirus. (Unstained; original magnification X200,000)
(Courtesy of B Getty)

Bacteria

Bacteria are single-celled organisms that are able to replicate independently from their host. They have larger and more complex DNA genomes in comparison to viruses, and therefore are able to produce a greater variety of cellular structures. In addition to nuclear DNA, some bacteria also have plasmids, which are circular arrays of DNA that can be transferred between bacteria of the same and different species. Plasmids can contain genes that confer resistance to one or more antimicrobial agents.

Bacteria are typically subdivided into Gram-positive and Gram-negative types. These terms refer to their appearance when stained with Gram stain and viewed under a light microscope (Figure 8.2). The structural relevance of this is that Gram stain clings to bacterial cell walls; Gram-positive bacteria have a thick peptidoglycan cell wall, whereas Gram-negative bacteria have a thinner cell wall, but a complex lipopolysaccharide cell envelope covalently linked to the cell wall.

A different classification of bacteria is also made on the basis of their morphological appearance on microscopy.

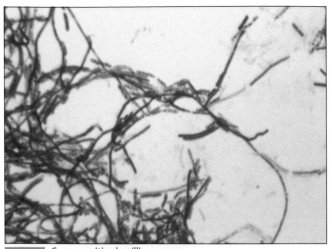

8.2 Gram-positive bacilli.
(Reproduced from the *BSAVA Textbook of Veterinary Nursing, 5th edition*)

Cocci are round, whereas bacilli are linear or sometimes spiral (spirochaetes) (Figure 8.3). Bacteria can also be classified according to the type of habitat they favour. Some bacteria flourish best in aerobic environments while others are adapted to survive in anaerobic conditions, and others can survive only in an intracellular environment. This has clear implications for where on or in the body each type of bacteria is likely to be found, and also for transmission – for example, bacteria surviving in the anaerobic environment of the gut are more likely to be transmitted via the faecal–oral route, and bacteria that survive only as intracellular pathogens (such as *Chlamydia felis*) are likely to require close body contact for transmission between individuals to occur.

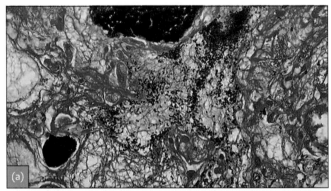

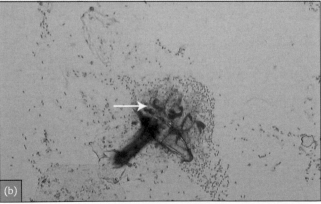

8.3 (a) Cocci seen in this smear are stained blue. (Diff-Quik® stain; original magnification X63) (b) Bacilli can be seen in this smear taken from a dog with otitis caused by *Pseudomonas aeruginosa*. Some of the bacteria have been taken up by neutrophils (arrowed). (Diff-Quik® stain; original magnification X63)
(a, Courtesy of L Grau Roma; b, © Jenny Stavisky)

Mycoplasmas

Mycoplasmas are another subset of bacteria, but are often regarded separately. They are small and fastidious, and lack a cell wall; as such they are unique among prokaryotes. They are relatively frequently identified as commensals in the upper respiratory and urogenital tract. They may act as primary pathogens in their own right, or as secondary invaders in complex multifactorial infections such as canine infectious respiratory disease and feline upper respiratory tract disease ('kennel cough' and 'cat 'flu'; see Chapters 14 and 15). Another example, *Mycoplasma haemofelis* (formerly *Haemobartonella felis*), can vary in its ability to cause clinically significant haemolytic anaemia, with flare-ups of clinical disease when an infected animal is stressed or immunocompromised.

Protozoa

Protozoa are among the simplest eukaryotes. Although they are single-celled organisms, they have organelles and their genetic material (DNA) is contained within a membrane-bound nucleus. Their structure is relatively complex compared with that of bacteria, and some species have structures for propulsion or other types of movement; for example, *Tritrichomonas foetus* is flagellated and highly motile (Figure 8.4). Protozoa are found worldwide and in most habitats. The majority are free-living but most higher animals, including mammals, are host to one or more species of protozoa, which cause infections ranging from asymptomatic to life-threatening.

The most common form of reproduction in protozoa is simple asexual binary fission. However, the pathogenic protozoans often have more complex life cycles that include both sexual and asexual multiplication. Typically, there will be stages of feeding and multiplication called trophozoites, although the terminology is different for some pathogenic species. Cysts are stages with a protective membrane, the thickness of which may depend on whether or not the cyst needs to survive outside a host species. The cystic stages are important in transmission from host to host, whereas non-encysted stages are generally associated with feeding and multiplication within a host.

Fungi

The fungi comprise a huge and diverse group of organisms, of which relatively few are of clinical importance. They range from single-celled organisms such as yeasts

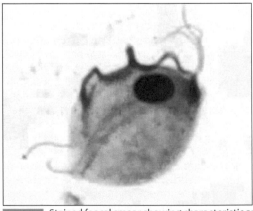

8.4 Stained faecal smear showing characteristic appearance of *Tritrichomonas foetus* with its long undulating membrane.
(Reproduced from the *BSAVA Manual of Canine and Feline Gastroenterology, 2nd edition*)

(Figure 8.5) to complex multicellular organisms such as mushrooms, and may reproduce sexually or asexually. Some species undergo both modes of reproduction depending on the environment in which they are growing; for example, *Candida* spp. grow as mycelia in the external environment, but become vegetatively reproducing ('budding') yeast in the body.

Mycoses (diseases caused by fungi) are classified by the site of infection (superficial, cutaneous, subcutaneous or systemic) and by whether the fungus is a primary or opportunistic pathogen. In the context of shelter medicine, the important diseases are generally superficial or cutaneous and are caused by primary pathogens, the most common being the dermatophytes. An outbreak of dermatophytosis can be challenging to manage and treat in the shelter environment (see Chapter 16).

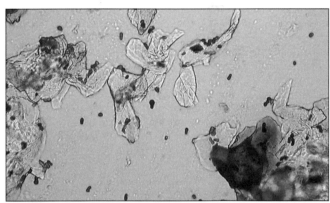

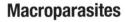 *Malassezia* in a smear taken from the ear of a dog with otitis. (Diff-Quik® stain; original magnification X63)

(© Jenny Stavisky)

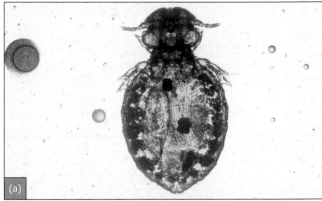

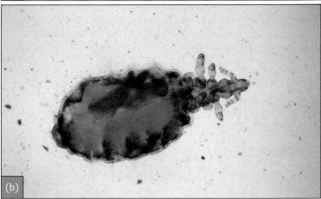

8.6 Microscopic appearance of ectoparasites. (a) The canine biting louse *Trichodectes canis*, suspended in liquid paraffin. (Original magnification X100) (b) The canine sucking louse *Linognathus setosus*, suspended in liquid paraffin. (Original magnification X100)
(Reproduced from the BSAVA Manual of Canine and Feline Dermatology, 3rd edition)

Macroparasites

Macroparasites are multicellular organisms that are, at least in some life stages, visible to the naked eye. They can be broadly categorized into ectoparasites (living on the outside of the body) and endoparasites (living inside the body) (see also Chapter 11).

Ectoparasites include fleas, lice, mites and ticks (Figure 8.6). They typically feed on debris of the skin and hair coat, secretions, and blood via skin puncture. They may cause disease syndromes directly – for example, a severe infestation of fleas can cause anaemia, most commonly seen in young kittens. Sometimes, ectoparasites will trigger an allergic reaction, producing disease indirectly, and some may act as a vector for another infectious agent; for example, ticks can carry *Borrelia burgdorferi*, the causative agent of Lyme disease (see Chapter 16).

Endoparasites include a variety of helminths, including roundworms, tapeworms and flukes. Several nematodes are commonly found in the gastrointestinal tract in cats and dogs, including *Toxocara* spp., *Toxascaris leonina*, and *Ancylostoma* spp. (see Chapter 11). All can be transmitted by the faecal–oral route, and also during lactation in both cats and dogs and transplacentally in dogs. These latter routes of transmission can lead to heavy infestations and severe disease in puppies and kittens.

Managing macroparasites in a shelter setting should be relatively straightforward, comprising the administration of broad-spectrum parasiticides as part of the admission protocol for new animals entering the shelter, and regular treatment at appropriate intervals (see Chapter 11).

Routes of transmission

A detailed description of the various routes of transmission for the vast array of infectious agents is outside the scope of this chapter and is covered elsewhere in this section of the manual.

In general terms, a useful option of looking at the ways in which infectious diseases are transmitted is in the context of an animal's 'journey' through the shelter.

What animals bring into the shelter

An asymptomatic animal can bring almost any infectious disease into the shelter. It is, therefore, prudent to have a separate area of the shelter for new arrivals where they can be quarantined from the rest of the shelter population. Clearly, any sick animals should be identified and treated on arrival, but some individuals may not be overtly ill on admission but develop clinical signs within a few days. The incubation period of the more important infectious diseases should be used to inform the period of quarantine. However, for many diseases carriage is possible, and so the absence of clinical signs does not always indicate absence of infection.

What animals pick up in the shelter

The environment in most shelters increases the risk for disease transmission. There are frequently relatively large numbers of animals of the same species in a relatively small, confined space and the environment can be stressful, compromising the animals' immunity.

What comes into the shelter from other sources

Other sources of infectious agents might include staff and volunteers working with the animals, visitors to the shelter, and pathogens carried by insect or other wildlife vectors.

What animals leave the shelter with

Ideally, infectious diseases are identified and treated, or prevented by vaccination or prophylactic parasite control, while the animal is in the shelter. However, this is not always the case, as being in a shelter environment typically increases the risk of acquiring an infection, which may be clinical or subclinical. This raises the questions of how much screening should take place for asymptomatic infectious disease, and what should be done with animals that are found to carry disease.

Risk factors for disease transmission, infection and outbreak

Some outbreaks of disease occur when a single pathogen emerges within a susceptible population. Recent examples of this include canine influenza in racing greyhounds, *Streptococcus equi* subspecies *zooepidemicus* in shelter dogs and virulent systemic FCV in cats. However, more commonly, outbreaks result from the interplay between a number of factors. Even relatively small changes in some of these factors can cumulatively lead to a tipping point where the pathogen overcomes the host's defences. These factors can be broadly separated into three categories: those relating to the pathogen, the host and the environment.

Pathogen factors

Virulence

Virulence, or the capacity of a pathogen to cause disease, is a key factor in determining the clinical outcome. From an evolutionary perspective, some organisms are adapted to cause very virulent disease, as this aids their transmission. An example of this is CPV. By causing acute profuse diarrhoea, the virus is excreted at high levels, maximizing its chances of being transmitted. For other diseases, low-grade long-term shedding is a more successful evolutionary strategy. Many feline viruses use this strategy, possibly because the ancestors of modern domestic cats lived largely solitary lives. Pathogens that evolved to cause infections that slowly 'smoulder' for long periods and emerge when the cat was likely to come into contact with conspecifics have persisted and retained their relationship with their host species. Hence, many feline diseases are either sexually or horizontally transmitted, or follow a pattern of chronic carriage followed by recrudescence under stress – and for a cat, close contact with other cats outside their social group is often a significant stressor.

Environmental persistence

The ability of a pathogen to persist in the environment is a key determinant of transmission route. If an organism cannot survive away from the host, it must rely on close contact for transmission. In contrast, spread via fomites is enhanced in organisms that can persist in the environment for long periods. As a general rule, many protozoa have good environmental persistence, and most helminths of dogs have a life stage with environmental persistence. There is variation between bacteria; for example, intracellular bacteria, such as *Chlamydia felis*, do not persist well outside the host, whereas clostridial species produce spores that are tough and can survive for long periods. Enveloped viruses, such as canine distemper virus and FeLV, generally do not persist in the environment, and are easily killed by most disinfectants, whereas non-enveloped viruses, such as CPV and FCV, are very successfully spread by fomites due to their greater environmental persistence.

Species tropism

Some organisms are highly species-specific, and will therefore infect only one species or closely related species. An example is feline immunodeficiency virus (FIV), which will infect only cats or related Felidae (Figure 8.7). Most pathogens are at least partially host adapted, but some are markedly less fussy, for example, *Microsporum canis*, which will readily infect cats, dogs and humans, as well as other species. In between these two extremes are organisms that have a general preference for one species, but have adapted to cross species boundaries. Examples include CPV and *Bordetella bronchiseptica*, both of which

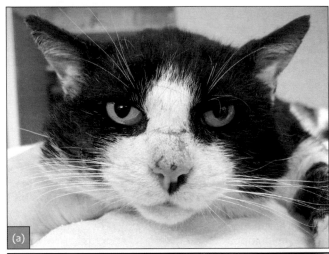

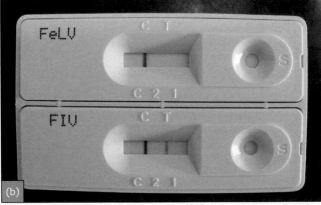

8.7 Feline immunodeficiency virus (FIV) is considered a relatively host-specific virus. (a) FIV is most commonly identified in feral or stray male cats and can be transmitted by deep bites. (b) Rapid diagnostic tests for FIV and feline leukaemia virus (FeLV), showing control (C) and test (T) bands in the window where the results are read. These samples are negative for FeLV and positive for FIV.
(Courtesy of R Elmore)

were initially thought to be restricted to dogs, but are now known to be transmissible to cats. This has clear implications for biosecurity (see Chapter 9) and population control measures, since isolation and quarantine must also be applied across species boundaries.

Host factors (individual and population)

Factors affecting individual host susceptibility include any process that impairs immune function. These factors include stress, nutrition, pregnancy, lactation, vaccination status, prior exposure and any concurrent infection, among many others. In a given population, therefore, the 'herd' susceptibility to disease will be determined by the proportions of immunocompetent and immunosuppressed individuals within the population.

The characteristics of the shelter population will affect the herd immunity. If a proportion of the population is resistant or immune to a disease, this will limit the number of animals that can be affected, and also reduce shedding and transmission. This provides a degree of protection to the population as a whole, and not just the immune individuals. Conversely, if the population is comprised of naive or immunocompromised individuals, this will raise the potential infectious burden throughout the whole population.

As an example, if a shelter has a large proportion of malnourished dogs that are largely unvaccinated, poorly socialized, poorly tolerant of kennelling and stressed, the population immunity against certain diseases is more likely to be low, and therefore there will be an increased risk of outbreaks (Figure 8.8). In contrast, if there is a high proportion of healthy, vaccinated, relinquished dogs, the population as a whole may show increased resistance to infection. These are generalizations – young, thin, stressed stray dogs will often be more susceptible to disease than relatively healthy, vaccinated owner-relinquished dogs. However, this is not a simple picture. Not all stray dogs are poorly socialized, and strays which have survived to adulthood in a disease-endemic environment may have a level of natural immunity. Some pet dogs that have lived only in a house with humans may find kennelling much more stressful than stray dogs. Additionally, although stray dogs may be more prone to having a low body condition score, obesity is much more prevalent in relinquished stray dogs, and this may also affect immune function. This means that careful consideration of the population entering the shelter, its composition and the likely impact on population immunity is essential in assessing the risk of infectious disease transmission and outbreaks.

The overall population make-up of a shelter will be governed by the organization's management practices and policies. Having a controlled intake will allow a degree of planning of resources and better utilization of quarantine facilities. However, some organizations cannot plan their intake, being tied to contracts (e.g. with local government) to house strays, or having large numbers of animals dumped or presented urgently. Management of intake, to protect incoming animals from endemic infections and resident animals from introduced infections, is of paramount importance. Further details can be found in Chapters 7 and 9. A brief summary of the interactions between management and environmental factors is provided below.

Environmental factors

The shelter environment should be considered, in the same way as any other animal housing. When working with a shelter it is important for the veterinary surgeon (veterinarian) to undertake a thorough visit and become familiar with the design features of the shelter such as ventilation, drainage and the presence of impervious surfaces for cleaning and disinfection (Figure 8.9). It is also important to take a full shelter history, playing close attention to biosecurity measures. Efforts to enrich the environment may compromise biosecurity, and decisions must be made according to the risks specific to the shelter population at that time as to whether to prioritize hygiene or stress reduction (Figure 8.10). For further detail, see Chapters 7 and 9.

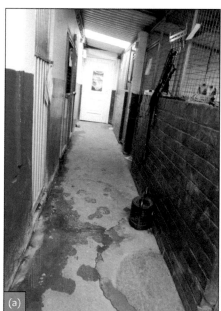

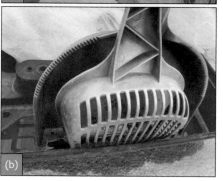

8.9 (a) Limited ventilation, cracked surfaces and poor drainage can contribute to disease persistence and transmission. If organic debris is not cleaned properly, disinfection will not be adequate. (b) This scoop was used for cleaning faeces from dog kennels, then left to soak in disinfectant without having been cleaned.
(© Jenny Stavisky)

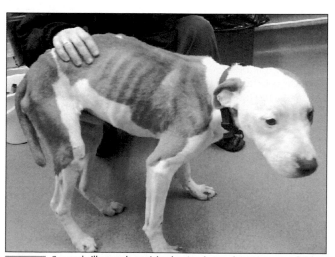

8.8 Severely ill or malnourished animals may be at increased risk of infectious disease.
(Courtesy of R Elmore)

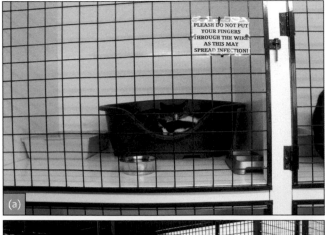

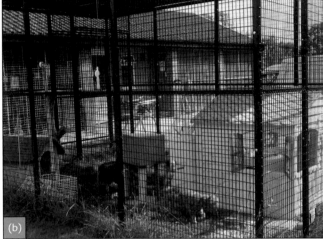

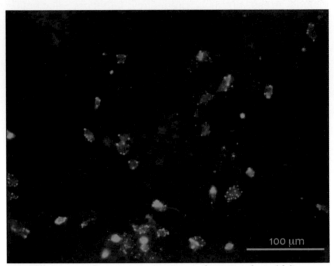

8.11   Immunofluorescent microscopy of FCV-F9 infected feline embryo A cells immunostained for FCV (green). FCV = feline calicivirus
(© A Radford and M Afonso)

8.10   (a) Barren environments are relatively easy to clean and disinfect. However, they can be highly stressful for residents. (b) Enriched environments are beneficial for reducing stress. However, in the event of an outbreak of disease, decontamination may be difficult.
(© Jenny Stavisky)

Diagnostic tests

Clinicians are often presented with animals showing a syndrome or collection of clinical signs rather than a single obvious diagnosis. Correspondingly, supportive symptomatic therapy is common, pragmatic and often the best course of action. However, diagnostic tests are a useful aid to decision-making where they are indicated. The converse statement is also true – that is, that a diagnostic test should be used only when its result will actually change a decision. This seems an obvious statement, but sometimes a diagnostic test is used in the hope of finding 'something' in a situation where a veterinary surgeon has reached a dead end on the basis of the clinical picture. Interpreting such a test, taken without a clear clinical rationale, can be difficult. It should also be remembered that a clinical history and a physical examination (whether of an individual or a population) are both types of diagnostic tests and are subject to the same strengths and limitations (such as sensitivity and specificity; see below) as laboratory procedures.

Immunoassays

Various types of immunoassays are available. These tests all rely on a simple basic principle – the specific selective binding that occurs between an antigen and its corresponding antibody. Some tests detect the presence of an antigen by presenting its matching antibody, while others detect the presence of antibody in a biological sample by providing an antigen within the test. The tests are designed so that if the target molecule is present and binding occurs, a signal is emitted, which can then be detected macroscopically. This signal may be a colour change, fluorescence or agglutination. Common types of test include immunofluorescence assays (IFA), enzyme-linked immunosorbent assays (ELISA), western blot and serum neutralization (Figure 8.11).

When interpreting an immunoassay, it is important to consider whether the test detects antigen or antibody. If antigen is detected, a positive result strongly suggests that the pathogen in question is present in the animal (although results should always be interpreted in the light of other clinical findings; see Sensitivity, specificity and predictive values, below). If the test detects antibody, this shows that the animal has been exposed to the pathogen in question. For some pathogens, such as FIV, this is diagnostic of current infection, since infection persists lifelong. Other pathogens, such as canine and feline coronavirus, are nearly ubiquitous, and therefore a single positive antibody test is typically unhelpful as it merely indicates that the animal has been exposed at some point in its life. Paired samples taken 2–4 weeks apart during the acute phase of infection, showing a greater than four-fold increase in antibody titre, are suggestive of active infection.

As for all other assays, false-positive results (cross-reaction with a molecule other than the target) and false-negative results (failure to detect the target when present) can occur (Figure 8.12).

Status	Test result	
	Positive	*Negative*
Animal is really infected	True-positive	False-negative
Animal is not really infected	False-positive	True-negative

8.12   Possible outcomes of diagnostic tests. When the test result is a real reflection of the status of the animal, the result is either a true-positive or a true-negative. Where the test result mistakenly identifies a non-infected animal as though it were infected, the result is termed 'false-positive'. Where the test fails to detect an infected animal, the result is termed 'false-negative'.

Polymerase chain reaction

Polymerase chain reaction (PCR) is a laboratory molecular diagnostic technique that has been developed relatively recently. It is very sensitive and versatile, and is based on a simple principle. PCR identifies positive samples by looking for a piece of genetic sequence that is uniquely present in the pathogen of interest. The assay identifies this piece of predictable target DNA, which will be present in every positive sample (Figure 8.13). A pair of primers, one targeted at each end of the target sequence, is added to the sample, along with a mixture of nucleotides, the building blocks for new DNA. The primers bind to the target sequence and a perfect copy of the target is created by nucleotides joining together. The reaction mixture is taken through a number of cycles of heating and cooling, during which the rounds of DNA replication occur. At the end of each cycle, if the target molecule is present, the number of copies doubles, giving an exponential increase in the quantity of a sequence of DNA of a very specific length. The reaction products are then introduced into one end of a gel made of agarose, separated out by applying an electric current across the gel (larger pieces of DNA move more slowly) and then stained with a chemical that binds to the DNA and enables it to be visualized (e.g. by fluorescence under UV light). If a band of DNA of the predicted size is present, the reaction is considered positive.

For viruses with an RNA genome, the process is similar, excepting that an initial step, called reverse transcription, is added to create a DNA 'mirror image' of the RNA molecule.

There are several adaptions of the conventional PCR method. 'Real-time' PCR, also known as quantitative PCR (qPCR), works on the same principles. However, instead of visualizing the product on a gel by staining it and examining the gel with the naked eye, which is a relatively crude and insensitive method, a fluorescently labelled dye is added to the mixture. The levels of fluorescence in the mixture are read by a machine at the end of each PCR cycle, allowing an assessment of the quantity of the target DNA in the initial mixture. This also provides the ability to detect samples at one-tenth, or even one-hundredth, the concentration of conventional PCR (Figure 8.14).

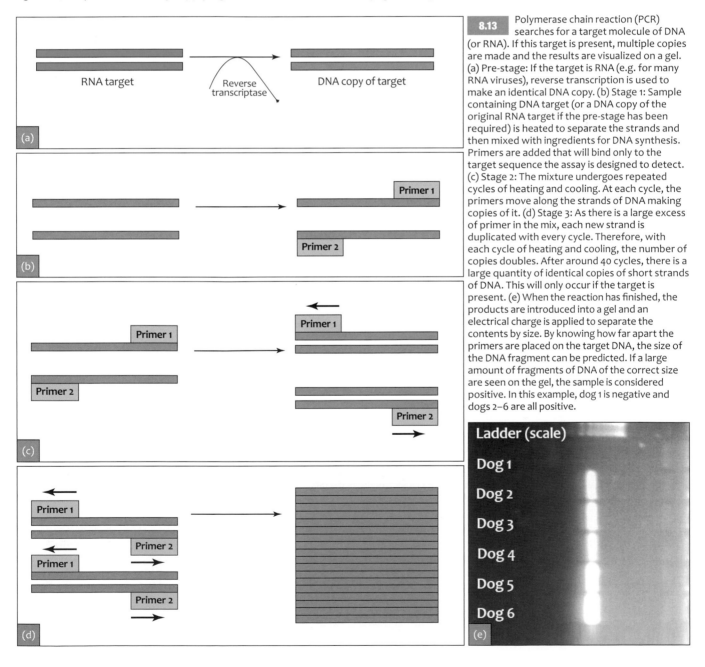

8.13 Polymerase chain reaction (PCR) searches for a target molecule of DNA (or RNA). If this target is present, multiple copies are made and the results are visualized on a gel. (a) Pre-stage: If the target is RNA (e.g. for many RNA viruses), reverse transcription is used to make an identical DNA copy. (b) Stage 1: Sample containing DNA target (or a DNA copy of the original RNA target if the pre-stage has been required) is heated to separate the strands and then mixed with ingredients for DNA synthesis. Primers are added that will bind only to the target sequence the assay is designed to detect. (c) Stage 2: The mixture undergoes repeated cycles of heating and cooling. At each cycle, the primers move along the strands of DNA making copies of it. (d) Stage 3: As there is a large excess of primer in the mix, each new strand is duplicated with every cycle. Therefore, with each cycle of heating and cooling, the number of copies doubles. After around 40 cycles, there is a large quantity of identical copies of short strands of DNA. This will only occur if the target is present. (e) When the reaction has finished, the products are introduced into a gel and an electrical charge is applied to separate the contents by size. By knowing how far apart the primers are placed on the target DNA, the size of the DNA fragment can be predicted. If a large amount of fragments of DNA of the correct size are seen on the gel, the sample is considered positive. In this example, dog 1 is negative and dogs 2–6 are all positive.

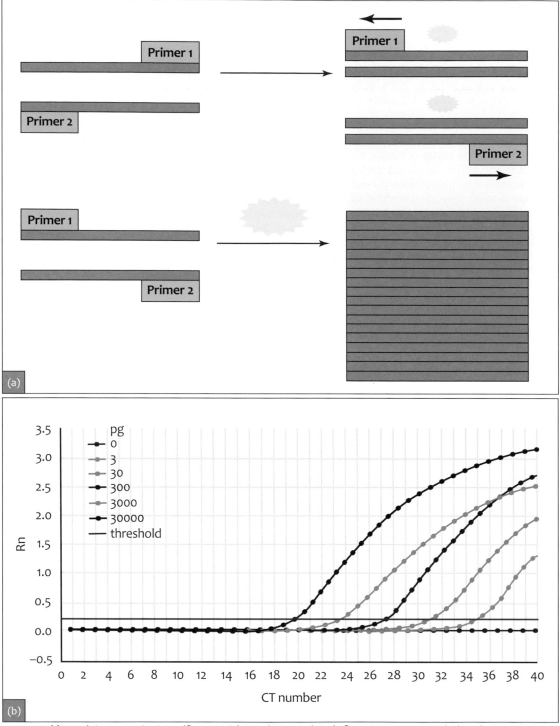

8.14 (a) In real-time, quantitative or 'fluorogenic' PCR, during each cycle fluorescence is emitted when the target sequence is duplicated. The amount of fluorescence generated in each cycle is proportional to the number of copies of the target present, and therefore increases with each cycle. (b) This fluorescence is measured by using a machine, rather than the naked eye, making real-time PCR 10–100 times as sensitive as conventional PCR. It is also possible to estimate the quantity of target that was present in the initial sample. This is because if more target is initially present, it will take fewer cycles of replication for the reaction to reach the threshold at which it can be detected. The number of cycles required to reach this is termed the cycle threshold (CT). Samples which have a larger amount of the target molecule will reach the threshold sooner and therefore have a lower CT number. Rn is a measure of the amount of fluorescence generated.

PCR is very sensitive and PCR tests are now the gold standard for detection for many infectious diseases. However, there are some limitations of using this method. When genetic material is detected at very low levels, it becomes difficult to be certain about the clinical relevance of a positive test. This is because PCR cannot differentiate live, viable infectious agents from dead material, so a positive PCR result does not always guarantee that the animal being tested has a viable infection.

False-positive tests can occur. The primers are highly specific, meaning they are unlikely to bind to anything but the target molecule. However, sample contamination, even on a microscopic level, can lead to a false-positive result. For this reason, good diagnostic laboratories should always run numerous negative controls to ensure any contamination is detected. False-negative results may also occur, especially with 'dirty' samples such as faeces, in which there are many other substances present that could degrade the target molecule. RNA is particularly sensitive to this type of degradation.

The final limitation is that, in order for PCR to function, the organism of interest needs to have a target region that is conserved – that is, a piece of genetic sequence common to every strain and variant. Whereas most organisms do have such conserved regions, there are a few, such as FCV, that are extremely genetically variable. This variability makes it difficult to design a consistent set of primers that will function with every positive sample. For such organisms, it is worth asking the diagnostic laboratory about their test sensitivity, and considering whether a different or additional type of test may be useful.

Bacterial culture and virus isolation

Bacterial culture is usually carried out on plates of growth media. If growth occurs on the plates, secondary testing, or culture on specific media, are carried out for typing. To determine antibacterial sensitivity, tiny discs impregnated with a series of different antibacterial agents are placed on the plate. The growth of susceptible bacteria will be suppressed by the relevant disc. The degree of sensitivity to each antibacterial is proportional to the amount of drug required to suppress bacterial growth, which corresponds to the size of the clear (bacteria-free) area around each disc (Figure 8.15).

Virus isolation works on similar principles. Viruses require living cells in order to replicate and, therefore,

virus culture is carried out on plates of cultured cells (or, occasionally, in organ culture). Viruses in a biological sample can be identified depending on which cell type they will grow in, and the pattern of cell death (cytopathic effect (CPE)) they produce (Figure 8.16). By attempting culture of serial dilutions of the sample, it is possible to obtain an estimate of the quantity of virus ('viral load') in the initial sample.

Both bacterial culture and virus isolation require there to be live, viable pathogen in the sample being tested. Therefore, if the test is positive, the result can usually be interpreted as reflecting a real, active infection (although this still does not necessarily mean the infection is the cause of the animal's clinical signs). However, some bacteria and viruses are not very environmentally resistant and may not survive well during transport of the sample to the diagnostic laboratory. This problem can be ameliorated to an extent by using appropriate transport materials (e.g. charcoal media when anaerobic infections are suspected; antibacterial viral transport media for viruses), carefully storing samples and ensuring they are not posted over weekends. However, some organisms can be damaged by transportation – for example, *Campylobacter* can enter a non-cultivable state, and many non-enveloped viruses can die quite quickly outside the host. Some organisms are fastidious and simply do not grow well in *in vitro* culture. In these instances, it is worth the veterinary surgeon discussing their clinical suspicions with the laboratory, to check whether additional or ancillary tests may be helpful.

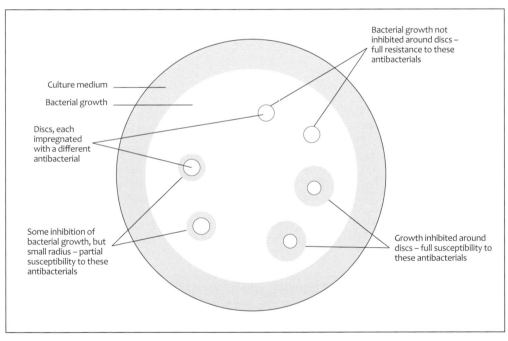

8.15 Bacterial culture and determination of antibacterial resistance.

Bacterial growth not inhibited around discs – full resistance to these antibacterials

Culture medium

Bacterial growth

Discs, each impregnated with a different antibacterial

Some inhibition of bacterial growth, but small radius – partial susceptibility to these antibacterials

Growth inhibited around discs – full susceptibility to these antibacterials

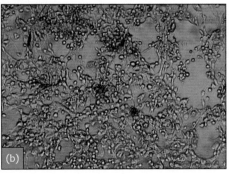

8.16 Virus growing in cell culture causes cell death, known as a cytopathic effect (CPE). (a) Healthy cell culture. (b) CPE caused by infection with feline herpesvirus.
(© A Radford and M Afonso)

(a)

(b)

Sensitivity, specificity and predictive values

Sensitivity and specificity are fixed properties of a test. Sensitivity is the likelihood that, if a sample is truly positive, a test will correctly identify it as such. If a test has 100% sensitivity, it will pick up every single positive sample. If a test has 100% specificity, it will always correctly identify a negative sample as being negative. However, it is very rare for real-life tests to have such high values, as increasing the sensitivity of a test compromises the specificity and *vice versa*. Therefore, care must be taken when interpreting the results of diagnostic tests, as false-positives and false-negatives occur as well as correct results (see Figure 8.13).

For example, if a test with 90% sensitivity is applied to 100 positive samples, it will identify 90 correctly as positive, and 10 incorrectly as false-negatives. If a test has a specificity of 90% and 100 negative samples are tested, 90 of them will be correctly identified as negative, and the other 10 will incorrectly give false-positive results.

There is a trade-off between sensitivity and specificity, which is intuitive. To ensure that an important pathogen (e.g. one that is zoonotic or highly contagious) is not missed, the test will be optimized to provide the highest sensitivity, which might mean that occasionally an animal which does not have the disease of interest, will have a positive test result. By contrast, in a situation where it is important to avoid classifying disease-free animals as positive – for example, because being identified as positive means that the animal will be euthanased – the test may be optimized to be highly specific, but will then inevitably occasionally miss a positive sample.

Although sensitivity and specificity are fixed for a given test, the way in which the test should be interpreted also depends on a third factor – the prevalence of disease in the population being tested. Where the disease in question is rare, even a small number of false-negative test results can complicate interpretation. For example, testing 100 animals for a rare disease with a prevalence of 1%, using a test with 99% sensitivity and 98% specificity, would give the following result:

- One diseased animal correctly tests as positive
- Two disease-free animals incorrectly test as positive
- Ninety-seven disease-free animals correctly test as negative.

The positive results in this example would correctly identify a diseased animal only one time in three. This means that a positive test is correct only 1/3 = 33% of the time; this is referred to as the positive predictive value (PPV) of the test. The negative predictive value (NPV) (i.e. the proportion of times that a negative test really is negative), is 97/97 = 100%, in this example – there are no false-negative results. It can be seen that in this example, a negative test result is much more 'trustworthy' than a positive test.

One way of increasing the reliability of positive test results is to choose the most appropriate subjects to test. By selecting animals that are more likely to have the disease of interest, the prevalence of disease in the test population is increased. Using the same test as before, the sensitivity and specificity of the test will not change, but the number of true-positives increases in proportion to the number of false-positives and therefore the results will be more reliable.

For instance, if the same test as above is applied to a population of 100 animals with a prevalence of the disease of interest of 20%, the results are likely to be:

- Twenty diseased animals correctly test as positive
- Two disease-free animals incorrectly test as positive
- Seventy-eight disease-free animals correctly test as negative.

The PPV would then become 20/22 = 91%; that is, a positive test would be correct 91% of the time. The NPV would be 78/78 = 100%.

By using clinical judgement to select those animals at increased risk of the disease of interest (whether due to their signalment, clinical signs or other factors), the prevalence of disease in the tested population is increased, which aids the interpretation of positive tests by increasing the PPV of the test.

Of course, once the prevalence of the disease of interest in the population tested reaches more than 50%, some of the issues outlined above with PPV and NPV will reverse. In populations with a very high prevalence of disease, the predictive values can again be low, just as with low prevalences. However, this example shows the general principle that selecting animals to test and considering which population they are representative of, preferably before the test results are available, will aid interpretation of the results (see Chapter 17 for more information).

How to decide when to use a test (and when not to)

Decisions around testing can be reduced to a single question: 'What will I do when I have the results of this test?' Each single test can be regarded as a fork in the path of a clinical investigation (see also Chapter 3). Each result should inform a decision; if this is not the case, do not carry out the test.

Reasons for testing are:

- To rule something in
- To rule something out
- To choose a direction for future testing
- To assess the risk to the population.

All clinicians occasionally reach a point in an investigation where they are tempted to use diagnostic tests 'just to see', because they have drawn a blank with their initial investigations. This is generally because the initial investigations were in the wrong directions, the test has not behaved in the way that was expected, or the disease is uncommon or the clinical picture is unusual for the disease. These are in order of decreasing likeliness.

Choosing which animals to test

When deciding which animals to test, it is important for veterinary surgeons to consider what they are trying to achieve by testing (see Chapter 3). The aim may be to look for the presence of a pathogen, or its absence, either in an individual animal or across a population. When trying to detect a pathogen, it is best to test animals that are likely to be in the acute, active phases of infection – that is, animals in the early stages of their clinical signs. For serological testing, the earliest IgM responses are likely to lag 5–7 days behind the initial infection, and IgG responses 1–2 weeks later (although a few organisms, including *Leptospira* spp., generate a faster antibody response).

If aiming to confirm the absence of a pathogen (i.e. that the population is clear of infection), using the most susceptible animals is recommended. Testing pooled samples (e.g. of serum or faeces, as appropriate, from a number of animals) may also be helpful, although it must be remembered that this can lead to a dilution effect. In such cases, it is useful to discuss the sensitivity of the assay in question with the diagnostic laboratory.

What to do with a positive test result

As this section has outlined, testing is not a simple issue of obtaining a 'black or white', yes or no answer. While diagnostic tests are extremely useful tools in clinical decision-making, every test must be interpreted in the clinical context, and no test should be used without a sound rationale. This maximizes the cost-effective use of resources, and also helps to avoid the awkward situation of having to interpret and act upon a test result that does not fit clinically, may be spurious and should not have been taken in the first place.

References and further reading

Clegg SR, Coyne KP, Dawson S *et al*. (2012) Canine parvovirus in asymptomatic feline carriers. *Veterinary Microbiology* **157**, 78–85

Cooper B, Mullineaux E and Turner L (2011) *BSAVA Textbook of Veterinary Nursing, 5th edn*. BSAVA Publications, Gloucester

Crawford PC, Dubovi EJ, Castleman WL *et al*. (2005) Transmission of equine influenza virus to dogs. *Science* **310**, 482–485

Dawson S, Jones D, McCracken CM *et al*. (2000) *Bordetella bronchiseptica* infection in cats following contact with infected dogs. *Veterinary Record* **146**, 46–48

Fabrizio F, Calam AE, Dobson JM *et al*. (2014) Feline mediastinal lymphoma: a retrospective study of signalment, retroviral status, response to chemotherapy and prognostic indicators. *Journal of Feline Medicine and Surgery* **16**, 637–644

Greene C (2011) *Infectious Diseases of the Dog and Cat, 4th edn*. Elsevier Saunders, St Louis

Hall E, Simpson J and Williams D (2005) *BSAVA Manual of Canine and Feline Gastroenterology, 2nd edn*. BSAVA Publications, Gloucester

Hurley KF, Pesavento PA, Pedersen NC *et al*. (2004) An outbreak of virulent systemic feline calicivirus disease. *Journal of the American Veterinary Medical Association* **224**, 241–249

Jackson H and Marsella R (2012) *BSAVA Manual of Canine and Feline Dermatology, 3rd edn*. BSAVA Publications, Gloucester

Pesavento PA, Hurley KF, Bannasch MJ *et al*. (2008) A clonal outbreak of acute fatal hemorrhagic pneumonia in intensively housed (shelter) dogs caused by *Streptococcus equi* ssp. *zooepidemicus*. *Veterinary Pathology* **45**, 51–53

Sykes JE (2014) *Canine and Feline Infectious Diseases, 1st edn*. Elsevier Saunders, St Louis

Villiers E and Ristić J (2016) *BSAVA Manual of Canine and Feline Clinical Pathology, 3rd edn*. BSAVA Publications, Gloucester

Chapter 9

Biosecurity in shelters

Emily Newbury and Lila Miller

Introduction to shelter biosecurity

What is biosecurity?

In the context of shelters, biosecurity refers to all the efforts made to control the incursion and spread of infectious disease. It can be divided into physical elements, for example, sneeze barriers between cat pens, and procedural elements. The latter refers to all of the ways in which people utilize the shelter facilities and how the animals within them are managed. This may also include preventive medicine interventions such as vaccination and disease testing (see Chapter 11).

Why worry about biosecurity?

Biosecurity is important for animal shelters because of the constant and often elevated risk of disease introduction and the multiple factors that contribute to disease spread. Animals arrive at shelters from diverse origins, frequently with little or no information about their health, previous vaccination history or disease exposure. Some animals may proceed rapidly to rehoming, while others may stay for a longer period, so because of the constant population turnover, the 'all-in, all-out' quarantine systems used in farming to minimize disease spread are impossible to implement in shelters. It is often necessary to house vulnerable groups such as puppies and kittens alongside adults, potentially exposing both groups to a higher disease risk. Finally, there are many opportunities for both direct and indirect transmission of disease in the typical shelter environment that must be considered and managed.

While control of disease is a vital component of animal welfare, any protocols that are developed must be practical, achievable and based on an informed risk/benefit evaluation. For example, enforcing a rigorous quarantine period, with no contact at all between animals, may limit direct transmission of disease, but it could also impede behavioural assessment (which involves handling and mixing the animals), slow rehoming (as potential adopters will not be able to view the quarantine population) and adversely affect the psychological health and wellbeing of animals unable to exercise or socialize in an already stressful environment. However, if there is an outbreak of a serious infectious disease or if the shelter accepts animals from a high-risk population, strict quarantine may be a vital control measure. Choosing a quarantine protocol is just one example of the

managerial decisions that must be made and can have wide-ranging impacts. It is therefore extremely important that the views and priorities of all parties (including veterinary, behavioural and animal care staff) are accounted for, to ensure practicality and encourage compliance. In addition, it is preferable for there to be a structure or decision tree in place before an outbreak occurs, as these situations are often fraught with emotions that can threaten to override the professional veterinary advice that may be difficult to accept and implement, but necessary to protect the health of the shelter population as a whole.

Visiting the shelter

It is not possible to fully appraise the biosecurity measures in place at a shelter without visiting it in person. Problems such as overcrowding, poor facility design and housing, and failure to properly clean and disinfect the housing and objects within it, and even a rough estimate of the prevalence of clinical disease, can often be identified by walking around the premises on a typical working day. Even though regular veterinary visits or rounds may be difficult to schedule and could be costly for the organization, they should be considered a critical component of a successful biosecurity programme. It may be more realistic for regular rounds to be performed by staff members who have been trained to observe the animals for signs of clinical disease (or for indirect indicators of disease, such as vomit, diarrhoea, blood, uneaten food, etc.) and can then report their findings to the shelter's veterinary surgeon (veterinarian).

In addition to information gained on visits, the animals seen at the practice can act as sentinels for possible changes in the burden of infectious disease. For example, if the number of presentations of a particular syndrome, or euthanasia or cremation requests, or the usage of particular medicines increases, a more in-depth investigation at the shelter should be arranged (see Chapter 7).

External influences on biosecurity

Local disease conditions

The environment in which a shelter operates will have an influence upon the biosecurity issues it faces. Urban, suburban and rural areas will each have their own intrinsic characteristics and their own disease problems.

Knowledge of local disease conditions can help to inform a biosecurity plan.

Factors likely to influence the prevalence of infectious disease among the owned animals in an area may include:

- Population density
- Animal population demographics – e.g. in an area with low neutering and vaccination rates and a large number of young animals, there may be a higher prevalence of certain diseases
- General health and resistance to disease of the animal population
- Use of preventive veterinary treatments, including vaccination and parasiticides
- Management choices – e.g. if cats are mainly kept indoors they will have less opportunity to come into contact with pathogens
- Presence of disease vectors.

Intake policy

The intake policy and population of each shelter will differ and will have an impact upon its biosecurity. Stray and neglected animals are an unknown entity and may be more likely to transmit or contract disease than owned animals. Studies in the USA have shown that a large percentage of animals admitted to some shelters are immunologically naive and thus vulnerable to diseases that are preventable by vaccination (Miller and Hurley, 2009). The current evidence for this is fairly sparse for shelters in the UK, and further research is needed. Open-intake facilities that accept all animals regardless of their 'adoptability', health or the shelter's capacity to care for them may also be expected to encounter more diseases compared with shelters that operate a selective intake policy. There is some suggestion that open-intake facilities are more concerned about infectious disease (Steneroden et al., 2011), but the evidence is insufficient to draw conclusions about the effect of intake policy relative to other influences on biosecurity.

Internal influences on biosecurity

General principles

Certain groups of animals within a shelter are considered to present a greater risk of either transmitting or contracting infectious diseases. These groups require careful management and would, in an ideal world, be segregated from the rest of the shelter population to facilitate disease control. The high-risk groups that will be considered in this chapter are:

- Newly arrived animals of unknown health or vaccination status
- Animals with clinical signs of, or recovering from, serious infectious disease
- Pregnant or lactating females
- Juvenile animals (<4 months of age).

Although these groups may present the most concern from a biosecurity perspective, all animals in a shelter are at risk of contracting or transmitting infectious diseases and, although this risk can be minimized, it can never be totally eliminated. For example, many common shelter syndromes such as canine and feline upper respiratory disease and diarrhoea are multifactorial and not entirely preventable by vaccination. Some organisms, such as feline herpesvirus, can be carried asymptomatically for long periods and recrudesce due to stress, even after a cat has undergone a period of quarantine. Other factors, such as an animal's nutritional balance, overall physical health, stress levels and psychological state, are also important in determining the animal's susceptibility to disease. In summary, the application of biosecurity principles will not result in a sterile environment but will hopefully reduce both the likelihood of an animal being exposed to infectious material and the dose received. Setting realistic goals will provide encouragement for frontline staff and volunteers (and veterinary surgeons) if it makes biosecurity efforts seem achievable and worthwhile even in the face of an overwhelming disease challenge.

Shelter design

While few shelters have the luxury of operating in ideal facilities, it can be worth reviewing the utilization and layout of buildings, especially if disease-related problems are worsening. In an ideal world there would be spatial or structural separation between animals in different disease risk groups. As well as having separate spaces, each animal housing area ideally requires space for storage, food preparation, hand-washing and cleaning. Foot traffic and all animal care activities should proceed from the most to the least healthy animals over the course of a day, and it should not be necessary for staff or visitors to walk through high-risk areas such as isolation to any other part of the facility (see Chapter 10).

Population density

The Association of Shelter Veterinarians (ASV), *Guidelines for Standards of Care* (Newbury et al., 2010) describe the concept of the 'capacity for care' of each shelter. Rather than simply looking at the maximum number of animals that can be accommodated by, for example, counting cages, the capacity for care combines other influential factors, including the number of staff needed to provide a good standard of care, the intake rate of the facility and the average length of stay of each animal. Housing too many animals in one place will facilitate disease spread by providing a greater number of susceptible hosts, increasing contact between them and inflicting greater stress, as well as affecting air quality and overwhelming cleaning and disinfection efforts. Assessing whether a high population density could be contributing to disease levels is another good reason for the veterinary surgeon to visit the shelter regularly.

Physical structure

The design of the shelter plays an important role in the ability of the staff to maintain a clean and sanitary facility. Diseases in shelters are transmitted via a variety of routes, but most frequently via fomites, direct contact or aerosols (Figure 9.1). In order to minimize disease transmission, it is important that all modes of transmission are addressed through a comprehensive management plan with good infection control and sanitation protocols, and ongoing staff and volunteer education and training.

In terms of the actual physical structure, all areas where animals are housed and the actual housing itself – that is, the primary enclosures and cages – should be constructed

Route	Description
Direct	Through contact with an infected animal
Indirect	Through contact with a contaminated object (fomite) or environment
Droplet	When one animal sneezes in close proximity to another, propelling infectious material on to the second animal
Airborne	If infectious organisms are carried through the air on particulate matter such as dust
Vector-borne	Via insects (e.g. mosquitoes) or ticks

9.1 Routes of infectious disease transmission.

of sturdy, non-porous materials that are impervious to liquids (Figure 9.2). This is particularly true of floors that are often subject to heavy foot traffic, repeated hosing with hot water and applications of cleaning and disinfecting chemicals that can compromise the integrity of the surface. Non-porous materials such as stainless or galvanized steel, fibreglass, polypropylene, plastic, glass, etc., can be easily cleaned and disinfected. The use of porous materials such as wood should be avoided in animal housing areas because it is impossible to effectively disinfect and can provide areas for harmful pathogens to lodge in and thrive. Although concrete is a popular floor material, if it is not treated, sealed and maintained properly, the surface will contain small crevices and may crack, providing areas that are difficult to disinfect. Although aesthetically pleasing and comfortable for humans, carpet should be avoided in animal areas. One of the drawbacks of non-porous surfaces is that they are usually cold, hard, slippery and uncomfortable. Bedding materials, such as shredded newspaper, blankets, towels or sawdust, are often used to increase animal comfort, but attention must be paid to cleaning or disposing of them promptly when soiled or whenever a new animal enters the enclosure.

Selection and placement of cages and primary enclosures are another important factor in maintaining a biosecure environment. In addition to being made of non-porous materials, cages should not be tiered if possible. If cages are small enough to be stacked they probably do not provide animals with enough space to perform their normal behaviour, exercise or stretch out. If cages must be tiered, urine, faeces, chemicals or contaminated water must not be able to pass from one cage to the cage beneath it, and the top cage must be accessible for cleaning.

Cages should be placed far enough apart and in a configuration that allows each animal access to adequate ventilation and natural light. Cat cages that are open in the front and the back allow better ventilation. Cat cages that face each other should be placed a minimum of 1.2 m apart so that respiratory diseases are not readily spread via sneezing. It may be necessary to place a physical barrier between cages to prevent animals from having physical contact with each other.

Double-sided enclosures (Figure 9.2) are the preferred type of housing for dogs and cats because the additional space reduces stress by providing animals with more choices and control over their movements. These enclosures also allow animals to move freely of their own accord from one side to the other during cleaning, decreasing the amount of handling needed; this in turn reduces their stress levels and opportunities for disease to be transmitted directly or via fomites. In addition, food and resting areas can be separated from the animal's toileting area, respecting the animal's behavioural preferences and increasing animal comfort. Finally, worker safety is increased because they do not have to handle potentially dangerous animals while cleaning their enclosures.

Ventilation

Good ventilation is essential for the maintenance of health in animals housed together, for a number of reasons (Figure 9.3). Besides providing oxygen and removing carbon dioxide, excessive moisture, ammonia and methane, proper ventilation also reduces odours, the spread of airborne pathogens and the incidence of respiratory disease. The ventilation requirements of animals will vary with the density of the population and the pollutants in the air. A higher ventilation rate will be required when the ambient temperature is high or when the shelter is crowded or over capacity, because animals themselves are a source of heat, carbon dioxide, water vapour and ammonia. Dust control is also

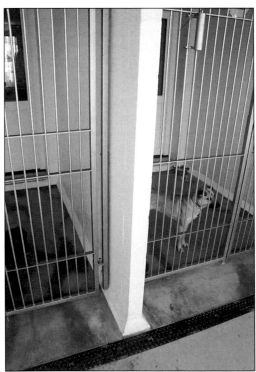

9.2 Double-sided dog housing with good ventilation, impervious surfaces, solid barriers between kennels and a covered external trench drain.
(© E Newbury and courtesy of Dogs Trust)

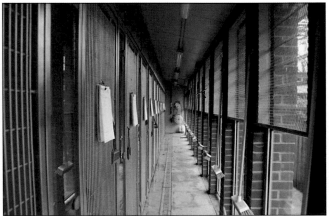

9.3 Passive ventilation achieved through open-fronted housing units and window grates. Note the dedicated, colour-coded equipment for each cat pen and the covered external trench drain.
(Courtesy of Cats Protection)

important because some bioactive aerosols, such as endo-toxins, can be transmitted via airborne particles. Good sanitation is thus essential to maintain good air quality.

The standard recommendation for ventilation in animal shelters is to have active ventilation that achieves a mini-mum of 10–14 complete air exchanges with outside air per hour. Because canine respiratory pathogens are aero-solized and more readily transmitted through the air than feline pathogens, which are spread by droplets, this type of separate air circulation system may be particularly recommended for areas housing dogs. The main draw-back is that these systems are expensive to install and require routine inspection and maintenance for efficient operation. High-efficiency particulate air (HEPA) filters can remove some viral particles and particulate matter, but appropriate commercial units are expensive to maintain and should not be relied upon as the sole means of achieving good ventilation.

Drainage

Adequate drainage must be provided. A variety of drains can be found in shelters, including single, group and trench drains. They may be constructed of stainless or gal-vanized steel or polyvinyl chloride (PVC), and should be at least 15 cm in diameter. They should have covers to prevent animals' feet and other objects from getting stuck in the drain (see Figures 9.2 and 9.3). The floor may be sloped to allow water to run off into the drain. Trench drains should be placed sufficiently far from the enclosure or covered so animals cannot touch contaminated water from another enclosure as it is flushed along the trench. Drains require proper maintenance to prevent the accumu-lation of pathogens, clogging, and stagnant water pooling around the surface. If drains are located in common areas, they should be cleaned and disinfected before allowing new animals to access the area.

Sanitation

Proper sanitation is a key element of an effective bio-security programme; its importance should never be underestimated. In addition to reducing the transmission of pathogens, it results in a cleaner and healthier environ-ment that increases the animals' comfort and helps to present a positive image of the shelter.

Identification of the pathogens most likely to be encountered and a thorough knowledge of their character-istics, that is, their incubation periods, resistance to deacti-vation, shedding pattern, modes of transmission, etc., are imperative to ensure that the cleaning methods and disin-fectants being used can destroy the pathogens and disrupt all modes of transmission. For example, it is essential to know that parvovirus can persist in the environment for several months under the right conditions and has been found to resist to many commonly used disinfectants such as quaternary ammonium compound-based products. The sanitation protocol should be documented, reviewed and updated periodically as needed, and made available to all staff and volunteers. Education and training are essential to ensure the protocol is being followed. Whenever there is a disease outbreak, one of the first control steps should be a thorough, first-hand review of sanitation procedures.

Proper sanitation involves both cleaning and disin-fection.

- **Cleaning** involves the physical removal of all soiled bedding and litter, dirt, and organic debris (i.e. urine and faeces) from all surfaces, in addition to washing with water (preferably hot) and a detergent with good degreasing properties. The result should be a visibly clean surface. Bedding, towels, uniforms, etc., should be carefully sorted and laundered in hot water, detergent and bleach, and dried in a commercial dryer. Care should be taken to avoid overloading the washing machine. The use of hot water at a temperature of at least 77°C for sanitizing water and food bowls will inactivate many organisms, and a commercial dishwasher that can achieve such temperatures is a labour-saving device that is often worth investing in. The use of mops and high-pressure hosing to clean enclosures should be avoided, especially during disease outbreaks, because mops can harbour organic material bearing pathogens, and the spray from pressure washing can spread organisms via the airborne route.
- **Disinfection** is a process that inactivates pathogens. Disinfection is most commonly achieved in shelters by the application of a chemical to the environment (Figure 9.4). Although some disinfectants can work in the presence of organic debris, effective disinfection requires proper preparation of the product in accordance with the manufacturer's instructions and application to a clean surface. Although it may be problematic for some shelters with minimal staffing to achieve, for the product to be effective, the recommended surface contact time must be allowed before the product is rinsed off (if necessary) and the surface dried. Surface contact times vary, usually between 5 and 10 minutes. Mixing different products together indiscriminately should be avoided to prevent the formation of toxic fumes and interactions that can interfere with their effectiveness (see QRG 9.1).

Every effort should be made to minimize stress and disruption of the animals' life and routine when cleaning and disinfecting. A study undertaken in a shelter found that rehousing cats during cleaning caused sufficient stress to induce herpesvirus activation and viral shedding 4–11 days after the stressor, with shedding continuing for 1–13 days. Stress levels can be reduced by keeping cats in the same cage for the duration of their stay and spot cleaning the cage daily, that is, removing visible dirt, soiled paper and bedding, litter trays, faecal material, etc., but not sanitizing the whole cage. Spot cleaning minimizes stressful animal handling and allows familiar scents that may be comforting to the animal to remain. In most cases,

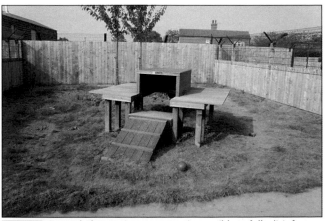

9.4 Some shelter environments are impossible to fully disinfect, such as this outdoor area with grass.

(© E Newbury and courtesy of Dogs Trust)

cages should be disinfected only when a new occupant is introduced, or on a weekly schedule as deemed necessary in accordance with disease conditions. This commonly recommended spot-cleaning protocol for sanitizing cat housing is being increasingly considered for maintaining dog housing as well in the USA. However, animals must be removed if the cage needs to be washed and disinfected, as cages should never be hosed down while the animals are still in them.

Sufficient staff should be assigned so that the shelter is cleaned in a timely fashion. Cleaning the shelter should not take all day. The National Animal Control Association and Humane Society of the United States recommend allowing 9 minutes per animal per day for routine cleaning. During disease outbreaks, it may be necessary to increase staff time devoted to cleaning and disinfection. Sanitation protocols should be reviewed with staff and volunteers periodically to ensure compliance.

Management of fomite spread – equipment and people

One of the most frequent and efficient routes of disease transmission in a shelter environment is via fomites. Any movable object, including people, can transfer infectious material between animals, so this route of transmission must be carefully managed. Figure 9.5 lists some common fomites to consider when devising disease management protocols. Cleaning and disinfection measures applied to animal housing should be expanded to include routine disinfection of objects such as litter trays and food bowls if disposable alternatives are not available or affordable (Figure 9.6). See QRG 9.1 for further information.

- Food and water bowls
- Litter trays
- Beds and other cage furniture
- Bedding
- Toys
- Collars, harnesses and leads
- Muzzles
- Veterinary equipment (e.g. stethoscope)
- Clothing and shoes
- Cleaning equipment
- People (staff, volunteers, visitors)
- Vehicles

9.5 Common shelter fomites.

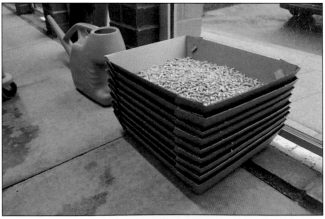

9.6 Using disposable items such as cardboard litter trays can help to minimize fomite spread.
(Courtesy of Cats Protection)

The order of cleaning areas in the shelter should be planned to protect the health of the most vulnerable populations, that is, puppies and kittens. Cleaning should commence in the area housing healthy puppies and/or kittens first, then healthy nursing bitches and queens, followed by healthy adult animals, and then finally unhealthy animals. Each area should have its own dedicated and labelled equipment. Colour coding, for example, having red squeegees and buckets in isolation, blue in quarantine and green in the nursery, is a constant visual reminder for staff and volunteers to maintain equipment in its designated area (Figure 9.7). If achievable, this separation of equipment should extend to all other objects in constant use such as bowls and litter trays. Animals should not share toys or other objects that cannot be effectively disinfected.

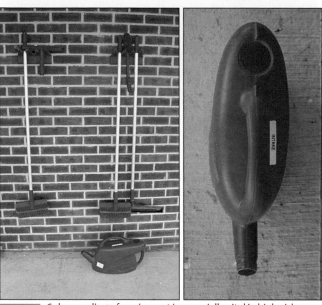

9.7 Colour coding of equipment is especially vital in high-risk areas such as quarantine.
(© E Newbury and courtesy of Dogs Trust)

Personal protective equipment (PPE) is a vital component of disease control both within the shelter and in the local community. As well as protecting animals, it is a key part of health and safety for shelter personnel given their potential exposure to zoonotic diseases. A minimum measure in a low-risk environment would be for staff and volunteers to change out of their work clothes and shoes before leaving the facility. This reduces the chance of infectious material from the shelter being transferred to their car, house and other places in their local area. Washing work clothes every day or as frequently as possible will also help to reduce the risk.

PPE should be readily available in shelters. Appropriate usage of PPE is even more important in a high-risk environment, such as areas where animals known to have infectious disease are housed (Figures 9.8 and 9.9). Applying barrier nursing principles when handling high-risk dogs and cats will help to prevent them from either transmitting or contracting an infectious disease. Options for PPE include overalls, gowns and scrubs (disposable options are available) with or without aprons, sleeve protectors, hats and masks. Considerations such as the diseases of concern, their zoonotic potential, cost and practicality will also affect the choice. The use of dedicated footwear or shoe covers when entering high-risk areas is preferable to foot baths, as the latter may be less

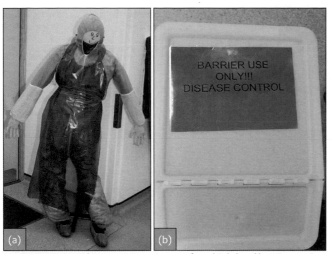

9.8 Personal protective equipment for a high-level barrier nursing environment includes (a) disposable overalls, sleeve protectors, gloves and shoe covers and (b) should be stored separately.
(a, courtesy of Cats Protection; b, © E Newbury and courtesy of Dogs Trust)

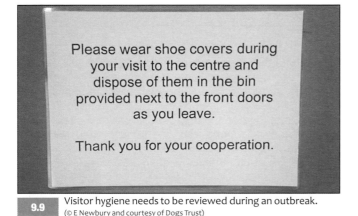

Please wear shoe covers during your visit to the centre and dispose of them in the bin provided next to the front doors as you leave.

Thank you for your cooperation.

9.9 Visitor hygiene needs to be reviewed during an outbreak.
(© E Newbury and courtesy of Dogs Trust)

effective in the face of challenge with organic material and insufficient contact time for disinfection. Colour coding by area should be extended to include PPE (e.g. having red scrubs and boots for the isolation area).

Hand hygiene is a hugely important part of biosecurity in both human and animal environments. Hand-washing facilities should be available in as many parts of the shelter as possible, and certainly in high-risk areas such as isolation. Commonly noted problems with hand-washing facilities include poor positioning, disrepair, a lack of soap or means to dry the hands and inappropriate water temperatures (too cold or too hot). Improper hand-washing techniques present another problem. (Proper hand-washing procedures are detailed at www.cdc.gov/handhygiene.) Several of the commonly available hand-washing products, including chlorhexidine- and triclosan-based products, have a limited spectrum of activity and will not kill some organisms of concern, such as non-enveloped viruses. However, good hand-washing practice, even with just soap and water, can reduce microbial loads by such a large degree that inability to provide more expensive hand cleaning products should not devalue its importance. This also serves to illustrate the importance of wearing gloves in very contaminated or high-risk areas or when handling obviously sick animals. Although unlikely to be effective if hands are visibly soiled, 70% alcohol-based hand gels may provide some additional decontamination after hand-washing or can be used in situations where washing is not possible. Signage and training can also be used to encourage compliance with hand hygiene protocols among staff, volunteers and visitors.

Principles of outbreak management

Details of the management of individual diseases are covered in the relevant chapters of this manual. One of the most important first steps in managing a disease outbreak is to identify the problem or pathogen and determine what signs constitute a clinical case. For example, not every case of diarrhoea is caused by parvovirus, especially in an adult dog with a strong history of vaccination.

The following represents an overview of aspects to consider in the event of a case or outbreak of a serious disease.

Outbreak management

1. Identify these three groups of animals:
   - Infected/affected – animals with clinical signs of the disease
   - In-contact – animals likely to have been exposed to the disease through direct contact with an infected individual or through contact with their secretions, discharges or excretions, contaminated surfaces or objects (fomites)
   - 'Clean' – animals that have not had contact with an infected individual or with any surfaces or objects likely to be contaminated.

In general, both the clinically ill and in-contact (exposed) animals will need to be considered as infected. The severity of the restrictions imposed on each group (see below) will depend on the disease concerned. If a highly pathogenic, highly infectious or zoonotic organism is involved, both the infected and in-contact animals will need to be carefully isolated and barrier nursed until they no longer present a risk. In extreme cases, if the shelter has the resources, a risk assessment can sometimes be performed for certain diseases via titre testing to determine whether each animal has a protective immune response. There may be some circumstances in which this is not possible and the only option is to euthanase infected animals with clinical illness.

Within the in-contact and 'clean' groups there may be subdivisions of risk depending on the disease concerned, the vaccination status of the animals and other factors affecting susceptibility, such as age. For example, an in-contact but properly vaccinated, apparently healthy adult dog would be considered low risk compared with a puppy still undergoing its primary vaccination course.

2. Implement heightened biosecurity protocols: ▶

Outbreak management *continued*

- Place clinically ill animals diagnosed with infection in isolation and restrict access to areas housing infected or in-contact animals – ideally designate specific staff to work in only these areas, and review the sanitation protocols and provide PPE (protective clothing, footwear and hand-hygiene facilities)
- As well as restricting access to animals at risk of transmitting the disease, it is essential to protect those animals most at risk of contracting it through the use of increased biosecurity (e.g. housing puppies and kittens at a distance away from the isolation area or sending them out of the shelter)
- Meet with staff and volunteers to review the characteristics of the disease, treatment options, barrier nursing protocols and all other outbreak measures to ensure that everyone is informed. Signage and written protocols can also be used to remind people of the required precautions
- Consider visitor hygiene and ensure that access to high-risk areas is restricted. It may be necessary to close the shelter to visitors for a period in severe circumstances.

3. Control animal movements:
   - Incoming animals – some organizations will choose to close to incoming animals, if this option is available, until either the disease outbreak is under control or the risk is lower. If animals are admitted, those least at risk of contracting the disease should be prioritized (e.g. older, vaccinated individuals)
   - Outgoing animals – in most cases, healthy 'clean' animals will be better off removed from the shelter as quickly as possible. This is especially true of puppies and kittens. Depending on the degree of risk, it may be necessary to inform the new owners about the outbreak and consider factors such as the presence of children or other animals in the household before deciding whether to rehome to them at that stage
   - Animal movements around the facility – until the outbreak is under control, it is best to keep animals in their current enclosure and with their current companion or group.

Staff and volunteer training in biosecurity

Almost 80% of people working in animal shelters in the UK are volunteers and, of those, the vast majority are part-time (Stavisky *et al*., 2012). While some volunteers may have extensive experience with animal care environments and infectious disease control, others will have none. Time to devote to training of volunteers is likely to be limited but should be considered an essential investment in preventing and managing disease outbreaks. This means that shelters have a lot of work to do to ensure that everyone is sufficiently informed in all relevant areas.

Production of standard operating protocols (SOPs) for the common animal care tasks is a useful first step in disseminating good practice. Involving staff and volunteers in the planning and revision of these SOPs will help to ensure that they are practical and accepted by everyone. Key areas to focus on may include some of the following, although every shelter will have its own priorities and ideas:

- Preventive medicine regimes (e.g. vaccination, worming and screening tests for certain diseases)
- Cleaning and disinfection protocols (e.g. disinfectant dilution, application methods, contact times, rinsing, etc.)
- Hand hygiene
- Use of PPE such as shoe covers and gloves
- Management of animals in quarantine
- Management of the nursery area
- Management of animals in isolation
- Visitor hygiene
- Flow of animals through the shelter.

Other methods of information transfer include 'on the job' training, group discussions and e-learning tools such as online videos and webinars (see Chapter 24 for further information). Training can be proactive with a structured curriculum or reactive in response to an event, such as a case of a particular disease. If a curriculum-based approach is used, it may be that new and existing staff require different information, but refreshers will still be useful and should be scheduled at set intervals (e.g. an annual review of barrier nursing methods). There is no limit to the topics and ideas that can be covered, and there are several different methods of training used in shelters already. For example, hand hygiene can be demonstrated with UV-luminescent gels that illustrate the commonly missed areas. Online videos that show optimal hand-washing techniques through dance or music are available (many originating from the human healthcare sector) and may work for some audiences. Combining different approaches will make it more interesting for everyone involved as well as helping to get the message across.

The relationship between stress and disease

'Stress' is a term loosely used to describe complex and incompletely understood somatic, emotional and cognitive responses to novel, challenging and threatening stimuli, as well as many other energy-demanding events. It is a normal part of the everyday life of all shelter animals, regardless of their background. When the stress response diverts resources from biological activities that are critical to wellbeing, including the immune system, the animal's capacity to cope is reduced and its susceptibility to disease increases. Repeated or chronic stress can also harm the gastrointestinal, cardiovascular, musculoskeletal, nervous, urinary, haemolymphatic and reproductive systems and contribute to detrimental metabolic responses that promote a range of health problems, including dehydration and depression. Some stressors encountered in shelters include pain, excessive cold or heat, sleep deprivation, disease, injury, anxiety, fear, lack of control of one's environment, confinement, isolation, boredom, and conflict with other animals.

Minimization of stress in the shelter is thus critical in helping to ensure the success of any biosecurity programme. Spot cleaning, leaving animals in the same enclosure for as long as possible during their stay, establishing routine schedules that use the same staff for sanitation and animal handling, minimizing unnecessary handling and noise (e.g. avoiding slamming stainless steel cage doors) are just some of the measures to be taken during cleaning procedures that can help to reduce stress (see Chapter 19).

Other measures that can help to reduce stress, minimize disease transmission and promote overall good health include:

- Environmental enrichment, including the provision of platforms, beds, hiding places, etc.
- Proper socialization with people and conspecifics
- Turning lights off at night so animals can sleep
- Prompt treatment of any medical and behavioural problems
- Maintenance of appropriate environmental conditions (heat, humidity and ventilation)
- Appropriate co-housing of behaviourally matched conspecifics
- Good nutrition that meets the needs of the individual animal
- Providing appropriate toys and exercise.

Management of specific populations

New animals

The constant introduction of new animals of unknown disease status presents a significant biosecurity challenge. An animal that is incubating or actively shedding a contagious virulent pathogen can obviously infect other susceptible individuals, and this is what is most feared in the shelter setting. For example, apparently healthy puppies that are incubating parvovirus can shed the virus before any clinical signs of the disease appear. However, there are other aspects to consider that may have effects long after the initial case is resolved. Even if no other animals are immediately infected, environmental contamination with a persistent pathogen can put future shelter inhabitants at risk. Staff and volunteers could also inadvertently carry infectious material from the shelter into the local area, leading to new cases there. Careful management of incoming animals can help to minimize these risks.

Intake examination

The point of intake is the ideal time to assess both the health status and the disease risk posed by an animal and to determine its subsequent management (Figure 9.10). There are obviously many things to consider when assessing the physical and mental well being of a new dog or cat. Each aspect has implications for biosecurity. It is advisable to create a standardized, systems-based intake examination form to ensure that all relevant information is recorded if it is not immediately entered on to a veterinary record system.

Quarantine

While 'quarantine' and 'isolation' are terms that are often used interchangeably, they are technically two separate concepts. Animals in quarantine are just *suspected* of carrying an infectious disease and may be apparently

Factor	Impact on biosecurity
Age	Younger animals are more susceptible to infectious disease
Origin	Stray animals may be more likely to carry, transmit and contract infectious disease than relinquished pets – care must be taken with initial management
Reproductive status	Neutering has been found to be associated with a positive antibody titre status, probably as a correlate of previous owner care that included vaccination
Body condition/weight	Poor body condition may increase disease susceptibility and also indicate a lack of previous owner care
Clinical examination	Are there any signs of infectious disease (especially those of zoonotic concern)?
Vaccination and other veterinary history	Useful if available; can inform management
Travel history	Which countries? Which areas within those countries? When? For how long? Were protective measures utilized?

9.10 Aspects of an intake examination relevant to biosecurity (see QRG 11.1).

healthy. They are there for their own benefit as well as for the benefit of the rest of the population, to limit their exposure to disease while they are observed, assessed and vaccinated if healthy (see Chapter 10). Animals in isolation are showing clinical signs of disease and very likely to be infectious to others. Most shelters will have facilities to isolate sick animals but not all will be able to routinely quarantine all incoming animals.

When considering implementing a routine quarantine period for new arrivals, it is important to balance the benefits against the costs for the individual organization (Figure 9.11). If animals arrive in or are housed in groups, come from areas with a high prevalence of disease or have frequent direct contact, quarantine of new animals may be particularly important.

The central decisions relating to quarantine are:

- Which animals will be placed into quarantine?
- How long will they be kept there?

Benefits
• Allows time for preventive healthcare measures such as vaccination and parasite treatment to take effect before mixing a new animal with the general population
• Allows time for diseases already incubating to emerge – for serious and environmentally persistent pathogens such as canine parvovirus this can be vital to minimize spread
• Screening tests (e.g. for feline immunodeficiency virus/feline leukaemia virus) can be carried out before mixing the animal with any others
• Behavioural assessment can also be carried out in this period to help to prepare a dog or cat for rehoming

Costs
• May extend the average length of stay and subject the animal to an even longer period in a stressful environment (increasing the incumbent disease risk)
• Quarantine is less likely to be effective for diseases with a long or variable incubation period, or for those with a high frequency of subclinical carriers in the general population, e.g. feline herpesvirus (increased stress may predispose to recrudescence)
• The physical facilities, equipment and staffing required may be unattainable for smaller organizations

9.11 The benefits and costs of instituting a routine quarantine period for new arrivals at a shelter.

It is preferable for all animals of unknown disease status to be quarantined for a period and prevented from being randomly co-housed with another animal or from accessing communal areas. If resources are limited, groups that are likely to present the highest risk (e.g. unvaccinated young strays) could be prioritized. There is probably less merit in including low-risk groups such as healthy vaccinated adults returned to the shelter. Ideally, a quarantine period should last as long as the maximum incubation time for the diseases of concern. If this is impractical, which it often will be, an average or 'typical' period can be used, especially if it is based upon data obtained from actual shelter cases. Details about the epidemiology of individual diseases can be found in other chapters of this manual.

Vaccination of new animals

Vaccination is an important aspect of biosecurity for both dog and cat shelters. To provide most biosecurity benefit and protection for the individual, vaccines should:

* Be administered to new animals on arrival
* Be administered only to healthy, immunocompetent individuals
* Provide rapid onset of immunity
* Cover all relevant diseases.

Vaccination on arrival will be difficult to achieve for many shelters unless they have an in-house veterinary team. According to the Royal College of Veterinary Surgeons, first vaccinations and boosters must be given under direct supervision from a veterinary surgeon, with an accompanying clinical assessment. This is also necessary to enable the issuing of a vaccination certificate. As a result, many shelters will batch their new animals for vaccination as and when their veterinary surgeon is available. This is less likely to be a problem in a low-risk environment, but it increases the risk of disease exposure for naive individuals in a high-risk environment.

Manufacturer advice states that only healthy dogs and cats should be vaccinated and that vaccination should not be combined with other procedures or medication. There is limited published evidence to inform decision-making in this situation, although elective surgical procedures, such as neutering, appear unlikely to affect vaccine responses in cats and dogs (Miyamoto et al., 1995; Fischer et al., 2007). Many shelter medicine experts believe that vaccination on intake is vital to protect animal health and that the benefits of vaccinating mildly ill and injured animals outweigh the risks of adverse side effects; this applies to all shelters, but particularly those with an open admission policy, shelters with a high prevalence of infectious disease, or in an outbreak situation.

Parasite treatment

As with the timing of vaccination, it is preferable to treat dogs and cats with a broad-spectrum anthelmintic as soon as possible after their arrival. Some worming preparations such as fenbendazole have the benefit of activity against Giardia, and these may be especially useful for young animals. Prompt deworming is important from a biosecurity perspective, as helminth ova and protozoal cysts can survive for long periods in the right environmental conditions, are resistant to many commonly used disinfectants, and some may also infect humans. Endoparasites can also lower disease resistance, rendering young animals even more susceptible to infectious diseases, particularly those that affect the gastrointestinal system. Minimizing the environmental parasite burden is another reason to consider implementing a quarantine protocol for new arrivals (see Chapter 11).

Screening tests

Screening for disease, especially in individuals that are not showing clinical signs, is a complex and controversial subject in both the human and veterinary medical fields. The reliability of any result obtained depends on the sensitivity and specificity of the test method but also on the expected prevalence of the disease in the test population (see Chapter 8). Unfortunately, prevalence data are not yet available for many common conditions of dogs and cats.

Sick animals

There are different ways in which sick and potentially infectious animals can be separated from the general population. Ideally, each shelter would have designated isolation facilities with sufficient capacity for their population and disease burden. In a 2010 survey of shelters in the UK, 73.8% of those housing dogs and 83% of those housing cats reported having isolation facilities, with a median proportionate capacity of 10% of total housing (Stavisky et al., 2012).

A decision has to be made, with veterinary advice being imperative, about which cases will be considered for isolation. There is no question that highly infectious conditions such as canine and feline parvovirus and dermatophytosis, and zoonotic pathogens such as Sarcoptes scabiei, merit careful barrier nursing. The management of respiratory disease or mild diarrhoea in dogs and cats is more uncertain and may depend on the design of the standard housing, shelter resources, and the prevalence and incidence of each syndrome.

Large shelters with an in-house veterinary team and good isolation facilities will be able to treat some infectious disease cases on site. Many smaller shelters with minimal resources will be forced to hospitalize their severely ill animals at an off-site location. This has the benefit of removing a source of infection from the shelter premises and reducing the workload of staff and volunteers who may not be experienced in nursing such cases. Unfortunately, it is also very costly. If specific isolation facilities are not available, animals can be barrier nursed in their enclosures, with strict biosecurity measures applied, but the lack of physical separation from healthy animals will greatly increase the risk of disease transmission and thus is not recommended.

Managing isolation facilities in a shelter setting requires that staff and volunteers receive specific training in barrier nursing. This is an excellent opportunity for veterinary involvement, but only 57% of shelters questioned in a recent survey reported asking their veterinary surgeon for advice about barrier nursing methods (Newbury, unpublished). This does not mean that the remainder were uninformed, but it is a topic that is worth reviewing with the shelter's veterinary surgeon. It is also advisable to produce a written barrier nursing protocol to ensure the information is communicated as broadly and as consistently as possible.

Recovering and recovered animals that have been hospitalized at a veterinary practice and are stable enough to return to the shelter may still be shedding pathogens and are therefore still infectious. Clear veterinary advice is important to ensure that these animals are isolated for the typical or maximum duration of shedding if a serious pathogen is involved (e.g. canine or feline parvovirus). Bathing animals that have recovered is essential to reduce the contamination of their coat and feet.

Pregnant/lactating females, puppies and kittens

As mentioned above, it is advisable to house pregnant/lactating females, puppies and kittens in separate nursery accommodation away from the other animals or off site if possible. Off-site options such as fostering may further reduce the disease risk and provide better socialization opportunities as long as sufficient training and support can be provided to the foster carers. In addition to having separate accommodation, larger organizations may be able to assign specific staff to work in the nursery area exclusively, which is likely to reduce the risk of disease transmission by the indirect or fomite routes. However, in the absence of these options, good biosecurity can still be achieved by:

- Cleaning and feeding in the nursery area first
- Minimizing foot traffic and ensuring that all visitors observe the biosecurity measures in place
- Wearing protective clothing and footwear when in the nursery area and changing it between litters to avoid cross-contamination (Figure 9.12)
- Good hand-hygiene provision – gloves, functioning sink, soap, alcohol gels, etc.
- Having dedicated equipment that is restricted to this area only.

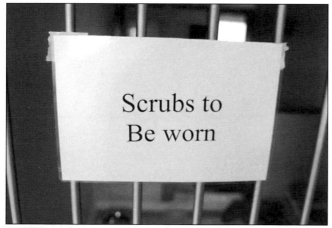

9.12 It is important to change the personal protective equipment (PPE) between the handling of different litters.
(© E Newbury and courtesy of Dogs Trust)

Several of the key organisms of concern for young animals are extremely environmentally resistant (e.g. *Giardia* spp., *Isospora* spp., feline and canine parvovirus). Issues of environmental contamination can arise quickly if the surfaces of the accommodation are not easily cleaned. Porous and damaged materials are impossible to disinfect and this can lead to recurrent disease problems in this very vulnerable population (Figure 9.13).

Issues of infection and re-infection with faecal–orally transmitted organisms can also arise due to the inherent messiness of puppies and kittens. While it may seem like an obvious point to make, frequent removal of faecal material and cleaning of litter trays can help to control infectious disease transmission. Ensuring that members of

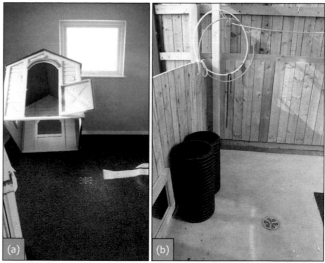

9.13 (a) A play area that is easy to disinfect. (b) A play area that is less easy to disinfect.
(© E Newbury and courtesy of Dogs Trust)

different litters are not housed together, splitting large litters post weaning, and cleaning the accommodation just before feeding may also make a difference. Lastly, bathing of puppies and kittens following treatment for organisms such as *Giardia* and *Isospora* spp. will help to reduce the likelihood of reinfection by removing infectious material from their coat and feet.

There will always be a degree of conflict between biosecurity measures and socialization when managing young animals. The crucial impact of early experience on the later behaviour of dogs and cats is widely acknowledged, and behavioural problems are commonly cited reasons for relinquishment and euthanasia in adulthood. Therefore, the management of puppies' and kittens' health must take account of this and provide for their socialization, mental stimulation and exercise as a priority. If possible, an area that is not used by any adult animals can be designated for outdoor exercise of puppies. This may eventually become contaminated through repeated use, and few outdoor substrates can be effectively disinfected, so care must be taken about which animals are allowed access (e.g. non-diarrhoeic animals only). Volunteer puppy and kitten socializers can be recruited who do not mix with any other animals on site and wear appropriate protective clothing. Individual puppies can also be carried to different locations to expose them to the sights and sounds of everyday life without increased disease risk. Disposable enrichment, such as food hidden in cardboard boxes, can be created for little cost and without risking cross-contamination between litters.

Vaccination of puppies and kittens

Puppies and kittens receive a certain quantity of maternally derived antibody (MDA) via the colostrum they consume in their first few days of life. The immunity conferred is dependent on the organisms to which their mother has been exposed or against which she has been vaccinated.

The MDA will also interfere with the efficacy of vaccination of puppies and kittens. Puppies and kittens are particularly susceptible to disease in the period when their MDA levels have fallen below that sufficient to offer protection but are still too high to allow vaccination to be effective. Vaccination protocols for these juvenile animals must take MDA into account in order to be effective (see Chapter 11).

Conclusion

Shelters should be proactive in developing a biosecurity plan to protect both animals and humans from potential infectious disease agents. Factors to be considered in the development of the plan include the design of the shelter, population management, and a healthcare programme including widespread examination, vaccination and de-worming of animals on intake, stress reduction, etc. For the biosecurity plan to be most effective, the pathogens most likely to be encountered in the environment should be identified and a risk assessment performed to deter-mine the probability of exposure to those pathogens. Veterinary surgeons, managers, and staff and volunteers who actually perform the procedures should work together to develop evidence-based, practical and feas-ible protocols that should be made available in writing to all staff. The protocols should be reviewed and updated periodically to make sure that the latest research in dis-ease control and sanitation methods is considered and the most effective products are being utilized. In addition, surveillance of staff while they carry out cleaning pro-cedures, ongoing training and enforcement of protocols by management are necessary to ensure compliance. The implementation of biosecurity measures is often labour-intensive, and higher upfront costs for testing for diseases (see Chapter 8) and purchase of PPE and more effective disinfectants are always a consideration for shelters that often have minimal resources. However, the return on the initial investment can be offset by the savings on the greater costs of isolating, quarantining, treating or euthanasing large numbers of ill animals. Failure to comply with biosecurity measures can contri-bute to very high intangible costs, such as animal suffer-ing and deaths, zoonosis, poor public relations for the shelter, and reduced staff morale that are likely to result from an outbreak of a preventable disease.

References and further reading

American Animal Hospital Association (2011) Canine vaccination guidelines. Available from www.aaha.org/public_documents/professional/guidelines/caninevaccineguidelines.pdf

Caveney L, Jones B and Ellis K (2012) *Veterinary Infection, Prevention and Control*. Wiley-Blackwell, Ames, Iowa

Dallas S (1999) *BSAVA Manual of Veterinary Care*. BSAVA Publications, Gloucester

Gore T, Headley M, Laris R *et al.* (2005) Intranasal kennel cough vaccine protecting dogs from experimental *Bordetella bronchiseptica* challenge within 72 hours. *Veterinary Record* **156**, 482–483

Fischer SM, Quest CM, Dubovi EJ *et al.* (2007) Response of feral cats to vaccination at the time of neutering. *Journal of the American Veterinary Medical Association* **230**, 52–58

Greene C (2011) *Infectious Diseases of the Dog and Cat, 4th edn*. Elsevier Saunders, St. Louis

Miller L and Hurley K (2009) *Infectious Disease Management in Animal Shelters*. Wiley-Blackwell, Ames, Iowa

Miller L and Zawistowski S (2013) *Shelter Medicine for Veterinarians and Staff, 2nd edn*. Wiley-Blackwell, Ames, Iowa

Miyamoto T, Taura Y, Une S *et al.* (1995) Immunological responses after vaccination pre- and post-surgery in dogs. *Journal of Veterinary Medicine and Science* **57**, 29–32

Newbury S, Blinn MK, Bushby PA *et al.* (2010) *Association of Shelter Veterinarians Guidelines for Standards of Care in Animal Shelters*. Available from www.sheltervet.org/assets/docs/shelter-standards-oct2011-wforward.pdf

Petersen CA, Dvorak G and Rovid Spickler A (2008) *Maddie's Infection Control Manual for Animal Shelters for Veterinary Personnel*. Center for Food Security and Public Health, Iowa State University, Ames, Iowa

Scherk MA, Ford RB, Gaskell RM *et al.* (2013) 2013 AAFP Feline Vaccination Advisory Panel report. *Journal of Feline Medicine and Surgery* **15**, 785–808

Stavisky J, Brennan ML, Downes M and Dean R (2012) Demographics and economic burden of un-owned cats and dogs in the UK: results of a 2010 census. *BMC Veterinary Research* **8**, 163

Steneroden KK, Hil, AE and Salman MD (2011) A needs-assessment and demographic survey of infection-control and disease awareness in western US animal shelters. *Preventive Veterinary Medicine* **98**, 52–57

Useful websites

ASPCA Pro:
www.aspcapro.org

University of California Davis Koret Shelter Medicine Program:
www.sheltermedicine.com

University of Florida Shelter Medicine program:
www.sheltermedicine.vetmed.ufl.edu/

QRG 9.1: A brief overview of disinfectants
by Emily Newbury and Lila Miller

Disinfection is defined as the destruction of the microorganisms in an environment through physical or chemical means. This differs from both cleaning, which is the physical removal of gross contamination, and sterilization, which eliminates all microorganisms.

Thorough cleaning must always precede disinfection or sterilization. Repeated vigorous physical cleaning of an environment may be the most important biosecurity measure that animal shelters can take. This is especially true when dealing with disinfection-resistant pathogens such as fungal spores.

In addition to all areas that animals live in or pass through, there are many other areas and objects in a shelter that must be disinfected.

Areas and objects to be disinfected
- All animal enclosures, including the floors, walls and cage handles
- Door knobs, light switches, air vents, etc.
- Bedding, clothing, carpet and other fabrics
- Food and water bowls
- Litter trays
- Toys
- Collars, leads, muzzles and other restraint equipment
- Grooming equipment
- Exercise areas – grassed areas, indoor exercise space

QRG 9.1 *continued*

Areas and objects to be disinfected *continued*
- Veterinary facilities, including medical (e.g. stethoscopes) and surgical equipment
- All non-housing areas (e.g. kitchens for preparing animals' feed, corridors)
- Staff areas (e.g. kitchens, break-rooms)
- Visitor facilities (e.g. reception area, toilets)
- Vehicles
- Equipment and food storage areas

Stages of cleaning and disinfection

Disinfection should take place as a step-by-step process, as outlined in the table below, in order to be both effective and safe for the humans and animals that will come into contact with the disinfected surfaces and objects.

Stage	Procedures
1. Cleaning	• Remove faecal material and any other visibly soiled materials, dirt and debris • Clean using a disinfectant with detergent properties or a detergent alone (if the latter is used, the surface should be rinsed before disinfection) • Cleaning should start in the cleanest and highest (ceiling) areas first and proceed to the dirtiest and lowest (floor) areas last
2. Disinfection	• Apply disinfectant to the clean surface at the correct concentration and allow it to remain for the recommended contact time • Products with claims to clean and disinfect in one step and to be effective in the presence of organic material should not be relied upon in high-risk situations • It is important to adhere to different dilution and application instructions that may apply to products that can be used to both clean and disinfect
3. Rinsing and drying	• Rinse the surface if indicated • Remove excess water or disinfectant (e.g. using a squeegee) from animal enclosures and always allow them to dry before animal contact is permitted

Stages of cleaning and disinfection.

Considerations for disinfectant use in animal accommodation

A wide range of disinfectants are commercially available. These contain different active ingredients (see table below) and have differential activity against the various types of pathogens encountered in the shelter environment. A number of factors should be taken into account in the choice and use of disinfectants.

- Choosing a disinfectant:
  - For effective disinfection, shelters should identify the pathogens of concern and verify that the disinfectant is efficacious against them. Pathogen identification and selection of the most appropriate disinfectant, where financially possible, is a critical step in controlling a disease outbreak.
- Health and safety issues:
  - Most disinfectants are hazardous to some degree and can cause irritation to eyes, skin and mucous membranes. Some products are particularly toxic to animals, such as phenol-based formulations (e.g. Dettol®), to which cats are very sensitive
  - For safety and efficacy, manufacturers' instructions for the preparation and application of their products should always be followed. Material safety data sheets (MSDS/SDS) that provide precautionary and first aid information are published online for most commercial disinfectant products. All organizations should also undertake Control of Substances Hazardous to Health (COSHH) assessments of the products they choose. The MSDS and COSHH documentation should be readily available to all staff
  - Personal protective equipment (PPE) including gloves, face masks and goggles should always be available and its use is strongly recommended.
- Factors that may affect disinfectant activity:
  - The presence of organic material
  - Exposure to light
  - Temperature (most products work best at a temperature above 20°C)
  - pH
  - Water composition (e.g. hard *versus* soft)
  - Mixing with other products such as detergents or ammonia
  - Stability and storage factors (check the shelf-life of concentrated and dilute products).
- Dilution:
  - The efficacy of a given disinfectant against certain organisms will depend on its concentration – check the manufacturer's test data for each group of pathogens
  - Higher concentrations may or may not be more effective against certain pathogens, but could be more toxic and expensive
  - It is useful to standardize the dilution process as much as possible, e.g. through the use of pre-mixed pumps or 'X pumps per bucket filled to the line'-type protocols.
- Application/distribution:
  - Mops and mop water can become very contaminated and so their use should be avoided, especially in high-risk environments; plastic brushes, hoses and squeegees are preferable (if suitable drainage is available)
  - Pressure washing can sometimes be useful, but can also aerosolize pathogens. It should be used with caution, and avoided in high-risk situations
  - Check whether rinsing of surfaces is required before allowing animal access to the disinfected area. Skin irritation, especially of the canine scrotum, eye ulcerations and other adverse effects can occur if manufacturers' instructions are not followed
  - Surfaces in animal accommodation must always be dry before animals are returned to these areas. Moist environments promote the growth of many pathogens and contribute to animal discomfort and stress.
- Contact time:
  - Most if not all disinfectants will have a recommended contact time that must be

QRG 9.1 *continued*

Active ingredient	Activity against					Notes
	Bacteria	*Non-enveloped viruses (e.g. parvovirus)*	*Mycobacteria*	*Fungi*	*Protozoal cysts*	
Sodium hypochlorite	Yes	Yes	Yes	Yes	?	Easily inactivated by organic material, detergent and light. Should be prepared fresh daily
Chlorine dioxide	Yes	Yes	Yes	Yes	Some	Easily inactivated by organic material, detergent and light
Quaternary ammonium compound (QAC) and biguanide blends	Yes	Typically not effective	Yes	Yes	No	Easily inactivated by organic material and soap. Has some detergent properties
Halogenated tertiary amine	Yes	Yes	Yes	Yes	No	Some efficacy in the presence of organic material. Has detergent properties
Dipotassium peroxodisulphate (potassium peroxymonosulfate)	Yes	Yes	Yes	Yes	No	Effective in the presence of organic material. Has detergent properties
Accelerated Hydrogen Peroxide®	Yes	Yes	Yes	Yes	No	Effective in the presence of organic material. Has detergent properties. Very safe; can be used on hands and on animals

Common disinfectant products suitable for use in animal shelters and their spectrum of activity. (Note: This table is intended for use as a general guide only. Disinfectants are often reformulated, so their properties may change. Always read the information provided by the manufacturer in detail before selecting a disinfectant.)

followed to avoid product failure. It is important to know and adhere to longer contact times if required to kill resistant pathogens such as fungal spores and mycobacteria.

- Assessing efficacy:
  - To verify that disinfection has been successful, cultures can be taken from a dry surface 2–3 days after disinfection to check for pathogen growth.

Adjunctive disinfectant techniques

- Steam:
  - Steam disinfection can have some efficacy against microorganisms (and specific life stages) that are difficult to kill with chemical disinfectants, such as protozoal oocysts
  - However, it requires the purchase of specialized equipment and may contribute to moisture build-up, especially in poorly ventilated facilities
  - There is little literature about its efficacy in a shelter setting.
- Disinfectant aerosols/canisters:
  - Some versions have a limited spectrum of activity – it is important to check and compare this when choosing a product
  - They are generally unsuitable for use in occupied areas, as the spray or 'fog' they produce is a respiratory and ocular irritant
  - Smoke detectors should be covered before use.

Other cleaning and disinfection targets

- Fabrics/bedding/clothing:
  - Many products can be used to soak bedding and other fabrics, but gross contamination with organic matter may compromise their efficacy. Heavily soiled materials or those contaminated with highly infectious material (e.g. parvoviral diarrhoea) are

best disposed of. Regulations for the disposal of clinical waste should be observed
- Most disinfectants (bleach is one exception) should not be mixed with laundry detergent as it may inactivate the disinfectant.
- The animals themselves:
  - Bathing animals after treatment for a faecal–orally transmitted infectious disease can help to reduce coat contamination and therefore the risk of the animal transmitting the infection to others
  - Some shampoos contain agents that may kill a percentage of pathogens (e.g. quaternary ammonium compound (QAC)/biguanide blends), but the act of physically cleaning the animal's coat and feet is most important
  - Antifungal shampoos containing agents such as enilconazole (Imaverol; Elanco) can also be used to treat the environment following a ringworm case/outbreak by misting pre-cleaned surfaces with a spray bottle. This is relatively expensive, however, and could be substituted for by using a standard disinfectant effective against fungi. (Note that the required disinfectant concentration may be higher if targeting fungal infection, and some products cannot kill fungal spores)
  - Never use any product on an animal that is not approved for that purpose.
- Outdoor areas:
  - It is obviously impossible to disinfect many of the outdoor substrates used in animal housing (e.g. grass, sand, gravel). Removal and replacement of the substrates may be the most effective method of decontamination
  - Ensuring that high-risk animals are prevented from accessing such areas can help to protect their health and minimize long-term environmental contamination. Rapid removal of faeces

QRG 9.1 *continued*

helps to prevent exposure to immediately infective pathogens and also prevents the environmental maturation of organisms (e.g. roundworm ova) that are not immediately infective

- Some disinfectants can be used to sluice down outdoor areas that have been occupied by an infectious individual. While efficacy on a porous, organic surface is likely to be compromised, their use may help a little. It is important to check the environmental safety profile of the disinfectant used and to consider the area in which it is discarded, as many products are toxic to aquatic life.

- Footwear:
  - Footbaths have limitations due to the inactivation of many disinfectant solutions by the organic material normally present on footwear, insufficient depth to cover shoe treads and inadequate contact time. Studies have shown that improper footbath use may actually contribute to disease transmission
  - Disposable shoe covers or dedicated footwear are both better options, especially in high-risk areas.
- Hands:
  - Thorough hand-washing with soap and water, and/or the application of an alcohol-based sanitizer, is a vital component of biosecurity. However, it is worth remembering that many of the commonly used hand-washing products and alcohol gels do not kill organisms of concern such as canine parvovirus
  - Broad-spectrum hand-washing products that contain a mixture of QAC and biguanide are available (e.g. F10® antiseptic hand soap)
  - Disposable gloves should be used whenever possible and certainly in high-risk situations.

Chapter 10

Shelter design and flow of animals through a shelter

Paula Boyden and Lisa Morrow

The appropriate design of a shelter is fundamental for providing facilities that optimize the physical and psychological health and welfare of animals that are in the care of a rescue organization. The shelter environment is far from 'normal' for dogs and cats. Shelters have a duty of care to meet the five welfare needs, as defined in the Animal Welfare Act 2006 (in England and Wales), the Animal Health and Welfare (Scotland) Act 2006 and the Welfare of Animals Act (Northern Ireland) 2011 (see Chapter 21).

Each shelter will inevitably have individual considerations relating to its specific circumstances and there are many design options. It is beyond the scope of this chapter to discuss all possible designs and so the aim is to outline the principles that should be incorporated into each individual design. All shelters need facilities that are ancillary to the animal accommodation for food preparation, laundry, cleaning and provision of healthcare. They also need public areas, such as a reception and facilities where the public can interact with the animals, as well as offices, staff rooms and, possibly, training facilities. Where a design principle is equally relevant to facilities that house cats and/or dogs, it will be discussed in general terms. If a concept is a specific consideration for either cats or dogs, it will be highlighted as such.

Principles of good shelter design

Good shelter design is crucial for directing the movement and flow of both people and animals around the shelter, and keeping different animals and/or different risk groups separate. This is an essential component of biosecurity and disease control. An example would be to have public areas in the most accessible part of the shelter but away from areas where sick animals are housed. Similarly, the various animal accommodation areas can be configured in such a way that staff or volunteers naturally move from areas with low risk of infectious agents being present to higher-risk areas. When animals are admitted to a shelter, they may well be of unknown disease status and, therefore, consideration must be given to where they are housed in order to avoid the spread of disease to existing inhabitants – that is, to having a quarantine facility for animals at intake (see Chapter 9). Isolation facilities are areas where known infectious disease is present. They should ideally be placed in a separate building and as far away from any other groups of animals as possible.

Siting of the shelter

The location of a shelter is important to its success as a rehoming facility. When setting up a new shelter, consideration needs to be given to accessibility and transport links, proximity to city centres, parking for vehicles and the size of the plot. It is also worth considering the location of other animal shelters in the vicinity. These factors will all have an impact on the success of the shelter; a shelter that is difficult to access risks becoming more of a sanctuary facility.

Before purchasing a site, further consideration should be made with regard to cost, the size of the plot, neighbours and obtaining planning permission. Informal discussions with prospective neighbours and the local planning authority before purchase might highlight any concerns that may need to be addressed.

The environment outside the facility is important. In terms of the positioning of the pen or kennel areas, consideration should be given to the effects of prevailing winds and weather, as this can affect the ability to maintain adequate temperature and ventilation inside the kennels and pens. The outlook beyond the pens or kennel units should provide the animals (cats in particular) with a view. For example, careful planting to encourage wildlife, such as planting buddleias to attract butterflies, will help to reduce cats' stress levels by providing them with mental stimulation. It is important that the animals cannot view other animals as part of their general outlook and that the 'flow' through the shelter avoids animals moving past multiple occupied pens or kennel units.

For dogs, sufficient land is required for walking and space for multiple exercise runs that are ideally separated into risk areas. It is beneficial to be able to have exercise areas with different substrates, such as grass, sand and concrete, and that exercise areas are allocated to particular risk groups of dogs (see Exercise areas; see also QRG 19.7). When planning to build a new shelter, the site and vicinity should also be considered in terms of the potential for noise from around the site that may cause anxiety for the animals in the shelter's care (Figure 10.1). This should be considered not only in terms of the volume of noise but also peaks in noise, or unpredictable variation, as well as familiar sounds that may be associated with an aversive outcome and likely to cause fear. These types of sounds are more likely to cause anxiety than constant and predictable noise. A site that is going to house dogs will also need to be assessed in terms of the impact that the noise made by the dogs will have on the surrounding area. A site that is going to house both dogs and cats requires careful

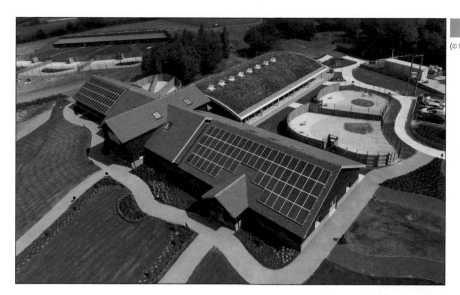

10.1 Arial view of a shelter showing the layout of the entire site.
(© Dogs Trust)

consideration in terms of design to ensure that the sound of dogs barking does not negatively affect the welfare of the cats.

Construction details and specifications

An animal shelter may be a new building designed specifically for that purpose or an adaptation of an existing structure. This will depend on the funds and facilities available; in most cases, a new build is preferable if funds allow.

The areas for housing cats may be contained within a building structure or may be composed of a series of stand-alone 'modules' of pens arranged within a garden setting. Stand-alone modules are preferable for cats because they meet more of the cats' behavioural needs (less visibility to other cats, improved outlook beyond the pen), have more natural ventilation and allow more flexibility in how the accommodation is used, especially in case of an outbreak of infectious disease (Figures 10.2 and 10.3).

A key element for dogs is to ensure that the kennel unit ideally consists of an indoor sleeping area with an adjacent outdoor run, the latter allowing toileting and movement. Ideally, dogs should have constant access to the run so that they are not forced to toilet in their sleeping area which can be particularly stressful for house-trained dogs (Figure 10.4).

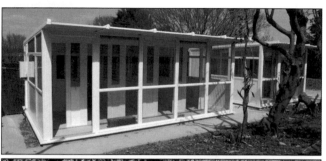

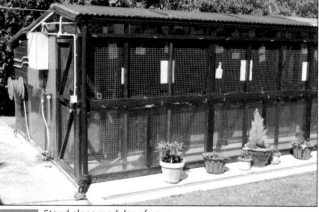

10.3 Stand-alone modules of pens.
(© Cats Protection)

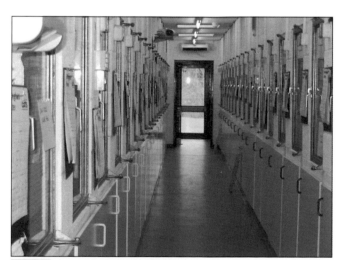

10.2 Accommodation in a building.
(© Cats Protection)

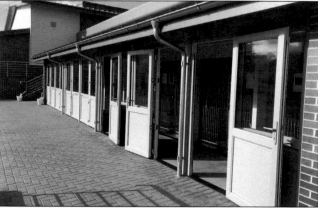

10.4 Stress abatement barrier: these barriers allow dogs constant access to all areas of their kennel unit and they also allow dogs to be walked without impacting kennelled dogs. In addition, they can aid with managing acoustics and ventilation.
(© Dogs Trust)

Materials

Materials used in the construction of a shelter should be durable, smooth, impervious and have waterproof surfaces that are resistant to degradation by disinfectants and steam. Examples include stainless steel, sealed tiles, sealed concrete, and fibreglass. Care should be taken with the use of polyvinyl chloride (PVC), as temperature, especially heat retention, may be a problem. Wood must not be exposed in areas where animals can come into contact with it, as it can harbour pathogens and cause splinters. If it is present in existing buildings it should be tanalized, rendered impervious and monitored carefully for any breaches of this. Alternatively, a wood-framed structure can be covered with a smooth impervious plastic such as melamine. Noise contributes to stress so materials that minimize noise levels should be considered. Junctions between horizontal and vertical must be coved or, if impractical, the joints sealed.

Ventilation

There should be separate air handling systems for the administration areas and the animal areas. Isolation should have a separate air source as well. It is ideal to change the air 100% with outside air rather than use recirculation or exchange. Ventilation with outside air is preferred over recirculated air because it is considered more effective at preventing spread of airborne pathogens, it provides higher quality air and costs less. Using mechanical ventilation to exchange air introduces problems with dust/dirt/fomite harbouring and requires regular cleaning. Often these systems are not in very accessible locations making cleaning difficult and compliance less likely. In addition, ongoing maintenance is required for this type of system and if it fails, the consequences can be serious in terms of not being able to supply adequate quality air to the animals and increasing likelihood of disease spread. Noise can be a problem for animals and people in facilities that have mechanical ventilation systems. When natural ventilation is used, the direction of prevailing winds and how the pens are sited in relation to that is very important; if this orientation in incorrect, it can result in too much air flow through pens and kennel units which can make it difficult to provide enough warmth or, conversely, it can restrict air flow to a degree that there is not enough fresh air for the animals.

For areas where air is recirculated or exchanged, there are various recommendations for the number of complete air changes that should be provided (Newbury *et al.*, 2010). If animals are segregated by age, air flow should be directed from young animals to adults. Draughts should be avoided.

Lighting

Natural light is preferable to artificial light, as the main light source and animals need to have a regular cycle of light and dark hours for their circadian rhythm. Adequate light must be available to allow inspection at any time.

Temperature

The temperature of a shelter is important for the comfort of the animals housed there and the humans working or visiting it. In a facility where the human and animal areas are all housed within one thermal building, the temprature should be maintained at 20–22 degrees Celsius (°C). In shelters with less building structure like facilities with banks of modular pens, covered walkways and overhead heaters can be used in areas where people work or view the animals.

Ideally the animals should have a choice of temperature in their environment. See General principles of kennel unit/pen design. The accommodation units should also be designed such that supplementary heat can be provided for litters of puppies or kittens, for nursing dams or queens and for elderly or sick animals that have difficulty maintaining body temperature. More detail on the specifications of these is described in the section on the design of animal accommodation areas.

Special consideration needs to be given to maintaining the temperature of a building which has tin/aluminium roof/sides or is made of PVC to ensure heat retention and overheating is not a problem (i.e. facilities for cooling as well as heating may be required). The ambient temperature should not exceed 26°C nor fall below 10°C, with an optimum range of 15–25°C. In addition, consideration should be given to the effects of prevailing winds and weather, as this can significantly affect the ability to maintain adequate temperature in a shelter.

Principles of design of specific areas of the shelter

Reception area

A shelter should have a reception area, separate from the animal accommodation area, where members of the public can engage with staff and volunteers (Figure 10.5). The reception should have sufficient space to be comfortable for visitors, and consideration should be given to providing seating for potential adopters to use while they wait to be shown around and meet animals, and while they complete the paperwork for adoption. If there is sufficient space, educational materials, video screens or goods for sale can be displayed.

Quiet/relinquishment room

Ideally, there should be a separate room, accessible from the reception area, that provides a private area for people to use when relinquishing animals, as they may be distressed (Figure 10.6). This room could also be used during the adoption process, to give staff the opportunity to impart important rehoming messages to adopters in a quiet environment where they are more likely to take in the information.

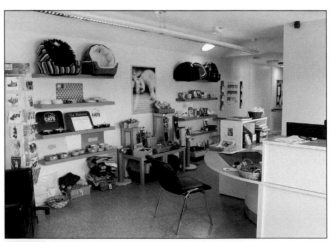

10.5 Reception area.
(© Cats Protection)

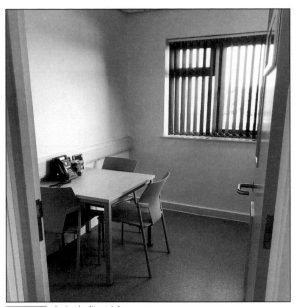

10.6 Quiet/relinquishment room.
(© Dogs Trust)

Veterinary facilities

All shelters should have an area away from the accommodation areas where animals can be examined. Depending on the organization's size, resources and activities, this might be a very basic examination area, a dedicated veterinary treatment room or even full veterinary facilities.

If veterinary medicines are to be stored at and supplied from the shelter (i.e. to be prescribed/dispensed, rather than only medicines that have been allocated to a specific animal), the premises must be registered as a 'Registered Veterinary Practice Premises'. This is administered by the Royal College of Veterinary Surgeons (RCVS) on behalf of the Veterinary Medicines Directorate (VMD).

A shelter may also wish to voluntarily register the veterinary facilities under the RCVS Practice Standards Scheme. This allows the RCVS to inspect the premises on behalf of the VMD.

Veterinary treatment and examination room

It should be possible to examine animals outside their kennel unit or pen in a safe and secure room. This examination room should be a separate, lockable room, situated where there is no need to enter an accommodation area to get to it, but relatively accessible from all areas of the shelter. The room may be used for veterinary examinations of animals within the shelter and, depending on the services offered by the shelter, for owners to attend for re-examination of their animals post adoption. Ideally, the room should have a small holding area or anteroom with adequate space to place cat carriers or for people to wait with dogs.

Ideally, the room should be equipped like a consulting room in a veterinary clinic. It should contain a sink, an examination table, weighing scales, clippers, a focal light source, a computer (if the shelter uses an electronic record system) and counter space (Figure 10.7). If veterinary medicinal products are to be stored there, the room must have lockable cupboards, a pharmaceutical fridge (which should maintain the temperature at 2–8°C), hazardous waste containers and the ability to maintain room temperature below 25°C. It may be useful to have a few stand-alone holding pens to facilitate routine treatments, such as

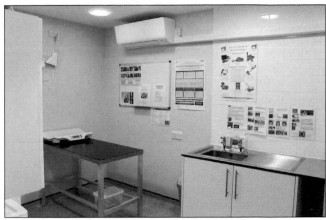

10.7 Examination room.
(© Cats Protection)

parasite control or initial health checks, before an animal is taken to its accommodation pen.

If the shelter has a surgical suite/veterinary clinic (see below), it is likely that the examination room would form part of this facility. In addition, the room may be multipurpose and used for other activities such as assessment of animals by shelter staff and grooming cats (note that separate grooming facilities are required for dogs to allow them to be bathed).

Surgical suite

Not all shelters will have this facility, and those that do not may use the services of local veterinary practices for surgical procedures. Some shelters will have facilities for a limited range of procedures, such as neutering, minor operations and dental treatment; others may have full veterinary facilities including X-ray, ultrasonography and the ability to hospitalize patients. If surgical facilities are available, there should be a separate room used only for this purpose, which should be equipped with an operating table, operating light, anaesthetic equipment, a scavenging system for removal of anaesthetic gases, an autoclave, and provision for storage of surgical instruments, gowns, gloves, suture material, etc. (Figure 10.8). The suite should also have an area for preparation of animals before surgery

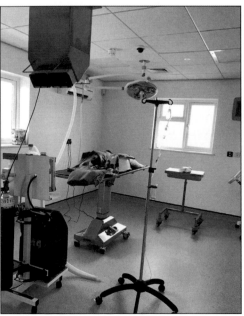

10.8

Surgical suite.
(© Dogs Trust)

and a recovery area. It is important that the recovery pens or kennels are used only for this purpose and not viewed as overflow pens/kennels by the shelter staff. Situating them within a lockable surgical suite or veterinary clinic will aid this differentiation.

Behaviour and 'real life' areas

Generally, a shelter needs to have one or more spaces where staff can work with adult cats or dogs that are bored or frustrated, for desensitization of fearful cats and dogs, or for kitten and puppy socialization. These are sometimes called behaviour or 'real life' rooms. A behaviour room provides an enriched environment for helping animals that are bored or frustrated (Figure 10.9). The aim is to habituate cats and dogs to that environment, helping them to overcome any particular behaviour problems that they may have.

The construction of an indoor behaviour or 'real life' room should be in accordance with the following general considerations:

* A separate room that is located near the rehoming area of the facility, if the public will have access to it
* Minimum room size approximately 5 m x 5 m
* A secure door
* Natural lighting
* A window so shelter staff can see in. This may be one-way glass
* Furniture that is made of material that is easy to clean and disinfect or change. Common items include a table, chairs, a sofa, a lamp, provision for a computer and play resources for cats and dogs. For cats, shelves and hiding places are also beneficial (Figure 10.10).

For more information about 'real life' rooms, see Chapter 19.

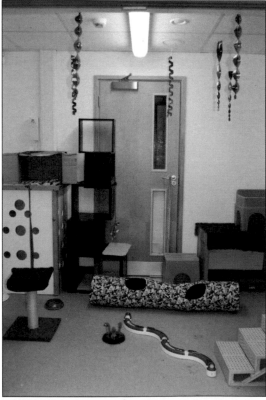

10.9 Behaviour room for cats.
(© Cats Protection)

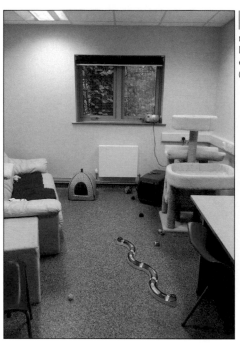

10.10 A 'real life' room looks more like a home environment.
(© Cats Protection)

'Meet and greet' areas

A 'meet and greet' area is for members of the public who wish to spend more time with an animal outside the pen/kennel unit environment.

For dogs, these activities can take place either indoors in a room or, for example, a large barn or in a secure outdoor area. This also allows space to facilitate the meeting of an existing family dog with a prospective new dog. Indoor facilities for dogs might also be used as enrichment areas and for activities such as training classes.

For cats, the 'meet and greet' area is generally a separate room within the shelter, ideally beside the reception and near the rehoming area. The 'meet and greet' and behaviour facilities for cats should be in separate rooms, but if this is not possible then one dual-purpose room will suffice.

It is important that these rooms are cleaned and disinfected between animals, and particularly between animals from different risk groups.

Exercise areas

For dogs, each kennel unit should consist of an indoor sleeping area and an outdoor run for toileting and movement. Additional exercise areas must be provided in order to allow increased levels of activity. These areas should consist of secure runs with different substrates on the ground, such as concrete, grass and sand (Figure 10.11). The areas can be enriched by providing the ability to climb (e.g. hillocks created by mounds of earth, wooden platforms), areas to forage (particularly grassy areas), water and toys. This enrichment is vital to provide stimulation for the dogs. It does not have to be expensive or manufactured; for example, straw bales or old tyres can be repurposed to provide enrichment (see QRG 19.7 for more ideas) (Figure 10.12). In addition, other areas should be identified where dogs can be walked; the ability to walk dogs on or off the lead will depend on the security of the area.

Some shelters may also have large indoor areas (sometimes referred to as training barns) that can be used for a variety of functions; for example, these can be used to provide enrichment and interaction for dogs, also as meet

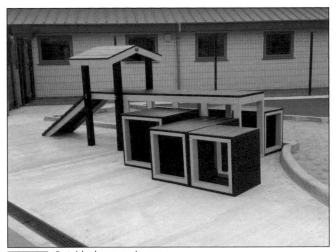

10.11 Outside dog exercise area.
(© Dogs Trust)

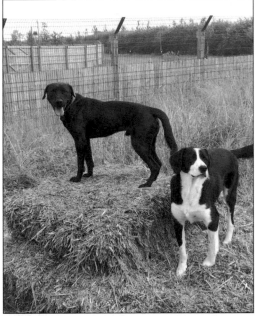

10.12 Hill straw bales (low cost enrichment).
(© Dogs Trust)

and greet areas and for assessments of dogs. They might also be used for external events such as training classes. Such facilities need to be secure, with a smooth, impermeable, non-slip floor that is easily cleaned and disinfected.

For cats, increasing exercise and activity can be achieved within the pen by making use of vertical space, for example, by providing shelves at different heights and/or artificial climbing trees, and by promoting play and hunting activities. Using puzzle feeders is an excellent way to encourage any cat (but especially overweight and obese cats) to get more exercise and stimulation. Some shelters will have the space to enhance and enrich a separate room that can be used to provide increased levels of exercise for cats. The design and layout of this room would meet the principles outlined above in the section on behaviour/ 'real life' areas. Cats must not be allowed to exercise in insecure areas such as corridors or open public areas within the facility. This is because there is increased risk of escape and of disease transmission, and, likely, higher stress levels for both the cat being granted more space and for other cats in the facility that can see the free-roaming cat (see QRG 19.8 for more detail).

Animal accommodation areas

Flow of animals from relinquishment to rehoming

An important element of biosecurity in shelters is housing animals according to their disease risk. For this strategy to be effective, it needs to be incorporated into the design of the facility. Other than moving animals in relation to their risk status, movements should be kept to a minimum, and good design can help with this.

If an animal shows signs of infectious disease on admission, or if it develops signs of infectious disease at any time while in the care of the shelter, it should be isolated. This can be achieved in a number of ways. Ideally, the animal is moved to a completely separate isolation facility. As an alternative, the section in which the animal is housed when the infectious disease is identified can itself become an isolation facility. If necessary, the animal can be moved, by agreement, to an isolation pen in a local veterinary practice. The decision to move the animal may be based on the health status or condition of the animal or the level of care or facilities available at the shelter.

Animals housed in isolation that have been given the 'all clear' by the attending veterinary surgeon (veterinarian) will either move to a rehoming section or, if not yet ready for rehoming, can be moved to a holding area while receiving any required treatment, such as vaccination.

Some shelters may also have an area for animals that have been chosen for adoption, but have not gone to their new home yet. Another use of this type of area is for animals that are ready for rehoming but are not coping well with exposure to the public in the rehoming area.

Animals that are pregnant on entry to the facility and young puppies/kittens should be housed in a maternity section at least until after they have received their first vaccination. This segregation serves to protect the most vulnerable animals from disease.

Animals are generally moved to the rehoming area (which is the only area to which members of the public should have access) a minimum of 48 hours after their first vaccination, and only after the veterinary surgeon has deemed them ready to be rehomed. This 48 hours may be part of, or in addition to, the 7-day intake assessment period.

General considerations for accommodation areas

As outlined above, shelters should ideally have at least four separate areas for housing animals, or the ability to provide the different types of housing (e.g. isolation, maternity) within the kennel/pen blocks. The basic principle for keeping animals in separate designated areas of a shelter is that they are kept in groups according to risk – both for transmitting disease and for contracting disease (Figure 10.13).

Animals must not be allowed to roam freely around the shelter because:

- Their movements are harder to track and trace
- Risk of escape or injury to themselves or others is increased
- It can be extremely stressful for animals – cats in particular – to be exposed to the constantly changing and often busy environment of a shelter; this includes seeing other animals not previously known to them and encountering lots of different people
- The risk of disease transmission is greater when free-roaming animals have access to various areas of the shelter.

Area	Purpose	Notes
Intake/admissions	A quarantine area and the area with highest risk of disease occurring. Animals are housed here for at least the first 7 days of their stay (see Chapter 9)	
Maternity	Area with animals most susceptible to disease, where pregnant and nursing animals are housed, as well as kittens and puppies that may not have been vaccinated	Young puppies or kittens of unknown origin may themselves be a disease risk and should therefore be kept separate from existing puppies/kittens on site until their disease status is known
Isolation	Area with highest risk of infectious disease being present, where animals that are ill and have a confirmed or suspected infectious disease are housed	Every shelter needs an isolation facility; however, how this is provided may vary. It can be: • A separate facility used specifically for this purpose • The ability to segregate certain units when required. Such units are often part of the admissions/intake area • Off site, e.g. by arrangement with a local veterinary practice. Prior agreement with the veterinary practice must be obtained if this is the case
Rehoming	Area with lower risk of disease occurring, where animals that are available for adoption are housed. Animals that came to the facility as a stray will have been in care for at least a predetermined number of days based on the stray policy of the organization. These animals will have had at least one vaccination and be deemed 'fit to home' by a veterinary surgeon	Some shelters have additional kennel or pen space that can be used for lower-risk animals such as: • Those that have been adopted (or reserved for adoption), but not yet left the facility • Animals that have been in care for more than 7 days, but do not fit the criteria to be housed in the rehoming area • When there are no pens available in the rehoming area • Animals that are not coping well with being exposed to the public in the rehoming area

10.13 Different types of accommodation areas in a shelter.

Dogs are often kept in pairs, or sometimes small communal groups, to meet their needs as social animals. Dogs must undergo behavioural assessment before being housed with others, and the introduction of one dog to another should be done safely and gradually.

Mixing of cats from different sources in communal accommodation is generally not recommended for disease control reasons, to facilitate monitoring and because of their solitary, territorial nature and general lack of need for the company of other cats. The stress-related effects of co-housing cats not previously known to each other are well documented; if cats are to be introduced to others, this integration must be done very gradually and extremely carefully, taking into account the personality of each of the cats in question.

There are many different layouts or orientations the pen/kennel areas can have in relation to each other, such as a circular, herringbone or U-shaped arrangement. The way they are laid out should take into consideration the following principles.

- For maximum biosecurity, each section should be completely separate from any other. If this is not possible then certain risk groups should not be adjoining (e.g. isolation or admissions should not be next to maternity).
- Each section should be self-contained, with its own ancillary facilities, if possible, and be able to operate independently of the others.
- Pens or kennel units should be oriented so that animals cannot see animals in other pens/kennels. If this is not possible, the animals should at least have the ability to hide or avoid visual contact with others.
- Internal corridors between rows of pens or kennel units should be wide enough that aerosols from coughing/sneezing cannot reach other pens or kennel units. An absolute minimum distance between rows is 1.2 m.
- Admissions/intake and isolation are areas that are not accessible to the public.

- Maternity is generally not accessible to the public, although it can be designed to facilitate viewing without compromising biosecurity. This also avoids moving vulnerable young animals around the shelter site. Access by the public is by invitation only.
- Members of the public should be able to access the rehoming area without passing through any of the other areas.
- There should be a door at the entrance to each different accommodation area of the shelter.
- The safety corridor (located at the end of the exercise or run area of the pens/kennel units in each accommodation area) must be securely meshed or enclosed to prevent escape. Safety corridors are not always present in kennel blocks for dogs. If this is the case, there should be a perimeter safety fence that encloses the accommodation.
- The viewing corridor, which may be the same as the safety corridor or may be at the opposite end of the pens/kennels where the sleeping area is, must also be secure to prevent escape.

Each area (admissions/intake, rehoming, maternity, isolation) should have its own food preparation area. In facilities housing cats, each area should also have a litter tray washing area that is separate from the food preparation area. The food preparation area and the tray washing area should each have dedicated sinks. This avoids cross-contamination between litter trays and food bowls and also encourages frequent hand-washing.

Laundry facilities should be available in each area if possible. If this is not feasible, bedding needs to be washed in separate loads by area and in order of increasing risk of infectious disease being present; thus, if there is only one laundry facility, the order of laundry batches should be maternity, then rehoming, admissions/intake and finally isolation. The use of an appropriate disinfectant as part of laundry procedures is also beneficial (see Chapter 9).

Because it is more likely for disease to be present in admissions/intake, and kittens/puppies are very susceptible to infection, the admissions/intake and maternity areas should ideally not share laundry, litter tray wash or food preparation facilities.

Drains in the animal accommodation areas should not allow contaminated material to pass from one pen/kennel unit to the adjacent one, and the animals should not be able to come in contact with the drain water. Drains should be easy to keep clean and free of debris. Hoses mounted on the wall in the safety corridor, or equivalent area, can be set up to deliver water mixed with disinfectant for deep cleaning the runs of each pen/kennel unit.

Specific considerations for intake/admissions areas

Animals housed in the intake/admissions area are usually the most stressed, as they are new to the shelter and are adapting to their new environment. For cats, this area should be quiet, with minimal human activity; places to hide within the pen and no lines of sight to other cats are extremely important to help them adapt and to reduce their stress levels as quickly as possible. For dogs, the intake/admissions area requires separate exercise areas to avoid potential spread of disease.

For shelters that lack a dedicated isolation area, the ability to segregate kennels in the intake/admissions area, while adhering to the specific considerations for isolation (see below), provides increased flexibility, should there be an outbreak of infectious disease.

Specific considerations for maternity areas

Ideally, the maternity section of a shelter should be built to the same specifications as the isolation area (see below), but in a small facility, or where the structure of the facility does not allow, as a minimum it should:

* Be a completely separate and self-contained area
* Have a built-in footbath at each entry/exit point; this will require frequent monitoring/changing of disinfectant to be effective. Provision of personal protective equipment (PPE) at entry/exit points is also necessary
* Have full-height sneeze barriers between pens/kennel units
* Contain a food preparation area, including a sink
* For cats, there should be a litter tray washing area, including a sink.

For individual pen design features, see the relevant sections below on cat and dog accommodation.

Specific considerations for isolation areas

The isolation area should be a separate and self-contained area of the shelter. It should have an exit to the outside of the building or be in a completely separate structure (Figure 10.14).

As this area is dedicated for animals that are sick, strict biosecurity measures are essential to stop the spread of disease to other parts of the shelter. It should have built-in footbaths at every entry/exit point; these will require frequent monitoring and changing of disinfectant to be effective. Provision of PPE at these points is also necessary. Each pen/kennel unit should have separate ventilation, and there should be full-height sneeze barriers between the pens/kennel units. The isolation facility also needs its own

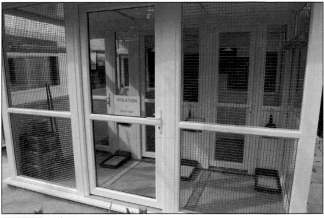

10.14 Isolation area.
(© Cats Protection)

food preparation area, including a sink. For isolation areas housing cats, it is good to have a separate litter tray washing area with a dedicated sink; alternatively, disposable litter trays and food bowls could be used.

Ideally, the isolation area would have its own laundry facilities, storage space, waste disposal facilities and a wider safety corridor. If space permits, it is also useful to have a small examination room within the isolation area.

Specific considerations for rehoming areas

These areas must be user-friendly for the general public and provide a place where people can see the animals, but not necessarily come into direct contact with them, so that each is protected from the other. Facilities for handwashing or use of alcohol hand-sanitizing gel should be provided.

Kennel unit/pen design

General principles of kennel unit/pen design

There are various recommendations regarding the size of cat pens or dog kennel units. While the ideal is 'the larger, the better', in practice space constraints are always present. As the main activity of shelters is usually to provide a temporary home for animals, guidelines are often given in terms of a minimum footprint (floor area) and/or a maximum number of animals per pen. Ideally, the animals will have two compartments within their accommodation so that they can have a warm, clean area for sleeping, eating and drinking and a cooler area where they can defecate and move about more. This 'run' or 'exercise' area is often separated from the sleep area by a pop hatch or cat flap to keep the heat in.

For pens that house single cats, the sleeping accommodation should have a minimum area of 0.85 m², with the smallest dimension being no smaller than 0.9 m (Chartered Institute for Environmental Health, 2013).

Defining specific kennel sizes for dogs is challenging owing to the wide variety of different shapes and sizes of dog breeds. As a general principle, a dog must be able to sit and stand at full height, stretch and wag its tail without touching the sides of the kennel unit. The floor area in the sleeping accommodation must be a minimum of twice the area required for a dog to lie flat. For two or more dogs sharing a kennel unit, the total area must be at least the sum of that required for each dog.

There must be no direct contact between animals in adjacent pens/kennel units or from the safety corridor. The walls of the pen/kennel unit should ideally be of solid construction and made from a material that cannot be seen through. If adequate light is a concern, then the top half of the barrier between pens/kennel units could be made of a solid but translucent material, to allow some light in and at the same time significantly reduce visibility between pens. If wire mesh is used to divide adjacent units, correctly fitted opaque (i.e. not transparent/clear, or frosted) sneeze barriers should be installed. These must be full width and can be full height or have a 10 cm gap at the top for ventilation. Typically, full-height sneeze barriers are used in pens designed specifically for isolation or maternity use.

All internal surfaces should be durable, smooth and impervious, avoiding cracks and gaps that could harbour infection. They should be able to be easily cleaned and disinfected with commonly used disinfectants. Steam treatment may also be used as a method of cleaning, so materials must be able to withstand this treatment without being damaged. Wood is not an ideal material; however, if used, any exposed wood on the inside of the pen must be suitably treated to conform to these specifications – that is, it should be rendered impermeable by chemical treatment or lining with an impermeable material such as plastic. All junctions should be sealed or, ideally, coved, and there should be no rough edges or projections that could cause injury. Where wire mesh is used, the wire diameter should not be less than 2 mm (14 standard wire gauge) for cat or dog accommodation. The size of the mesh opening must not be less than 16 mm, and should not exceed 25 mm for cats and small dogs/puppies and 50 mm for large dogs. Gaps between openings (e.g. between a door and its frame, or between the door and floor) must be less than 25 mm to avoid trapping injuries. For pens or kennel units that are not inside a thermally insulated building, the roof should be capable of filtering ultraviolet (UV) light and providing shade; it is recommended that double roofing (mesh and a waterproof layer) be installed to prevent escape of cats should the structure be damaged by extreme weather.

Flooring should be installed such that adequate drainage is achievable from each pen separately, with no communication of water between pens and no pooling of water. To avoid pooling, floors should be laid to a minimum slope of 1 in 80, leading to a shallow drainage channel or an effectively covered deep drainage channel that sits outside the pen. The floor itself should be an impervious surface capable of withstanding commonly used disinfectants, smooth enough to allow for squeegees to be used yet textured enough to avoid shelter staff slipping.

The temperature in the sleeping area should ideally be maintained at between 15°C and 18°C, with an absolute minimum of 10°C and maximum of 26°C. Fireproof thermal insulation can be incorporated into the roof and sides of the sleeping area if necessary. There should be provision for ambient and safe heating if temperatures fall below 15°C, and the ability to cool the pens/kennels to avoid the temperature exceeding 26°C. The animal should always be able to remove itself from a source of heat. If there is no central heating system, sleeping accommodation should have a separate source of warmth, such as tube or panel heaters. These heaters need to be safe – they must not pose a risk of burning the animal, should be waterproof and should be placed in such a way that the cables cannot be chewed. The material and design of the heat source should be such that it is easy to disinfect. Thermometers should be in place to allow the maximum and minimum temperature of the pens/kennels to be easily checked.

The design of the pen or kennel unit should ensure there is permanent ventilation to prevent humidity and manage smells, and also control the spread of airborne disease, without incurring draughts. It is best to have 100% air exchange with outside air rather than recirculation of air within the accommodation; if this is not possible to achieve with natural ventilation, mechanical forced ventilation should be employed. For areas where air is recirculated or exchanged, there are various recommendations for the number of complete air changes that should be provided:

- The Universities Federation for Animal Welfare recommends 10–12 air changes per hour
- The Humane Society of the United States recommends 8–15 air changes per hour
- The Association of Shelter Veterinarians recommends 10–20 air changes per hour.

Natural light is preferable and a diurnal cycle of light and dark periods is required. Skylights can be used to facilitate this.

Ideally, each pen or kennel unit should have covered electrical sockets for diffusers/heat pads, etc. These should be rated as water safe.

Design details for cat accommodation

Cats should be housed either individually, in groups of a maximum of two adult cats from the same source, or as a family group of one queen and her litter of kittens. Cats operate in terms of three-dimensional space, feel safer in elevated spaces, and must have choice of areas in which to spend time. Multiple shelves and perches at various heights should be provided in both the sleeping area and exercise area. This will allow the cat to have different vantage points from the pen; in addition, increasing the use of vertical space will effectively increase the footprint of the pen. Corner shelves are good because the cat cannot be approached from behind, which will make the cat feel safer. Access to shelves should be designed so that even less agile cats can use them; for example, ladders, ramps, extra shelves or a Feline Fort® can be used (see also QRG 19.8) (Figure 10.15).

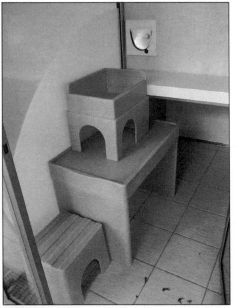

10.15 The Feline Fort® increases vertical space and provides places to hide.
(© Cats Protection)

All cats need a place to hide, regardless of whether they show obvious signs of stress or hiding behaviour. A balance should be struck between allowing the cat to be seen by visitors and ensuring that its welfare needs are met. Provision of adequate hiding places has been shown to speed up rehoming. The cat hide component of the Feline Fort®, the Hide, Perch & Go™ box, igloo beds and cardboard boxes are all suitable examples of pen equipment that will provide the cat with a place to hide while remaining partially visible (Figure 10.16).

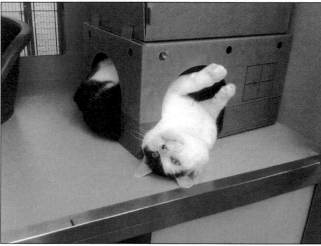

10.16 The Hide, Perch & Go™ box provides cats with a place to hide.
(© Cats Protection)

All pens should have a private location in the exercise/run area where litter trays can be placed. In a walk-in style pen, cat flaps should be positioned in the door between the sections, to allow a litter tray to be placed in a private part of the exercise and toileting section without blocking the door.

Where two cats are housed in the same pen, there must be enough space to provide more than one of each essential resource. When cats are housed together it is important to provide beds in places that allow them to maintain a distance of 1 m from each other. If the sleeping area is full height instead of a cabin (see below for more detail) then this area must have a sleeping shelf provided at a height of 0.9 m from the ground. The shelf needs to be large enough for safe placement of a cat bed, covered hiding box or the cat hide component of the Feline Fort®.

Cat flaps should have as large an opening as possible to accommodate the variety of sizes of cats that the pen may house. Flaps with a rectangular opening will provide a larger effective area than those with a curved bottom section. Ideally, a pen will have multiple cat flaps at different levels with easy access to each one – especially in larger pens that are more likely to have more than one cat in residence. This will facilitate easy manoeuvring of cats around the pen and help prevent resource blocking.

It is also desirable to include windows in the sleeping area, with access to them (e.g. provided by shelving), to provide a stimulating and interesting view. Ideally, the outside environment should be designed to provide visual interest.

Overall, the shelves, sleeping area and the area where litter trays are placed should be oriented so that they are not overlooked by cats in neighbouring pens.

Different designs of pens for cats

There are many different designs of cat pen available. The most common type seen in shelters in the UK consists of a raised, heated cabin area for sleeping, eating and drinking,

and a larger, cooler run area with shelves where the cat can move around and where the litter tray can be placed in a private location under the cabin (Figure 10.17). The cabin section may be at the back or the front of the exercise area; the former provides more privacy for the cat as it increases the distance to the point from which the cat may be observed. Walk-in style, full-height designs are becoming more popular owing to human health and safety considerations (Figure 10.18); these can be fitted with shelving or other furniture, such as a Feline Fort®, to create the different functional areas and provide enrichment for the cat.

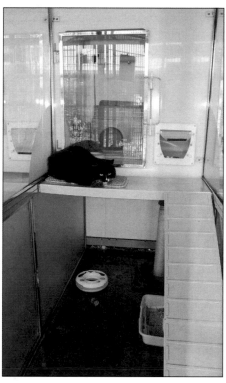

10.17 Two-compartment cat pen with a raised cabin area and a larger 'run' area where the cat can move more and toilet in private.
(© Cats Protection)

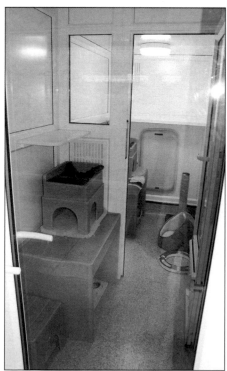

10.18 Two-compartment walk-in style pen for cats.
(© Cats Protection)

Walk-in style pens can be configured as two compartments or as one. In addition, some shelters will use pens that consist of a cabin only (like the recovery pens used in veterinary practices) to house rescue cats, but these have very limited space and it is difficult to fit all of the cat's essential resources (see below) into the space available. The main disadvantages of one-compartment pens are that they provide the cat with less choice, it is more difficult to provide areas of different temperature and ventilation tends to be more limited. In a one-compartment pen, the cat's litter tray, food and water are in the same air space; this can be aversive and cause stress, unless the pen is very spacious. In addition, some potential difficulties arise for both the cat and the caregiver with one-compartment pens, because the cat needs to be removed from the pen or temporarily placed in a carrier while the pen is cleaned and disinfected. In two-compartment pens, the cat can be encouraged to move through a cat flap into the other section to facilitate cleaning, whereas in a one-compartment pen they will always need to be handled during the pen cleaning process.

It is possible to use a single design of pen that accommodates the needs of all cats housed in the shelter; however, some pens designed for a specific application may be considered and are described as follows.

Isolation pen: This may be the same as a standard two-compartment pen with a smaller sleeping/cabin area relative to the exercise and toileting area; it may be a two-compartment pen with the space split equally between the sleeping area and the exercise/toileting area; or it may be a one-compartment pen. Splitting the space equally between two compartments allows for a larger sleeping area to be provided, so that cats can be confined to the sleeping area if necessary. Whichever design is used, the pen still needs to provide a place for the cat to hide and three-dimensional spaces for enrichment. Separate ventilation should be provided for each isolation pen.

Maternity pens: These are specially designed pens that have an extra sleeping area, or extra shelving within the sleeping area, that only the queen is able to access. This allows the queen to have a break from rearing her kittens if she chooses, and will assist the queen in self-weaning the kittens. The pen and its furniture must be arranged so that kittens cannot fall from a height (Figure 10.19).

Larger pens: Larger pens can be used for housing cats that have come from a large multi-cat household, for cats that are showing signs of frustration as a result of being confined in a standard-size pen for a long time, or for a cat that simply does not cope with the limited amount of space a standard pen provides. It is not recommended to use these large pens to mix cats from different social groups, for disease control and behavioural reasons.

There are various designs of larger pens; their main feature is usually that they have more floor area than a standard pen. They can be constructed as a larger fixed-size pen, separate from the standard pens in the facility. This allows greater numbers of cats to be housed, and this type of pen is often used when a large group of cats is taken in from the same household. The simplest way to create a 'larger' pen is to make greater use of the vertical space available in a standard pen (e.g. by adding more perches or shelves). A more flexible design for creating larger pens is to have a removable partition in the wall of the exercise area between two adjacent pens in a bank of standard pens; if more space is required, the partition can be removed to effectively create a double-sized pen.

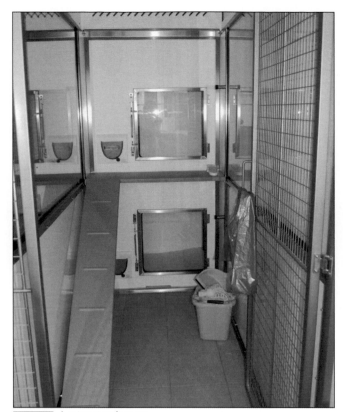

10.19 A cat maternity pen.
(© Cats Protection)

Feral enclosures: A feral cat is a cat that was not socialized to a domestic environment when it was between 2 and 7 weeks of age (see Chapter 4). As a result, it is fearful of humans and is very unlikely to adapt to a domestic home. The welfare needs of feral cats are best met by living in an outdoor, free-roaming environment. Keeping feral or poorly socialized cats confined in a shelter is extremely stressful for the cats and is not recommended. Some animal organizations that work specifically with feral cats in trap-neuter-return programmes may have a feral enclosure that they use to house cats that need to be kept for a short time after neutering, before relocation if they cannot be returned to their site of origin (see QRG 5.1). A feral enclosure is not a pen *per se*, but a much larger, escape-proof fenced area, ideally with long grass and small cabins or huts where the cats can shelter from the elements and maintain a distance from each other (Figure 10.20).

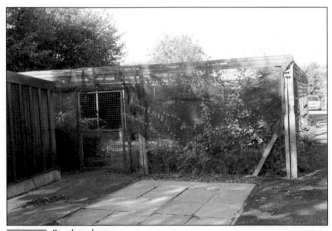

10.20 Feral enclosure.
(© Cats Protection)

Essential resources for cat pens

Regardless of the structure and design of the pen, there are some essential items that need to be provided in order to meet cats' welfare needs. For cats coming into an unfamiliar environment, it is important that they have the ability to make choices and that they have a sense of being in control of the space to which they have access. For the majority of cats, the space provided in a shelter pen is considerably more restricted than they are accustomed to, and so it is important to maximize the available space (e.g. by using perches or shelves) and provide enrichment.

Essential resources for a cat pen:
* Beds
* Separate food and water bowls
* Scratching posts
* Litter trays
* Places to hide
* Places to get up high
* Toys.

Note: Cats need **choice** and **control**

Enrichment for cat pens

When cats first enter a shelter environment they undergo a period of acute stress while they adapt to the novel surroundings. The duration of this period is variable depending on the cat's personality, their previous experiences and the environment that is provided for them. There is much that can be done to ease the settling-in process for them and help them adjust quickly (see Chapter 19). The pen environment that is provided can have a big impact on how well cats cope and how quickly they adapt. It is, therefore, critical that all pens have the essential resources described above, especially places to hide and get up high. In the first few days after entry into a shelter, keeping the cat's environment consistent is key to helping it settle in, and the number, location and type of items in the pen needs to be kept the same. If a cat shows a preference for its resources to be placed in a certain way in the pen, shelter workers need to be responsive to this and place the items where the cat would like them to be.

After a cat has made the initial adjustment to the pen, enrichment of the environment should be approached in a different way, in order to avoid or reduce boredom and frustration that can occur in cats kept in pens. The type of enrichment that works best will vary with the individual cat, but the general principle is to vary the types of toys and play activity and the daily routine that the cat experiences. Puzzle feeders are an excellent way to stimulate the cat; there are many different kinds available, from a simple pyramid made out of cardboard tubes from toilet rolls (Figure 10.21) to advanced toys that require the cat to use various sensory and motor skills (Figure 10.22). Some cats will need more ability to see the area outside their pen or the outdoors over time. Others will need more time with people. QRG 19.8 outlines some key concepts for providing environmental enrichment in a pen environment.

Design details for dog accommodation

Ideally, dogs are housed in pairs or small groups, because they are social animals that require companionship and interaction. It is important that dogs are assessed behaviourally before being mixed. Dogs, unlike cats, may not

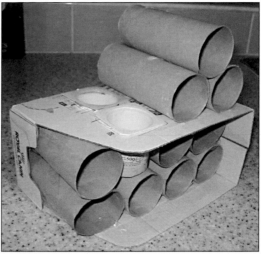

10.21 Low-cost homemade puzzle feeder.
(© Cats Protection)

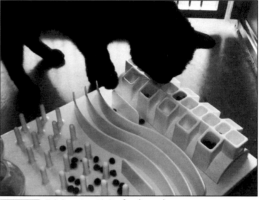

10.22 Trixie cat activity fun board.
(© Cats Protection)

routinely be considered as operating in a three-dimensional space; however, the provision of items, such as chairs and bunk beds in kennel units increases the options available to them.

Kennel units, which may be of a standard size within a shelter, are often divided into an indoor sleeping area and a (preferably outdoor) 'run' area designed for movement and toileting. If the run area is open to the elements, at least 50% of it should be covered to provide protection from extremes of weather, including UV light. Kennel units should be positioned such that there is natural ventilation without draughts, or provision should be made to address any draughts.

An access door for caregivers into each end of the kennel unit (i.e. allowing direct access to both the sleeping area and the run area) is recommended for safety reasons. Having a pop hatch rather than an open aperture between the sleeping and run areas will allow a dog access to all areas of the kennel unit while maintaining the temperature within the sleeping area. Provision of a solid door on a pulley will facilitate remotely operated isolation of the resident dog(s) to a particular area of the kennel unit should this be necessary.

The siting of a third access door for caregivers, between the sleeping and run areas of the kennel unit, should also be considered. This will allow all kennel routines, such as feeding, cleaning and taking the dog(s) out for exercise, to be undertaken from a single ('routine') side of the kennel. This is of welfare benefit to the dogs in that they will soon recognize that people approaching from the 'non-routine' side of the kennel will not access the kennel or be a threat. This is particularly useful in kennel units that are used to house dogs ready for rehoming. The side to which the general public have access is designated the 'non-routine' side of the kennel unit. Therefore, the approach of an unknown member of the public should not pose a perceived threat, as the dog learns that no direct contact is made from that side of the kennel unit.

Consideration must also be given to the fact that it is likely that dogs will be resident for much longer than the average 1- to 2-week stay in a boarding establishment. While some boarding establishments may have a dedicated run area that is located away from the sleeping accommodation, it is preferable in the shelter environment for the kennel units to have two compartments (sleep and run/activity). This gives the dogs more choice, particularly as they will spend a significant proportion of their day in this accommodation. The kennel unit must be of a sufficient size for the number of dogs it is intended to house (see 'Size' below). In addition, kennel units should be designed in such a way that a dog has the ability to remove itself from the line of sight of a dog in a different kennel.

Considerations for designs of kennels for dogs

Based on a standard format for a kennel unit consisting of a sleeping area and an adjoining run, there are several design considerations to be made.

Materials: Traditionally, the doors of dog kennels have been constructed of metal bars or mesh. This can be a significant safety concern in terms of visiting members of the public attempting to touch the dogs; this also has an impact on the dogs from the threat of a stranger impinging into their kennel space. The use of glass-fronted kennels removes any perceived threat from the dog's perspective and is a much safer environment for visitors. The provision of facilities such as 'sniff holes' in the glass can allow interaction between a potential adopter and dog in a controlled manner (Figure 10.23).

Size: Kennel units would normally be built to a standard size within the shelter according to whether they are to house single or multiple dogs. Multiple-dog housing is preferable to encourage co-housing of dogs wherever

possible. It also provides much more flexibility; for example, it may allow three small dogs to be housed in an area designed for two larger dogs. Defining specific sizes of kennel for dogs is challenging due to the wide variety of shapes and sizes of different breeds. As a general principle, a dog must be able to sit and stand at full height, stretch and wag its tail without touching the sides of the kennel. The floor area of the sleeping accommodation must be a minimum of twice the area required for a dog to lie flat. For two or more dogs sharing a kennel, the total area must be at least the sum of that required for each dog.

Layout: The way in which the kennel units are arranged in the shelter requires careful consideration. Dogs do need to be able to have control over their visual access to other dogs, and must have that ability within the kennel unit. Kennels that are opposite each other, or in a horseshoe shape, must be arranged with sufficient distance between them such that if non-desirable interactions occur they are not aggravated by the dogs being in close proximity.

Isolation pen: An alternative approach for isolation of sick dogs is to have kennel units designated for isolation purposes that could be part of the general kennels (specifically, the intake/admission kennels) but, for example, sited at the end of a row of kennels, with a means of separating them (e.g. by the use of a secure door) when isolation is required. These kennels could then be utilized for the majority of the time, allowing greater efficiency of use of kennel space. Such kennel units must have their own adjoining run in order to reduce as far as possible the risk of disease spreading around the shelter site.

Maternity pens: These are specially designed kennel units designed to facilitate whelping and accommodate puppies in a safe environment for the first 2–3 months of life (Figure 10.24). The kennel unit is divided into two compartments that are separated by a low door, so that the bitch can separate herself from her puppies as required. As the puppies grow and are weaned, the larger space can house them until adoption.

If the maternity kennel units are glass fronted, it may be possible to provide a viewing area for potential adopters. This ensures that viewing of puppies occurs in a controlled environment; this is particularly useful from a disease control perspective as it means that puppies do not need to be moved around the site.

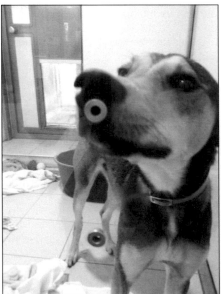

10.23 Sniff holes in a glass-fronted kennel unit.
(© Dogs Trust)

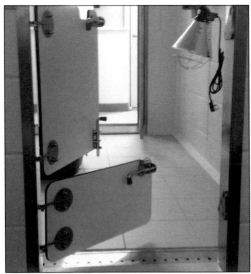

10.24 A whelping pen.
(© Dogs Trust)

Versatile spacing: Rather than having brick partitions between the sleeping areas of adjacent kennel units, if funds allow, installing opaque glass doors between one or two pairs of kennels should be considered. Having these doors means that if a particularly large breed of dog is in the shelter, two adjacent kennels can be opened up to provide the dog with a bigger living space. When these pens are in 'closed' mode, the door seal needs to be sufficient to prevent wash-down water leaking between units. The door and its seal must also prevent nose-to-nose contact of residents in adjacent kennels.

Larger pens: Larger kennel units may be used for dogs that are long-term residents of the shelter. In addition to having more space, these units may also provide direct access to a dedicated run area with environmental enrichment (Figure 10.25).

Dogs that have specific behavioural problems may also benefit from being housed in an area that provides more space. If site space and funds allow, it is recommended to have some kennel units away from the main shelter accommodation where dogs can be housed in a 'self-contained' manner. This will provide a quiet, calmer environment where individual dogs' needs can be met and behavioural problems addressed.

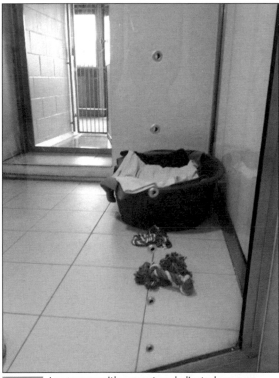

10.25 Larger pen with access to a dedicated run area.
(© Dogs Trust)

Communal dog enclosures: Some dogs may not tolerate the kennel environment well. At a heightened level of stress, a dog's behaviour may be unpredictable and it may not respond to training or behavioural rehabilitation. For such dogs, the opportunity to reside in a less enclosed environment may be beneficial. A communal dog enclosure is a large enclosure designed to house several dogs, with an inside area providing basic accommodation while protecting the dogs from extremes of weather. As the dogs are not walked in the traditional fashion, it is important that such enclosures have sufficient environmental enrichment.

Care must be taken when selecting dogs to live in such a group. It is important that any dogs selected to enter a communal enclosure can be sufficiently handled to ensure both the safety of the handlers and adequate monitoring of the dogs' health and welfare.

Essential resources for dog pens

Irrespective of how well designed and equipped a kennel unit is, it is not the same as a home environment and is likely to be a source of stress for many dogs. Shelter proprietors have a duty of care to ensure the dogs' welfare needs are met.

> Essential resources for a dog pen:
> * Beds
> * Food and water bowls
> * Place to hide
> * Enrichment – e.g. toys.

Enrichment for dog kennel units

Like cats, dogs also experience acute stress on entering a shelter environment, particularly for the first 2 weeks. Dogs respond well to routine and, given that they will spend a significant part of the day in their kennel unit, activities such as feeding become a focus and highlight of the day. For some dogs, the act of eating can be over in seconds; the use of items such as puzzle feeders can prolong this activity and provide enrichment. Toys can help to alleviate boredom, but must be able to be disinfected, or disposable, and rotated in order to remain novel.

Kennel units can be further enriched by giving dogs choices such as a variety of beds (for example, 'bunk beds' that allow dogs to rest at an elevated point). See QRG 19.7 for further information.

References and further reading

Chartered Institute of Environmental Health (2013) *CIEH Model Licence Conditions and Guidance for Cat Boarding Establishments 2013* (updated June 2016). Available at www.cieh.org/WorkArea/DownloadAsset.aspx?id=59750

Chartered Institute of Environmental Health (2016) *CIEH Model Licence Conditions and Guidance for Dog Boarding Establishments 2016*. Available at www.cieh.org/WorkArea/DownloadAsset.aspx?id=59652

Feline Advisory Bureau (2002) *Boarding Cattery Manual*, ed. C Bessant. Feline Advisory Bureau, Tisbury

Key D (2006) *Cattery Design: The Essential Guide to Creating Your Perfect Cattery*. David and Kay Key Kennel & Cattery Design, Chipping Norton

Key D (2008) *Kennel Design – The Essential Guide to Creating Your Perfect Kennels*. David and Kay Key Kennel & Cattery Design, Chipping Norton

Newbury S, Blinn MK, Bushby PA *et al.* (2010) *Guidelines for Standards of Care in Animal Shelters*. Association of Shelter Veterinarians. Available at: www.sheltervet.org/assets/docs/shelter-standards-oct2011-wforward.pdf

Useful websites

Association of Charity Vets (ACV):
www.associationofcharityvets.org.uk

Association of Shelter Veterinarians:
www.sheltervet.org

Royal College of Veterinary Surgeons, Information regarding veterinary practices:
www.rcvs.org.uk/registration/register-of-veterinary-practice-premises/
www.rcvs.org.uk/practice-standards-scheme/

Universities Federation for Animal Welfare:
www.ufaw.org.uk

United States Humane Society:
www.humanesociety.org

Chapter 11

Preventive medicine in the shelter environment

John Helps and Rachel Dean

> *Preventive medicine focuses on the health of individuals, communities, and defined populations. Its goal is to protect, promote, and maintain health and well-being and to prevent disease, disability, and death.*
>
> American College of Preventive Medicine,
> www.acpm.org

Preventive medicine is a cornerstone of shelter medicine. The population of animals in a shelter environment is dynamic, with individuals of different immune and disease status constantly entering and leaving. This environment is often and unavoidably emotionally and psychologically stressful. This, combined with the high stocking densities that are often encountered in shelters, means that the continual flux of animals considerably increases the risk of infectious disease.

The focus of this chapter is the control of infectious and parasitic diseases with the use of vaccines and pharmaceutical products, with particular attention paid to flea control and the rational approach to endoparasites. These forms of disease control, alongside biosecurity measures, good management practices and population control, are vital to the reduction of morbidity and mortality due to infectious pathogens (see Chapter 9 and QRG 9.1).

The UK is fortunate to be free of rabies and a number of globally important parasites, such as heartworm (*Dirofilaria immitis*) and established populations of ticks, such as *Rhipicephalus* spp. Such additional risks of exotic disease can have a significant impact on the approach taken to preventive health measures within a shelter. For guidance on such threats, the reader is encouraged to seek further information about the additional risks that are relevant to their geographical location, for example, from the professional guidelines listed in the Useful websites section at the end of the chapter (see also Appendix 1 at the end of the manual). QRG 16.3 provides a brief overview of some of these pathogens.

Vaccination

Principles of vaccination

Shelter kennels and catteries provide a unique set of challenges for the control of infectious disease. The rapid turnover of animals of different ages and variable health status, with potentially unknown prior vaccination history, inevitably results in the regular reintroduction of new potential pathogens into a population of individuals that may be immunologically susceptible. Other factors, such as shelter design, ventilation and hygiene (see Chapter 10), stress levels, mixing of animals and variable levels of biosecurity (see Chapter 9) can all significantly affect the risk of infectious disease.

Having an understanding of the principles of vaccination allows the veterinary surgeon (veterinarian) to deploy them to the most appropriate effect. It is, however, important to remember that vaccines do not provide full protection in all circumstances, and their use is no substitute for adequate biosecurity and infection control measures within the shelter. The use of a range of such measures is paramount in maintaining effective overall disease prevention against a far wider range of contagious threats than those covered by vaccines. So, while the strategic use of vaccines is essential in reducing the number of immunologically naive individuals, vaccination forms only one element of the disease prevention strategy.

What is a vaccine?

Vaccines are antigenic products typically derived from, or synthesized to immunologically imitate, the causative agents of diseases (Figure 11.1). Vaccination is a form of active immunization that involves administering an antigen

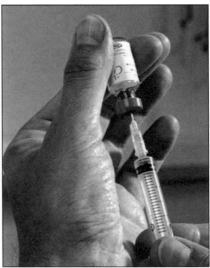

11.1 Vaccines are a vital part of preventive medicine. (Reproduced from the *BSAVA Textbook of Veterinary Nursing*, 5th edition)

product in a way that leads to the development of acquired immunity and, therefore, immunological memory. Administering vaccines for certain pathogens may stimulate both branches of the acquired immune system (see Principles of immunology), leading to a variable expectation of immunity, depending on the pathogen and the vaccine.

Why do we use vaccines?

The routine and strategic use of vaccines can:

- Reduce or prevent the risk of infection and/or clinical signs in an individual animal following exposure
- Reduce the risk of shedding and transmission of infection from vaccinated animals
- Reduce the risk of transmission of zoonotic infections (e.g. leptospirosis, rabies) to humans.

Importantly, within the shelter environment, appropriate use of vaccines may:

- Deny the pathogen access to susceptible hosts that allow continued propagation of infection in a disease outbreak. If a sufficient proportion of animals is vaccinated, this can curtail the outbreak and help drive a pathogen towards extinction – this is the principle of 'herd immunity'
- Substantially reduce the economic and reputational consequences of disease outbreaks
- Be an important factor in protecting and promoting animal welfare.

Limitations of vaccination

The level of protection achieved by vaccination may be incomplete. Therefore, it must not be assumed that a cat or dog is totally protected from disease if it is vaccinated.

The efficacy of a vaccine is affected by a range of factors:

- The vaccine must be sufficiently antigenic to elicit an immune response (see Licensing of vaccines)
- A fully competent immune system is needed for the animal to mount an appropriate immune response (see Principles of immunology). Some young, old and/or sick animals may have impaired immune systems; this does not preclude them from being vaccinated but may affect the efficacy of vaccination. Parasitism, genetic factors, stress and immunosuppressive diseases and medications may negatively affect the response
- The presence of maternally derived antibodies (MDAs) can interfere with the immune response in young animals, so this should be considered when vaccinating kittens and puppies (see Maternally derived antibodies)
- Appropriate storage and mixing and correct administration of the vaccine are necessary to ensure the maximum possible efficacy.

Even when an immunocompetent animal is correctly vaccinated, it may still show some clinical signs and shed infectious pathogens following field exposure. This is dependent on both the biology of the pathogen and the expected level of efficacy of the vaccine. Whereas some vaccines can prevent both clinical signs and shedding of the pathogen (e.g. canine parvovirus (CPV), feline panleukopenia virus (FPV)), others can only reduce clinical signs and mortality associated with infection (e.g. feline herpesvirus (FHV), canine parainfluenza virus (CPiV), *Bordetella*

bronchiseptica), thus decreasing the effects of infection for the individual animal and the risk of transmission to other animals.

Vaccines
Valency

Most vaccines for small animal use are made up of combinations of antigens, so that a range of diseases is covered in each dose. These are typically termed **multivalent** vaccines. Sometimes, vaccines may contain a single antigen (**monovalent**) or two antigens (**bivalent**). Vaccines may also be defined by the method of manufacture of the antigens they contain. An understanding of what any given vaccine contains is helpful, since it can inform expectations and appropriate vaccine use.

Route of administration

Most vaccines licensed for companion animals are given by subcutaneous or sometimes intramuscular injection to stimulate a systemic immune response (Figure 11.2). In some cases, however, alternative routes for vaccines may have immunological advantages. For example, intranasal vaccines can rapidly trigger mucosal immunity; this is an effective approach to immunization that does not appear to be impaired by MDA, and which addresses respiratory pathogens, such as *B. bronchiseptica* in dogs and cats, at the site of infection (Figure 11.3). Vaccines based on other routes of administration are used in small animals in some parts of the world. For example, oral vaccination against

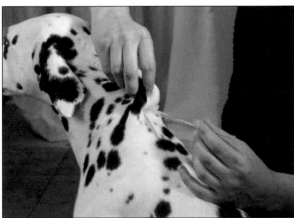

11.2 Most vaccinations for companion animals are given subcutaneously.
(Courtesy of MSD Animal Health)

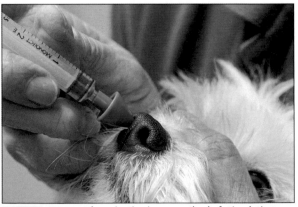

11.3 Intranasal vaccination is one method of stimulating mucosal immunity.
(Courtesy of MSD Animal Health)

Bordetella is available in the USA, and in some regions of the world oral bait vaccines are used to vaccinate stray dogs and wildlife against rabies.

Types of vaccine

Figure 11.4 gives some expected features and expectations of different vaccine types.

Live vaccines: The vaccines most often used in cats and dogs are most commonly based on live antigens. These types of viral vaccines are sometimes referred to as modified live virus (MLV) vaccines. Such formulations are typically based on attenuated (weakened) strains of pathogens; these are developed by repeated passage in cell culture until their virulence is lost but sufficient immunogenicity is maintained to stimulate effective immunity. Intranasal vaccines for *B. bronchiseptica* are also live vaccines, based on a naturally avirulent strain of the bacterium.

Live vaccines may more closely mimic natural infection than killed or inactivated vaccines, in that they typically are able to stimulate both humoral and cell-mediated immune responses. They tend to trigger a rapid immune response, providing a good chance of early protection following vaccination. A single dose of vaccine may be effective provided that MDA has declined to non-interfering levels (see Maternally derived antibodies). Evidence suggests that the priming immune response induced by MLV vaccines is less likely to be affected by MDA (DiGangi *et al.*, 2012).

These immunological advantages mean that, where available, live viral vaccines are often the preferred approach in the shelter situation, where a rapid onset of immunity after a single dose is critical. However, this does not preclude the use of other vaccine products where appropriate.

Inactivated vaccines: Some pathogens are problematic to attenuate safely, and in such cases killed or inactivated strains of the pathogen may be used to produce vaccines. Examples include vaccines used for protection against feline leukaemia virus (FeLV), canine leptospirosis and rabies. Many (but not all) inactivated vaccines incorporate a chemical adjuvant. An adjuvant is a non-specific stimulant that 'alerts' the immune system to the presence of the vaccine. The adjuvant triggers the innate immune response and helps to promote an appropriately protective

immunity. The principal advantage of using an inactivated vaccine is that it is easy to avoid the risk of residual virulence of the pathogen, which may be a theoretical concern with a live vaccine, particularly in relation to significant immunosuppressive disease. Because live vaccines against FPV are contraindicated in pregnant queens, an inactivated vaccine (if available) may be the preferred option, if a pregnant queen needs to be vaccinated in a high-challenge environment such as a shelter.

Subunit and vector vaccines: Improvements in molecular biological techniques have brought innovative ways of formulating vaccines, and some of these approaches are used in small animal vaccination. Vaccine antigens based on **subunits** (a small immunogenic part of the pathogen) are sometimes used in veterinary vaccines. When purified, the subunits may stimulate an immune response that is more focused on key antigens shown to be important for protective immunity. Such an approach may minimize additional unnecessary extraneous material in the vaccine, although, as with some inactivated vaccines, subunit-based products may require the inclusion of an adjuvant.

Some vaccines are genetically engineered; these may be described as **recombinant**. Other subunit vaccines are synthesized. When the vaccine's immunizing antigen is produced by expression of genes spliced into the genetic material of a harmless vector virus, this is termed a **vector vaccine**. This strategy combines some of the immunological advantages of both live and killed vaccines. Feline leukaemia is an example of a disease for which this technology has been employed to good effect; a vector vaccine has been developed that contains a recombinant canarypox vector virus carrying genes that code for FeLV envelope antigen.

Vaccination protocols

When deciding on a vaccination protocol for a shelter, it is important to understand the shelter's working environment. This includes the husbandry and management practices, the aims of the organization and the budget available for preventive medicine. A good understanding of the population of animals in the shelter is also needed, with a focus on their ages and origin (e.g. privately owned, stray cats, dogs from a pound), as well as knowledge of the diseases prevalent in the shelter.

Parameter	Live vaccines	Inactivated/subunit vaccines	Vectored vaccines
Primary course	Single dose may prime immunity in the absence of maternally derived antibody (MDA) Better response expected than to inactivated vaccines in the presence of MDA	Two or more doses required for optimum efficacy High levels of MDA may affect the efficacy of a primary course if the first dose is blocked	Response expected to be similar to that for a live vaccine
Onset of immunity	Rapid onset of immunity – immune response expected within a week	Slower onset of peak immunity is expected after an anamnestic response [a]	Response expected to be similar to that for a live vaccine
Induced immune response	Broad cell-mediated and humoral (antibody) immune response	Humoral immunity – in the case of purified subunit products this will be highly specific to the included antigen(s)	Cell-mediated and humoral responses expected to both the vector virus and the immunizing antigen it expresses
Adjuvant	Requires no adjuvant	Adjuvant can be required to promote local and systemic innate immune responses	Requires no adjuvant
Residual virulence	Theoretical concern of reversion to virulence	No concern of residual virulence	Avirulent vector virus means that reversion to virulence should not be a concern

11.4 Expected features of live, inactivated, subunit and vectored vaccines. [a] Renewed, rapid production of an antibody on the subsequent encounter with the same antigen.

Principles of immunology

To understand the principles of vaccination, it is important to understand some basic immunology. The immune system has three main 'arms': physical barriers, innate immunity and acquired immunity.

Physical barriers

The physical barriers of the immune system stop pathogens entering the body in the first place. These constitute the constant and immediate response of the immune system. The skin is one of the most effective aspects of this arm of the immune system – if the surface is breached infection can occur, but the skin heals rapidly, re-sealing the defences. Vomiting, diarrhoea, coughing and sneezing are all part of the physical arm of the immune system, as are the beating cilia and flow of mucus in the respiratory tract. All of these mechanisms 'flush' invaders out of the body. In addition, there are bacteria that live on the skin and in the digestive tract that are the natural (commensal) flora of these surfaces and block infection by potential pathogens. Vaccination has no effect on the physical barriers of the immune system.

Innate immunity

Innate immunity is the rapid response of the body when a pathogen breaches the physical barriers. The innate immune system is able to recognize that the pathogen is biochemically different from the host cells. It is a non-specific response that has no 'memory'. If an animal is unable to mount an effective innate immune response, overwhelming infection will rapidly result. The innate immune response is the same every time, regardless of the nature of the pathogen. It protects the body until the more specific, but slower to respond, acquired immune response becomes effective.

The innate immune response is most easily recognized as inflammation – the non-specific response of the host to microbial invasion and tissue damage. The initial response promotes increased blood flow to the affected tissue, which attracts cells and immunochemicals to the centre of the invasion. Neutrophils and macrophages are the cell types involved in inflammation, and they destroy microorganisms, limiting the spread of infection within the host. There are many immunochemicals (e.g. cytokines, inflammatory proteins, etc.) of the innate immune system, including those of the **complement** system – this is a 'cascade' of proteins that can bind to and destroy microorganisms. The administration of a vaccine will elicit an innate immune response as a 'foreign' antigen is introduced to the body.

Acquired immunity

The acquired immune response is the slowest arm of the immune system to become mobilized but is the most sophisticated. It is highly specific and is able to actively adapt when the body is exposed to novel pathogens. The acquired immune system can identify, target and neutralize pathogens in a highly specific manner. Following a repeat challenge, the body can recognize the pathogens, triggering a very rapid protective response. This 'memory' is what makes the acquired immune system so powerful and vital in the maintenance of long-standing immunity.

There are two branches of the acquired immune system, which enable the body to protect itself against both intracellular and extracellular pathogens:

- **Humoral immunity** – this involves B cells that differentiate into plasma cells producing antibodies against extracellular pathogens
- **Cell-mediated immunity** – this involves T cells of various types. Cytotoxic T cells destroy cells infected with intracellular pathogens.

The two branches of acquired immunity are closely interrelated, with T helper cells required for B cells to produce humoral immune responses, and regulatory T cells keeping inappropriate responses to self-antigens (i.e. the body's own tissues and proteins) at bay. To remain healthy and be able to deal with all types of pathogens, both branches of the acquired immune system need to be fully competent.

With an increasing number of vaccine antigens available for use, various national and international professional groups have developed vaccine guidelines to aid practitioners in decision-making around vaccination (see Vaccine guidelines, below). These guidelines, which have been devised using a mixture of evidence and expert opinion, provide broad guidance on the use of vaccines in small animal practice. They should not be seen as a set of rules that need to be followed for all cases, and they need to be applied to the local setting carefully. All of the guidelines currently available make the recommendation that the decision on which vaccines are used routinely (core vaccines) and which are not (non-core vaccines) should be based on a risk:benefit analysis.

If there is a good working relationship between the shelter and the veterinary team, this is one situation where it may be possible to carry out a well understood risk:benefit analysis as well as a cost:benefit analysis for vaccination. This is because the environment of the shelter is relatively constant and the contacts between animals are known. The diseases that each animal entering the shelter harbours may vary, but often the animals come from the same known populations outside the shelter, so the diseases that commonly enter the shelter are predictable. The future population to which the cats and dogs will be rehomed is also often known. It may, therefore, be possible to use this information to understand the vaccine needs of the animals in the shelter and weigh these needs against the risks and costs of vaccination. In most situations, the benefit of vaccinating an animal in a shelter completely outweighs any perceived risk (see Side effects and putative risks associated with vaccination), but the use of certain non-core vaccines may be precluded due to financial cost.

Some of the guidelines include specific recommendations for shelters. This is an important acknowledgement of the fact that vaccination of cats and dogs in a shelter environment is different from that in private practice, where vaccination tends to be applied on an individual rather than a 'herd' basis. It is important to be aware of the implications of deviating from the product data sheet/ Summary of Product Characteristics (SPC) when altering the protocol used to vaccinate pet cats and dogs. It is also very important to inform the new owners of which vaccines a cat or dog has received, as the animals' vaccination needs may change as soon as they leave the shelter.

General recommendations for the vaccination of animals in shelters can be divided into the following topics:

- Vaccinating on entry to the shelter
- Vaccinating dogs
- Vaccinating cats
- Vaccinating puppies and kittens
- Effects of disease status.

Vaccinating on entry to the shelter

- As a general rule, all animals should be vaccinated as soon as possible after entry to the shelter, unless there is a well evidenced up-to-date vaccination history. In an ideal world, all dogs and cats would be fully vaccinated and adequate time elapsed to allow immunity to develop before entry to a shelter. In reality, this is not usually the case, and animals without a recent vaccination history will need to be vaccinated on entry to the shelter.
- Ideally, effective quarantine of newly vaccinated individuals for a period of at least 7–10 days should be in place, to allow for incubating infections to become apparent and for vaccine-induced active immunity to become established. In many shelters this is not possible because of space or resource constraints, but it is important to recognize that an animal that has just arrived at a shelter could still develop infectious disease despite being vaccinated. Shelter workers should be made aware of this issue and the animals managed in the best way possible with the facilities available.
- For all new animals with an unknown previous vaccination history, it is necessary to commence a primary vaccination course on entry.
- Previously vaccinated animals that have lapsed from the recommended vaccination schedule, can present a dilemma. Recent key guidance suggests that a single dose is all that is required to restart a vaccination schedule in an individual whose immunity has previously been adequately primed, regardless of the time elapsed since the last vaccination. Such advice is based on the principle of persisting immunological memory, but it falls outside the licensed recommendations for use of the products, which are largely based on priming immunity for puppies and kittens. On a technical basis, the majority of live vaccines require only a single dose for immunization once MDA is no longer a problem. However, inactivated vaccines require at least two doses to induce an optimum primary response. Key opinion in recent years has been inconsistent in providing specific advice on this issue, and there is an absence of good evidence for individual products to back up such general advice. A common pragmatic approach taken by some veterinary practices to 'restart' vaccination for dogs and cats is to administer a single dose of multivalent vaccine to individuals that

have lapsed for <15–18 months; for pets that have lapsed longer than this, the vaccine course is restarted as per the SPC or data sheet recommendations for adult animals. While this possibly risks giving additional unnecessary doses, it has the advantages of simplicity, ensuring compliance with the licensed use and removing any doubt as to the vaccination status of animals – all important considerations in a high-risk environment.

Vaccinating dogs

- For dogs, routine vaccination against canine distemper virus, canine adenovirus-2 and CPV is recommended. These infectious diseases all continue to occur in shelters, with CPV being by far the most likely to be encountered. Maintaining high levels of vaccinal immunity in the dog population is essential to keep these diseases at a low level. Shelters may be vulnerable to introductions of disease in new intake, especially where the ability to quarantine the dogs is limited and there is a risk of transmission to other susceptible individuals before the onset of vaccinal immunity.
- Canine leptospirosis vaccines should be strongly considered, as the disease is potentially zoonotic and also endemic to the UK and other European countries. Transmission of leptospirosis is most often dependent on exposure to damp environments and waterways contaminated with the urine of infected rodents. The risk of disease transmission within the shelter should be low, but this will depend on the dogs' access to outdoor space, the adequacy of the drainage in the accommodation and exercise areas, whether rats are a problem in the facility and whether the dogs are exercised in a high-risk area. It is also possible that dogs may be exposed before admission. A survey of kennelled dogs of unknown vaccine status in Ireland demonstrated that asymptomatic shedding of leptospires by dogs may be surprisingly common, with around 7–8% of urine samples testing positive by polymerase chain reaction (PCR) (Rojas et al., 2010). Given the zoonotic potential and the unknown future risk of exposure to leptospires, leptospirosis vaccination is often included in vaccine protocols for shelter dogs.
- Vaccines against pathogens that cause canine infectious respiratory disease ('kennel cough'), such as B. bronchiseptica and CPiV, are often recommended because the kennel environment provides an increased risk of disease and broad coverage by vaccination reduces the risk of transmission. Vaccines provide effective immunity in individuals that are vaccinated before field infection occurs. However, in some shelters with a low prevalence of respiratory disease, these vaccines are not given as part of the routine protocol – in such circumstances, because of the very rapid onset of immunity (from 72 hours post vaccination), they can still be used in a more targeted way in the event of an outbreak, where the pathogens covered by vaccination are considered the likely cause.

Vaccinating cats

- For cats in shelters, routine vaccination against FPV (also known as feline parvovirus or feline infectious enteritis), feline calicivirus (FCV) and FHV is strongly recommended, as clinical disease and death due to these three pathogens is far more prevalent among shelter cats than the owned cat population.

- In shelters that have a known problem with conjunctivitis and upper respiratory disease due to *Chlamydia felis*, vaccination against this pathogen is recommended. In shelters where the pathogen has either not been detected or where there is a low rate of ocular disease, the use of this vaccine may not be warranted. *C. felis* does not survive well in the environment and so is more likely to be a problem in cats housed in groups. A similar approach may be used for *B. bronchiseptica* vaccination of cats.
- If cats are housed individually, the risk of transmission of FeLV is very low except between a queen and her litter. This is because the virus is rapidly inactivated outside the body and close contact is required for transmission. The use of FeLV vaccines within the shelter is, therefore, unlikely to be of immediate benefit except in a group housing situation. However, many shelter cats will be rehomed to multi-cat environments, and this should be considered when designing a vaccine protocol.

Vaccinating puppies and kittens

- The youngest animals in the shelter are the most susceptible to infection and therefore will potentially benefit the most from vaccination. The immunological status of each kitten or puppy, the amount of MDA (see Maternally derived antibodies) and the degree of exposure to infectious pathogens will be very variable. In many shelters, the routine vaccination protocol for puppies and kittens (two doses 2–4 weeks apart, from 8–10 weeks of age) will provide sufficient protection. However, where disease prevalence is high, some shelters will need to start vaccinating kittens and puppies younger, more frequently and/or for longer. In the case of young puppies or kittens that may not have received sufficient colostrum from their dam and/or may be at heightened risk of early exposure to disease, administering an additional vaccine dose from 4–6 weeks of age may be considered. Vaccine SPCs allow for earlier licensed use of some parvovirus vaccines from as early as 4 weeks of age, and for some multivalent products for dogs and cats from 6 weeks of age. Provided the level of MDA is sufficiently low, a response to this early vaccination is likely, giving a reasonable chance of early protection where increased risks are anticipated.
- An additional dose of vaccine after 10 or 12 weeks of age – ideally from 16 weeks, when MDA has declined to low levels – has been recommended by professional guidelines due to the persistence of high levels of MDA, which interfere with the response to vaccination, in a small proportion of individuals. Although the proportion of individuals that would benefit from this practice may be low, the value of an additional vaccine dose may be significant in circumstances where a high risk of exposure to disease is anticipated or high morbidity and mortality (e.g. due to CPV) is being experienced.
- Should the decision be made to give additional vaccine doses, on a precautionary basis a minimum of a 2-week interval between different vaccine doses is often advised, although the evidence base for this remains unclear.

Effects of disease status

- Vaccine safety and efficacy are assessed in healthy, immunocompetent individuals. However, this introduces a number of dilemmas in the typical shelter environment, such as the vaccination of animals with concurrent disease or at the time of surgery. While vaccination of a sick animal falls short of the ideal, proceeding with vaccination may well still be the appropriate decision in shelter situations, except in the case of animals with acute febrile illness or (with live vaccines) pregnant animals.
- The decision whether to vaccinate a sick animal should be based on a careful and informed risk:benefit analysis, taking into account the local environment within the shelter. The increased risk of infectious disease in shelters means that use of vaccines is likely to provide considerable benefit in many scenarios. When there is doubt as to whether to vaccinate, the manufacturer may have additional data or be able to provide some further guidance on the safe use of a specific vaccine product.
- Severely immunocompromised animals may not respond appropriately to vaccination, and in some cases, vaccination may be explicitly contraindicated on the label – e.g. they are not suitable candidates for vaccination against *B. bronchiseptica*.
- Professional guidelines indicate that the use of an inactivated vaccine is preferred over live attenuated products to avoid any risk of residual virulence in at-risk immunocompromised patients, if such an option exists, although such use is always considered extra-label use and requires a careful assessment of the relative risks and benefits.

Vaccine formulations for dogs and cats commonly used in animal shelters

Figures 11.5 and 11.6 offer broad guidance to the features of different small animal vaccines in common use in shelters in the UK at the time of writing. It is essential to consult appropriate SPCs or data sheets to verify the indications, claims and appropriate use for the brand of vaccine being used, as specific claims will vary from the generic advice given here. Rabies vaccination is included for reference purposes but would normally be pertinent only to shelters outside the UK or in situations where quarantine was being practised. Note that other UK-licensed vaccines for Lyme disease (borreliosis), leishmaniosis and canine herpesvirus are not listed.

Summary

In summary, vaccination of any individual is an active medical intervention to provide immunizing protection. Vaccination brings many benefits and as with other medicines may be associated with a low level of of adverse risk. However, active surveillance reveals that the incidence of serious adverse signs triggered by the appropriate use of vaccines is very small and is far outweighed by the medical benefits in terms of disease prevention gained, and this is nowhere more so than within the shelter environment.

Pathogen	Abbreviation used in table	Vaccine type	Marketed combinations	Route of administration	Formulations	Presentation	Reconstitute with	Typical primary course	Recommended minimum revaccination interval
Canine distemper virus	D	MLV	DAP / DAPPi (with L2 or L4) / DAPi (with PL2)	s.c.	Multivalent only	Freeze-dried plug for reconstitution	Liquid L2/L3/L4 or R or vaccine solvent	Two doses 2–4 weeks apart, from 6 weeks of age with a minimum finishing age of 10 weeks	Up to 4 years after first annual booster, depending on label advice
Canine adenovirus-2	A	MLV	As above	s.c.	Multivalent only	Freeze-dried plug for reconstitution			
Canine parvovirus	P	MLV	As above and P only / PL2	s.c.	Multivalent or monovalent / Multivalent	Freeze-dried plug for reconstitution / Liquid	Freeze-dried DAPi	(Stand-alone parvovirus dose from 4 weeks of age where needed)	
Canine parainfluenza (injectable)	Pi	MLV	Pi / DAPPi (with or without L4) / DAP1 (with PL2)	s.c.	Monovalent or multivalent	Freeze-dried plug for reconstitution	Liquid L2/L3/L4wi vaccine or vaccine solvent		Annual for all dogs at risk
Canine leptospirosis	L2 L3 L4	Inactivated with or without adjuvant	L2 / L4 (with or without DAPPi) / PL2 (with DA2Pi)	s.c.	Bivalent (two serovars), trivalent (three serovars) or tetravalent (four serovars) / Bivalent combined with canine parvovirus	Liquid suspension for injection / Liquid suspension for injection	Freeze-dried options as shown above / Freeze-dried DAPi	Two-dose primary course, 2–4 weeks apart (NB. 3–4 weeks for L3/L4 vaccines) from 6 weeks of age or more, finishing from 10–12 weeks	
Bordetella bronchiseptica	Bb	Avirulent live	Bb only / Bb with Pi	Intranasal	Monovalent and bivalent with Pi	Freeze-dried plug for reconstitution	Intranasal vaccine solvent	Single intranasal dose from as early as 3 weeks	
Canine parainfluenza (intranasal)	Pi	MLV	Bb with Pi	Intranasal	Bivalent with Bb	Freeze-dried plug for reconstitution	Intranasal vaccine solvent	Single intranasal dose from as early as 3 weeks	
Rabies	R	Inactivated with adjuvant	R	s.c.	Monovalent only available in the UK	Liquid suspension for injection	Not required, but some may be mixed and given with other vaccines before administration	Earlier use possible but a single dose from 12 weeks of age required for the pet travel scheme	Every 3 years depending on label advice

11.5 Summary of the main canine vaccine options available in the United Kingdom at the time of writing. It is essential to consult the appropriate SPC or data sheet for the chosen vaccine brand before use, because the exact label advice will vary. MLV= modified live virus; s.c.= subcutaneous.

Pathogen	Abbreviation used in table	Vaccine type	Marketed combinations	Route of administration	Formulations	Presentation	Reconstitute with	Typical on-label primary course advice	Recommended minimum revaccination interval
Feline herpesvirus (viral rhinotracheitis)	H	MLV	HC HCP HCPCh	s.c.	Bivalent (HC) or multivalent	Freeze-dried plug for reconstitution or liquid all-in-one inactivated	Liquid vaccine solvent or FeLV vaccine	Two doses 3–4 weeks apart from 8–9 weeks of age with a minimum finishing age from 11–12 weeks	Annually or every 1–3 years depending on label and level of risk
Feline calicivirus	C	MLV or inactivated	HCPFeLV HCPChFeLV	s.c.	Bivalent (HC) or multivalent				
Feline panleukopenia virus	P	MLV		s.c.	Multivalent				Annually or up to every 3 years depending on label advice
Feline Chlamydia	Ch	Attenuated live	HCPCh with or without FeLV	s.c.	Multivalent				Annual for all cats at risk
Feline leukaemia virus	FeLV	Inactivated/subunit adjuvanted or non-adjuvanted vector vaccine	FeLV only or with HCChP or HCP	s.c.	Monovalent or multivalent	Liquid	Freeze-dried multivalent options as shown		
Bordetella bronchiseptica	Bb	Avirulent live	Bb only	Intranasal	Monovalent	Freeze-dried plug for reconstitution	Vaccine solvent	Single intranasal dose from 4 weeks	
Rabies virus	R	Inactivated + adjuvant or recombinant	R only	s.c.	Monovalent	Liquid	Not applicable	One dose, finishing from 12 weeks of age	1 year or 3 years depending on label advice

11.6 Summary of the main feline vaccine options available in the United Kingdom at the time of writing. It is essential to consult the appropriate SPC or data sheet for the chosen vaccine brand before use, because the exact label advice will vary. MLV= modified live virus; s.c.= subcutaneous.

Licensing of vaccines

As with all licensed veterinary medicines, veterinary vaccines are closely regulated. To obtain a marketing authorization within the European Union (EU), and to allow specific claims and warnings to be applied, biological products have to satisfy a series of defined tests of safety, efficacy and quality in trials undertaken in accordance with strict guidelines meeting the requirements of good laboratory practice, as defined by the regulatory authorities of the EU's various member states. Specific statements and guidance in the supporting literature for any product, for both efficacy and safety, are based on the data generated from such carefully controlled studies. For example, safety for live viral vaccines must be demonstrated in the minimum age of species for which they are labelled, at a 10-fold overdose and with repeated use. Furthermore, they must also demonstrate an inability to revert to virulence with repeated transfer (termed 'back-passage') between animals.

The efficacy and safety of vaccines is assessed in healthy individuals, and in particular in the youngest and most susceptible age group for which they are indicated. While residual virulence is a theoretical concern with live vaccines, modern vaccine technology and the safety trials that back the regulatory approval of such products lead to a high level of confidence in their use in the field. As with all pharmaceuticals, the properties of a vaccine are defined by the studies that support its marketing authorization and are laid out in the official Summary of Product Characteristics (SPC); in the UK, this is distilled into the familiar product leaflet and National Office of Animal Health (NOAH) data sheet. Further information is published and available online in the form of European Public Assessment Reports (EPARs). These valuable documents define the product's composition, pharmaceutical form, indications, appropriate use, precautions, expected adverse reactions, interactions with other vaccines and pharmaceuticals, as well as pharmacological and immunological properties. Careful reading of product SPCs and data sheets will reveal a great deal of additional information about a product, including the expected level of efficacy and the likely frequency of adverse event reports. Product data sheets are published annually but, especially in the case of recently launched products, information may be updated regularly based on pharmacovigilance reports from the field. It is therefore also important to look out for regular updates from the manufacturer and, if in doubt, always refer to the most recent version (available online at www.noahcompendium.co.uk).

While the SPC provides a great deal of information, the information it contains is dependent on the regulatory process and studies that support the product's marketing authorization. The advice contained within the SPC is therefore constrained in scope and cannot necessarily account for all situations or questions that might arise. It is important to remember that in circumstances where there is a need to consider the use of any vaccine outside its licensed use, the manufacturer may, on request, be in a position to give additional supporting information to the prescribing veterinary surgeon.

Vaccines have a powerful role in the prevention of a number of key infectious diseases. Specific claims in the SPC and data sheet may vary depending on the vaccine. At best, a vaccine may fully prevent clinical signs and shedding following challenge; however, the claim to efficacy against a pathogen is often based on a significant reduction of clinical signs compared with unvaccinated controls.

At the time of writing, the UK is approaching the exit of the EU. Although much remains unclear, including the changes in the licensing process, the principles which underpin the marketing authorization of veterinary medicines and vaccines are likely to remain.

Maternally derived antibodies

Maternally derived antibodies (MDAs) are passed from the dam to her offspring, principally in colostrum. This passive antibody transfer provides early protection, but this wanes exponentially to non-protective levels within a period of weeks (Figure 11.7). The quality and quantity of colostrum and the amount ingested by each neonate varies; this means that the level of MDA transferred to a newborn puppy or kitten varies a great deal between litters and even between individuals within a litter. The timing of when puppies and kittens become susceptible to disease and when they become able to respond to vaccination is therefore also variable and not possible to predict for individual animals or litters with any degree of certainty.

Higher levels of MDA are able to block the immune response to vaccination. The lag period between a young animal becoming susceptible to disease and being able to mount a response to vaccination is often known as the 'immunity gap'. This period is a weak point of any programme of vaccination for puppies or kittens, because exposure to the diseases covered by vaccines during this period may result in clinical disease.

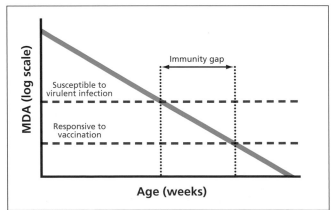

11.7 The fall in maternally derived antibodies (MDAs) is depicted by the solid line. As MDA interferes with the response to vaccination, the final vaccination is timed to coincide with the expected decline in MDA to a point where a response is possible. The period between the decline in MDA to non-protective levels and vaccinal immunity developing is known as the **immunity gap**. Animals exposed to infection during this period will not be protected.
(Reproduced from the *BSAVA Textbook of Veterinary Nursing, 5th edition*)

Vaccine guidelines

A number of professional bodies have published guidelines to aid veterinary practitioners' decision-making in the vaccination of cats and dogs. These include:

* Advisory Board on Cat Diseases (www.abcdcatsvets.org)
* American Animal Hospital Association (www.aaha.org)
* American Association of Feline Practitioners (www.catvets.com)
* International Cat Care (http://icatcare.org)
* World Small Animal Veterinary Association (www.wsava.org)
* Association of Shelter Veterinarians (ASV) (http://www.sheltervet.org/assets/docs/shelter-standards-oct2011-wforward.pdf)

The aim of this guidance is to provide broad information on the use of vaccines. The guidelines are based on a combination of available evidence and academic opinion. The evidence base for these guidelines varies from one vaccine to another and between species, so considerable care is needed in adapting such guidance into day-to-day practice. It is important to remember that guidelines are there to *guide* decisions and are not a rulebook. The guidelines do not always agree with each other, and it is important to consider the local environment in which the vaccines are being used before implementing any recommendations; the majority of the guidelines still state that a risk:benefit assessment is appropriate for all individuals and a single protocol may not suit all circumstances.

Guidelines often make recommendations outside the licensed use of a vaccine. While off-licence use can be considered, it is always important that appropriate justification can be made by the responsible veterinary surgeon, that informed consent is given (where an owner is involved) and that appropriate consideration of the prescribing cascade has been made. However, for shelters, another possible limitation is that local authorities may have specific requirements in relation to vaccination, which are likely to require the use of vaccines in accordance with their licensed use.

Some of these guidelines provide recommendations specific to the shelter situation. This is an important acknowledgement that vaccination of cats and dogs in a shelter environment is different from that in private practice, where vaccination is applied on an individual rather than 'herd' basis.

Adverse effects and putative risks associated with vaccination

Following vaccination, innate immunity is stimulated. As a result of this, certain transient and self-limiting adverse effects are expected. Adverse effects are far less significant in terms of morbidity and mortality than the diseases that are vaccinated against, so for most individuals in a shelter, the benefits of vaccination far outweigh the risks. Examples of types of adverse event reports include:

* Systemic reactions, such as malaise, inappetence or mild pyrexia
* Local reactions at the site of injection, with a subcutaneous swelling of variable size and local discomfort or pain
* Occasionally, local swellings relate to the occurrence of infection and abscessation at the site of injection; this may be suspected when a local inflammatory reaction progresses over several days. Rigorous quality control procedures typically ensure sterility of the vaccine itself and when such issues rarely arise, they are most likely to represent inoculation of bacteria that were present on the skin surface at the time of vaccination. While the use of surgical spirit or other clinical disinfection of the skin is usually not recommended before vaccination, because it may interfere with the viability of live vaccines, it is important that injectable vaccines are administered in as hygienic a manner as is possible
* Transient acute type I hypersensitivity reactions are occasionally reported related to a component of the vaccine. Depending on the species, these may manifest as angioedema and urticaria, agitation and gastrointestinal signs, such as diarrhoea, and anaphylactic shock with circulatory collapse may be seen. Suspicion of hypersensitivity should prompt emergency treatment, which, depending on the severity and response to therapy, may include oxygen, fluids, antihistamines, corticosteroids and adrenaline
* Clinical signs of infectious disease are sometimes noted in recently vaccinated animals. For example, kittens may present with signs of feline upper respiratory tract disease and/or shifting lameness soon after vaccination. While the improper administration of live attenuated feline vaccines by aerosol, or orally, may lead to respiratory signs, thorough investigation of such reports reveals, in the overwhelming majority of cases, evidence of field infection
* Shedding of vaccine virus can occur, but reversion to virulence of a live vaccine is neither a likely nor an expected syndrome when products are used as indicated. When clinical signs are observed in the post-vaccine period, clinical infection with field agents is overwhelmingly the most likely explanation
* A range of other clinical immune-related syndromes are sometimes reported, e.g. polyarthritis and immune-mediated haemolytic anaemia, although the role of recent vaccination may be hard to establish given that spontaneous cases occur
* Feline injection site sarcomas (FISS) have been associated with vaccination in cats, although a simple causal association has still not been proven. The number of vaccines administered, the type of antigen and the vaccine formulation (e.g. adjuvanted *versus* non-adjuvanted) administered have all been suggested as factors contributing to FISS formation. However, the evidence on this subject is sparse and contradictory. These tumours are very rare in the vaccinated cat population and the risk of infectious diseases that are vaccinated against in shelters is much higher. Therefore, the possible risk of FISS is not a reason to avoid vaccination of cats in shelters.

Ectoparasite control

The presence of ectoparasites on animals entering a shelter is commonplace. It is important to control these parasites for the benefit of the shelter population as a whole as well as individual health. In many situations, where affordable, it is advisable to treat all animals on entry to the shelter, whether ectoparasites are seen or not. Many of the products available not only kill any parasites present, but also protect the animal against reinfestation for a period, and potentially during the animal's stay in the shelter. The risk of reinfestation will vary depending on the environment, for example, inside *versus* outside, whether the animal accommodation has hard or soft furnishings, and whether animals are housed individually or in groups. Retreatment of animals that stay for longer periods is an important part of prevention of ectoparasites and must not be ignored.

Why control ectoparasites?

A wide variety of ectoparasites can infest dogs and cats, and their satisfactory control is vital to ensure the animals' health and welfare. Appropriate management is important for a number of reasons:

- External parasites may cause significant disease, in particular skin lesions and eruptions, which may trigger immunological reactions such as flea allergic dermatitis (see Chapter 16). Consequent pruritus and self-inflicted trauma is a significant welfare problem, and may predispose to bacterial or fungal (e.g. *Malassezia* spp.) infections
- Heavy infestations of blood-sucking arthropods, such as ticks or fleas, can lead to anaemia, particularly in young animals
- Ectoparasites can also transmit important pathogens to their hosts, including humans. In the case of fleas, examples include the flea tapeworm (*Dipylidium caninum*) and zoonoses such as 'cat scratch fever' (bartonellosis) and cat flea typhus due to *Rickettsia felis*
- Failure to deal with an infestation adequately may also negatively impact on the human–companion animal bond once the animal is rehomed and, potentially, the reputation of the shelter.

An essential part of the health check on entry to the shelter is a thorough examination of the skin and hair for evidence of external parasites. Consideration of any available history relating to disease or pruritus and examination of the hair coat and skin can prompt suspicion of an existing parasite problem. In some cases where there is a clinical suspicion, collection of coat brushings for examination can be helpful. This is a cheap and quick diagnostic test that facilitates the diagnosis of any parasites present. However, in many cases where time is limited, blanket treatment of all animals entering a shelter is advisable.

Which ectoparasites?

There is a broad choice of effective ectoparasiticidal products available for use in cats and dogs. Their residual activity means that most can be used both therapeutically to treat a pre-existing problem and prophylactically to prevent infestation. The approach will vary depending on the parasite being considered and particular needs of the shelter.

- **Lice and mites:** For external parasites that spend the major part of their life cycle on the animal, such as lice and most mite species, transmission typically requires close direct or indirect contact with other pets or wildlife species. A therapeutic approach to manage such problems on entry to the shelter is usually appropriate since it is unlikely that animals will become reinfected during their stay.
- **Fleas, ticks and harvest mites:** For parasites where significant parts of the life cycle are completed in the environment, such as fleas, ticks and harvest mites, a preventive approach is preferable where there is a significant risk of infestation. Good hygiene and environmental decontamination are important components of infestation control (see QRG 9.1).
  - With the exception of the brown dog tick (*Rhipicephalus sanguineus*) and related species chiefly found in southern Europe and not endemic to the UK, dogs and cats are unlikely to be reinfested with ticks during their stay in a shelter unless they have access to outdoor exercise in parks, woodland, scrub and moorland. Hence, a therapeutic approach using a product that covers for ticks on initial entry to the shelter is likely to be adequate in almost all instances.
  - Harvest mites are the parasitic larval stages of free-living mites and are likely to be encountered seasonally in animals that have access to woodland and scrub habitat. While animals that are admitted to the shelter during the summer or autumn may require treatment if affected, a year-round preventive strategy is unlikely to be needed.
  - Fleas, particularly the cat flea, *Ctenocephalides felis*, are particularly common and successful parasites in humid and temperate climates, as in the UK. Fleas are likely to be the most common ectoparasites encountered in animals entering into and resident in shelters. Many of the available products will treat any existing infestation, but protection against reinfestation is also important. Flea allergic dermatitis is one of the most commonly diagnosed conditions in pruritic cats and dogs, and has significant morbidity in shelters. To control clinical signs, it is vital to prevent further flea bites. Therefore, if at all possible, preventive treatment should be given to all cats and dogs entering the shelter, and should be continued for the duration of their stay.

Since fleas are the most commonly encountered ectoparasites, and their control underpins the routine preventive use of ectoparasiticides within the shelter, the life cycle of fleas and their effective management with ectoparasiticides will be reviewed below (see Chapter 16).

Flea biology and life cycle

Understanding the flea life cycle (Figure 11.8) is vital in order to get the best results from any flea control strategy.

The time taken from egg to adult flea depends very much on the prevailing environmental conditions, and varies between 2 and 20 weeks in usual circumstances. It is important to understand that a significant proportion of the environmental flea burden is likely to be the pupae, which are resistant to the use of insecticides and may lie dormant for weeks or months. Even if adult fleas, eggs and larvae are treated effectively, pupae may remain unaffected and may need to emerge as adults before they can be

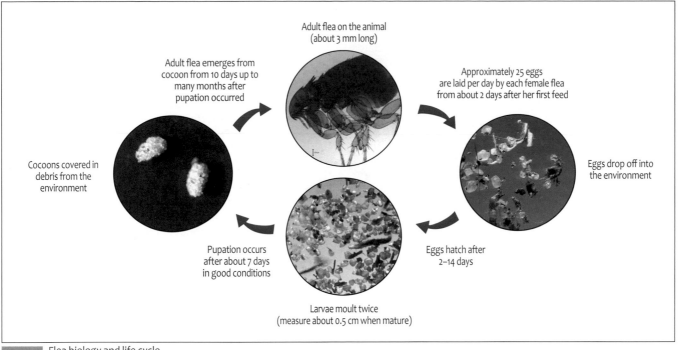

Adult flea on the animal
(about 3 mm long)

Adult flea emerges from
cocoon from 10 days up to
many months after
pupation occurred

Approximately 25 eggs
are laid per day by each female flea
from about 2 days after her first feed

Cocoons covered in
debris from the
environment

Eggs drop off into
the environment

Pupation occurs
after about 7 days
in good conditions

Eggs hatch after
2–14 days

Larvae moult twice
(measure about 0.5 cm when mature)

11.8 Flea biology and life cycle.
(Reproduced from the BSAVA Textbook of Veterinary Nursing, 5th edition)

affected by treatment. This lag phase is termed the **pupal window effect**. This means that effective treatment of animals and the environment may need to be sustained over a number of weeks or months before an infestation can be fully cleared.

Untreated dogs, cats and potentially mammalian wild-life species may act as reservoirs of fleas. Adult fleas occasionally transfer from one animal to another, but for the most part infested animals 'seed' the environment with flea eggs.

The flea life cycle is ideally suited to the indoor environment, which provides the warm and humid conditions that favour the development of the immature stages. While carpets and soft furnishings provide a safe harbour for flea eggs, larvae and pupae, development can occur readily on other surfaces, if levels of hygiene, temperature and humidity allow.

Controlling fleas in the shelter

A reactive approach to flea control – relying on regular grooming and examination with appropriate treatment of any observed infestation – may be appropriate for animals kept individually in low-risk domestic situations, but the multi-animal environment of the shelter presents a very different risk profile. The potential for frequent reintroduction of fleas means that there is a need to reduce the risk of flea populations establishing in the shelter environment to an absolute minimum. For the shelter, therefore, a sustained integrated approach to controlling fleas on an ongoing basis needs to be implemented.

Comprehensive long-term control of fleas in the shelter depends on:

- Adequate control of adult fleas
- Appropriate consideration of the environmental stages of the flea life cycle.

In the shelter environment, regular administration of effective registered insecticidal treatments on dogs and cats should be combined with appropriate cleaning and vacuuming of cages, beds and bedding. Products administered to dogs and cats should ideally directly impact on the environmental flea burden and, where appropriate, this treatment should be combined with a separate environmental treatment too.

Flea products

There is a wide choice of effective ectoparasiticidal products authorized for the control of fleas, and each year it seems as if an ever-increasing number of new formulations and combinations becomes available. Many modern flea control products licensed for use in dogs and cats also address the environmental flea burden in some way, as well as simply killing the adult fleas on the animal. There is also an increasing number of novel and potent active formulations; these can have a lower risk of resistance or tolerance, which may occur with older insecticides, and provide innovations in terms of convenience, duration of action and speed of flea kill.

Modes of action: Almost all flea control products that are applied or administered to dogs and cats primarily exert their action by killing adult fleas. Fleas take up topical treatments by a combination of ingestion and, to a variable extent, exposure of the flea's impervious chitinous exoskeleton. In contrast, systemic products require a blood meal containing the active agent(s) to be ingested by the flea.

Flea control products for dogs and cats can be differentiated on the basis of mechanisms by which they address the environmental flea burden.

Ovicidal and larvicidal effects: Some products, such as those that contain imidacloprid or indoxacarb, are able to act to reduce environmental flea burdens because dander or dirt falling from the treated animal's skin and coat contains sufficient active agent to kill flea larvae and/or eggs in the animal's immediate environment.

Insect growth regulator activity: Some products that are applied to dogs and cats are combined with an insect growth regulator, for example fipronil combined with the growth regulator (S)-methoprene. The growth regulator inhibits larval development in the environment, which interferes with the flea life cycle beyond the product's direct action on adult fleas.

Chitin synthesis inhibition: Oral or injectable systemic products based on lufenuron have no direct effect on adult fleas but nonetheless prevent the development of fleas in the environment. Regular use of such products in all animals prevents the establishment of infestations in the environment, although a separate adulticide treatment may be needed to manage adult fleas.

Rapid speed of kill: Systemic products, such as those that contain spinosad, or the isoxazolines (afoxolaner, fluralaner or sarolaner), exert a rapid killing action after the flea has fed on a treated animal. These products work quickly enough to render female fleas unable to lay eggs before they die. When this effect persists for the full treatment interval, egg laying from all fleas feeding on a treated animal is abolished, blocking the flea life cycle and driving the infestation to extinction within a few weeks or months.

All products are likely to require regular re-administration at the licensed interval to ensure that effective cover continues beyond the pupal window effect period in the environment, to deal with existing infestation and also to maintain effective long-term prevention. For this reason, ensuring good compliance with the chosen product is important.

Route of administration: The route of administration of ectoparasiticidal products is an important factor in the choice of product(s) for a shelter. The amount of handling of an animal on admission to a shelter may need to be kept to a minimum for animals with behavioural problems. This can have a bearing on treatment choices. In addition, the resources available in terms of time and staff may often be limited. Therefore, product convenience, the time taken to correctly apply or administer each treatment, and the length of time for which each treatment is efficacious are important considerations.

Topical flea products:

- **Spray products**, whether in aerosol or pump form, were once widely used and have some advantage in that they potentially achieve a more even distribution of product over the skin. Nevertheless, they may be difficult to directly apply at skin level, the animal may resent treatment, the cosmetic effect may be poor and human exposure to the product is more difficult to avoid. The wide availability of more convenient alternative treatments means that sprays are much less commonly used than in the past.
- **Preventive flea collars** are an inexpensive way of providing longer-term treatment. They also have the advantage that, should an adverse reaction occur, the product can be removed. Many traditional collars rapidly decline in efficacy, although modern prescription products appear to maintain efficacy well during the treatment period. Correct fitting in line with label advice is vital for optimum efficacy – all collars need to be fitted closely enough to create adequate friction with the coat to allow the product to release

the active constituent(s). The collar must not, of course, be too tight and constricting, while allowing it to be too slack risks poor efficacy and injury to the animal.
- **Spot-on flea control products** are popular due to their ease of application. In many cases, they are dosed at monthly intervals, although longer efficacy up to 12 weeks is available. When applying a spot-on product, it is important that the correct technique is used according to the specific product leaflet instructions. These products are usually well tolerated when applied correctly at the skin surface. However, it is important not to allow them to be ingested by the animal; this is particularly important in cats, which appear more sensitive in this respect. In some cases, individuals may experience adverse reactions to topically applied products associated with sensitivity to the active ingredient or excipient; these reactions may occur either locally, at the application site, or systemically, associated with inappropriate ingestion.

The efficacy of some topical products such as sprays, collars and spot-ons can be reduced by swimming, shampooing and moulting. It is recommended to consult the relevant data sheet where this is a concern, since tolerance to these effects is variable between products. For a shelter, this may be an important consideration in the choice of product(s) if, for example, regular bathing of some animals is needed to manage a skin condition.

With the exception of one flea collar that contains flumethrin and is licensed for cats, extreme care must be exercised to ensure that pyrethroid-containing products are not applied to cats.

Systemic flea products:

- **Oral insecticides.** In recent years, a number of chewable tablet formations have become available. Particularly for dogs, such products offer a convenient alternative route of administration, with a rapid kill of the fleas and a systemic mode of action that avoids any of the 'wash-off' concerns of topically administered products. These oral products have spectra of activity that can include ticks and dosing intervals ranging from 1 month to 12 weeks. Like topical products, oral flea products are usually well tolerated. When adverse reactions do occur, they most commonly involve transient gastrointestinal signs, such as vomiting, diarrhoea or inappetence, following administration.
- **Oral and injectable lufenuron.** Lufenuron, an inhibitor of chitin synthesis and deposition, is the active ingredient in some non-insecticidal flea products for dogs and cats. An oral suspension with monthly dosing and a long-acting 6-month injectable formulation are available for cats. For dogs, oral monthly tablets are available with or without the inclusion of the anthelmintic agent milbemycin (see below). While lufenuron has no action against adult fleas, this approach ensures that the production of viable environmental flea life stages is blocked. Regular treatment of all in-contact animals thereby prevents the establishment of environmental infestations.

Figure 11.9 lists available veterinary ectoparasiticides with claims of efficacy against fleas, with formulations organized into 'families' of products that contain common active agents.

Active ingredients	Species	Form	Mode of action versus fleas	Typical dosing interval	Legal category	Effective against immature fleas	Other parasite efficacy (on-label)	Earliest onset of action (fleas)	Typical minimum age/weight (dogs)	Typical minimum age/weight (cats)	Use in pregnancy (on-label)
Topical flea control products based on fipronil											
Fipronil	Dog, cat	Spot-on, spray	Topical	1–2 months	NFA-VPS, AVM-GSL	No	Ticks, lice	Within 24 hours	8 weeks, 2 kg	8 weeks, 1 kg	Some formulations
Fipronil/(S)-methoprene	Dog, cat	Spot-on, spray	Topical	4–8 weeks	NFA-VPS	Yes	Ticks, lice	Within 24 hours	8 weeks, 2 kg	8 weeks, 1 kg	Some formulations
Fipronil/(S)-methoprene/amitraz	Dog	Spot-on	Topical	5 weeks	POM-V	Yes	Ticks, lice	Within 24 hours	8 weeks, 2 kg	n/a	Yes
Fipronil, (S)-methoprene, eprinomectin, praziquantel	Cat	Spot-on	Topical	1 month	POM-V	Yes	Ticks, tapeworms, roundworms, hookworms, heartworm, vesical worms	24 hours	n/a	7 weeks, 0.6 kg	Not established
Topical flea control products based on imidacloprid											
Imidacloprid	Dog, cat	Spot-on	Topical	4 weeks (dogs), 3–4 weeks (cats)	NFA-VPS	Yes	Lice (dogs)	Within 1 day	8 weeks	8 weeks	Limited data
Imidacloprid/moxidectin	Dog, cat	Spot-on	Topical	Up to monthly application	POM-V	Yes	Heartworm, hookworms, roundworms, whipworms, Demodex, Otodectes, Sarcoptes, Notoedres, Trichodectes	Not stated	7 weeks, 1 kg	9 weeks, 1 kg	Not established
Imidacloprid/permethrin	Dog	Spot-on	Topical	Up to monthly application	POM-V	Yes	Ticks, sandflies (2–3 weeks), mosquitoes (2–4 weeks), stable fly	Within 1 day	7 weeks, 1.5 kg	n/a	Yes
Imidacloprid/flumethrin	Dog, cat	Collar	Topical	8 months	POM-V	Yes	Ticks, lice	Not stated	7 weeks	10 weeks	Not established
Topical flea control products based on indoxacarb											
Indoxacarb	Dog, cat	Spot-on	Topical	4 weeks	POM-V	Yes	No	4–48 hours	8 weeks, 1.5 kg	8 weeks, 0.6 kg	Not established
Indoxacarb/permethrin	Dog	Spot-on	Topical	4 weeks	POM-V	Yes	Ticks	Up to 48 hours	8 weeks, 1.2 kg	n/a	No
Systemic adulticidal flea control products											
Afoxolaner with or without milbemycin	Dog	Chewable tablet	Systemic	Monthly	POM-V	No	Ticks ± worms with milbemycin combination	8 hours	8 weeks, 2 kg	n/a	Not established
Fluralaner	Dog, cat	Chewable tablet (dog) or spot-on (dogs, cats)	Systemic	12 weeks	POM-V	No	Ticks	8 hours	8 weeks, 2 kg	n/a	Yes (dogs only)

11.9 Prescription flea control formulations for dogs and cats. This figure offers broad guidance to features across the range of small animal ectoparasiticides with licensed claims of efficacy against fleas. Products are listed by active ingredient(s) and represent a range of brands. It is essential to consult the appropriate SPC or data sheet for the chosen brand before use, because the exact label indications, claims and appropriate use may vary across brands for any given formulation. AVM-GSL = authorized veterinary medicine – general sales list; NFA-VPS = non-food animal – veterinarian, pharmacist, suitably qualified person; POM-V = prescription-only medicine – veterinarian. (continues) ▲

Systemic adulticidal flea control products continued

Active ingredients	Species	Form	Mode of action versus fleas	Typical dosing interval	Legal category	Effective against immature fleas	Other parasite efficacy (on-label)	Earliest onset of action (fleas)	Typical minimum age/weight (dogs)	Typical minimum age/weight (cats)	Use in pregnancy (on-label)
Sarolaner	Dog	Chewable tablet	Systemic	Monthly	POM-V	No	Ticks, Otodectes, Sarcoptes, Demodectes	8 hours	8 weeks, 1.3 kg	n/a	Not established
Sarolaner with selamectin	Cat	Spot-on	Systemic	Monthly	POM-V	No	Ticks, biting lice, Otodectes, and worms (see Figure 11.11)	Up to 24 hours	n/a	8 weeks, 1.25 kg	Not established
Selamectin	Dog, cat	Spot-on	Systemic	Monthly	POM-V	Yes	Heartworm, Otodectes, Sarcoptes, biting lice (and hookworms and roundworms in cats)	Not shown on label	6 weeks	6 weeks	Yes
Lotilaner	Dog	Chewable tablet	Systemic	Monthly	POM-V	No	Ticks	4 hours	8 weeks, 1.3 kg	n/a	Not established
Spinosad	Dog, cat	Chewable tablet	Systemic	Monthly	POM-V	No	No	4 hours (cats, 24 hours)	14 weeks, 1.3 kg	14 weeks, 1.2 kg	Caution in breeding females. Not evaluated in breeding males

Oral and injectable products based on lufenuron

Active ingredients	Species	Form	Mode of action versus fleas	Typical dosing interval	Legal category	Effective against immature fleas	Other parasite efficacy (on-label)	Earliest onset of action (fleas)	Typical minimum age/weight (dogs)	Typical minimum age/weight (cats)	Use in pregnancy (on-label)
Lufenuron (with or without milbemycin in dogs)	Dog, cat	Suspension and injection (cats), tablet (dogs)	Systemic (not adulticidal)	Monthly or 6-monthly (injection)	POM-V	Yes	(Gastrointestinal nematodes and heartworm efficacy) (tablets for dogs)	24 hours (immature stages)	2.3 kg	4 kg	Not established

Topical flea control products based on other active agents

Active ingredients	Species	Form	Mode of action versus fleas	Typical dosing interval	Legal category	Effective against immature fleas	Other parasite efficacy (on-label)	Earliest onset of action (fleas)	Typical minimum age/weight (dogs)	Typical minimum age/weight (cats)	Use in pregnancy (on-label)
Dinotefuran, permethrin, pyriproxyfen	Dog	Spot-on	Topical	Monthly (3 weeks for Dermacentor spp. ticks)	POM-V	Yes	Ticks, stable fly, sandflies, mosquitoes	12 hours	7 weeks, 1.5 kg	n/a	Not established
Pyriprole	Dog	Spot-on	Topical	Monthly	POM-V	No	Ticks	24 hours	8 weeks, 2 kg	n/a	Not established

11.9 (continued) Prescription flea control formulations for dogs and cats. This figure offers broad guidance to features across the range of small animal ectoparasiticides with licensed claims of efficacy against fleas. Products are listed by active ingredient(s) and represent a range of brands. It is essential to consult the appropriate SPC or data sheet for the chosen brand before use, because the exact label indications, claims and appropriate use may vary across brands for any given formulation. AVM-GSL = authorized veterinary medicine – general sales list; NFA-VPS = non-food animal – veterinarian, pharmacist, suitably qualified person; POM-V = prescription-only medicine – veterinarian.

Environmental treatment

For heavy flea burdens, to speed up resolution of an infestation or when needed for use alongside products that do not necessarily directly reduce the environmental burden, separate treatment of the environment is necessary. Environmental treatments include foggers and sprays. A number of such products contain insect growth regulators in combination with a synthetic pyrethroid. When using such products, it is important to bear in mind that care is required in their use, especially in the vicinity of cats, which are susceptible to the effect of pyrethroids. In particular, the environment must be thoroughly ventilated and the product allowed to dry before animals are allowed to return to the treated area.

Endoparasite control

A wide range of helminth parasites may be harboured by dogs and cats entering shelters (see Chapters 12 and 13). While young animals frequently have heavier burdens of intestinal roundworms than older animals, few infections are strictly age related, so the need to control worms continues throughout life.

Almost all worms are transmitted by the passage of eggs or larvae in faeces. A key objective of preventive worm control is to break the life cycle to ensure that contamination of the environment (and, in some cases, zoonotic risk) is minimized. This is achieved through good hygiene and the picking up and appropriate disposal of faeces. Provided commercial diets are fed, within the well run shelter kennel or cattery, there should be no likelihood of transmission of worms via contaminated raw meat or the carcases of rodents or livestock.

Why control endoparasites?

As with ectoparasites, helminth parasites may be responsible for disease in their own right, and, in some cases, present zoonotic risks, which may be potentially serious.

Which endoparasites?

Major groups of helminth parasites include:

- Intestinal roundworms, including ascarids (*Toxocara canis*, *T. cati* and *Toxascaris leonina*), hookworms (e.g. *Uncinaria stenocephala*) and whipworms (*Trichuris vulpis*), and tapeworms (including *Dipylidium* spp., *Taenia* spp. and *Echinococcus granulosus*)
- Non-intestinal worms including the French heartworm (often referred to colloquially as 'lungworm') *Angiostrongylus vasorum*, and the lungworms (*Oslerus osleri* and *Crenosoma vulpis*)
- Helminths, such as heartworm (*Dirofilaria immitis*), the tapeworm *Echinococcus multilocularis*, subcutaneous worms (*Dirofilaria repens*) and eyeworms (*Thelazia* spp.), are particular considerations in dogs imported into the UK; although, in the case of *Echinococcus*, treatment with praziquantel is required 1–5 days before importation.

Endoparasites that are particularly pertinent to routine worming within the shelter include:

- *Toxocara* spp.
- Tapeworms
- *A. vasorum*.

Toxocara species

The prepatent period of *T. canis* is just over 4 weeks. In situations where there is high risk of exposure, for example where predation of potential paratenic hosts occurs or there is a shared common use of a potentially contaminated green space or contact with children, monthly retreatment would effectively prevent patent infections. This level of control of roundworms is often not needed in shelters, as exposure to reinfection or children is reduced in many environments. Quarterly treatment is currently thought to be a useful compromise for such lower-risk situations.

Tapeworm species

The tapeworm species *E. granulosus* and *E. multilocularis* (outside the UK, in endemic areas of central and eastern Europe) are the species of major zoonotic concern (Figure 11.10). Dogs are potentially final hosts and may transmit the parasite to humans. In the UK, fresh infections are unlikely to be acquired in the shelter environment without access to sources of infection such as raw meat or the carcases of fallen livestock. However, it is important to treat older puppies and adult dogs for tapeworms on entry to the shelter with a product containing praziquantel, to ensure this parasite is eliminated if present. This approach, applied to both dogs and cats, will effectively control other species of tapeworm such as *Dipylidium caninum* acquired from ingestion of infected fleas or canine chewing lice, and *Taenia* spp. from the ingestion of infected intermediate hosts, such as infected meat and the carcases of rabbits and rodents.

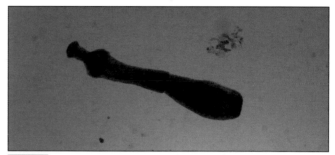

11.10 *Echinococcus* tapeworm.

Angiostrongylus vasorum

In recent years, the French heartworm *A. vasorum* has increasingly been diagnosed beyond traditionally endemic areas in the UK. Treatment of dogs against *A. vasorum* is recommended in areas endemic for this parasite where exposure to the risk of ingestion of infected slugs and snails (the intermediate host of the parasite) is likely.

Anthelmintic products

Treatment with a broad-spectrum product that provides effective control of both roundworms and tapeworms is appropriate for both dogs and cats on entry to the shelter (Figure 11.11). Specific prevention of *A. vasorum*, where there is judged to be a probable ongoing risk of exposure, is likely to require monthly administration of licensed products that contain either milbemycin or moxidectin. A number of the flea products considered above also have anthelmintic activity but, with the exception of one broad-spectrum spot-on product for use on cats, none provides extended activity against all the significant feline endoparasites.

Active ingredients	Formulation	Legal category	Species	Earliest age/weight	Use in pregnancy indication	Toxocara canis (adults)	Toxocara cati (adults)	Toxascaris leonina	Uncinaria stenocephala	Ancylostoma caninum	Ancylostoma tubaeformae	Trichuris vulpis	Oslerus osleri	Aelurostrongylus spp.	Angiostrongylus vasorum	Dirofilaria immitis	Taenia spp.	Dipylidium caninum	Echinococcus spp.	Giardia	Other parasites
Benzimidazoles																					
Fenbendazole	Granules, liquid, paste	NFA-VPS	Dog, cat	2 weeks (dogs)	Y	Y	Y	Y	Y	Y	Y	Y	Y	Y						Y	
Praziquantel/pyrantel and combinations																					
Praziquantel	Tablets, spot-on	AVM-GSL	Dog, cat	2.5 kg	Y												Y	Y	Y		
Emodepside/praziquantel	Spot-on	POM-V	Cat	8 weeks, 0.5 kg	Y		Y	Y			Y			Y			Y	Y	Y		
Pyrantel/oxantel/praziquantel	Tablets	POM-V	Dog	2 months, 1 kg	N	Y		Y	Y	Y		Y					Y	Y	Y		
Pyrantel/praziquantel	Tablets	NFA-VPS	Cat	6 weeks	N		Y	Y			Y						Y	Y	Y		
Pyrantel/febantel/praziquantel	Tablets	NFA-VPS	Dog	2 weeks, 3 kg	Y	Y		Y	Y	Y		Y					Y	Y	Y		
Pyrantel/febantel	Oral suspension	NFA-VPS	Dog	2 weeks	N	Y		Y		Y		Y									
Milbemycin/praziquantel	Tablets	POM-V	Dog, cat	1 kg (dogs), 6 weeks, 0.5 kg (cats)	Y	Y	Y	Y	Y	Y	Y	Y			Y		Y	Y	Y		Crenosoma vulpis, Mesocestoides spp., Thelazia callipaeda
Macrocyclic lactones combinations																					
Milbemycin/afoxalaner	Tablet	POM-V	Dog	8 weeks, 2 kg	N	Y		Y	Y	Y		Y			Y	Y					Fleas, ticks
Moxidectin/imidacloprid	Spot-on	POM-V	Dog, cat	7 weeks (dog), 9 weeks (cat), 1 kg	N	Y	Y	Y	Y	Y	Y	Y		Y	Y	Y					Ectoparasites (see Figure 11.9) Spirocerca lupi
Milbemycin/lufenuron	Tablets	POM-V	Dog	2 weeks, 1 kg	Y	Y		Y	Y	Y		Y				Y					
Milbemycin/praziquantel	Tablets	POM-V	Dog, cat	1 kg (dog), 6 weeks, 0.5 kg (cats)	Y	Y	Y	Y	Y	Y	Y	Y			Y		Y	Y	Y		Crenosoma vulpis, Mesocestoides spp., Thelazia callipaeda
Selamectin	Spot-on	POM-V	Dog, cat	6 weeks	Y	Y	Y				Y					Y					Ectoparasites (see Figure 11.9)
Selamectin + sarolaner	Spot-on	POM-V	Cat	8 weeks, 1.25 kg	N		Y				Y					Y					Fleas, ticks, ear mites, biting lice
Spinosad/milbemycin	Tablets	POM-V	Dog	3.9 kg	N	Y		Y	Y	Y		Y				Y					Fleas
Other anthelmintic products																					
Nitroscanate	Tablets	AVM-GSL	Cat	2 kg	Y	Y	Y		Y	Y							Y	Y	Limited efficacy		
Piperazine	Tablets, cream, syrup	AVM-GSL	Dog, cat	2 weeks	–	Y	Y														
Piperazine/dichlorophen	Tablets	AVM-GSL	Cat	6 months	–	Y	Y										Y				

11.11 On-label indications and licensed spectra of activity of selected anthelmintic formulations. This figure offers broad guidance across the range of small animal endoparasiticides. Products are listed by active ingredient(s) and represent a range of brands. It is essential to consult the appropriate SPC or data sheet for the chosen brand before use, because the exact label indications, claims and appropriate use may vary across licensed brands for any given formulation. Legal categories: AVM-GSL = authorized veterinary medicine – general sales list; NFA-VPS = non-food animal – veterinarian, pharmacist, suitably qualified person; POM-V = prescription-only medicine – veterinarian.

Fenbendazole

Fenbendazole is a benzimidazole anthelminthic with broad-spectrum activity against canine and feline helminth parasites, with the particular exception of *Dipylidium* and *Echinococcus* spp. tapeworms. It is effective for both adult and immature stages of roundworms, making it an appropriate choice for young puppies and kittens. In pregnant bitches, daily administration of a fenbendazole product from day 40 of pregnancy to 2 days postpartum will prevent the transplacental transfer of immature *T. canis* larvae and help to prevent prenatal infection of puppies. For treatment of puppies and kittens, or for animals with known infections, a 3-day course is recommended.

Fenbendazole is also used to help manage a number of specific helminth infections as well as the protozoan parasite *Giardia*, although for these infections more extended courses of treatment may prove necessary. Although Fenbendazole is sometimes used in the management of clinical cases of angiostrongylosis, it remains unlicensed for this indication and is not an appropriate choice for the routine prevention of *A. vasorum*.

Praziquantel and combinations

Praziquantel is an effective agent for all key tapeworm species. It is available on its own or in a variety of combinations with pyrantel ± febantel or oxantel to provide a broad spectrum of activity against roundworms and tapeworms. When these products are combined with milbemycin, the spectrum is extended even further to cover a number of other helminths, including *A. vasorum*. Treatment with a tapeworm product that contains praziquantel is recommended for all dogs and cats on entry to the shelter to ensure reliable broad-spectrum cover against these important endoparasites.

Macrocyclic lactones and combinations

The macrocyclic lactones include milbemycin, selamectin and moxidectin. As well as combination products with praziquantel, milbemycin is also available in tablet form in combination with agents active against fleas, such as spinosad, lufenuron and afoxalaner. In addition, moxidectin is available in combination with imidacloprid as a spot-on product to give an extended spectrum of activity, including cover for *A. vasorum*. If using this extended-spectrum product, cover against tapeworms can be provided by using an additional product containing praziquantel. In designing a shelter control protocol, it is important to consider potential incompatibilities between the products chosen. It is always wise to check the SPC or data sheet

for each product to ensure warnings and contraindications are fully understood. An important example relates to incompatibilities between certain macrocyclic lactones – in particular, commonly used milbemycin products should not be given to animals receiving moxidectin, since they have similar modes of action.

Route of administration

While most anthelmintic products are administered via the oral route, as a tablet, chewable tablet, liquid or paste, topical (spot-on) routes of administration can be more convenient. Options include preparations for cats based on:

* Praziquantel in combination with emodepside
* Praziquantel in combination with fipronil, (S)-methoprene and eprinomectin.

A number of endectocides contain single active agents or combinations designed to provide wider coverage of dogs and cats against fleas, other key ectoparasites and a range of helminth parasites. These include macrocyclic lactone-based products either available as spot-on formulations including:

* Moxidectin + imidacloprid
* Selamectin

or oral tablet formulations based on:

* Milbemycin + lufenuron
* Milbemycin + afoxalaner.

References and further reading

Bond R, Riddle A, Mottram L, Beugnet F and Stevenson R (2007) Survey of flea infestation in dogs and cats in the United Kingdom during 2005. *Veterinary Record* **160(15)**, 503–506

Churchill AE (1987) Preliminary development of a live attenuated parvovirus vaccine from an isolate of British origin. *Veterinary Record* **120**, 334–339

Cooper B, Mullineaux E and Turner L (2011) *BSAVA Textbook of Veterinary Nursing, 5th edn*. BSAVA Publications, Gloucester

DiGangi BA, Levy JK, Griffin B *et al.* (2012) Effects of maternally-derived antibodies on serological responses to vaccination in kittens. *Journal of Feline Medicine and Surgery* **14(2)**, 118–123

Moore GE, Desantis-Kerr AC, Guptill LF *et al.* (2007) Adverse events after vaccine administration in cats: 2,560 cases (2002–2005). *Journal of the American Veterinary Medical Association* **231**, 94–100

Moore GE, Guptill LF, Ward MP *et al.* (2005) Adverse events diagnosed within three days of vaccine administration in dogs. *Journal of the American Veterinary Medical Association* **227**, 1102–1108

Rojas P, Monahan AM, Schuller S *et al.* (2010) Detection and quantification of leptospires in urine of dogs: a maintenance host for the zoonotic disease leptospirosis. *European Journal of Clinical Microbiology and Infectious Diseases* **29**, 1305–1309

Worming puppies and kittens

Puppies may be heavily infested by *T. canis* as a result of infection acquired either transplacentally *in utero* or through the dam's milk. Serious illness may result from heavy infestations. Routine treatment of puppies with appropriate anthelmintics is necessary from 2 weeks of age. Dosing at fortnightly intervals until 2 weeks post weaning and then monthly intervals to 6 months of age is recommended.

Intestinal ascarids are important considerations in kittens. However, in this case prenatal infection does not occur, so dosing at fortnightly intervals can commence from 3 weeks of age until 2 weeks post weaning; subsequent doses at monthly intervals to 6 months of age are recommended.

Nursing bitches and queens may have patent infections while lactating and should be treated at the same time as the initial treatment of their puppies/kittens. The use of an anthelmintic with activity against both larval and adult stages of ascarid, such as fenbendazole, is recommended to ensure that migrating and intestinal stages are covered with each treatment. Treatment of pregnant bitches from day 40 of pregnancy to 2 days postnatally with a 25 mg/kg daily dose of fenbendazole should prevent the prenatal transmission of *T. canis*.

Useful websites

Advisory Board on Cat Diseases:
www.abcdcatsvets.org

American Animal Hospital Association:
www.aaha.org

American Association of Feline Practitioners:
www.catvets.com

ESCCAP Guidelines
GL1: Worm control in dogs and cats
GL3: Control of ectoparasites in dogs and cats
www.esccap.org

International Cat Care:
https://icatcare.org

World Small Animal Veterinary Association:
www.wsava.org

QRG 11.1: Intake assessment for animals entering shelters

by Rachel Dean and Jenny Stavisky

It is important that animals go through an intake process when they enter a shelter, or as soon as possible afterwards. It is vital that as much information as possible is obtained from the person relinquishing or who has found the animal, so that any relevant history is available to the organization. Some of the assessment can be undertaken by the staff of the shelter, but some requires veterinary input. The intake process should encompass the legal aspects of acquiring animals, as well as assessment of the mental and physical health of each individual.

It can be helpful to standardize the intake assessment within a shelter so that it becomes part of the routine for every new arrival. Formalizing what is recorded (on paper or computer system) for each animal on arrival, and what procedures have been completed can help ensure that communication about the needs of each individual is clear. Each organization needs to create their own documentation that is suited to their setting and the types of animals they care for.

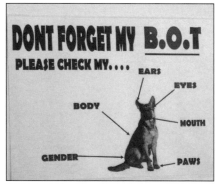
New arrivals waiting to be assessed by shelter staff.

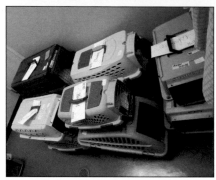
Posters can be a handy reminder of the important health checks that should be completed as part of the intake process.

Intake assessment form

The following is a basic guide to what information could be included on an intake assessment form:

- General information and history
- Legal requirements and ownership
- Health
- Preventive healthcare
- Behavioural assessment.

General information and history

The signalment, including age, sex, breed and neuter status, of the animal should be recorded. If the animal is being relinquished by an owner, any relevant medical/vaccination history, along with pedigree papers (if relevant), microchip details, pet passport and information about their diet, temperament, likes and dislikes should be obtained. If the animal is a stray, it is useful to know where it was found and whether there were any sightings prior to collection and, if so, over what time period.

Legal requirements and ownership

If the animal is being relinquished, it is important to get the owner to sign a 'change of ownership' document. If the animal is a stray, scanning for a microchip may provide information about potential owners. The presence of tattoos or ear tipping may suggest that previous organizations have administered healthcare to the animal.

If the animal does not match the description of anything on your lost and found register, it is worth contacting other rescue organizations and veterinary practices in the area and visiting local websites to see whether anyone has reported the animal missing. Providing information on the shelter's website or through social media may be successful in reuniting a lost pet with their owner.

Before doing anything with a stray animal, the minimum legal holding period (currently

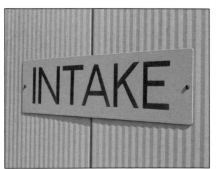
Every animal admitted to a shelter should go through an intake process.

QRG 11.1 *continued*

7 days for dogs in the United Kingdom; no regulation for cats) or the policy of the organization should be followed (see QRGs 21.1 and 21.2 for further information on dealing with stray dogs and cats).

Health

All animals entering a shelter should be examined by a veterinary surgeon or veterinary nurse, if possible, at the earliest opportunity following admission. A full health check should be undertaken to look for signs of infectious disease and other health disorders. Any animal suspected of having an infectious disease should be isolated.

A pragmatic approach to individuals should be borne in mind at all times; for example, rather than

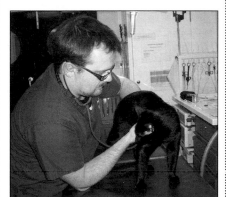

All animals should be thoroughly examined by a veterinary surgeon or nurse upon entering a shelter.
(© Rachel Dean)

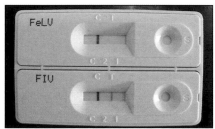

Test kits, such as these for feline leukaemia virus (FeLV) and feline immunodeficiency virus (FIV), can be used to screen for infectious diseases in animals being admitted to the shelter.
(© Rachel Dean)

obtaining blood samples from every thin cat, the staff should provide adequate nutrition and observe them for a number of days to see whether they put on weight or have any other signs of disease (see Chapter 3). Particular attention should be paid to the skin for signs of ectoparasites or ringworm. A Wood's lamp examination can be a useful screening test in these cases. If there is suspicion of ringworm, the patient should be isolated and further diagnostic tests or treatment undertaken.

It is always important to check the neuter status of each individual and carefully examine intact female animals for signs of pregnancy. All animals should be weighed and have their body condition assessed (using a consistent scale that staff are familiar with).

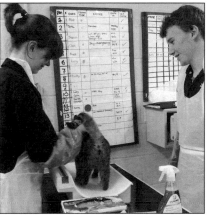

The bodyweight and body condition of animals upon arrival should be assessed and recorded as part of the intake process.
(© Rachel Dean)

Preventive healthcare

It is important to follow the shelter policy for cats and dogs with regard to vaccination, parasite control, neutering and microchipping. All products used and any follow-up treatments required should always be recorded. If possible, newly admitted animals should be housed in an admissions or quarantine area, so further observations can be undertaken before the animal is ready to be rehomed (see Chapter 9 and main text).

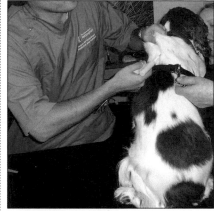

A microchip being implanted in a dog prior to rehoming.
(© Rachel Dean)

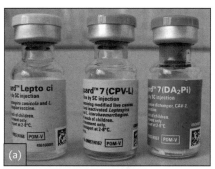

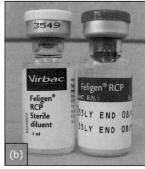

Vaccinations for (a) dogs and (b) cats should be administered in accordance with practice policy.

Behavioural assessment

Often animals need some time to settle into their new environment, so it may be best to leave a full behavioural assessment for a few days. However, any immediate concerns about aggression should be clearly noted for health and safety reasons (see Chapter 19 and Appendix 1).

Chapter 12

Diarrhoea in the dog in the shelter environment

Jenny Stavisky and Runa Hanaghan

Diarrhoea is a common presentation in dog shelters and can range from occasional low-level 'grumbling' problems to outbreaks with high mortality. This chapter will explore the management of diarrhoea with consideration of morbidity levels, aetiology, environmental management and the potential for cross-species transmission, including zoonosis.

Definition of diarrhoea

Diarrhoea is defined as an increase in the water or nutrient content of the faeces, which are generally characterized by a softer or more liquid consistency than is usual (Figure 12.1). Clinically, diarrhoea can be subcategorized in a number of ways:

- Based on presentation (mild, moderate, severe; acute, chronic)
- Based on anatomical location (small intestinal, large intestinal)
- Based on the underlying physiological process (osmotic, secretory, increased intestinal permeability, changes in intestinal motility).

Each of these approaches can be used, alone or in combination, when considering the possible aetiology, likely course of disease, most appropriate intervention and biosecurity measures to use.

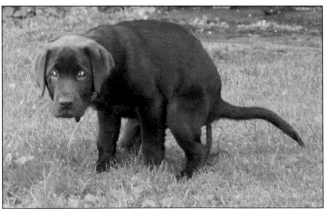

12.1 Diarrhoea is characterized by increased frequency, volume or urgency of defecation.
(Courtesy of C Westgarth)

Presentation

Diarrhoea can be classified most simply according to the clinical presentation. Mild diarrhoea, where the animal is otherwise well and has a good appetite and no other clinical signs, will often resolve with dietary rest and no further treatment. This is a common presentation in shelters, and it may be useful to educate the animal care staff and provide a protocol so that every single dog with mild diarrhoea is not immediately flagged for veterinary attention. A questionnaire study of dog owners revealed that around 15% had observed their dog to have diarrhoea in the previous 14 days, whereas only 2–7% of veterinary presentations typically involve diarrhoea (Marshall *et al.*, 1987). This illustrates the fact that not every case of canine diarrhoea is of veterinary concern. However, in the shelter environment, where dogs may be very closely monitored by staff, a triage system will help to manage the caseload (Figure 12.2). Moderately or severely affected dogs clearly need to be recognized more urgently and treated more intensively.

As well as acute diarrhoea, chronic diarrhoea is not uncommon in shelter dogs. Many of these cases appear to be stress related, and if the animal is otherwise well and maintaining (or, if appropriate, gaining) weight, the diarrhoea may resolve once it is rehomed. Weight loss or failure to gain weight, persistent severe diarrhoea or additional clinical signs such as vomiting are all indications for pursuing ancillary testing.

Anatomical location

The small and large intestine have different, although slightly overlapping, physiological functions. The small intestine is the primary site of digestion and nutrient absorption, whereas the large intestine recovers electrolytes and water, being able to absorb 90% of the fluid content from the lumen. Additionally, some important fat-soluble vitamins are recovered in the large intestine.

This difference in function results in some important variations in clinical presentation between large and small intestinal diarrhoea, as shown in Figure 12.3. However, it is important to remember that some disease processes may affect both sites, resulting in a mixture of clinical signs.

Underlying physiological processes

By considering the physiological processes that underlie the production of normal or abnormal faeces, the veterinary surgeon (veterinarian) can gain clues to the likely cause of

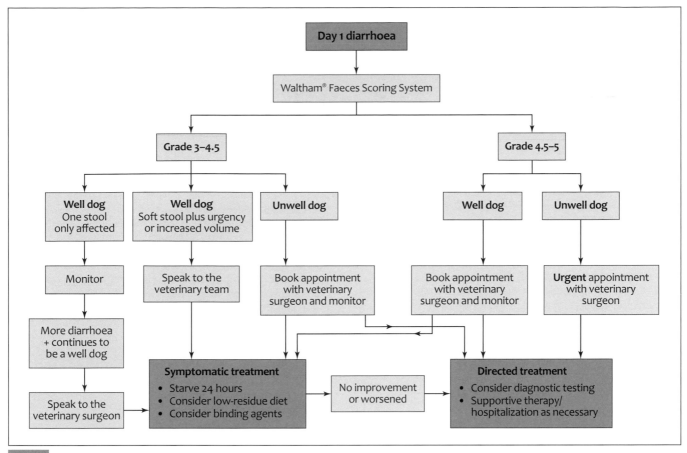

12.2 Sample triage chart to enable animal care staff to determine when to seek veterinary attention.

Characteristic	Small intestinal diarrhoea	Large intestinal diarrhoea
Frequency	Mildly increased	Markedly increased
Faecal volume	Increased	Normal/decreased
Tenesmus/urgency	Rare	Common
Faecal mucus/blood	Rare	Common
Melaena	May be present	Rare
Weight loss	Common	Rare

12.3 Characteristics of small and large intestinal diarrhoea.
(Data from McCann and Simpson, 2006)

the process – and also to the most effective treatment. Diarrhoea occurs when an excess of fluid passes onwards from the small intestine, overwhelming colonic absorptive capacity, or when colonic absorption is decreased (e.g. in colitis). Elements of both of these processes may occur simultaneously. There are broadly four mechanisms by which this can occur, so that on a physiological basis, diarrhoea can be categorized as: osmotic; secretory; abnormal permeability of the mucosa; and changes in gastrointestinal motility.

Osmotic

The contents of the intestine are hypertonic, resulting in a tendency to draw water into the lumen down an osmotic gradient. When there is an excess of osmotically active particles present in the lumen, this will cause an influx of fluid into the lumen. This will result in diarrhoea if it overwhelms the capacity for reabsorption in the remainder of the gut. Common causes of this type of diarrhoea are scavenging or other dietary indiscretion, disorders of digestion and absorption, such as exocrine pancreatic insufficiency, or inflammatory bowel disease. Osmotic diarrhoea generally resolves with fasting (although if there is an underlying cause, such as exocrine pancreatic insufficiency, the diarrhoea will recur when the animal resumes eating).

Secretory

Stimulation of enterocytes by bacterial toxins (such as those of *Salmonella* spp.) causes them to actively secrete anions into the intestinal lumen. Sodium ions then follow along the gradient of electrical charge and fluid, in turn, follows down the resulting osmotic gradient, thus increasing the fluid in the lumen. When the absorptive capacity of the distal intestine is exceeded, diarrhoea will result. Unlike osmotic diarrhoea, secretory diarrhoea will not respond to fasting.

Abnormal mucosal permeability

Enterocytes are joined together by tight junctions, which regulate the movement of fluid and solutes into the intestinal lumen. If these are disrupted, the mucosa becomes 'leaky', allowing solutes, fluid and even, in severe cases, protein to cross into the lumen. This can occur with severe inflammatory disease, gastrointestinal ulceration and other processes where the normal mucosal architecture is disrupted, including lymphangiectasia, neoplasia and portal hypertension.

Abnormal motility

Diarrhoea is, counterintuitively, relatively rarely the result of increased gut motility. The gastrointestinal tract has two main types of motility. **Peristalsis** occurs when longitudinal contractions of the smooth muscle propel ingesta along the tract. **Segmental contractions** occur when the smooth muscle effectively divides the intestine into small, temporary churns, where digestive enzymes mix with and break down ingesta. A reduction in segmental contractions results in a decrease in the capacity of the gut to break down and absorb nutrients; the result is that fluid is drawn into the lumen along an osmotic gradient. Inflammatory and infectious (including viral) diseases can cause a reduction in contractions, which may progress to (at the most severe) complete ileus.

Although the underlying reasons are different, all of these processes result in an excess of fluid in the intestinal lumen (Figure 12.4). Nutrient absorption can also be affected to a varying degree. Although one of these processes may predominate, in an individual patient several of these processes may occur at once. For example, a dog infected with parvovirus will have damage to the intestinal villi (thus losing absorptive capacity), may also have ileus secondary to the severe inflammation, and may have secondary bacterial infection with toxic secretory diarrhoea.

Clinical approach to diarrhoea

Taking a history

Taking the history is divided into two parts:

- Shelter history and examination. It may be helpful to ask some or all of the questions shown in Figure 12.5. Often, the questions are best combined with a visit to the premises to walk around the kennels and other areas and, where possible, to observe cleaning and biosecurity practices in action
- Dog's history (may be a single animal or, in the case of an outbreak, a group).

A shelter history is essential to elucidate the routes of entry and transmission of diarrhoea-causing pathogens, the impact of existing management controls and to allow understanding of how further management methods for control can be implemented. For an individual animal, signalment is clearly very important, given that some diseases are highly associated with particular age groups. If the affected animal is a puppy, it is important to ascertain whether it was orphaned or hand-reared, the condition of the dam and the size of the litter, as these have clear implications for the likely levels of maternally derived antibody (MDA) present in the puppy. If not already specified in the shelter history, ask whether the puppy was born on

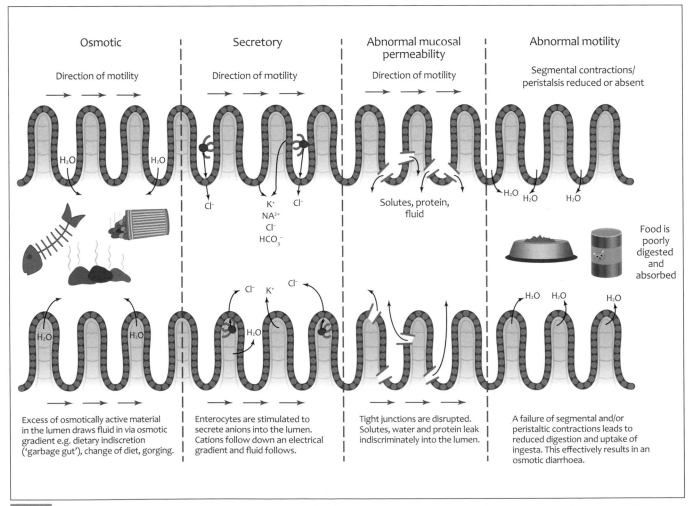

12.4 A variety of physiological processes can cause diarrhoea. Cl^- = chloride; H_2O = water; HCO_3^- = bicarbonate; K^+ = potassium; Na^{2+} = sodium.

Shelter information	
Management protocols	
Who is in charge of biosecurity at the shelter?	Is there a dedicated protocol? If so, what does it cover? Does everyone know about it?
Where do the dogs come from?	Is there a contract to deal with stray dogs? Are they transferred from 'pound' kennels? What proportion is owner-relinquished? Is intake controlled, or are a large number of animals 'dumped'? Do animals trickle in or enter in batches? Are any animals imported from overseas?
Risk-based separation of animals	Is there a quarantine facility? Do all dogs enter it? How long do they stay for? Is there a quarantine/isolation facility for sick animals? How is it equipped and used?
Population density	What is the capacity of the unit? Is it exceeded? If so, how often and by how much?
Cleaning protocols	Is there a cleaning protocol? Are staff trained to understand and use it? Is there sufficient staffing, and do staff practise good biosecurity? Is there adequate equipment for each area? Is the equipment shared? How are faeces and contaminated waste disposed of?
Disinfection	What disinfectant is in use? Is it appropriate (e.g. parvocidal)? Is it made up to the appropriate concentration? Is all organic debris cleaned away before disinfection?
Kennel design	
Is there appropriate drainage?	Are the drains inside or outside the kennel? Are they covered? Is there an appropriate gradient to the floor?
Can the surfaces be adequately cleaned?	Are the surfaces non-porous and easy to clean? Are there cracks or maintenance problems?
What opportunities are there for direct contact between dogs?	Is there communication between kennels, e.g. wire fencing rather than a solid wall? Where are the entrance and exit points? Are there shared exercise areas that cannot be decontaminated (e.g. grass)?
General hygiene and waste disposal	Is there standing water or watercourses? How is rubbish disposed of? Is vermin control necessary/in place?
Stress management	Are the kennels full of noisy barking dogs? Is there some form of visual obstruction so dogs cannot look straight at each other? What breeds or types are predominantly present? What enrichment is provided?
Nutrition	
What is the standard kennel diet?	Is a set brand fed? If so, is it a fixed formula? If not, is the diet variable or a 'kennel mix' of donated food? Is out-of-date food used?
How is feeding regulated?	Is the food weighed or measured? How often are animals fed? Are they fed from bowls or toys or scatter fed?
Is there a chance of feed contamination?	How is the food stored? Are raw foods, rawhide or bones fed? Are homemade diets fed?
Are other diets available?	For example, variety of brands; life-stage, sensitive, prescription diets
Is the weight/body condition score of the dogs monitored?	If yes, how often?
Veterinary protocols	
Vaccination protocols	What (estimated or known) proportion of animals has already been vaccinated on entry? Are all animals vaccinated? When are they vaccinated, in relation to entry to the kennel? Is a live or a killed vaccine used? How many doses are given? At what age does the primary course begin? At what age is the primary course concluded?

12.5 Questions to ask when taking a history in a shelter with diarrhoea. (continues) ▶

Shelter information	
Veterinary protocols continued	
Control of endo- and ectoparasites	Are animals routinely treated for endoparasite control? Does the protocol cover all agents to which the dogs are likely to be exposed? Is ectoparasite control routinely required (i.e. for transmission of tapeworm due to fleas)?
Control of protozoal disease	Is there known or suspected contamination of the site with protozoal or other infectious agents? Is there any routine treatment for protozoal infection?
General information	
Dog history	
Signalment, e.g. is it a puppy?	Hand-reared? Orphaned? Condition of the bitch? Size of the litter? Is the puppy likely to have acquired maternally derived antibody? Born on site or brought in?
Vaccination history	Has vaccination been started? Within what timescale? With what vaccine?
Background	Did the dog come from a pound? Does it have any behavioural issues that could contribute to stress levels?

12.5 (continued) Questions to ask when taking a history in a shelter with diarrhoea.

site or brought in, and whether it has been transported, fostered or otherwise potentially exposed to pathogens by either direct or fomite transmission.

Vaccination history (if administered, when, whether a full course was given, and use of live *versus* killed vaccine) is also essential information, as are details of other preventive medicines given. It is important to remember that protocols are not always rigidly adhered to, so when treating an individual animal, it is still worth checking its records even if the protocol says it 'should' have received a certain treatment. In addition, it can be worth checking whether the treatment prescribed has actually been administered or, for example, was mixed with food that was not eaten and then discarded.

Presentation and clinical signs

Details of the specific clinical history should include the duration of clinical signs, severity of diarrhoea (Figure 12.6) and presence of blood, mucus or tenesmus, as well as other clinical features including the presence of vomiting or regurgitation and whether the dog is interested in food. A lethargic, pyrexic dog is clearly of more immediate concern than an otherwise healthy, bright and active dog that is eating well and has mild to moderate diarrhoea.

The WALTHAM® Faeces Scoring System

Grade 1
Hard dry and crumbly; 'Bullet-like'
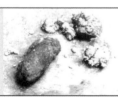

Grade 1.5
Hard and dry
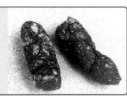

Grade 2
Well formed; does not leave a mark when picked up; 'kickable'
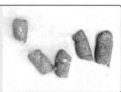

Grade 2.5
Well formed, with a slightly moist surface, which leaves a mark when picked up; almost sticky to touch
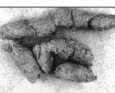

Grade 3
Moist beginning to lose form, leaving a definite mark when picked up
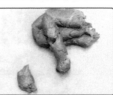

Grade 3.5
Very moist, but still has some definite form
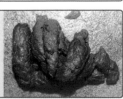

Grade 4
The majority, if not all the form is lost; poor consistency; viscous
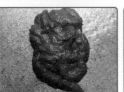

Grade 4.5
Diarrhoea, with some areas of consistency
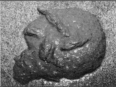

Grade 5
Watery diarrhoea
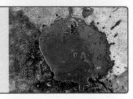

Reference: Moxham, G. (2001) Waltham feces scoring system – A tool for veterinarians and pet owners: How does your pet rate? WALTHAM® Focus, 11, 2, 24–25

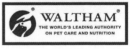
WALTHAM®
THE WORLD'S LEADING AUTHORITY
ON PET CARE AND NUTRITION

12.6 Waltham® Faeces Scoring System.
(Reproduced with permission from Waltham® Centre for Pet Nutrition)

Differential diagnoses

Non-infectious

There are many non-infectious causes of diarrhoea. In a shelter, stress is often implicated as a contributing factor; this may be definitively realized only when a dog with diarrhoea is rehomed and the problem resolves. Likewise, the change in diet when entering the shelter may cause diarrhoea in some dogs. Although some shelters feed a fixed-formula diet, many rely heavily on donations of food, meaning that the dogs' diet is inconsistent. Some shelters address this by mixing together all the donated food to give a 'kennel mix', which all dogs (or all adult dogs) are fed, to provide less variability; however, dogs with dietary sensitivities may be affected by such an approach and develop diarrhoea.

In addition to the more shelter-specific factors, all of the causes of diarrhoea that are seen in owned dogs may be differential diagnoses in the shelter environment. Therefore, while stress, diet and infectious causes will often be uppermost in the mind of a veterinary surgeon faced with investigating cases of diarrhoea in a shelter environment, individual animals may exhibit diarrhoea with many other causes, such as inflammatory bowel disease or neoplastic disease (e.g. lymphosarcoma). Additionally, diarrhoea may be multifactorial; consequently, where diagnostic tests are used, care must be taken to avoid focusing on the presence of a potential pathogen, and test results must be interpreted in the light of clinical findings.

Infectious

The major differential diagnoses for infectious causes of diarrhoea are shown in Figures 12.7 and 12.8.

While there is an exhaustive list of differential diagnoses for dogs presenting with severe acute diarrhoea and associated systemic signs, the most common infectious cause is likely to be canine parvovirus (CPV). However, other relatively common causes of severe diarrhoea, and a presentation including sick, pyrexic dogs with or without vomiting or haematochezia, include salmonellosis and virulent canine enteric coronavirus (CECoV). Confirming the diagnosis can therefore be useful, owing to factors such as the zoonotic potential of *Salmonella* and the relative difficulty in decontaminating the premises after an outbreak involving an environmentally resistant organism, such as CPV or *Giardia*.

Diagnostic testing

Diagnostic tests should be carried out when they will affect decisions regarding case management or environmental control measures. It is important to remember that for many cases of diarrhoea, especially if mild to moderate, testing may be relatively unrewarding. Many of these cases are likely to be caused by management factors such as stress or diet. It is also worth noting that while there are many organisms known to be associated with diarrhoea, not all of them can be tested for commercially. Additionally, for some organisms, such as *Campylobacter*, many dogs can be infected and shed the organism without showing clinical signs. This makes the role of these organisms in disease unclear – even if they are identified, they may not necessarily represent the cause of the diarrhoea. This can make the interpretation of test results difficult, and deciding what – and whether – to treat even more so.

Financial considerations

The shelter's finances may dictate the level of testing that can be used. The benefit of testing samples from individual dogs is that treatment and specific management practices can be directed to that particular case. Even within a block of kennels, cases of diarrhoea may have different or multifactorial aetiologies, and if only one case is tested it may not represent the others sufficiently. However, testing every individual case can be a very costly exercise, and this may be a reason to consider testing pooled samples instead.

Pooled samples (i.e. amalgamated faeces from several affected dogs) can be useful in an outbreak situation if finances are limited. Testing of pooled samples can indicate the background levels of infection and can be less costly than individual testing of each case presented. While testing of pooled faecal matter can lead to an understanding of the outbreak from a 'herd' perspective, it will not be possible to identify specifically which individuals are shedding pathogens. Using pooled samples may also result in dilution of the overall sample (e.g. if samples from six dogs, only one of which is shedding, are combined), thereby reducing test sensitivity (see Chapter 8). It is important to consider what type of pathogen is suspected, and to choose an appropriate test accordingly.

External laboratory tests are available for many potential pathogens; these range from faecal flotation tests to highly sensitive polymerase chain reaction (PCR) assays (see Chapter 8). However, it is often possible to perform basic screens for many pathogens using cheap and immediate in-house tests.

In-house testing

In-house tests are useful, quick and cheap screens for many intestinal parasites. However, they are of limited sensitivity and so, while a positive result is useful in ruling in an infection, a negative result cannot necessarily rule it out. Repeat samples or alternative testing methods should be used for confirmation in such cases.

Faecal smear: These can be used for detecting protozoal oocysts. Place a drop of saline on a slide, add a thin smear of fresh faeces and cover the sample with a cover slip, and examine microscopically (Figure 12.9). Low light levels may help with visualization, as many parasites will be translucent. Alternatively, Ziehl-Neelsen, Diff-Quik® or fuchsin stain can be used.

Faecal flotation: When faeces are mixed with a hypertonic solution, eggs and oocysts will rise to the top of the suspension. Saturated saline or sugar solutions are cheap and easy to prepare by simply adding salt or sugar to water and allowing it to dissolve. The salt/sugar is added until no more will dissolve and a residue sinks to the bottom – at this point, the solution is fully saturated. These solutions can be kept as stock solutions and reused, although they should be discarded once they begin to crystallize.

To carry out the test, add the faecal sample to an equal volume of saturated solution and mix well. Leave the mixture to stand for 15 minutes, to allow eggs and oocysts to rise to the top. Gently skim the top with a slide or coverslip and examine microscopically (Figure 12.10). Alternatively, ensure the mix of faeces and saturated solution fills its container to produce a slight positive meniscus and balance a cover slip on top while the oocysts rise – they will then cling to the cover slip.

Pathogen	Incubation	Pathogenesis	Shedding/carrier status	Diagnostic tests	Common clinical features
Viruses					
Canine parvovirus (CPV)	Typically 3–6 days, occasionally up to 14 days	• DNA virus – mutations uncommon; however, some small but significant mutations have occurred since 1978 • CPV replicates initially in the lymphoid tissue of the oropharynx, then replicates in thymic and mesenteric lymphoid tissue • Viraemia follows 1–5 days post infection, and the virus localizes preferentially to rapidly dividing cells in the bone marrow and endothelial crypts of the small intestine • Immunosuppression, breakdown of the mucosal barrier and secondary septicaemia follow	• Affected dogs shed for 7–12 days post exposure • Viral shedding may occur before clinical signs are seen	• Patient-side ELISAs generally perform well (see below for limitations) • Haemagglutination/ haemagglutination inhibition – sensitivity of these tests is relatively poor • PCR/real-time PCR widely available; most sensitive test	Often haemorrhagic diarrhoea, leukopenia, pyrexia, vomiting, collapse. In neonates, myocarditis and cerebellar hypoplasia may be seen (cerebellar disease is rare in dogs and more a feature in feline parvo)
Canine enteric coronavirus (CECoV)	1–3 days	• RNA virus – two biotypes (type I and type II) but clinically indistinguishable • Damages cells at tips of villi	• Shedding commences 3–14 days post infection • Dogs shed for a variable period after infection, but can be weeks or months	• Real-time RT-PCR • Serology is of limited use unless paired titres are taken as exposure is very common	Generally mild and self-limiting diarrhoea (if any clinical signs are seen). Occasionally, severe disease with haemorrhagic vomiting and diarrhoea is seen due to spontaneous mutations and emergence of virulent strains in susceptible individuals, usually young puppies
Canine distemper virus (CDV)	1–5 weeks	• RNA virus – multiple strains but a single serotype • Replicates in lymphoid tissues causing immunosuppression (often lymphocytopenia) • Initial viraemia is then followed by massive cell destruction and release of virus • Virus locates to respiratory and GI tracts, CNS and other organs, resulting in secondary bacterial respiratory infections, which may be severe, and the wide range of additional clinical signs	• 25–75% of infected animals may show no clinical signs • Recovered animals may shed for up to 4 months on recovery	• RT-PCR on blood, faeces, conjunctival swab, cerebrospinal fluid • Immunohistochemistry/ immunofluorescence on conjunctival swabs • Serology (paired samples needed, hard to interpret in vaccinated animals)	Haemorrhagic vomiting and diarrhoea; pyrexia; bronchopneumonia; conjunctivitis; neurological signs (which may be acute or delayed); hyperkeratitis. Enamel hypoplasia may be seen in dogs infected during dental eruption. Old dog encephalitis may occur months or have progressive neurological impairment, possibly due to virus persistently sequestered in the CNS
Bacteria					
Campylobacter	1–7 days	• Infection is faecal–oral, may be from contaminated food or water source • Releases enterotoxins	• Shedding for several weeks has been reported • Shedding may be intermittent • Shedding can occur in around 40% of non-diarrhoeic dogs	• Rectal or faecal swab, fuchsin, X400–X1000 magnification required. Motile, darting rods, often with spiral or 'gull-wing' morphology. • Culture (bacteria can be fastidious and enter non-cultivable state during transport) • PCR helpful if available	May be asymptomatic. Clinically, often mild and self-limiting diarrhoea. More severe diarrhoea with mucoid or bloody faeces and lethargy more likely in co-infections or young puppies

12.7 Clinical details of major infectious causes of diarrhoea. CNS = central nervous system; GI = gastrointestinal; ELISA = enzyme-linked immunosorbent assay; PCR = polymerase chain reaction; RT/PCR = reverse transcriptase PCR. (continues)

Pathogen	Incubation	Pathogenesis	Shedding/carrier status	Diagnostic tests	Common clinical features
Bacteria continued					
Salmonella	Typically <48 hours	• Invasion of enterocytes leads to massive inflammatory response, which may be enhanced by endotoxins • Damage to epithelium may be severe and lead to mucosal sloughing • Invasion of the local lymphoid tissue allows evasion of the host immune response	• Evasion of host immune response can lead to persistent shedding, with recrudescence following stress	• Culture	Asymptomatic carriage is possible. Diseased animals are often pyrexic, with haemorrhagic diarrhoea. Sepsis and consequent severe systemic illness can occur
Clostridium (*C. perfringens*)	Typically within <24 hours of eating contaminated foods. Nosocomial infections in humans typically occur within 5–10 days of commencing antimicrobial therapy	• May be secondary to other infectious agents or dietary change • Overgrowth and production of cytotoxins causes hypersecretion of fluid into the intestinal lumen (Toxin A), inflammation and death of enterocytes (Toxin B)	• Studies have reported a prevalence of >80% in non-diarrhoeic dogs	• Rectal or faecal swab, fuchsin staining, X400–X1000 magnification required. Spore-forming rods. However, value of this is disputed as these are common commensals • ELISA for enterotoxin • PCR/real-time PCR for enterotoxin	Large intestinal diarrhoea with mucus, tenesmus and haematochezia
Protozoa					
Giardia	5–14 days	• After ingestion of cysts, exposure to digestive enzymes causes release of Trophozoites, which adhere to the mucosa, replicate and encyst • This causes damage to tight junctions allowing secretion of fluid and solutes into the intestinal lumen • Microvilli are truncated, causing maldigestion and malabsorption	• Prevalence of shedding is 5–20% in healthy dogs	• Patient-side ELISAs • PCR/real-time PCR • Faecal smear/zinc sulphate microscopy	Chronic diarrhoea and weight loss
Cryptosporidium	3–7 days	• Ingested oocysts release sporozoites, which attach to intestinal epithelial cells • Mucosal infiltration causes inflammation, resulting in hypersecretion and malabsorption	• Asymptomatic carriage has been reported at a prevalence of 2–8% • Immune response determines whether clinical signs are seen	• Faecal smear (Ziehl–Nielsen stain) • Faecal flotation – may be hard to detect as small size and often low numbers • Immunofluorescence assays for faecal oocysts • PCR (faeces)	Watery small intestinal diarrhoea. Intestines may feel thickened on palpation
Isospora	Prepatent period for shedding is 6–12 days. Clinical signs occur variably, and sometimes not at all, post infection	• Ingested oocysts are stimulated by bile to release sporozoites • These invade enterocytes and replicate, and eventually the merozoites produced in this process rupture the cells, causing villus atrophy, inflammation, malabsorption • Some sporozoites may encyst in the mesenteric lymph nodes, allowing chronic relapsing infection	• Age-related immunity occurs. Most infections are seen in puppies <4 months of age • Recrudescence at times of stress can occur • Infection in dogs >1 year old is rare	• Faecal flotation – shedding may be intermittent, so repeat samples may be required	Infection may be asymptomatic. Vomiting, inappetence and watery diarrhoea, occasionally bloody, may be seen. Severe infestations may cause failure to gain weight, anaemia and hypoproteinaemia

12.7 (continued) Clinical details of major infectious causes of diarrhoea. CNS = central nervous system; GI = gastrointestinal; ELISA = enzyme-linked immunosorbent assay; PCR = polymerase chain reaction; RT/PCR = reverse transcriptase PCR. (continues)

Pathogen	Incubation	Pathogenesis	Shedding/carrier status	Diagnostic tests	Common clinical features
Nematodes					
Toxocara canis	Most dogs infected within first 3 weeks of life. Development of disease depends on infectious burden	• These helminths can grow to 18 cm in length and cause intestinal obstruction, intussusception and, occasionally, obstruction of bile or pancreatic ducts or intestinal rupture • Milder signs are due to an immune-mediated (mainly eosinophilic) inflammatory response	• Most dogs will acquire a degree of immunity at around 6 months of age • However, infection with arrested larvae is extremely common • Even in adult dogs, shedding has been reported in up to 15% of dogs	• Adult worms may occasionally be seen in vomit or faeces • Faecal flotation in saturated salt or zinc sulphide (X40 magnification)	Potbellied appearance of puppies, failure to thrive. Vomiting and diarrhoea due to mucosal irritation and obstruction. More severe signs if total obstruction or intussusception occur
Cestodes					
Dipylidium caninum	Once infected, segments may be shed within 2–3 weeks	• Attachment of the tapeworm scolex within the intestine may cause mild inflammation • Passage of segments may cause perianal irritation	• Shedding continues until treatment occurs • Reinfection is common	• Faecal flotation – characteristic egg packets	Clinical signs are uncommon, beyond the passage of disturbing wriggling proglottids. Exceptionally heavy burdens may cause anaemia and hypoproteinaemia
Taenia	Once infected, segments may be shed within 6–9 weeks	• Attachment of the tapeworm scolex within the intestine may cause mild inflammation • Passage of segments may cause perianal irritation	• Shedding continues until treatment occurs	• Observation of motile gravid segments in faeces	Generally asymptomatic. Severe infections can cause intestinal obstruction and diarrhoea
Echinococcus	Once infection occurs, cysts can be shed within 4 weeks		• Shedding continues until treatment occurs	• Faecal flotation	Generally asymptomatic

12.7 (continued) Clinical details of major infectious causes of diarrhoea. CNS = central nervous system; GI = gastrointestinal; ELISA = enzyme-linked immunosorbent assay; PCR = polymerase chain reaction; RT/PCR = reverse transcriptase PCR.

Pathogen	Vaccine	Immunity	Zoonotic/cross-species potential	Transmission route	Other relevant information
Viruses					
Canine parvovirus (CPV)	Modified live	• Immunity following infection is likely good but there is no data on whether this immunity is lifelong • Vaccinal immunity is considered sterilizing • It has been suggested that a degree of age-related immunity occurs in unvaccinated dogs, possibly due to low-grade natural challenge	• Transmission between cats and dogs is well-established	• Faecal–oral • Non-enveloped virus, survives for weeks or months in the environment • Resistant to many disinfectants	• Current circulating strains in the UK are CPV-2a and CPV-2b. CPV-2c is circulating in Europe and likely to enter the UK. These strains are not clinically distinguishable, and all can infect cats • Vaccines are based on CPV-2b or CPV-2 (the latter being extinct in the field). However, all vaccines appear to confer good protective immunity when used appropriately
Canine enteric coronavirus (CECoV)	Inactivated attenuated	• Immunity following natural infection does not necessarily provide cross-protection for all strains; therefore reinfection is possible • At the time of writing, there is no coronavirus vaccine available in the UK, but vaccines are available elsewhere	• Transmission to cats occasionally reported • Experimental intraperitoneal infection of cats caused feline infectious peritonitis (FIP)-like signs	• Faecal–oral • Enveloped virus, therefore relatively environmentally labile, although can persist for several weeks in ideal conditions	• Synergistic co-infection with other viruses (e.g. CPV) can cause enhanced severity of disease • Genetically distinct from canine respiratory coronavirus (CRCoV)

12.8 Vaccination and transmission information for major infectious causes of diarrhoea. (continues)

Pathogen	Vaccine	Immunity	Zoonotic/cross-species potential	Transmission route	Other relevant information
Viruses continued					
Canine distemper virus (CDV)	Modified live only in the UK at time of writing. Vectored subunit vaccines also available elsewhere	• Recovery from infection provides lifelong immunity • Live vaccines provide sterilizing immunity; inactivated vaccines do not and are therefore not recommended	• Ferrets and other mustelids • CDV has been implicated in Paget's disease in humans, but link remains controversial	• Shed in all body secretions • Enveloped virus, therefore survives poorly in environment – direct and aerosol transmission most important • Transplacental transmission can occur	• Take care with vaccines – if at room temperature for >2–3 hours vaccine will inactivate • Recent administration of a live vaccine may give false-positive test results – this can be differentiated from field infection by real-time PCR, which is commercially available as a diagnostic test.
Bacteria					
Campylobacter spp.	n/a	• May be a degree of short-term immunity to the infective serotype, but unlikely to be lifelong or apply to other Campylobacter serotypes	• Potentially zoonotic – observe good hygiene (most human cases are from contaminated foodstuffs) • Spread to cats and possibly other species, depending on infectious serotype	• Faecal–oral • Can survive for long periods (weeks/months) in the environment, especially in water	• Commonly isolated from healthy as well as diarrhoeic dogs • Role in disease remains poorly understood and controversial
Salmonella spp.	n/a	• There is some evidence of a degree of mainly cell-mediated immunity; however, relatively little data available	• Potentially zoonotic – observe good hygiene	• Faecal–oral • Can survive for weeks to years in the environment, so fomite transmission is important • Feeding of raw meat and hide products has been associated with several outbreaks	• Due to intermittent shedding, it is recommended that three negative faecal cultures are required to ensure eradication has occurred
Clostridium spp.	n/a	• Unknown	• C. difficile is an important pathogen of humans • However, dog to human transfer has not yet been established	• Spores highly environmentally resistant, may persist for years • Outbreaks most likely to result from contaminated food or soil • May be nosocomial following antimicrobial use.	• Although C. difficile has been isolated from dogs with and without diarrhoea, its role is unclear • Even the enterotoxic forms are common in healthy dogs and cats • High levels of enterotoxin with an appropriate history and clinical signs are suggestive
Protozoa					
Giardia	n/a	• Not reported	• Dogs may shed species potentially infectious to humans; therefore care, especially for immunocompromised people, is recommended • Cross-species infection is possible between dogs and cats, and likely other animals, but reports are so far uncommon	• Faecal–oral • Oocysts are highly environmentally resistant, and remain viable for weeks under cool, damp conditions	• There are a number of Giardia biotypes, known as 'assemblages' • Each assemblage appears to have a relatively strong host-range tropism • However, assemblages have been found in non-associated hosts, making the host ranges hard to predict unless molecular methods are used
Cryptosporidium	n/a	• Not reported. However, infected immunocompromised dogs may exhibit clinical signs	• C. canis and C. felis are unlikely to cause disease in humans • However, care, especially in immunocompromised individuals, is sensible	• Faecal–oral • Contaminated food, water or other forms of fomite spread	n/a

12.8 (continued) Vaccination and transmission information for major infectious causes of diarrhoea. (continues)

Pathogen	Vaccine	Immunity	Zoonotic/cross-species potential	Transmission route	Other relevant information
Protozoa continued					
Isospora	n/a	• Age-related immunity • Infection uncommon in adult dogs	• Most *Isospora* spp. are considered highly host-specific, therefore zoonotic or other cross-species transfer is unlikely	• Faecal–oral • Ingestion of sporulated oocysts • Infection may also occur by ingestion of infected prey (e.g. rodents)	n/a
Nematodes					
Toxocara canis	n/a but perinatal anthelmintic treatment of the bitch will help to limit transmission	• Immunity results in larvae remaining in arrested stages within body tissues. These then become reactivated during pregnancy • Disease due to *T. canis* infection is uncommon in dogs over 6 months of age	• Risk to humans of visceral larval migrans – uncommon but potentially severe, observe good hygiene	• Infestation most commonly transplacental or transmammary during pregnancy and suckling • Infection can also be acquired via ingestion of embryonated eggs or a paratenic host (e.g. mice, rabbits)	• Environmentally highly persistent but degrade on exposure to sunlight or desiccation • Eggs require 2 weeks to become embryonated; therefore, good environmental hygiene is likely to be effective in limiting transmission
Cestodes					
Dipylidium caninum	n/a	• No residual immunity; reinfection common • Control depends on control of ectoparasites	• No zoonotic/cross-species risk	• Infection via fleas or biting lice – the dog ingests these while grooming	• Classic grain of rice segments may be seen around the anus
Taenia spp.	n/a	• Age-related immunity has not been demonstrated • Control depends on access to intermediate hosts	• Dogs are important in the spread of *T. hydatigena* on pastures, resulting in infection of livestock • Zoonotic transmission has occasionally been reported	• Dogs shed proglottids in their faeces. These are consumed by an intermediate host. Infection in dogs then occurs by ingestion of the intermediate host • If the dogs do not have access to intermediate hosts, reinfection is unlikely	• Good hygiene, especially in dogs with access to livestock pasture, is important • The main significance of this pathogen is its impact on intermediate hosts
Echinococcus	n/a	• Experiments to determine immunity post infection have given conflicting results • Attempts to develop a vaccine against *Echinococcus* spp. in dogs, in order to control hydatid disease in humans, have shown some promise	• Infection of livestock, especially sheep, on contaminated pastures, is a public health risk • Hydatid cysts in humans are relatively uncommon, but can cause severe and even fatal disease • Humans can acquire infection from ingestion of eggs in dog faeces or contaminated meat	• Infection most commonly acquired from ingestion of cysts from infected sheep carcases	• Control measures for *E. granulosus* are periodically instigated in affected areas, such as South Wales • *E. multilocularis* is not currently established in the UK. Tapeworm treatment immediately before import is an important control measure in preventing importation of this pathogen to the UK

12.8 (continued) Vaccination and transmission information for major infectious causes of diarrhoea.

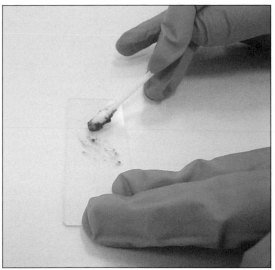

12.9 Faecal smear technique. Apply a thin layer of faeces to a slide with a drop of saline. Apply a cover slip and examine under X20 and X40 magnification.

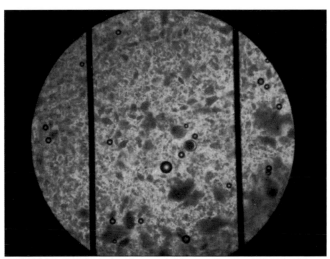

12.10 Faecal floatation demonstrating common parasite eggs/protozoa.

Testing for CPV

A number of 'cage-side' or 'patient-side' tests for CPV are available; these are cheap, convenient and an excellent first port of call when CPV infection is suspected. They detect CPV antigen in the faeces by binding to a corresponding CPV-selective antibody that is contained within the test. This causes a colour change, which is seen as the positive line or dot on the test. However, occasionally these tests can give unexpected results. Figure 12.11 provides a brief guide to interpreting these tests.

CPV infection is suspected, but the test is negative

In this case, the options are:

* To retest immediately with the same kind of test – this will rule out some causes of test failure, although if the failure is due to, for example, the tests having been incorrectly stored, the next test will fail too
* To retest with an alternative form of test, such as PCR (see Chapter 8), which is likely to require a minimum of 24–48 hours for a result and may be more costly. The advantages are that PCR will rule out failure of the patient-side test, is more sensitive and will detect virus even if it is bound to antibody
* To retest with the same kind of test 12–24 hours later – this will show if the dog has now started shedding viral antigen.

In any of these cases, if there is a clinical suspicion of CPV, biosecurity protocols should be instigated regardless of whether the test is positive or negative, as spread of the virus would be the worst outcome.

CPV infection is not suspected, but the dog has tested positive

The key point here is, unless there is a clinical suspicion of CPV, why would the test be used?

Figure 12.11 shows the rare reasons why a dog might test positive when it is not infected with CPV. The difficulty in interpretation tends to occur when a dog has moderate diarrhoea within a few days of entering a shelter and being vaccinated; in this situation it is difficult to state with confidence whether the dog has CPV or the test has detected the vaccine virus.

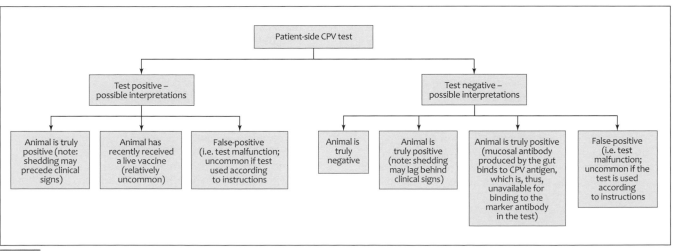

12.11 Interpretation of patient-side canine parvovirus (CPV) tests.

Diagnostic testing with low-grade or background diarrhoea

In this situation, the question is whether diagnostic tests are required at all, and what the results of any test will change. With low-grade diarrhoea, the veterinary surgeon will always be faced with the conundrum that there may be an infectious element but, even if a potentially infectious cause is identified, it can be difficult to decide whether this is the primary pathogen or part of the normal gut micro-biota for that individual. If an infectious cause is identified, particularly if it is potentially zoonotic, this raises the questions of whether the dog's eventual adopter can manage with the clinical signs at home; whether there is a risk to human and/or other animal members of the household; and whether this might contribute to re-relinquishment of the dog if the adopter is not fully appraised of the situation and expectations set (Wells and Hepper, 1999).

Treatment and management considerations

Treatment will need to be tailored, with consideration given to both the individual dog and the 'herd' environment. By using the Waltham® faeces scoring system (see Figure 12.6), staff can help to describe the level of diarrhoea among dogs in the shelter, to facilitate decision-making regarding case management. Combined with the clinical history and examination, faecal scoring can help to determine the list of differential diagnoses. Often, using a logical staged approach, with symptomatic treatment for most cases, will prove to be most efficacious and cost-effective.

Approach to the treatment of low-grade diarrhoea

Most shelter environments will have a background level of diarrhoea; the very nature of the environment, in which many different dogs from differing backgrounds and ages are brought together, will provide the opportunity for diarrhoea to occur.

- Confidence in the shelter's biosecurity is essential in order to manage diarrhoea effectively. If there is a failure of biosecurity at any point, there is a potential for low background levels of pathogens to take hold and provide a perfect environment for a disease outbreak (see Chapter 9).
- It is helpful to understand the layout of the kennels, to piece together potential routes of contact between individual cases that may present with low-grade diarrhoea. This can help when considering the underlying reasons for individual cases and will also help to inform testing for a specific infectious cause. For example, higher than normal rainfall can lead to more standing water in the environment, providing greater opportunity for the persistence and transmission of *Giardia*, with a resulting increase in cases of typical watery diarrhoea.
- If noise-sensitive or frustrated dogs are affected with diarrhoea, reducing their stress as much as possible may help to improve the diarrhoea. Although the optimum situation for these dogs may be rehoming them into a suitable home environment, pending rehoming, factors such as relocating them to a less busy kennel and placing visual barriers to block the view of other kennels may help to reduce stress levels (see Chapter 19).

Symptomatic treatments may be suggested or used according to experience and judgement and within financial limitations. It is worth considering products not just on their cost but also with compliance in mind. A formulation that is easy for the kennel staff to administer is more likely to be adhered to in their busy schedule.

Dietary considerations: Understanding how these dogs are fed can help the veterinary surgeon and shelter staff put methods in place to limit the occurrence of diarrhoea in the first place. The ideal situation would be for the shelter to have a good-quality food that is fed consistently. This may not always be possible depending on the resources available, as outlined earlier in this chapter. Food spoilage needs to be considered, as this can also lead to problems, and it is best to adhere to sell-by or use-by dates (Wilson *et al.*, 2014).

General management principles such as withholding food for 12–48 hours (depending on signalment) and feeding a low-residue diet can be helpful in certain cases of diarrhoea, but will not resolve all of them (Wilson *et al.*, 2014).

Other symptomatic treatments: Administering binding agents (clay-based products), such as kaolin, may be considered in managing low-grade diarrhoea within a shelter. Commercial products are commonly used; however, there are many formulations and subsequently a cost element must be considered but the choice will be largely related to individual preference. Evidence of efficacy is lacking for many of these products, because they largely fall outside the classes of medication specified by legislation. Empirically, however, a binding element can be provided by using proprietary kaolin (Grellet *et al.*, 2014), which can be very cost-effective. Some commercial products also have varying amounts of prebiotics and probiotics in their formulations. If costs prohibit the shelter from purchasing these, prebiotics can also be provided via the diet in the form of mannan and fructo-oligosaccharides, and probiotics could be provided by adding plain 'live' yoghurt to the dogs' food to provide a quantity of commensal bacteria (Wilson *et al.*, 2014).

Approach to more severe infectious diarrhoea if treated at the shelter

The primary concern is normally with the unwell dog. However, the shelter staff may urgently want guidance and advice to prevent transmission of disease (see Chapter 9). Combinations of viral disease and secondary bacterial infection plus the implications of stress and immune system impairment can contribute to a fatal outcome.

- All faeces can contain potentially pathogenic organisms, so all staff should be aware of general biosecurity, e.g. cleaning up after all dogs and washing hands after handling any dog or faecal material, and also before eating (Perez *et al.*, 2014; Filipov *et al.*, 2016).
- Viral causes of diarrhoea can produce very severe disease, and affected dogs will require supportive therapy and hospitalization. If these cases are to be managed within the shelter, essential decisions include: who is to direct the management; care of affected dogs; limiting as far as possible the number of staff responsible for the kennel block the infected dogs came from; how to increase biosecurity appropriately; how to identify any failures in procedures. Staff should have clear guidance on the risk of transmission within the shelter and also, where appropriate, on any possible risks to their own pets. Advice on appropriate biosecurity to minimize these risks (e.g. use of overalls, changing and/or disinfecting footwear, etc.) should be provided.

- Zoonotic infections, whether bacterial (*Campylobacter*, *Salmonella*, etc.) or protozoal (e.g. *Giardia*) will need to be handled carefully within the shelter to limit spread. It is understood that a high proportion of asymptomatic dogs can carry organisms such as *Campylobacter* and *Clostridium* spp., so testing dogs after a course of treatment may be costly and of little benefit. Protocols for biosecurity and reducing the risk of spread within the shelter will be critical, and environmental factors are important to appreciate in this respect – for example, keeping the environment as dry as possible will help to control *Giardia*.

Approach for dogs being treated at the practice for suspected parvovirus

If managing one or more cases of severe enteritis or suspected CPV from a shelter at the practice, it is helpful to discuss with veterinary colleagues the factors that may limit the available treatment options. Providing fluids and pain relief is the first priority. Good nursing care will greatly improve the welfare and prognosis of dogs under treatment. Some charitable organizations will struggle to fund more expensive interventions, and it may be necessary to view each case pragmatically, primarily addressing the animal's welfare. Suspected secondary infections may need to be treated along with maintaining hydration, rather than getting a full diagnostic picture of the case that has been presented. It is best to choose diagnostic tests by weighing up the information that may be gained and the cost that the test involves. For example, a simple blood smear may indicate if the patient has no or very few white blood cells, indicating a poor prognosis; this option would both give an instant answer and be relatively inexpensive. Decisions may include recommending euthanasia for a case where welfare is poor and treatment options restricted.

There are a number of adjunctive therapies available for the treatment of CPV in particular. Interferon omega is licensed and has shown improved survival rates when used early in the course of disease (Wang *et al.*, 2012). However, it is expensive and consideration should be given to the shelter and practice having a policy regarding whether the shelter is willing to fund this treatment. Alternative treatments, such as hyperimmune plasma and oseltamivir (Tamiflu®), have been suggested, but at the time of writing there is little evidence to encourage their use. Care must also be taken when considering the use of products usually reserved for human healthcare (Allison *et al.*, 2012).

Being involved in setting an expected time frame within which the case would be expected to improve is crucial. This allows all parties (the veterinary surgeon, the veterinary team and the shelter team) to reconsider how the case is progressing if improvement is not seen over the agreed period of time.

Rehoming dogs with diarrhoea

Diarrhoea occurs in all shelters – it would be very unusual for it not to. Many owned dogs have occasional gastrointestinal upset without being presented at a veterinary surgery, so such occasional, self-resolving cases of diarrhoea are clearly considered incidental by owners much of the time. It is not ideal for the new owner to manage diarrhoea in a dog they have just adopted from a shelter. However, where stress is a major causative factor, many dogs with low-grade diarrhoea will improve after rehoming, as their stress levels decrease once they settle into their new home.

Where potential adopters are considering rehoming a dog with a recent history of, or ongoing, diarrhoea, it is helpful for the shelter to have as much information as possible, to make sure that appropriate advice and guidance can be given, especially with respect to any potentially zoonotic pathogens. However, **any** faeces can contain pathogens that could potentially infect other animals (including humans) and cause mild or severe disease. This is dependent on the pathogen, but also on the individual's susceptibility.

It is important, where possible, to be aware of the presence of potentially immunocompromised individuals (e.g. very young children, very old people, individuals with a chronic disease) within a household. Obtain informed consent, without causing undue anxiety. Practising basic hygiene, such as avoiding letting dogs lick people's faces, and hand washing following handling of dogs or faeces, should be sufficient to manage risk in most cases, as these pathogens are almost universally transmitted by the faecal–oral route.

Guidance notes or advice sheets for new owners can help to communicate the salient points about the management of these dogs and related hygiene issues. Support from the shelter team can help settle these dogs into their new homes, and this support can be strengthened by a good relationship with the shelter's veterinary surgeon. The aim is to ensure that the relationship between the dog and its new home is secured and the dog is not re-relinquished (Wells and Hepper, 1999). If adopters' expectations are managed and sensible hygiene precautions taken, the presence of diarrhoea should not necessarily be a barrier to rehoming.

Approach to an outbreak of severe diarrhoea

Many of the veterinary team's decisions and solutions will be dependent upon the information gained from the history. It is important to have a broad view of the shelter and its management, as this will help with decision-making in the face of a disease outbreak. Having a good working relationship with the shelter team is key and will help to limit the spread of disease and manage the consequences of the outbreak. Veterinary protocols and biosecurity systems will limit the incidence of disease, and careful negotiation with the shelter on how to develop these can be helpful – as can any contributions that the veterinary surgeon can make to improve them, for example, during regular visits to the shelter.

The main aims of this collaborative approach to a disease outbreak are as follows.

1. **Identify the disease.**
   If an outbreak of severe disease occurs, it is often helpful to identify the primary pathogen, in order to instigate the most appropriate control measures. As there may be a delay while results of confirmatory tests are awaited, it is sensible to approach the application of control measures using the worst-case scenario. If the shelter's finances prohibit definitive diagnosis, it is wise to proceed according to the worst-case scenario on the list of likely differential diagnoses, and manage the outbreak accordingly.

2. **Identify in-contact animals.**
   Identification of potential in-contacts is an essential step. To do this successfully requires a good understanding of the workings of the shelter and also a strong relationship with the shelter staff. Timing of subsequent isolation measures for in-contact animals should be guided by the incubation period of the suspected causative agent. Knowledge of the pattern of movement of dogs around the shelter will help here – for example, when are dogs moved between blocks of kennels? Where are they walked? Do they cross paths with other dogs?

3. **Minimize the spread of disease.**
   Effective biosecurity measures should be instigated at the earliest opportunity. Isolation and 'lockdown' options for groups of kennel units, movements of people around the site, and cleaning and disinfection plans should be implemented and scaled up as appropriate (see Chapter 9).

4. **Appreciate shelter pressures and logistics.**
   There may be difficult negotiations required to take into account the competing demands of the organization. For example, in a rehoming charity, can rehoming continue while efforts to control the outbreak are ongoing? What concerns may there be, and what risks or benefits are there to this approach?

5. **Communicate.**
   - It is important to set out timelines and monitor progress.
   - Regular contact with the shelter is essential – the shelter staff will often need to put in many hours and work incredibly hard to help contain the disease and nurse the dogs affected.
   - Be prepared to change the timeline and approach depending on the results of initial management measures.
   - Ensure communication is clear to all involved.

Veterinary surgeons in charge of their practice's work with a shelter may find that they are juggling many factors – sick animals at the practice being treated by colleagues; contact with the shelter's management as often as once or twice per day; providing biosecurity advice and education for shelter staff as necessary; and managing public expectations (e.g. if the shelter has put a temporary 'lockdown' in place).

Knowledge of the disease involved and its methods of transmission will allow appropriate advice to be given and used to limit the spread of disease if it occurs. It may be important to stop all movement of dogs in and out of the shelter – restriction periods should be decided taking into account the incubation period of the pathogen in question. For example, the typical incubation period for CPV is 4–7 days, although occasionally it may be up to 14 days. Therefore, a restriction period of at least a week, and possibly up to 14 days, would be sensible. If circumstances permit, it may be wise for the shelter to consider fostering out dogs that may be most vulnerable, for example, puppies; as well as avoiding exposure to the pathogen that may be circulating at the shelter, these animals may thrive better in a low-stress home environment, which would strengthen their immune system in general. Limiting access of the general public to come and see the animals, and possibly issuing public awareness notices for display at the shelter entrance, or as press releases to local media, can help to minimize any concerns that the local community may have in relation to the disease spreading beyond the premises.

Prevention

There are many clinical measures available for the prevention of diarrhoeal disease, depending on the organism in question. In addition, the appropriate storage of foodstuffs to avoid spoiling or contamination is an important preventive measure that should not be ignored (Figure 12.12). Biosecurity measures (which are covered in more detail in Chapter 9) are also clearly essential to limit the introduction and transmission of disease.

From a medical perspective, the two main preventive treatments that are commonly utilized are vaccines and parasiticides. Strictly speaking, the administration of parasiticides is generally therapeutic rather than preventive in this context, as at the time of writing there are no endo-parasiticides with residual action. However, parasiticides are used in the context of preventing disease, by reducing the infectious burden, and so are, therefore, included here.

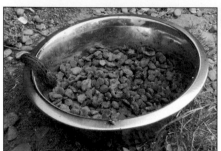

12.12
Contamination of foodstuffs is a potential aetiological factor in cases of diarrhoea among shelter dogs.

Vaccines

Vaccines are available for the important enteric viruses of dogs; that is, CPV, canine distemper virus (CDV) and CECoV. CPV and CDV vaccines are universally regarded as 'core' for both owned and shelter dogs. Vaccination against CECoV may prove useful in some populations, as CECoV outbreaks can have high morbidity; however, since the disease is most commonly mild, CECoV vaccination is not specifically indicated in most circumstances.

Using vaccines within shelters often requires altering the strategy used for pet dogs. This is particularly a concern with CPV, as its long period of environmental persistence means that most shelters can be regarded as high-challenge environments. Conversely, puppies in such high-challenge environments may be considered likely to have obtained high levels of MDA from their dam. This will persist for a longer period than in puppies with lower levels of MDA, suggesting that vaccination should be delayed to ensure an adequate response. However, puppies born to a sick dam, or orphaned puppies, may have very low levels of MDA, necessitating an early start to a vaccination programme. Without performing repeat serology, it is not possible to accurately predict when a given puppy's MDA will decline sufficiently to allow it to respond to vaccination (see Chapter 11).

Therefore, in a shelter situation, particularly where there is a high disease burden or an active outbreak, off-licence use of vaccines may be considered in order to protect the animals most at risk. This may include vaccinating puppies (and kittens) from 4 weeks of age and repeating doses at 2-week intervals until 16–18 weeks of age (Figure 12.13). Whether to vaccinate bitches when pregnancy status cannot easily be established is another cost–benefit decision that must be made. Although a live vaccine is traditionally recommended in a shelter environment, due to the faster onset of immunity provoked, consideration

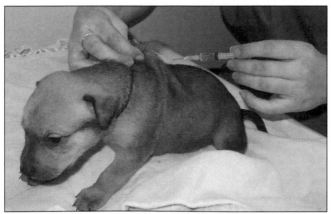

12.13 In some situations, commencing vaccinations from 4 weeks of age may be appropriate.

should be made as to whether a killed vaccine (if available) is appropriate for bitches that may be pregnant. This decision should be taken with a careful balancing of the potential risks and benefits, also taking into account whether the shelter's policy would be to allow a bitch to carry a pregnancy to term or to neuter the bitch while pregnant.

Again, in conventional practice, vaccines are often withheld from animals compromised by poor body condition, stress, concurrent injury or disease. Each shelter's policies must be carefully considered to determine what is appropriate for that environment, and clearly, management practices, such as appropriate use of isolation or fostering, are also important. However, considered in terms of a risk–benefit calculation, a vaccine is unlikely to harm the individual (beyond the occasional reaction of fever and malaise) and may at least partially protect it from disease and reduce shedding of the pathogen, therefore, better protecting the herd. Infectious diseases are much more common than severe reactions to vaccines. In terms of the effect of compromising factors on vaccine efficacy, studies in feral cats have shown that vaccination at the time of neutering induces a protective antibody response in the majority of cases. This suggests that stress and surgery may not inhibit animals' immune response to vaccines (Fischer *et al.*, 2007).

Endoparasite treatment

Many dogs entering a shelter will present with various endoparasites. Figure 12.14 shows the spectra of activity of some common anthelmintics. Anthelmintic treatment should cover nematodes (including *Angiostrongylus*) and cestodes. Cesticide treatment is particularly important in individuals presenting with large flea burdens, as the tapeworm *Dipylidium caninum* can be transmitted by fleas. Unless there is a reliable recent history of administration, it is sensible to undertake endoparasite treatment of all shelter dogs at intake (Figure 12.15).

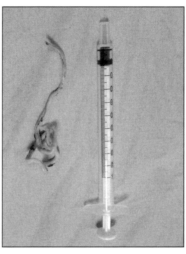

12.15 Many dogs entering a shelter will be infested with a variety of endoparasites, such as *Toxocara* spp.

Product category	Nematodes	Heartworms and lungworms	Cestodes	Protozoa	Comments
Benzimidazoles (e.g. fenbendazole, febantel)	*Toxocara* spp. (all stages), hookworm, whipworm	*Oslerus (Filaroides) osleri, Angiostrongylus vasorum, Crenosoma vulpis*	*Taenia* spp., *Dipylidium caninum* (partial efficacy)	Yes	• Concerns about resistance • Febantel is metabolized to fenbendazole and oxfendazole in the body • Fenbendazole is licensed for pregnant and lactating bitches
Macrocyclic lactones – avermectins (e.g. selamectin)	*Toxocara* spp. (adulticide only)	Prevention of *Dirofilaria immitis*	No	No	• The margin of safety in certain dogs, such as Collie or Collie crossbreeds, is less than in other breeds – read the data sheet for more guidance • Care will need to be taken in dogs that might have originated or travelled to an area where *D. immitis* is present as testing for exposure will be important before using this product
Macrocyclic lactones (e.g. milbemycin, moxidectin)	*Toxocara* spp. (adults and L4 larvae), hookworm, whipworm	*A. vasorum* (reduction of the level of infection by immature L5 and adult parasite stages), *C. vulpis* Prevention of *D. immitis*	No	No	
Nicotinic anthelmintics (pyrantel, febantel, oxantel)	*Toxocara* spp., hookworm, whipworm	No	No	No	• Febantel and oxantel are derivatives of pyrantel with increased activity against whipworms
Praziquantel	No	No	*D. caninum, Taenia* spp., *Echinococcus* spp.	No	• Kills all intestinal stages of *Echinococcus* – useful in control programmes or imported animals
Piperazine	*Toxocara* spp. (adults only), hookworm (high doses required)	No	No	No	• Piperazine is readily absorbed from the GI tract and care needs to be taken in dogs with renal impairment or epilepsy

12.14 Spectrum of activity of commonly available anthelmintics.

Chronic protozoal infections are a problem in some shelters, especially those with grassed or muddy shared exercise areas, as cysts can persist for extremely long periods in these environments. In recognition of this, some organizations will treat dogs with benzimidazoles at intake to limit shedding (however, this treatment will not eliminate shedding) and thereby reduce contamination of the environment.

References and further reading

Allison AB, Harbison CE, Pagan I et al. (2012) Role of multiple hosts in the cross-species transmission and emergence of a pandemic parvovirus. Journal of Virology 86, 865–872

Bowman DD (2013) Georgis' Parasitology for Veterinarians, 10th edn. Elsevier, St Louis

Filipov C, Desario C, Patouchas O et al. (2016) A ten-year molecular survey on parvoviruses infecting carnivores in Bulgaria. Transboundary and Emerging Diseases 63(4), 460–464

Fischer SM, Quest CM, Dubovi EJ et al. (2007) Response of feral cats to vaccination at the time of neutering. Journal of the American Veterinary Medical Association 230, 52–58

Greene C (2011) Infectious Diseases of the Dog and Cat, 4th edn. Saunders, St Louis

Grellet A, Chastant-Maillard S, Robin C et al. (2014) Risk factors of weaning diarrhea in puppies housed in breeding kennels. Preventive Veterinary Medicine 117, 260–265

Marshall JA, Kennett ML, Rodger SM et al. (1987) Virus and virus-like particles in the faeces of cats with and without diarrhoea. Australian Veterinary Journal 64, 100–105

McCann T and Simpson JW (2006) Pathophysiology of diarrhoea. Companion Animal 11, 31–88

Perez R, Calleros L, Marandino A et al. (2014) Phylogenetic and genome-wide deep-sequencing analyses of canine parvovirus reveal co-infection with field variants and emergence of a recent recombinant strain. PLoS One 9, e111779

Sykes JE (2014) Canine and Feline Infectious Diseases, 1st edn. Elsevier, St Louis

Tupler T, Levy JK, Sabshin SJ et al. (2012) Enteropathogens identified in dogs entering a Florida animal shelter with normal feces or diarrhea. Journal of the American Veterinary Medical Association 241, 338–343

Wang J, Cheng S, Yi L et al. (2012) Evidence for natural recombination between mink enteritis virus and canine parvovirus. Virology Journal 9, 252

Wells DL and Hepper PG (1999) Prevalence of disease in dogs purchased from an animal rescue shelter. Veterinary Record 144, 35–38

Wilson S, Illambas J, Siedek E et al. (2014) Vaccination of dogs with canine parvovirus type 2b (CPV-2b) induces neutralising antibody responses to CPV-2a and CPV-2c. Vaccine 32, 5420–5424

Case example 1: Parvovirus at the local rehoming shelter

Following examination of Micky, a 3-month-old Collie cross with severe haemorrhagic diarrhoea, lethargy and vomiting, and a patient-side test, parvovirus infection was confirmed. Micky had recently been accepted into a local shelter along with six other adolescent dogs from the local pound and, on initial examination 4 days previously, while all dogs were in poor body condition, they were otherwise clinically unremarkable. Micky is now hospitalized at the veterinary clinic and not very well; she is being supported with intravenous fluid therapy and nursing care but still seems quiet. The shelter contacted the pound to advise of the suspected parvovirus outbreak; staff at the pound said that many dogs from the same group of adolescents had died after showing previous haemorrhagic diarrhoea.

The shelter staff have asked for advice on how to manage the rest of the dogs they have at their premises. They are concerned about both this dangerous infection and all the other dogs at the shelter – they have puppies and some older residents, as well as 40 dogs that are in the various stages of rehoming.

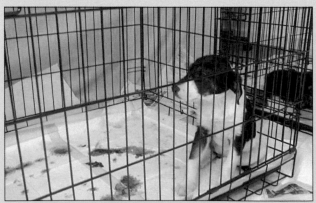

Micky, a 3-month-old Collie cross presented with severe haemorrhagic diarrhoea, lethargy and vomiting.

HOW TO IDENTIFY IN-CONTACT DOGS

The manager, who is most familiar with the layout and management of the shelter, should be asked to find out where the dogs from the pound have been housed since they arrived; this will determine if and where they have been walked on site, as well which staff have been involved in their care. Piecing this information together would help to ascertain the risk to other dogs in the shelter from contact. Fortunately, the pound dogs were housed in a kennel block separate from the rest of the shelter. However, as the shelter was short staffed when the dogs arrived, a member of staff who had been working in this block had also been helping to care for a litter of 7-week-old puppies that have been on site since birth.

WHAT MEASURES DOES THE SHELTER NEED TO TAKE TO MINIMIZE THE RISK OF SPREAD?

- **Adequate disinfection procedures** – On checking with the manager what dilution the disinfectant is being used at, and how much contact time is allowed when disinfecting surfaces and other materials, it comes to light that the shelter staff have been using the disinfectant at half the manufacturer's recommended concentration and using a contact time of only 10 minutes during routine cleaning. It is essential that disinfectants are used at the correct concentration and left in contact with the cleaned surfaces for the time recommended on the product label.
- **Specific members of staff to deal with the infected kennel block** – The newly arrived dogs with suspected parvovirus are housed in a block separate from the rest of the kennel. This block can be treated as an isolation facility, with one or two members of staff being dedicated to this block during the lockdown period. The shelter has provided

→ CASE 1 CONTINUED

disposable overalls, overshoes and footbaths at the entrance to the block. Footbaths must be maintained appropriately; however, on inspection those at the shelter were found to be not clean. It is important to ensure that the manager understands that the staff working in this kennel block cannot cross-cover other parts of the shelter because of the risk of transmission of infection.

- **Exposure of puppies by a member of staff** – There is a high risk that the puppies cared for by the staff member who had been working in the infected kennel block have been exposed. Vaccinations at the shelter begin at 6 weeks of age, and the manager feels that these puppies should be perfectly safe as they received their first vaccination a week ago, before potential exposure. However, even with vaccination, there is still a risk, as the puppies' response to vaccination is affected by their previous health status and MDA – this may limit the effectiveness of the vaccine. As the risk is still present, these puppies should be barrier nursed and ideally fostered in a local home with their dam while being monitored. One of the volunteers offers to take them and monitor them over the next 7–10 days. The volunteer will not come on site during this period and has been trained in appropriate biosecurity measures for the puppies while they are in the foster environment.

WHAT INFORMATION CAN BE GIVEN TO REASSURE THE SHELTER TEAM AND MANAGE THEIR CONCERNS?

The manager should be made aware that Micky is not very well but that supportive care has started and it is hoped that improvements will be seen over the next few days.

The problem has been identified quickly and appears to be a single case at the moment; this, plus the quick and strong response by the shelter team to implement the recommended biosecurity measures, will help to minimize the effects. All shelter staff and volunteers should be made aware of the circumstances and measures in place.

PRIORITIES: PREVENTING FURTHER SPREAD; TREATING EXISTING CASES; TREATING NEW CASES THAT ARE CURRENTLY INCUBATING

The next morning there are concerns about two other dogs from the same group as they are lethargic, anorexic and pyrexic. They are housed together, and at least one of them has produced grade 5 diarrhoea overnight. They are admitted to the veterinary clinic and started on treatment, with a presumptive diagnosis of CPV.

IDENTIFICATION OF CAUSE: OPTIONS FOR DIAGNOSTIC TESTING

Micky's condition has become slightly worse overnight. The options for further testing are discussed with the shelter's management; however, costs are a problem for the shelter at the moment and the primary concerns are in relation to other infections, due to the clinical picture of the inpatient.

- The dogs were treated for roundworm/tapeworm and *Giardia* on intake, as well as being vaccinated, so it is not necessary to look for these pathogens at this stage.
- Empirical antibacterial cover is being provided due to evidence of breach of the intestinal mucosa (costs limit the option of bacteriology).
- The practice team is supporting Micky with pain relief, nursing and fluids.
- A colleague has concerns about other viral causes. (The snap test could be confirmed with PCR testing, but this is not practicable for financial reasons; further virology for coronavirus/distemper is probably not definitively indicated in the absence of other clinical signs or an outbreak situation, so is not performed, especially in view of the cost limitations.)

Micky's condition worsens during the day. A blood smear shows virtually no white cells, indicating poor immune function and a very guarded prognosis. Euthanasia of the dog is recommended as she is unlikely to recover. The other dogs that have been admitted are still quiet and inappetent. A post-mortem examination to understand more about the outbreak is an option. However, the manager declines this due to funding restrictions; it has cost more than anticipated to manage this case and the shelter would struggle to cover this extra expense.

DECISION ON SHELTER ISOLATION OR SHUTDOWN LENGTH

Following the two additional cases, it should be recommended that the shelter closes, with a suggested shutdown period extending to 7 days following the last known case of parvovirus. The manager has concerns, as the shelter is in the middle of a busy period at the moment and is trying to raise funds to build a further block of kennels to replace some older facilities, but agrees that the kennels should be 'locked down' to visiting dogs or further intake.

IMPACT ON THE SHELTER WITH RESPECT TO PUBLIC PERCEPTION AND OWNED DOGS

The shelter has a shop and tea room on site, and is under pressure to continue raising funds, so wants to keep these facilities open to visitors. However, members of the public have been bringing their own dogs into the shelter site when visiting. Notices should be put up in the public areas of the shelter to inform people of the risk, emphasizing that only dogs that have been vaccinated are allowed to visit. A regular visitor, who normally visits the tea shop two or three times per week with their elderly dog, becomes upset when they see the notices. They speak briefly to a member of the shelter team and decide to call the local radio station to inform the public that there is an outbreak of parvovirus at the shelter. Unfortunately, this results in local panic. The shelter becomes involved in reassuring the public about the measures put in place to limit the disease, as well as spreading the message that vaccination can help to reduce the risk for pet dogs. The shelter veterinary surgeon could offer to speak on local radio and use this opportunity to explain that the other two dogs that were admitted to the veterinary practice have made a full recovery and that there have been no further cases.

→ **CASE 1 CONTINUED**

HANDLING DOGS FROM A POUND: ANY LESSONS TO LEARN?

At a follow-up visit the following week, the shelter manager advises they plan to reopen the shelter in a few days' time. They realize how important it was to contain the disease, even when faced with a staff shortage; had the infection not been contained, the impact that it would have had on the entire shelter could have been much worse. On the day of the visit, the pound dogs that brought in the infection are due to be moved from the separate block into regular kennels, to make space for another group of dogs to come in. However, it would be better to postpone the movement of these dogs for perhaps a few more days, to make sure that they are well before they move out of the separate block. The ideal situation would be for pound dogs to be vaccinated before arrival at the shelter, and the manager agrees to put this proposal forward to the committee at their next meeting.

Case example 2: Rehoming a *Campylobacter*-positive dog

The local shelter is visited by a veterinary surgeon twice a week. It has had a low-level ongoing problem with diarrhoea. Laboratory results have come back (*Campylobacter* positive) from a sample of faeces taken from Spud, a 2-year-old male neutered Jack Russell Terrier in the rehoming section that has been particularly badly affected by diarrhoea.

RELEVANT HISTORY AND BACKGROUND

Spud came in with a group of dogs that have been managed with dietary therapy; the diarrhoea began to settle down but Spud has produced grade 3.5 diarrhoea every day or every other day.

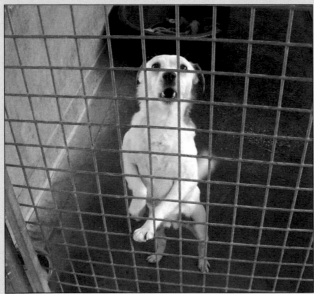

Spud, a 2-year-old Jack Russell Terrier with diarrhoea potentially partially attributable to *Campylobacter* infection. He is otherwise healthy and, with monitoring, may be rehomed with consideration to the zoonotic potential.

SHOULD SPUD BE REHOMED?

Spud has been in the shelter for 10 days and a suitable family has come forward looking to rehome him. The shelter has completed all the paperwork with the family, and are just waiting for approval before his adoption. It is explained to the manager that *Campylobacter* can be found in a proportion of normal dogs, and that there are no concerns that this is the sole cause of Spud's diarrhoea. The shelter manager is worried and would like him to be treated – the shelter has had *Campylobacter* in other dogs in the past, and treatment seemed to be effective in those cases. The manager is also concerned about rehoming Spud while he is *Campylobacter* positive, as it is a zoonotic pathogen and the new adopters may contract it.

HOW WOULD YOU COMMUNICATE THIS?

It may be a good idea for the veterinary surgeon to speak with the potential adopters, to explain that the chances are that Spud is exhibiting signs of this disease because he is in a shelter environment, and reassure them that it is common for a proportion of dogs to shed *Campylobacter* while remaining healthy. Settling into a good home and being fed a sensible diet should help to manage him, as will removing him from the potentially high-burden environment of the shelter. The veterinary surgeon could offer to see Spud after a few days with his new family to see how they are getting along; if there are still problems at this stage other options can be explored if necessary.

WHAT MIGHT HELP IMPROVE KNOWLEDGE FOR THE FAMILY?

Providing the adopters with a guidance sheet about adopting dogs with particular diseases will help to explain the issues the family will need to be careful with. It should detail the disease and the steps that adopters can take to reduce the risk of transmission to humans, such as washing their hands after handling the dog and also before eating. The shelter includes a copy of the guidance with the rehoming pack that is provided to Spud's new owners when he goes to his new home. His diarrhoea settles, and when he is seen again he is healthy and active, and is getting on very well with his new family.

Chapter 13

Diarrhoea in the cat in the shelter environment

Allison German and Lisa Morrow

Diarrhoea is a frequent presenting or developing problem in cats at shelters, especially on or soon after arrival. The World Health Organization defines diarrhoea as the passage of three or more loose or liquid stools per day, or more frequent passage than is normal for the individual. It involves an increase in the water content and sometimes the solid content of faeces. Diarrhoea is described as acute if the duration is less than 14 days and chronic if of longer duration. Diarrhoea ranges from mild and self-limiting to severe and fatal; the development of dehydration in young kittens in particular can be rapid and severely debilitating. Adopting a sensible tiered approach to diagnosing and treating diarrhoea in the shelter is important for its management. Cases may need to be considered on an individual basis or as a population. Knowing the underlying cause of the diarrhoea and treating it effectively can save costs in the long term, help to prevent disease spreading through a centre, and can prevent the development of antimicrobial resistance as a consequence of indiscriminate use of antibiotics.

Normal faecal patterns and diarrhoea

As part of being able to recognize when there are one or more cases of diarrhoea among cats in a shelter, it is important to understand what is normal for a shelter cat, both on an individual basis and on a population basis. In addition, it is important to ensure adequate monitoring to detect diarrhoea in its early stages or determine when the problem has resolved. At any time point within a rescue cattery, there will be cats that are not defecating, cats with normal faeces, cats with constipation and cats with diarrhoea. Adult cats tend to defecate once a day, although there is a subpopulation that defecates every other day. Kittens tend to defecate more frequently, and passing two to four stools in a day may be normal. Faecal scoring charts are a very useful way of recording defecation of an individual cat within a shelter, and also of monitoring the population. One example of the type of scoring chart available is the Cats Protection Faeces Grading System (Figure 13.1), which is adapted from the Bristol Stool Chart originally devised for people. This system grades cat faeces from 1 (watery) to 6 (hard and dry). Monitoring faeces by grade allows the caregiver to know whether the cat is actively passing faeces, when to intervene if constipation

Grade	Appearance	Description
1		Liquid, watery faeces
2		Mostly unformed stools; watery faeces with lumps
3		Approximately 50% formed stools in softer stools
4		Mostly formed stools with a very small amount of softer stool
5		All firm, well-formed stools
6		Small, very hard faecal pellets

13.1 The Cats Protection Faeces Grading System.
(© Cats Protection)

or obstipation is a concern, and when to intervene with dietary management or veterinary care if faeces are loose.

Despite defecation being an essential bodily function, little is known about what the defecation profile should be for the average population of cats in a shelter. In a cross-sectional study of 1686 faecal samples (graded according to the Cats Protection Faeces Grading System) from cats and kittens housed in 25 Cats Protection Adoption Centres in the UK in 2012, 5.6% were grade 6 (dry, hard), consistent with constipation, and 11.9% were grade 3 or lower, consistent with diarrhoea (Figure 13.2) (German *et al.*, 2017). The cat population was considered healthy, with no centre reporting an outbreak of diarrhoea. This indicates that in these rescue catteries, at any one time, 12% of cats may have diarrhoea; this information can help veterinary surgeons (veterinarians) to define when an outbreak occurs. In this study population, diarrhoea was more likely to occur in kittens and in pens with more than one cat housed in them. Less than 1% of the residual variance was associated with the adoption centre; this indicates that good management routines and hygiene standards are effective in confining infection and preventing its spread through a shelter (see Chapter 9).

Diarrhoea in context of the shelter environment

The shelter environment provides lots of opportunities for the transmission of diarrhoea-causing pathogens and outbreaks of diarrhoea. Shelters are frequently high-throughput units with many cats under one roof. These units will vary from foster homes to communal pen units and individual accommodation within shelters. Being relinquished or stray and entering a new environment (such as the shelter) is very stressful for cats and may result in a reduced immune response, allowing infection with novel pathogens or recrudescence of low-grade or latent infection. There are many infectious agents that cause diarrhoea, and cats may also develop diarrhoea secondary to a change in diet or the presence of stressors in their new environment. In addition, cats may present with diarrhoea related to non-infectious causes, such as irritable bowel syndrome, lymphoma, inflammatory bowel disease, hyperthyroidism, disorders of the liver, pancreas or kidney and adverse drug reactions.

Distinguishing between infectious and non-infectious causes is clearly an important starting point when dealing with diarrhoea in a shelter environment where there are other cats at risk. It is a key part of the initial assessment of a cat with diarrhoea, where a judgement must be made on whether a cat is potentially infectious to others (cats and people) and, thus, whether it needs to be isolated and barrier nursed. This decision is generally based solely on the history and clinical signs. The rest of this chapter will focus on infectious causes of diarrhoea in the cat.

History taking

For cats entering a shelter, there is often very little historical information available, and this is especially true in terms of information relating to the nature of their pattern of defecation and typical grade of faeces. Even if the relinquisher is aware of a problem with diarrhoea, they may not disclose this through fear that their cat will not be accepted by the shelter. If the cat has been relinquished by an owner, it is often useful to contact the previous veterinary surgeon (veterinarian), where possible, to obtain any medical history. Many shelters make detailed recordings of cats' urination, defecation, and eating and drinking habits (Figure 13.3). This information can be extremely useful to the practitioner presented with a cat with diarrhoea, as it helps to determine the onset and duration of the diarrhoea, the type and character of the faeces, and the general demeanour of the cat; it is particularly useful in identifying patterns over time. It is often worth asking the shelter staff or volunteers what they have observed about the cat, as sometimes this will elicit key information.

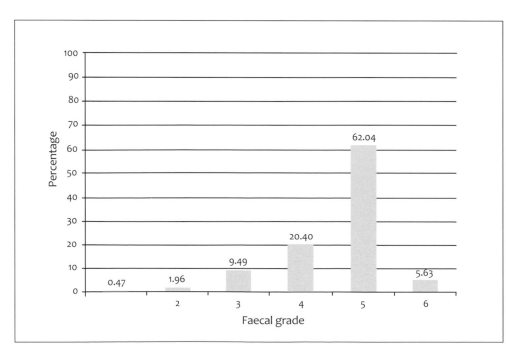

13.2 Profile of faecal consistency in a UK shelter cat population. Data are from a cross-sectional study of 1686 faecal samples scored using the Cats Protection Faeces Grading System. (Data from German *et al.*, 2015)

Observation sheet

Start date: ....

CATS PROTECTION

Cat name: .... Pen: ....

Start weight: .... End weight: ....

Cat ID: .... Age: .... Sex: .... Colour: ....

Reason for observation: ....
(e.g. admission, ill, under/overweight, food monitoring, water intake etc.)

Diet: Wet/Dry (delete as appropriate)

Comments: ....

Faecal grade: 1 – Watery   2 – Sloppy   3 – Soft   4 – Semi-solid   5 – Solid   6 – Hard-dry

* = Tick/cross/? In box then add comments if needed

Date	Time	Eating*		Drinking	Urination		Faecal grade		Comment	Initial
		Wet	Dry		Inside	Outside	Inside	Outside		
	AM									
	Noon									
	PM									
	AM									
	Noon									
	PM									
	AM									
	Noon									
	PM									
	AM									
	Noon									
	PM									
	AM									
	Noon									
	PM									
	AM									
	Noon									
	PM									
	AM									
	Noon									
	PM									

Ensure admissions form is updated at the end of the observation period.

13.3 Cats Protection observation sheet.
(© Cats Protection)

Veterinary surgeons attending a shelter on a regular basis (or employed by the shelter organization) will be familiar with any housing, feeding or other environmental considerations that might have an impact on the diarrhoea. For veterinary surgeons who see the animal at their practice, it is prudent to ask questions about the environment the cat is living in. This type of questioning is helpful in determining whether there could be significant stressors or dietary-related factors involved in the presentation, and helps to assess the likelihood of the diarrhoea being infectious or not. If multiple cases are present in the shelter, it is useful to look at a plan of the cattery layout and mark the cases by date of identification on the plan to see whether there is any pattern that might indicate the spread of an infectious agent. Figure 13.4 illustrates the type of information that can be helpful in assessing diarrhoea in a cat shelter.

Cat history	
General information	
Background	• Stray? Single or multi-cat household? • How long has the cat been in the facility? Has it been moved from one area to another within the facility? • Has it mixed with other cats or spent time in areas where other cats have been? • Does the cat have any known pre-existing behavioural issues, or experienced recent life events that could influence stress levels? For example, has any building work been going on at the shelter; has there been a marked change in the weather for cats housed in outdoor units; have public visits been busy recently or has the cat had a socialization event recently? • Do other cats in the shelter have diarrhoea? If so, what proportion of the cats is affected and where are they located? • Are there currently cats with diarrhoea in the isolation unit? • Are multiple accommodation areas of the shelter affected?
Signalment (e.g. age, sex, breed)	• For kittens: hand-reared? Orphaned? Condition of queen? Size of litter? Born on site or brought in?
Demeanour	• Withdrawn? Seeking attention? • Bright and active? Quiet and subdued? • Any change in interaction with other cats or people?
Diet history	• Any recent diet changes? If so, what did the change involve (e.g. feeding frequency, diet type)?
Vaccine history	• Has vaccination been started? • Within what time scale? • With what vaccine?
Anthelmintic treatment history	• When was the last worming treatment? • What product was used?
Other treatment history?	• Have antibiotics been prescribed recently?
Nature of the diarrhoea (as reported by shelter staff)	• Appearance: colour, grade, volume, presence of mucus, blood or worms • Number of stools passed per day • Faeces passed inside or outside the litter tray? • Is the cat straining to pass faeces? • Do faeces drip from the anus? • Is there faecal staining around the perineum or on the hindlegs? • Does the anus/perineum appear sore?
Other relevant clinical signs (reported by shelter staff)	• Any increase in drinking or changes to pattern of eating? • Is there any vomiting? If so, record the frequency, volume and content
Shelter history	
Management protocols	
Who is in charge of biosecurity at the shelter?	• Is there a dedicated protocol? • If so, what does it cover? • Does everyone know about it?
Where do the cats come from?	• What proportion is owner-relinquished? • Is intake controlled, or are a large number of animals 'dumped'? • Do animals trickle in or enter in batches? • Are animals transferred from other shelters? • Are any animals imported from overseas?
Risk-based separation of animals	• Is there a quarantine unit? • If so, do all cats enter quarantine? • How long do they stay in quarantine for? • Is there an isolation unit for sick animals? • Are kittens and queens housed in a separate maternity unit? • How are the different areas equipped and used? • Which areas do the public have access to? • Do the units have dedicated staff members or do staff cross/work between units?
Population density	• What is the capacity of the unit? • Is this capacity exceeded? • If so, how often and by how much? • Are cats housed individually or in groups from different sources?
Cleaning protocols	• Is there a cleaning protocol? • Are the staff trained to understand and use it? • What is the litter tray cleaning routine? Are cats given the same litter tray back after cleaning? • Is there sufficient staffing and do staff practise good biosecurity? • Is there adequate equipment for each area? Is equipment shared? • How are faeces and contaminated waste disposed of? • Have there been any recent changes to the protocols or new staff members?
Disinfection	• What disinfectant is in use? • Is it appropriate (e.g. parvocidal)? • Is it made up to the appropriate concentration and is contact time adequate? • Is all organic debris cleaned away before disinfection? • Have there been any recent changes to the protocols or new staff members?

13.4 Information that can be helpful in assessing diarrhoea in a cat shelter. (continues) ▶

Shelter history *continued*	
Pen design	
Is there appropriate drainage?	• Are the drains inside or outside the pen? • Are they covered? • Is there an appropriate gradient to the floor?
Can the surfaces be adequately cleaned?	• Are the surfaces non-porous and easy to clean? • Are there cracks or maintenance problems?
What opportunities are there for direct contact between cats?	• Is there communication between pens (e.g. wire fencing rather than a solid wall)? • Where are the entrance and exit points? • Are there shared exercise areas that cannot be decontaminated (e.g. grass)? • Are there shared facilities that cannot be or are not regularly decontaminated, e.g. scratch posts in an exercise area? • Are there open drainage channels that run between outdoor or isolation pens?
General hygiene and waste disposal	• Is there standing water or watercourses? • How is rubbish disposed of? • Is vermin control necessary/in place?
Stress management	• Are the cats given a place to hide within their pen? • Is there some form of visual obstruction so cats cannot see other cats? • What enrichment is provided?
Nutrition	
What is the standard diet?	• Is there a set brand fed? • Is donated food used? • Are cats fed according to life stage? • Is out-of-date food used? • Are other diets available (e.g. sensitivity or prescription diets)?
How is feeding regulated?	• Is the food weighed or measured? • How often are animals fed? • Are they fed from bowls or is enriched feeding used (e.g. puzzle feeders or scatter feeding)?
Is there a chance of feed contamination?	• How is the food stored? • Are raw foods fed? • Are homemade diets fed?
Are weight and body condition scores of the cats monitored?	• If yes, how often?
Veterinary protocols	
Vaccination protocols	• What (estimated or known) proportion of animals has already been vaccinated on entry? • Are all animals vaccinated? • When are cats vaccinated in relation to entry to the shelter? • Is a live or a killed vaccine used? • How many doses are given? • At what age do kittens start their primary course? • At what age do kittens complete their primary course?
Control of endo- and ectoparasites	• Are animals routinely treated for endoparasites? • Does the protocol cover all agents to which the cats are likely to be exposed? • Is ectoparasite control routinely used (i.e. to prevent the transmission of tapeworm through flea bites)?
Endemic infections	• Is there any known contamination of the site with protozoa or other infectious agents, resulting in low grade continuous infection?
Control of protozoal infection	• Is there any routine treatment for protozoal infection?

13.4 (continued) Information that can be helpful in assessing diarrhoea in a cat shelter.

Clinical signs

The clinical signs will vary subtly between the different causes of diarrhoea. The first assessment to make is whether the diarrhoea is acute or chronic and then whether the diarrhoea is small intestinal, large intestinal or mixed (Figure 13.5). Cats with large intestinal diarrhoea may not always show as clear clinical signs as dogs. They may also demonstrate pain on defecation and defecate outside the litter tray. Vomiting may occasionally be associated with small intestinal diarrhoea. Cats with diarrhoea may also be polyphagic and polydipsic due to nutrient malabsorption and fluid loss.

The clinical examination should make note of whether the cat is dehydrated, the intestines are gassy and dilated,

Characteristic	Small intestinal	Large intestinal
Volume	Large	Small
Frequency	Mild increase from normal	Large increase from normal
Weight loss	Common	Rare
Inappetence	Can occur	Rare
Mucus	Rare	Common
Blood (if present)	Melaena	Haematochezia
Tenesmus	Rare	Common
Colour	Variable	Normal
Gas	Sometimes	Absent

13.5 Comparison of the clinical signs associated with small and large intestinal diarrhoea.

the abdomen is painful (diffusely or focally), faeces can be palpated in the colon or not, the perineum is stained and whether there is an offensive odour or halitosis. In adult cats, examination should also include a physical check for systemic disease: the thyroid glands should be palpated, heart auscultated, lymph nodes palpated and the abdomen examined for any masses. Kittens should be assessed for intestinal intussusception. All cats should be weighed and body condition scored.

Specific clinical signs for infectious diseases

Parasites

Protozoa: The clinical signs associated with protozoal infections are shown in Figure 13.6.

Helminths: These are covered in more depth in Chapter 11, but their role in diarrhoea is briefly considered here.

- **Roundworms (*Toxocara cati* and *Toxascaris leonina*):** Clinical signs are more common in kittens and include diarrhoea, poor coat quality, a distended abdomen and failure to thrive. Heavy infestations may lead to intestinal obstruction, intestinal perforation and intussusception. Heavy burdens may also cause pneumonia in kittens.
- **Hookworms (*Uncinaria stenocephala*):** In small kittens, a heavy infestation can cause anaemia,

melaena and haematochezia. *U. stenocephala* is relatively non-pathogenic, but a heavy infestation can cause diarrhoea.
- **Tapeworms (*Dipylidium caninum* and *Taenia* spp.):** Infestation is usually associated with no clinical signs. Very rarely, diarrhoea, weight loss or failure to thrive may be seen.
- **Whipworms (*Trichuris campanula* and *T. serrata*):** Infestation in cats is rarely symptomatic.

Viruses

For information on the clinical signs associated with feline leukaemia virus and feline immunodeficiency virus, the reader is referred to Chapter 17. The clinical signs associated with feline coronavirus are discussed in Chapter 18.

Supplementary information on the pathophysiology, diagnosis, treatment and management of feline parvovirus can be found in Morrow and German (2018).

Bacteria

- **_Salmonella_ spp.:** Clinical signs vary depending on the host's immune status, concurrent infections and the infectious dose. Clinical syndromes may include gastroenteritis, septicaemia, signs based on organ localization or an asymptomatic carrier state. Cats may show pyrexia, diarrhoea, vomiting, conjunctivitis, abortion and septicaemia. Clinical signs can mimic disease associated with feline parvovirus (FPV).

Pathogen	Population affected	Presence and nature of diarrhoea	Other clinical signs	Exacerbating factors	Additional points
Isospora spp.	Mostly young kittens. Infection in adults is of questionable significance	Asymptomatic to transient watery diarrhoea, to severe mucoid or haemorrhagic diarrhoea	Vomiting can occur	Stress Malnutrition Immunosuppression	Infection can become enzootic in a shelter
Cryptosporidium spp.	Infection more likely in kittens and shelter cats	Asymptomatic to small intestinal diarrhoea	Anorexia and weight loss can be observed	Often presents as a coinfection with other parasites or other debilitating disease (irritable bowel disease, lymphoma, feline immunodeficiency virus (FIV))	
Giardia spp.	Prevalence is higher in kittens and shelter cats	Often asymptomatic, but may be acute or chronic small intestinal diarrhoea (self-limiting, mild or severe). Faeces are usually malodorous, mucoid, pale and soft. *Giardia* can also colonize the colon in cats, so large intestinal or mixed-pattern diarrhoea may be observed	Severe or chronic cases can be associated with weight loss	Immunodeficiency	Infection may self-limit in 27–35 days or may be recurrent
Tritrichomonas foetus	Usually seen as a clinical problem in cats under 2 years of age. More common in multi-cat environments	Asymptomatic to chronic or recurrent large intestinal diarrhoea. *T. foetus* colonizes the ileum, caecum and colon and causes a neutrophilic and lymphoplasmacytic colitis. Diarrhoea can worsen without an increase in the number of trophozoites. Mucus, tenesmus and haematochezia can occur. Defecation frequency is increased and cats can become faecally incontinent (a constant dripping of yellow foul-smelling faeces). Clinical signs may wax and wane	The anus can become sore and oedematous due to increased frequency of defecation and grooming. Generally, the cat remains bright and alert and the appetite is not affected	Stress Coinfections	Check for coinfection with *Giardia duodenalis*, feline leukaemia virus (FeLV), FIV and feline coronavirus (active shed)

13.6 Clinical signs associated with common protozoal infections in cats.

- **Clostridia:** *Clostridium perfringens* is a commensal organism and infection is usually associated with no clinical signs, although in some circumstances, with certain toxin-producing strains, it can cause diarrhoea (usually large intestinal). Diarrhoea can be either acute or chronic. Acute infection is short-lived and self-limiting. In chronic infection, diarrhoea is intermittent, recurring every 4–6 weeks and otherwise the cat shows little sign of being unwell. Very rarely, acute haemorrhagic gastroenteritis has been reported. *C. difficile* is more often associated with diarrhoea than asymptomatic infection in cats; diarrhoea is acute and watery, sometimes with vomiting, abdominal discomfort and fever.
- **Campylobacter:** Campylobacteriosis is usually asymptomatic. Large intestinal diarrhoea (mucoid, watery or haematochezia) may occur and is more commonly seen in kittens than adults. Clinical signs are more common with coinfections.

Diagnosis

A specific diagnosis is not always needed for cats with diarrhoea in a shelter environment. The history, including any observations since the cat's entry to the shelter, clinical signs and response to treatment are the main tools used to assess diarrhoea. This approach is commonly used because it often leads to a successful outcome (i.e. the diarrhoea resolves) in a relatively short period of time and it incurs minimal cost.

As mentioned previously, the first stage of diagnosis is to identify whether the cause of the diarrhoea is infectious or not, given that diarrhoea due to stress or dietary change is considered to be common in cats newly admitted to a shelter. In larger facilities operating under a high level of organization and structure, staff will often assist with this first stage by following a dietary management and monitoring protocol for 3 days if the cat is (and remains) otherwise clinically well. If the cat has not responded, or if it is very young or shows signs of illness, the cat will be seen by a veterinary surgeon.

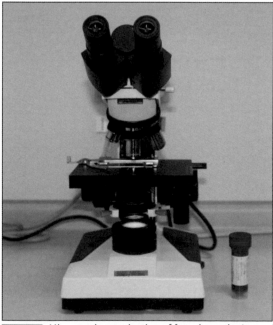

13.7 Microscopic examination of faecal samples is a rapid, inexpensive and informative assessment tool.

There are times when testing of faecal samples will be necessary. Of the many tests available, microscopic examination (Figure 13.7) is often the most informative, inexpensive, rapid and easiest to interpret. The speed of assessment can be increased greatly if the shelter has provision for microscopic examination on site. Cage-side tests for FPV and *Giardia duodenalis* are readily available, as are polymerase chain reaction (PCR) tests for many agents, but these must be interpreted with caution. Many agents can be detected in faeces, but the identification of an agent does not always mean it is the cause of the clinical signs observed. Nor do such tests indicate whether or not a cat is infectious to others. This is particularly true for cats that are not showing clinical signs of diarrhoea. For these reasons, screening all cats for faecal parasites on intake is not recommended, and faecal testing should be done only in cats that have diarrhoea and have not responded to dietary and/or medical management. Faecal testing can be useful when an outbreak of infectious diarrhoea is occurring in a shelter because knowing what organism is involved can help with management of the population of cats in terms of treating those that are affected, the possibility of prophylactic treatment for others at risk and reducing contamination of the environment to reduce spread of disease. More information on the approach to diagnostic testing in the shelter environment can be found in Chapter 3.

Specific diagnostic tests for infectious diseases
Parasites

Figure 13.8 lists the characteristics of infectious protozoa and helminths that commonly cause diarrhoea in cats, along with the diagnostic tests available. For practical guidance on faecal flotation and microscopic diagnosis of common parasites, the reader is referred to Chapter 12.

Viruses

Figure 13.9 lists the characteristics of viruses that commonly cause diarrhoea in cats, along with the diagnostic tests available for these pathogens.

Feline rotaroviruses may cause diarrhoea in individual cats but they are not epidemiologically associated with diarrhoea. Feline astrovirus, reoviruses, caliciviruses, enteroviruses, torovirus and FHV-1 have all been implicated as playing a potential role in diarrhoea, although the significance of their role is yet to be determined. They will not be considered further in this chapter.

Bacteria

Figure 13.10 lists the characteristics of bacteria that commonly cause diarrhoea in cats, along with the diagnostic tests available. Faecal cultures are often difficult to interpret, as, while many bacteria can be identified, most will be normal commensals. Kittens are more commonly affected than older cats. Bacterial enteritis can occur secondarily to existing gastrointestinal disease. Faecal bacterial culture is often poorly informative and money may be better spent on other diagnostic tests. Selection of cases for faecal culture should be based on:

- Diarrhoea that persists after evaluation and treatment for parasitic disease
- Acute haemorrhagic diarrhoea and septicaemia
- Outbreaks of diarrhoea
- Screening for bacteria with zoonotic potential.

Common species	Incubation/ prepatent period	Pathogenesis	Identification	Diagnostic tests	Shedding	Carrier status	Epidemiology	Notes
Isospora spp. (Coccidia)								
I. rivolta and I. felis	Prepatent period 4–11 days depending on species. Maturation of cysts in the environment takes 8–36 hours and requires humidity and temperatures of 20–37°C	Single-celled, spore-forming intracellular parasites that infect the intestinal tract. Some sporozoites may penetrate the intestinal wall and set up cysts in extraintestinal tissue such as lymph nodes.	Thin-walled oocysts in faeces. Some oocysts exist in a two-celled stage	ZnSO₄ faecal flotation test. May also be diagnosed on direct examination of a faecal smear. Usually high levels if significant	Intermittent. Can be asymptomatic. Can be shed for up to 9 weeks after treatment	Yes	Prevalence of 3% in laboratory-submitted diarrhoea samples from UK pet cats. Prevalence is higher in kittens than adults. Prevalence is higher in shelter cats, stray and feral cats. Prevalence of over 80% has been reported in stray populations	Can be incidentally acquired/passed through from ingested prey (Eimeria spp.). Concurrent infections make clinical signs more likely
Cryptosporidium spp. (Coccidia)								
C. felis most common. C. parvum seen less frequently. C. parvum has at least 21 genotypes	Oocysts are immediately infective when passed in faeces (3–6 days after infection), infect in low numbers and are environmentally resistant	Small protozoan parasites that replicate in the intestinal border, protected by the host cell membrane	Oocysts in faeces	Faecal smear stained with Giemsa or modified Ziehl–Neelsen (oocysts are very small and intermittently shed); direct immunofluorescence; faecal ELISA; PCR. Can be seen in intestinal biopsies on histopathological examination	Intermittent. Can be asymptomatic	Corticosteroid treatment may induce oocyst shedding in subclinical carriers	Prevalence is reported at 3–20% in cats with diarrhoea; higher in kittens and shelter cats	Most tests are designed for C. parvum, so may have lower sensitivity for other species
Giardia spp.								
G. duodenalis (syn G. lamblia and G. intestinalis), assemblage F (occasionally A and B)	3–25 days (usually 7–10). Cysts are passed in faeces and are immediately infective; they can survive in the environment for months. The infective dose is low (10–100 cysts)	Consumed in contaminated water/ food; excystation in the duodenum stimulated by gastric acid and pancreatic enzymes; trophozoites attach to intestinal epithelium; multiplication and then encystation occur. Clinical signs are caused through intestinal malabsorption and hypersecretion	Trophozoites (short-lived) or cysts in faeces. Trophozoites are teardrop-shaped, with two nuclei, eight flagella (six emergent), a concave ventral disc and 'falling leaf' motility. Cysts are ellipsoid and environmentally resistant	Microscopic analysis is currently the gold standard. Trophozoites: direct faecal smear (observe for 'falling leaf' motility); cysts: ZnSO₄ faecal centrifugation test. As shedding is intermittent, it is best to process three samples over 1 week. Faecal antigen ELISA, IFA (PCR is available but is mainly a research tool and should be used only in cats with diarrhoea)	Intermittent. Can be asymptomatic. Reinfection is rapid, which presents difficulties in differentiating chronic infection from reinfection	Yes. Corticosteroid treatment can reactivate a latent infection	Prevalence in the UK cat population is approximately 4%, with up to 15% reported in cats with diarrhoea. Prevalence is higher in kittens, immunodeficient cats, diarrhoeic cats and shelter cats. A meta-analysis of 68 studies during the period 2001–2014 of G. duodenalis in cats reported an overall prevalence of 12% (Bouzid et al., 2015). Prevalence varies depending on the diagnostic method used (6.5% by microscopy compared to 15.9% by ELISA/IFA/PCR)	Antigen detection tests should be used only for cats with diarrhoea, as the significance of an antigen-positive, cyst-negative healthy cat is unknown. Similarly, use only faecal flotation tests rather than antigen detection tests if doing post-treatment testing, as it is unknown how long antigen persists after infection has cleared

13.8 Common protozoa and helminths that cause diarrhoea in cats. ELISA = enzyme-linked immunosorbent assay; IFA = immunofluorescence assay; PCR = polymerase chain reaction; ZnSO₄ = zinc sulphate. (continues) ▲

Common species	Incubation/ prepatent period	Pathogenesis	Identification	Diagnostic tests	Shedding	Carrier status	Epidemiology	Notes
Tritrichomonas								
T. foetus	8–10 days	Flagellated protozoan that colonizes the ileum, caecum and colon	Trophozoite (short-lived). No cyst stage. Spindle-shaped, single nucleus, three anterior flagella, long undulating membrane, jerky forward trajectory of movement	Direct faecal smear (sensitivity 14%, survive 2 hours); faecal culture 'InPouch™ TF' system; faecal PCR (susceptible to false negatives but is the most sensitive and specific test); colonic/ileal biopsy	Intermittent. Can be asymptomatic. Reactivation can be triggered by environmental stressors, diet change or immunosuppressive medication	Yes	Young cats are primarily affected (median 9 months), although infection has been reported in cats aged up to 13 years. The parasite is mostly seen in multi-cat (particularly pedigree) households and shelter cats. There has been one report of T. foetus in an immunosuppressed person, so there is a potential zoonotic risk	
Roundworms								
Toxocara cati, Toxascaris leonina	In cats the prepatent period is approximately 13 weeks for T. leonina. For Toxocara cati, it is more variable, but usually around 6 weeks after ingestion of eggs. The patent period for both species is 4–6 months	T. cati has a similar life cycle to T. canis, but kittens are not infected prenatally	Large ova (80 μm) with thick walls	Faecal flotation				See Chapter 11 for more detailed information
Hookworms								
Ancylostoma tubaeforme (mild pathogen), A. braziliense (tropics and subtropics) and Uncinaria stenocephala (Europe, UK?, North America)	Prepatent period is 15–17 days	Adult worms attach to the small intestinal mucosa and feed on blood	Ova (75 × 45 μm)	Faecal flotation				Very rare in cats in the UK. See Chapter 11 for more detailed information

13.8 (continued) Common protozoa and helminths that cause diarrhoea in cats. ELISA = enzyme-linked immunosorbent assay; IFA = immunofluorescence assay; PCR = polymerase chain reaction; $ZnSO_4$ = zinc sulphate.

Common species	Incubation period	Pathogenesis	Diagnosis	Diagnostic tests	Shedding	Carrier status	Epidemiology	Notes
Feline panleukopenia virus (FPV)								
FPV	FPV replicates in oropharyngeal lymphoid tissue 18–24 hours after infection, followed by a disseminating viraemia for 2–7 days. Virus can be detected in faeces within 24 hours post infection.	Small icosahedral single-stranded DNA virus that actively targets dividing cells. • Has an affinity for lymphoid cells, bone marrow and the intestinal crypt epithelium • In pregnant cats in early to mid-gestation, the virus targets the fetus and can lead to fetal death, resorption or abortion • If the queen is infected in late gestation onwards, kittens may be born with cerebellar hypoplasia, hydranencephaly, optic nerve atrophy and retinopathy	History, clinical signs, vaccination status and leukopenia (Note, leukopenia does not occur in all cases, but usually the degree parallels clinical signs), viral antigen, viral nucleic acid, histopathological changes	• CPV faecal ELISA (faecal shedding of FPV is short and variable, sometimes only 24–48 hours post infection. The ELISA also detects CPV in cats, which is often asymptomatic) • Faecal PCR (more sensitive and can identify viral strains). • Histopathology: intranuclear inclusion bodies in the small intestinal crypt epithelium • Other tests: *in situ* hybridization, immunohistology and electron microscopy of faeces or intestinal biopsies for viral particles and inclusion bodies	• Virus shedding period 1–2 days, although sometimes up to 6 weeks post recovery	• Asymptomatic infected cats shed infectious virus particles and therefore can act as carriers	• Few data exist to indicate the prevalence of FPV; serosurveys show exposure in excess of 90% • A kitten mortality study (Cave *et al.*, 2002) showed that FPV was responsible for 25% of sudden death post-mortem submissions • Prevalence is higher in shelter environments • Prevalence has subjectively decreased over recent years, likely due to widespread vaccination and cross-protection from CPV-2 infection	• Leukopenia does not occur in all cases • Secondary bacterial infections and endotoxaemia may arise from enteric microflora
Feline coronavirus (FCoV)								
FCoV – enteric variants	Virus is shed in faeces 2 days following infection	Large, enveloped, positive-stranded RNA virus that infects enterocytes. • The primary site of viral replication is the small intestinal epithelial cells (Type II) and likely the ileum and colon (Type I) • Early in infection, replication can occur in the tonsils and oropharynx with a brief period of shedding in saliva • Virus may also be shed in respiratory secretions and urine	Diagnosis is rarely performed as diarrhoea is self-resolving or responds quickly to supportive care	• Serology (antibody titre) indicates exposure (ELISA) • Antibodies raised against enteric pathotypes are indistinguishable from those raised against FIP pathotypes	• Continuous • Can be asymptomatic • Length of shedding variable depending on environment/reinfection rates • 65% of Type I infected cats shed for 2–3 months or longer	• Yes; 13% of naturally infected cats become lifelong carriers	• High prevalence in the cat population. See Chapter 18 for more information	Has potential to cause FIP through *de novo* mutation within an individual or through infection with a highly pathogenic FIP field strain. Refer to Chapter 18 for information on FIP

13.9 Common viruses that cause diarrhoea in cats. CPV = canine parvovirus; ELISA = enzyme-linked immunosorbent assay; FIP = feline infectious peritonitis; PCR = polymerase chain reaction.

Agent	Identification	Pathogenic or not?	Diagnosis
Escherichia coli	Gram-negative rods	Common isolate from faeces; virulent forms exist, which may be pathogenic	Diagnosis requires determination of virulence, which necessitates biochemical assays or PCR
Salmonella spp. (*S. typhimurium* most common)	Gram-negative rods	Pathogenic, but 18% of healthy cats are reported to carry *Salmonella* spp. in their faeces. In cats, infection is dependent on a high infective load and may be aided by gastrointestinal compromise due to another cause or immunodeficiency	Dedicated culture. Toxic neutrophils may be seen in cases of sepsis. If septicaemia is suspected, culture of *Salmonella* spp. from sites other than the gastrointestinal tract can help the diagnosis
Clostridium perfringens	Gram-positive, spore-forming, obligate anaerobic rods	Commensal, but may become a pathogen secondary to antibacterial therapy, diet change or intestinal disease. *C. perfringens* enterotoxin is the virulence factor produced by sporulating rods and is associated with diarrhoea	Light microscopy of rectal swab for a high number of sporulating rods, combined with assay for clostridial enterotoxin. ELISA is the traditional diagnostic test; however, it is not validated for cat faeces, so the results should be interpreted with caution. A PCR assay also exists to distinguish toxigenic strains
Clostridium difficile	Gram-positive, spore-forming, obligate anaerobic rods	Sporadic reports in cats. *C. difficile* causes diarrhoea or may occur alongside antibiotic therapy. Asymptomatic infection is also reported	Isolation of *C. difficile* should be accompanied by faecal ELISAs for toxin A and toxin B or a PCR for toxigenic strains should be performed. Clinical cases in cats are usually positive for toxin A
Campylobacter spp.	Microaerophilic Gram-negative curved rods	Normal finding in healthy cats. In some studies, there is no difference between the isolation rate of *Campylobacter* spp. from diarrhoeic cats and healthy cats. *C. upsaliensis* has been isolated from 50–60% of normal cats. *C. jejuni* is less frequently identified. Concurrent infections or immunosuppression enhance the risk of disease	Observation of S-shaped organisms on a faecal smear alongside culture. Faecal samples or swabs should be placed in anaerobic transport medium and refrigerated to enhance isolation. PCR tests are also commercially available. They are more sensitive than other tests and may allow typing of the organism

13.10 Common bacteria that cause diarrhoea in cats. ELISA = enzyme-linked immunosorbent assay; PCR = polymerase chain reaction.

Treatment

The approach to veterinary treatment of diarrhoea in the shelter environment follows the pragmatic approach outlined in Chapter 3. Using response to empirical treatment with minimal diagnostic testing is a very useful and practical approach. There are two main drivers for this: time and money. Cost limitations will always exist in the shelter environment, and the more efficiently a shelter uses its financial resources, the more animals it can help. Sick animals in shelters need to recover as quickly as possible to reduce the chance of spread to others – and also because this means that the cat has a better chance of leaving the shelter sooner. This is not just good for the individual cat's welfare; it also results in more pen space being available so another cat can be taken in.

Treatment of an isolated case of diarrhoea will generally start with dietary management (this is also part of the diagnostic process, described above) and selected use of other non-specific and supportive therapies. Where a causative agent is known, pathogen-specific therapy may also be appropriate (Figure 13.11).

Treatment of multiple concurrent cases may involve further investigative work, diagnostics and possibly prophylactic treatment, as outlined later in Approach to an outbreak of diarrhoea.

Initial on-site management

Often, shelter staff are very observant and proactive in managing faecal health in the cat population. If an otherwise healthy cat passes stools graded 3 or lower (scored using the Cats Protection Faeces Grading system) for 3 days, staff should implement dietary management at the same time as notifying the shelter manager and/or the veterinary surgeon. Cats should be fed a proprietary highly digestible, high-quality protein diet, or a home-cooked chicken/fish meal for 3–5 days. If daily faecal monitoring charts are not already being completed, staff should start to use them (see Figure 13.3). Hygiene measures and biosecurity should be increased. If diarrhoea persists or worsens 3 days after instituting these interventions, veterinary attention should be sought. Veterinary care should be sought sooner if:

- The number of cases increases
- There is other evidence that an infectious agent may be the cause
- The cat is unwell as well as having diarrhoea
- The cat is very young
- The cat is pregnant
- The cat has another disease/medical problem
- There is blood in the faeces.

Non-specific and supportive therapies

- **Dietary management:** For cats over 8 weeks of age, feed a highly digestible low-fat food, such as a white meat diet (chicken/fish), or an appropriate commercial diet for 3 days. This should be provided in frequent small amounts (e.g. four feeds per day). Gradually reintroduce the normal diet and feeding interval once faecal grade has returned to normal. It is mused that villus recovery may be more rapid if enteral nutrition is provided rather than starving the gut. However, there is currently no published evidence to support this in cats.
- **Anthelmintics:** Fenbendazole at 50 mg/kg orally q24h for 3–5 days to cover for *Giardia duodenalis* and helminths.
- **Supportive care:** Intravenous fluid therapy, antiemetics and nutritional support. Glucose infusions or oral glucose gel may be required in kittens to prevent hypoglycaemia. If severe hypoproteinaemia is diagnosed, colloids or a plasma transfusion may be

Agent	First-line treatment	Second-line treatment	Notes
Protozoa			
Isospora spp. (Coccidia)	• Sulfadimethoxine at 50 mg/kg orally q24h for 10–14 days • Trimethoprim/sulphonamide at 15 mg/kg orally q12h for 10–14 days	• Toltrazuril at 30 mg/kg orally single dose or 15 mg/kg orally q24h for 3 days, repeat in 10 days. **Off label, dose accurately**	• Often self-limiting, but treat if clinical signs warrant or to manage potential spread within an establishment • Treatment can also be given prophylactically in kittens and to direct contacts to reduce spread • Treatment may reduce shedding in subclinically affected individuals but may not always be curative
Cryptosporidium spp. (Coccidia)	• Azithromycin at 10 mg/kg orally q24h for a minimum of 10 days has variable response	• Tylosin at 10–25 mg/kg orally q12h for 14 days minimum helps infected cats recover, although it does not necessarily treat *C. felis* • Nitazoxanide at 25 mg/kg orally q12h for at least 5 days is being evaluated. Side effects of vomiting. Treats dual infection with *Giardia duodenalis*	• Drugs are mostly ineffective or toxic • Paromomycin use has been reported, but efficacy is questionable and it may cause acute renal failure
Giardia spp.	• Fenbendazole at 50 mg/kg orally q24h for 3–5 days	• Metronidazole at 25 mg/kg orally q12h for 7 days • Febantel at 56.5 mg/kg orally single dose or q24h for 5 days	• Treatment failures may occur and there is no permanent immunity. Dual therapy with fenbendazole and metronidazole can help with resistant cases. • High doses of metronidazole may cause neurological side effects in cats • Treat in-contact as well as infected animals. Reinfection is the most common reason for treatment failure • Other drugs that have been used to treat giardiosis: paromomycin, nitazoxanide, tinidazole, ronidazole, quinacrine
Tritrichomonas foetus	• Fenbendazole at 50 mg/kg orally q24h for 5 days + metronidazole at 10 mg/kg orally q12h for 14 days • Combine with environmental and dietary management (see Notes)	• Ronidazole at 30 mg/kg orally q24h for 2 weeks is the only treatment for which efficacy has been demonstrated. Longer or higher doses are NOT more efficacious. Not licensed. Care needed: possible neurological side effects. Bitter. Approximately 60% of cats respond to treatment and 5% develop side effects (anorexia or neurological signs). Do not use in kittens less than 12 weeks of age	• Infections may wax and wane despite medication and diarrhoea can sometimes be refractory • Reduce environmental stress, treat or isolate in-contact animals and use a high-quality single-source protein or hydrolysed protein diet • Many cases clear spontaneously within 9 months of onset of clinical signs • Probiotics may be useful as a supportive treatment
Helminths			
Roundworms	• Pyrantel at 20 mg/kg orally single dose, repeated after 3 weeks • Fenbendazole at 50 mg/kg orally q24h for 3 days • Selamectin at 6 mg/kg topical application monthly • Moxidectin minimum dose 0.1 mg/kg topical application monthly • Milbemycin minimum at 2 mg/kg orally, single dose	• Refer to Chapter 11 for more in-depth information on treatment of helminth infestations	• Given the absence of transplacental migration, there should be no need to commence treatment until 3 weeks postpartum. *Toxascaris leonina* is also not acquired prenatally, and even heavy infestations are unlikely to cause significant clinical disease. The treatment protocols that treat *Toxascaris canis* and *Toxocara cati* will adequately treat *Toxascaris leonina* • Treatment at least four times a year is advised to make a significant impact on preventing patent infection in the population. Kittens should be treated every 2 weeks until 2 weeks after weaning. Queens should be treated in parallel with the first kitten treatment. In high-risk situations, treatment of adults every 4 weeks is recommended
Hookworms	• Fenbendazole at 50 mg/kg orally q24h for 3 days or a single dose of 100 mg/kg orally • Pyrantel at 10 mg/kg orally single dose • Selamectin at 6 mg/kg topical application monthly • Moxidectin minimum dose 0.1 mg/kg topical application monthly • Milbemycin minimum 2 mg/kg orally, single dose	• Refer to Chapter 11 for more in-depth information on treatment of helminth infestations	

13.11 Pathogen-specific treatment of diarrhoea in cats. (continues)

Agent	First-line treatment	Second-line treatment	Notes
Viruses			
Feline panleukopenia virus (FPV) (also called feline parvovirus)	• Supportive treatment with intravenous fluid therapy, correcting electrolyte imbalances	• Treatments may include dextrose solution (2.5–5%) or 40% oral glucose (dextrose) gel for hypoglycaemia; plasma or colloids for hypoproteinaemia; antiserum (from vaccinated or recovered cats, given after exposure but before clinical signs develop); broad-spectrum antibiotics if neutropenic or pyrexic; antiemetics for nausea or vomiting; gastric protectants if oesophagitis develops; vitamin B_{12} and thiamine; intravenous recombinant interferon omega; nutritional support (as soon as can be tolerated)	• Cost–benefit must be considered in the choice of second-line treatment in the shelter situation
Feline coronavirus (FCoV)	• Usually resolves spontaneously. May occasionally need supportive care. Reduce stress		• Refer to Chapter 18 for information on treatment of feline infectious peritonitis (FIP)
Bacteria			
Escherichia coli	• Treat only if clinical signs are severe, other pathogens are eliminated and there are signs of systemic involvement	• Enrofloxacin and potentiated amoxicillin can be used for treatment of septicaemia	
Salmonella spp.	• It is controversial to treat infection unless infection is systemic	• Base choice on results of culture and sensitivity testing. Potentiated amoxicillin can be used while antibiotic sensitivity results are awaited	
Clostridium perfringens	• Tylosin at 7–11 mg/kg orally q8–12h or amoxicillin at 11–22 mg/kg orally q8–12h for 10–14 days, or longer term. Either have tylosin compounded or put it into gelatin capsules as it is very bitter • Metronidazole is not always effective in all cases		• Very rarely causes clinical disease in cats • Fermentable fibre (e.g. psyllium) can be added to the diet, which is thought to alter the faecal microenvironment and reduce toxin production
Clostridium difficile	• Treatment may not be necessary as cats that test positive are not usually ill • Prior exposure to antibiotics is a risk factor for developing clinical disease	• Metronidazole at 10–20 mg/kg orally q12h for 7–14 days	
Campylobacter spp.	• Even in symptomatic cases, there may be an alternative cause of the diarrhoea, so the use of antibiotics should be approached with caution • In mild cases, treatment may not be necessary. Otherwise, use antibiotics and supportive treatment including fluid therapy if the cat becomes dehydrated • Treatment with antibiotics may increase the chance of faecal shedding • Antibiotics should be used on the basis of culture and sensitivity results. Common choices include tetracyclines, erythromycin and clindamycin	• Tetracyclines and fluoroquinolones are effective but resistance may be mutationally acquired	• Penicillins, cephalosporins and trimethoprim are considered ineffective

13.11 (continued) Pathogen-specific treatment of diarrhoea in cats.

required. A blood transfusion may be required in cats with panleukopenia or salmonellosis if anaemia is severe.

- **Probiotics:** The use of probiotics and prebiotics (e.g. oligofructose and inulin) remains controversial. There have been few peer-reviewed scientific studies looking at probiotic (or prebiotic) use in cats. Most information available comes from manufacturers of these products or is extrapolated from other species. The use of enterococci is reportedly beneficial in certain conditions and in certain species, but they are also reported to be opportunistic pathogens and carriers of drug resistance genes. A study by Waltham Centre for Pet Nutrition (Marshall-Jones et al., 2006) showed that Lactobacillus acidophilus probiotic supplementation in cats was beneficial for intestinal health and positively influenced the colonic microflora. Prebiotics are thought to act by increasing the numbers of Bifidobacter spp. and decreasing the numbers of pathogenic microorganisms. Increased numbers of Bifidobacter spp. are seen in healthy cats compared with cats with diarrhoea.
- **Adsorbents:** Kaolin can be used as an adsorbent to reduce the number of pathogens in the intestinal lumen that are free to bind to the epithelium. Again, there are no convincing studies confirming the benefit of this treatment, though anecdotally it is said to help. Conversely, it is possible that it may increase morbidity by enhancing faecal sodium excretion. An alternative is bismuth, which has antimicrobial properties and may have an anti-inflammatory/anti-secretory role.
- **Opiate antidiarrhoeals (diphenoxylate and loperamide):** These can reduce the severity of diarrhoea by reducing water excretion and enhancing adsorption by the villi. However, reduction of motility is not necessarily a benefit, as sometimes diarrhoea is hypomotile.
- **Cobalamin:** Cobalamin (Vitamin B_{12}) supplementation may be warranted in more refractory/chronic cases. This vitamin is required for DNA replication in the intestinal crypts and depletes with diarrhoea.
- **Environmental management:** Practices that can help to contain and reduce the spread of diarrhoea-causing pathogens include: isolation of problem cases to halt outbreaks; good hand hygiene in between contact with different cats; appropriate disinfection routines, e.g. sodium hypochlorite at 1:32 dilution; and careful and appropriate disposal of faeces and good litter tray hygiene.

Pathogen-specific treatment

Pathogen-specific treatment (see Figure 13.11) should be based on the diagnosis. Antibiotics should be used only if there is a specific indication based on faecal analysis or systemic signs. Small intestinal bacterial overgrowth is rarely seen in cats compared with dogs. Faecal cultures are difficult to interpret due to the presence of commensal organisms that can be opportunistic pathogens. Generally, isolation rates for putative bacterial enteropathogens are similar between healthy and diarrhoeic cats. Pyrexia may be due to non-bacterial causes. Performing a rectal smear and looking for neutrophils on cytology may help determine whether there is a bacterial component to the diarrhoea. Antibiotics may prolong recovery if they deplete the normal commensal flora.

Post-treatment management and follow-up

Generally, treatment is considered to have been effective when clinical signs resolve. Following treatment, and before rehoming or moving the cat, it is prudent to ensure that clinical signs have resolved for a reasonable amount of time (e.g. 3–7 days) to reduce the chance of relapse occurring. Many of the infectious agents that can cause diarrhoea in cats may be shed for long periods of time after treatment, and shedding may be continuous or intermittent. Repeated post-treatment diagnostic testing to determine whether a cat has cleared the infection can be time-consuming and expensive if the first post-treatment test result is positive. Multiple tests may have to be carried out before a negative result is obtained. This can result in a clinically well cat being in care for a longer period of time than is necessary. For these reasons, post-treatment diagnostic testing is generally not recommended for a cat where diarrhoea has cleared. However, for microorganisms that have a significant zoonotic potential, such as Campylobacter spp., some shelters have a formal policy of not rehoming the animal until one negative test result has been obtained.

Management and prevention

There are four main categories to consider when managing diarrhoea in the shelter environment:

- Surveillance
  - Ensure all staff are aware of the signs of diarrhoea
  - Record and report observations. Using a scoring system to grade and record faecal quality is useful
  - Ensure all members of the team are aware if a cat is affected
  - Report outcome back to staff to help with compliance
- Reduction of infectious organisms
  - Quarantine new admissions and isolate sick cats
  - Control the number of admissions to ensure a manageable population density, and have the cattery split into zones or wings to help manage disease spread
  - Ensure adequate and appropriate hygiene and disinfection protocols are followed
  - Implement appropriate treatment and active management programmes as soon as possible after diarrhoea is identified
- Optimizing host resistance
  - Maximizing the wellbeing of the cats will make them more resistant to contracting disease by optimizing the health of their immune system. Reducing stress, optimizing nutrition, providing a vaccination programme and taking time for social activities (e.g. grooming and attention) will aid this
  - Consider prophylactic treatment for problem organisms
- Reducing exposure of cats to disease
  - Ensure adequate quarantine measures are in place for new admissions and sick cats, and modify cattery pen design if necessary to improve barrier protection between cats
  - The majority of infectious agents in a cattery are spread by fomites, so the use of personal protective equipment (PPE) by workers is recommended to limit spread across the premises.

Quarantine

A quarantine wing or zone is most effective if staff know for how long cats should be isolated and if they understand how particular diseases are spread. Staff should be aware of the incubation periods, shedding patterns, duration of shedding and routes of shedding of common diarrhoea-causing organisms. Diseases that have a carrier state should be monitored carefully. Overgarments (i.e. PPE) and cleaning equipment should preferably be restricted to each pen. Alcohol hand sanitizers are not effective against all pathogens, so the use of disposable gloves may be preferable; these should be changed between contact with different cats. Thorough cleansing of surfaces before disinfection is important to remove organic matter and enable optimum penetration of disinfectant (see QRG 9.1).

Hygiene

The choice of disinfectant should be based on which agents are being targeted for control (see QRG 9.1). When using disinfectants, allowing the recommended contact time with surfaces and materials is important to ensure effective action. Faeces should be removed from cages as frequently as possible. Placing a queen's litter tray out of reach of her kittens and placing a height-restriction cover over the kittens' litter tray can help to minimize potential disease transmission. Figure 13.12 provides further details on the appropriate choice of disinfectant and environmental control methods for each infectious agent.

Zoonoses

The cat is not often thought of as being a major source of zoonotic organisms, but there are a number of pathogens of cats that could be a potential risk to human health (Figure 13.12). Risk is often heightened in people who are immuno-suppressed, sick, young or old. These risks can be kept to a minimum with the use of good facility and personnel hygiene protocols. Current understanding of which feline pathogens truly represent a risk to human health is incomplete, but improvements in knowledge are being made on the basis of advances in molecular techniques and performing appropriate epidemiological studies to investigate risk.

Approach to an outbreak of diarrhoea

All shelters should have biosecurity and hygiene protocols in place to contain and prevent the spread of infectious disease within the facility. All staff and volunteers should be trained in disease control so they can identify and isolate potentially infectious sick cats. Shelter workers should practise good hygiene and disinfection, and be particularly aware of their role in fomite spread.

Even in ideal conditions (advanced facility design; risk-segregated housing; physical barriers to disease spread; stress-reduction measures for the animals in the shelter; thorough veterinary examination; regular observation of animals; preventive treatments; good nutrition; scrupulous hygiene and high levels of biosecurity) disease outbreaks cannot always be avoided. This is one of the strongest arguments for having disease outbreak protocols in place before such an event. Protocols can help to reduce morbidity and mortality and reduce the impact on shelter operations.

It is useful to have a predetermined definition of what an 'outbreak' is, so that the actions outlined in the protocol can be undertaken once this threshold has been reached. An outbreak is commonly defined as evidence of disease spread within a facility. An outbreak can also be defined as occurring when a certain proportion of the cats housed in the facility are affected. If faecal consistency is regularly recorded, a baseline diarrhoea prevalence for the facility can be calculated. A UK study of shelter cats in centres not reporting a problem with diarrhoea calculated an acceptable level of diarrhoea as 12%, with intervention being required at 15%, and an optimal target of 5% prevalence. This study took into account diarrhoea arising in all age groups, from admission to rehoming, including any cats in the isolation facility (German et al., 2017).

General considerations

Some key questions that will need to be answered when an outbreak of diarrhoea occurs are:

* What actions must be taken to prevent further spread?
* Is there a blanket treatment that can be given to all at-risk cats to prevent more illness? For example, early vaccination of kittens in the face of a FPV outbreak
* What diagnostic tests are needed to identify the causative agent and monitor disease levels? For example, faecal testing, serology, post-mortem examination
* Are PPE or footbaths required, and if so, where?
* Does the shelter need to close?
* When can the outbreak be considered to be over, and when can the shelter's normal activity resume?

General approach

All cats should be carefully observed for any sign of illness, with new cases isolated and treated immediately. If most cats in a section of the facility or in the facility as a whole are affected, it is usually best to not move the cats but to consider the section (or whole facility) as being infected and treat it as an isolation facility.

Use the shelter's records and review all current processes to help establish whether the cases are originating outside the centre, inside it, or both. This is where, aside from a thorough clinical examination of affected cats, knowledge of the incubation periods, pattern, duration and route of shedding, and the carrier status can be very helpful in narrowing down the list of possible causative agents. It will also clarify a pragmatic diagnostic approach for identifying the causative agent, monitoring the outbreak and, sometimes, determining when the outbreak is over. Knowledge of where cases originated and how the disease was able to spread is important not only for managing the current outbreak, but also in informing prevention strategies for a future outbreak. Biosecurity needs to be at a heightened level during an outbreak of diarrhoea and may be further refined if a specific agent is identified.

* Disinfection protocols will need to be reviewed to ensure an appropriate disinfectant is being used at the correct dilution and for an adequate contact time.
* Depending on the severity of the clinical disease and the proportion of cats affected, strict cleaning and disinfection protocols normally reserved for the isolation unit may need to be applied across all areas of the facility.

Agent	Transmission route	Environmental control	Vaccine available?	Immunity (reinfection possible?)	Cross-species infectivity	Zoonotic potential?
Protozoa						
Isospora spp.	Infection usually occurs after consumption of a paratenic host (e.g. mouse); direct faecal–oral spread; reactivation of infection from extra-intestinal cysts	• Resistant • High heat/steam cleaning or 10% ammonia solution • Frequent litter tray change (organism takes 8–36 hours to become infective) • Insect control (mechanical vectors) • Clean infected cats' coat/perineum	No	Reinfection possible	Potential – *I. rivolta*	It is possible that people could serve as paratenic hosts for *I. rivolta*, but no cases of human infection have been recorded
Cryptosporidium spp.	Faecal–oral spread and contaminated food or water	• Resistant • Resistant to sodium hypochlorite • Use formol saline (10%) and ammonia (5%) with contact time 18 hours • Clean bowls and trays with boiling water	No	Reinfection possible	Potential – *C. parvum*	Low risk as most cats are infected with *C. felis*, not *C. parvum*
Giardia duodenalis	Ingestion of cysts shed in faeces, or contaminated food and water	• Cysts are immediately infective and can survive in the environment for months • Use quaternary ammonium compounds (QACs) or sodium hypochlorite diluted 1:32 • Ensure treated areas are allowed to dry • Litter trays should be changed regularly and disinfected daily • Bathe individual cats to remove cysts from the coat • Treat in-contact as well as infected animals • Isolate cats with diarrhoea	No	No permanent immunity; infection may self-limit in 27–35 days or may be recurrent	Potential is debated, and depends on the molecular biology of the sub-assemblages	People are primarily infected with assemblages A (35%) and B (6%). 38.5% of cats are infected with assemblage A. Although the World Health Organization considers *G. duodenalis* to be zoonotic, the molecular relationship between human and animal A assemblages is unclear
Tritrichomonas foetus	Faeces	• Only survives 2 hours in the environment • Use good litter tray and equipment hygiene, isolate infected individuals and keep their coat/perineum clean	No	Reinfection possible and relapses occur, but usually once recovered and over 2 years of age, cats rarely relapse	Unknown. Potential to cows?	Potential in immunosuppressed people
Helminths						
Roundworms	Larvae pass to kittens through the queen's milk after reactivation of infection during pregnancy. Alternatively, ingestion of embryonated eggs shed in faeces will cause infection	• Long-lived in the environment (>1 year) • Susceptible to extremes of temperature, desiccation and ultraviolet light • Use preventive medicine programmes and dispose of faeces/litter appropriately • Use impermeable surfaces in catteries and avoid soil or sand. If there is a high worm burden, overlay or cover areas of soil/sand with impermeable substrate • Quarantine incoming animals and monitor faeces at regular intervals	No	Reinfection common	*Toxascaris leonina* – potential to dogs	Yes – ocular and visceral larval migrans
Hookworms	Faecal–oral spread of third-stage larvae (L3). L3 can also pass to kittens through the queen's colostrum	As for roundworms	No	Reinfection occurs	*Uncinaria stenocephala* – potential to dogs	Yes – cutaneous larval migrans

13.12 Transmission, prevention and control of common infectious agents that cause diarrhoea in cats. (continues)

Agent	Transmission route	Environmental control	Vaccine available?	Immunity (reinfection possible?)	Cross-species infectivity	Zoonotic potential?
Viruses						
Feline panleukopenia virus (FPV) (also called feline parvovirus)	Contact with contaminated environment. Cat-to-cat transmission may occur during the shedding period. The virus is present in all secretions, especially faeces. In utero infection occurs. Fomite transmission is common and insects may act as mechanical vectors	• Resistant • Survives in the environment for up to 1 year • Use 6% sodium hypochlorite, inorganic peroxygen compounds (e.g. Virkon®), 4% formaldehyde and 1% glutaraldehyde; contact time of 10 minutes is required	Yes (see main text)	Long-term immunity post infection or vaccination	Yes – dogs and foxes	No
Feline coronavirus (FCoV)	Faecal–oral spread and possibly by inhalation. Care should be taken with litter tray hygiene, fomites, shared food bowls and mutual grooming	• Survives for only a few hours in the environment • Use good litter tray hygiene • Susceptible to most disinfectants, e.g. sodium hypochlorite	Not in the UK	Reinfection likely in multi-cat environments	No	No
Bacteria						
Escherichia coli	Faecal–oral spread and contaminated food, water or soil	• Usually survives approximately 1 week but can be considerably longer • QACs, inorganic peroxygen compounds or bleach are effective	No	Reinfection possible	Yes, dependent on strain	Yes, some strains
Salmonella spp.	Faecal–oral spread, contact via infected food/raw meat or via birds and bird faeces ('song bird fever'). Cats shed the organism in their saliva and faeces	• Environmental disinfection should be performed using sodium hypochlorite or QACs	No	Reinfection possible	Yes, dependent on serovar	Yes, but transmission from cats to people is rarely documented
Clostridium perfringens	Faecal–oral spread and contaminated food, water or soil	• Spores last a long time in the environment • Use bleach diluted 1:10, steam cleaning	No	Reinfection possible	Possible	Unknown
Clostridium difficile	Faecal–oral spread, ingestion of spores, and contaminated food and water	• Spores last a long time in the environment • Use bleach diluted 1:10, steam cleaning	No	A small percentage of healthy dogs and cats carry C. difficile asymptomatically in their intestine. Prevalence is higher in kittens and breeding colonies. Reinfection possible	Possible	Potentially, but not proven
Campylobacter spp.	Contact with undercooked/raw food, particularly chicken, contaminated food and water, and via the faeces of infected animals	• Relatively hardy bacterium, which survives well in water and resists freezing • Survives well in faeces • QACs, inorganic peroxygen compounds or bleach are effective	No	Some cats may remain colonized and become persistent shedders despite antibiotic treatment. Reinfection is possible.	Yes	Yes – the infective dose for people is low. However, infection is species-dependent. The most common zoonotic strains in people are C. jejuni and C. upsaliensis

13.12 (continued) Transmission, prevention and control of common infectious agents that cause diarrhoea in cats.

- Footbaths will need to be put in place and changed regularly.
- Gloves should be worn when cleaning cat accommodation and handling cats. Gloves should be changed or hands should be washed between contact with different cats.
- Movement of both animals and people around the shelter should be minimized. This means:
  - Move cats to different areas only when absolutely necessary
  - Do not rehome cats during an outbreak of disease
  - Do not admit new cats during an outbreak
  - Recommend that staff/volunteers work in only one area of the shelter, if possible, and do not enter other areas unless absolutely necessary
  - Access to the infected area must be strictly limited – ideally only one person should enter it
  - Do not permit members of the public into the infected area. In some cases, if the disease is present in multiple areas of the facility, it may be necessary to prevent any public access to the shelter until the outbreak has resolved.

References and further reading

August JR (2006) *Consultations in Internal Medicine, Vol 5.* Elsevier Saunders, St Louis

August JR (2010) *Consultations in Internal Medicine, Vol 6.* Elsevier Saunders, St Louis

Bouzid M, Halai K, Jeffreys D and Hunter PR (2015) The prevalence of *Giardia* infection in dogs and cats, a systematic review and meta-analysis of prevalence studies from stool samples. *Veterinary Parasitology* **207(3–4)**, 181–202

Cave TA, Thompson H, Reid SW *et al.* (2002). Kitten mortality in the United Kingdom: A retrospective analysis of 274 histopathological examinations (1986 to 2000). *Veterinary Record* **151**, 497–501

Ettinger SJ and Feldman EC (2010) *Textbook of Veterinary Internal Medicine: Diseases of the Dog and Cat, 7th edn.* Elsevier Saunders, St Louis

German AC, Cunliffe NA and Morgan KL (2015) Faecal consistency and risk factors for diarrhoea and constipation in cats in UK rehoming shelters. *Journal of Feline Medicine and Surgery* **19(1),** 57–65

Greene C (2011) *Infectious Diseases of the Dog and Cat, 4th edn.* Elsevier Saunders, St Louis

Marks SL, Rankin SC, Byrne BA and Weese JS (2011) Enteropathogenic Bacteria in Dogs and Cats: Diagnosis, Epidemiology, Treatment, and Control. *Journal of Veterinary Internal Medicine* **25(6)**, 1195–1208

Marshall-Jones, Baillon ML, Croft JM and Butterwick RF (2006) Effects of *Lactobacillus acidophilus* DSM13241 as a probiotic in healthy adult cats. *American Journal of Veterinary Research* **67(6)**, 1005–1012

Miller L and Hurley K (2009) *Infectious Disease Management in Animal Shelters.* Wiley-Blackwell, Ames, Iowa

Miller L and Zawistowski (2013) *Shelter Medicine for Veterinarians and Staff, 2nd edn.* Wiley-Blackwell, Ames, Iowa

Morrow L and German A (2018) Infectious enteritis in cats. *Companion*, February 12–14

Ramsey I and Tennant B (2001) *BSAVA Manual of Canine and Feline Infectious Diseases.* BSAVA Publications, Gloucester

Useful websites

European Advisory Board on Cat Diseases Vaccination guidelines: www.abcdcatsvets.org/

International Cat Care Cat health advice sheets: www.icatcare.org/

European Scientific Counsel Companion Animal Parasites guidelines: www.esccap.org

Chapter 14

Respiratory disease in the dog in the shelter environment

Shaun Opperman and Joe Brownlie

Canine infectious respiratory disease (CIRD), commonly referred to as kennel cough, is a highly contagious respiratory infection in dogs that is frequently seen in shelters and which is prevalent worldwide. It is a complex disease, with several causal agents, which in part accounts for its variable clinical picture. While mortality rates are low, the disease can nevertheless be debilitating and patients can be ill for long periods of time. In addition to the obvious welfare considerations, there are many other costs to the shelter resulting from CIRD:

- It delays throughput of dogs by increasing the average length of stay in the shelter
- Investment in treatment/isolation facilities is required
- Cost of staff time, medicines and treatment
- Delays to surgical procedures
- Management of CIRD necessitates an adjustment to working practices
- Increased length of stay can result in a deterioration in behaviour for some dogs
- Risk of infecting other dogs in surrounding areas and also those in potential new homes
- Effect on staff morale.

As with most infectious diseases, prevention of CIRD is key. However, this can prove surprisingly difficult to achieve for a number of reasons.

- Dogs at intake may already be incubating kennel cough. For shelters that take in significant numbers of dogs from local authority or other kennels, this is particularly likely to be the case, as the dogs will already have been housed with others for variable periods of time before intake and so may already have been exposed to the causative pathogens.
- While it seems obvious to recommend quarantine of new arrivals, and it is certainly desirable, in practice this can be difficult to achieve. Most centres run at full (or close to full) capacity and are often under a lot of pressure to take in new arrivals.
- Vector transmission – many shelters have (necessary) working practices that inevitably assist in the spread of disease (e.g. behavioural assessments, introductions to potential owners and their own dogs, interactions with volunteers and members of the public).
- A naive population with high stress levels and consequent compromised immunity, such as frequently exists in shelters, is particularly susceptible to infection.

- Comorbidity frequently aggravates the condition, especially with other infectious diseases that are commonly encountered in shelters.
- The complex nature of the disease – not all causative agents have a vaccine, and vaccination can rarely be achieved before a dog's admission to the shelter.

Pathogenesis

The nature and recovery of causal microbial agents can vary between different outbreaks and shelters, and at different stages of the infection. For this reason, CIRD represents a considerable challenge for both diagnosis and control despite the availability of multivalent vaccines targeting several of the viral and bacterial pathogens implicated in the syndrome (Chalker et al., 2003; Erles and Brownlie, 2005). As one of the major health and welfare issues affecting kennelled and pet dogs, CIRD has attracted considerable interest in recent years. Consequently, a number of novel viral agents thought to be involved in the pathogenesis of CIRD, have been identified (Priestnall et al., 2013), and characterization of these is vital for improving disease control.

With a growing understanding of the infectious causes of CIRD, a hypothesis has been established for the likely order of events that proceed to clinical disease. The oral, nasal and pharyngeal mucosa are 'bathed' in many viruses, bacteria (including mycoplasmas) and other microbial agents. Most of these are commensal and are well controlled by innate immune mechanisms that, in turn, can be strengthened by adaptive immune responses (see Chapter 11). Through a detailed series of field studies and, later, experimental research (Priestnall et al., 2013), it has been shown that the initial challenge to the respiratory mucosa is invariably viral and occurs in the upper airway (see Pathogenesis of CIRD, below). This viral challenge disables the innate immune response to varying degrees; most typically, it reduces the ciliary action of the respiratory epithelium, thus reducing mucus clearance in the upper airways. This permits local invasion by 'bystander' bacteria, often of low virulence, beyond the upper airways to cause further infection and damage. It has been suggested that mycoplasmas often fulfil this niche, particularly *Mycoplasma cynos* (Chalker and Brownlie, 2004; Chalker et al., 2004). By this time, the upper airways are further compromised and allow greater penetration of bacteria into the lower airways. These lower regions are normally sterile and less adapted to rapid protective immune responses against microbial challenge. It is now that more pathogenic bacteria, such as streptococci, can colonize these deeper tissues and evoke inflammatory reactions. These reactions include increased cellularity

and oedema in these tissues, in turn, compromising lung function.

A number of microbial agents have been identified as important causes of CIRD. The pathogenesis of these agents is outlined in Figure 14.1 and their transmission and impact is shown in Figure 14.2.

Pathogenesis of CIRD

- CIRD is a complex disease with a dynamic aetiology
- Initially, an infectious agent (or agents) will compromise the innate immune response, particularly in the upper airways, such as canine respiratory coronavirus (CRCoV)
  - Such infectious agents will have rapid aerosol transmission
  - Such agents may themselves not cause severe pathology
  - These agents may or may not give rise to protective immunity to subsequent infection
- Compromise of the innate immune response facilitates secondary infections with bacterial/viral species (e.g. *Mycoplasma cynos*)
  - These secondary invaders may have high aerosol transmission and, with deeper access to the airways, cause further damage
- Finally, bacteria capable of causing severe pathology can now invade the deep lung tissue (e.g. *Streptococcus equi* ssp. *zooepidemicus*).

Microbial agent	Type	Tropism	Clinical disease	Shedding of pathogen	Carrier reservoirs	Diagnostic tests[a]
Viruses						
Canine distemper virus (CDV)	ss RNA (distemper) morbillivirus	Systemic	Mild to fatal	1–3 weeks, occasionally prolonged	Dogs, wildlife	Antibody ELISA Virus PCR
Canine adenovirus-2 (CAV-2)	ds DNA adenovirus	Respiratory	Respiratory – mild	1–3 weeks	Dogs	Antibody/antigen ELISA Virus PCR
Canine herpesvirus-1 (CHV-1)	ds DNA herpesvirus	Mucosal, systemic	Respiratory, genital (severe in puppies)	1–3 weeks, establishes latent infection	Dogs	Antibody/antigen ELISA Virus PCR
Canine parainfluenza virus (CPiV)	ss RNA parainfluenza virus	Respiratory	Respiratory – mild	1–2 weeks	Dogs	Antibody/antigen ELISA Virus PCR
Canine respiratory coronavirus (CRCoV)	ss RNA coronavirus	Respiratory	Respiratory – mild to moderate	1–2 weeks	Dogs	Antibody/antigen ELISA Virus PCR
Canine influenza virus (CIV)	ss RNA influenza virus	Respiratory	Respiratory – mild to severe	1–3 weeks	Dogs, potentially horses	Antibody/antigen ELISA Virus PCR
Canine pneumovirus (CnPnV)	ss RNA pneumovirus	Respiratory	Respiratory – mild to moderate	1–2 weeks?	Dogs	Not available in the UK
Bacteria						
Bordetella spp.	*B. bronchiseptica*	Respiratory	Respiratory – mild to moderate	1–3 weeks and persistent	Dogs, cats and others	Bacterial culture PCR
Streptococcus spp.	*S. canis*	Respiratory	Respiratory – mild to moderate	1–3 weeks	Dogs	Bacterial culture PCR
	S. equi ssp. *zooepidemicus*	Respiratory	Moderate to severe	1–3 weeks	Dogs, horses, cats and others	Bacterial culture PCR
Mycoplasma spp.	*M. canis*	Respiratory	Mild to moderate	1–3 weeks and persistent	Dogs	Bacterial culture PCR
	M. cynos	Respiratory	Mild to moderate	1–3 weeks and persistent	Dogs	Bacterial culture PCR

14.1 Pathogenesis of microbial agents associated with canine infectious respiratory disease, as currently understood. [a]Other diagnostic assays such as virus isolation, virus neutralization assay and immunohistochemistry may be available for some viruses. DNA = deoxyribonucleic acid; ds = double-stranded; ELISA = enzyme-linked immunosorbent assay; PCR = polymerase chain reaction; RNA = ribonucleic acid; ss = single-stranded.

Microbial agent	Type	Transmission routes	Impact	Cross-species transmission?	Vaccine available?	Zoonotic?
Viruses						
Canine distemper virus (CDV)	ss RNA (distemper) morbillivirus	Aerosol Direct contact Faeces, urine	Highly transmissible Potentially fatal	All canine and feline, including wild species	Yes	No
Canine adenovirus-2 (CAV-2)	ds DNA adenovirus	Aerosol	Low	No	Yes	No
Canine herpesvirus-1 (CHV-1)	ds DNA herpesvirus	Aerosol	Low	No	Yes	No
Canine parainfluenza virus (CPiV)	ss RNA parainfluenza virus	Aerosol	Low	No	Yes	No
Canine respiratory coronavirus (CRCoV)	ss RNA coronavirus	Aerosol Possibly fomites	Low to moderate	No	No	No
Canine influenza virus (CIV)	ss RNA pneumovirus	Aerosol Oral Possibly fomites	Low to high	Horse, dog Possibly feline species	Yes	No
Canine pneumovirus (CnPnV)	ss RNA pneumovirus	Aerosol	Low to moderate	Dogs	No	No
Bacteria						
Bordetella spp.	*B. bronchiseptica*	Aerosol Direct contact	Low to high	Dog, cat and others	Yes	Yes, low risk
Streptococcus spp.	*S. canis*	Aerosol Direct contact	Low	Dog	No	No
	S. equi spp. *zooepidemicus*	Aerosol Direct contact	Moderate to high	Dog, horse and others	No	Yes, low risk
Mycoplasma spp.	*M. canis*	Aerosol Direct contact	Low	Dog	No	No
	M. cynos	Aerosol Direct contact	Low to high	Dog	No	No

14.2 Transmission and impact of microbial agents associated with canine infectious respiratory disease, as currently understood. DNA = deoxyribonucleic acid; ds = double-stranded; RNA = ribonucleic acid; ss = single-stranded.

History taking

While history taking and a thorough clinical examination are, of course, important with regard to the diagnosis and treatment of the individual dog, of equal or greater importance is to view the shelter dog population as a whole. The multiple interactions that exist in a busy shelter and the environment itself will affect all aspects of the disease and must therefore be taken into account. Unless proper consideration is given to the prevention of disease spread, shelter workers can find themselves merely 'firefighting' in the face of continuous disease and using up precious resources. It is easy to get caught up with individual clinical cases, and serious or continued outbreaks can become quite overwhelming for veterinary surgeons (veterinarians) and lay staff alike. At some point, it becomes necessary to take a step back and look at the bigger picture. Above all, clinicians should not be afraid to ask for help from other organizations that may have had long experience in dealing with CIRD or from the veterinary schools, which, similarly, may have a wealth of data gleaned from investigations and collaborations with other shelters. The investigation of CIRD at Battersea Dogs & Cats Home (see box) is an example of this type of collaborative work.

Some of the questions that should form part of an assessment of the picture of CIRD in a shelter are listed below.

Investigation of CIRD at Battersea Dogs & Cats Home

In 1999, Battersea Dogs & Cats Home was concerned by the recurring incidence of 'kennel cough' within its kennel units. A concerted vaccination programme was not preventing the problem. The organization approached Professor Joe Brownlie at the Royal Veterinary College to undertake an investigation of this respiratory disease. Although kennel cough is an endemic problem in many, if not most, large kennels, it had now become more severe and refractory to both treatment and vaccination. Thus began a 6-year programme into the nature and dynamics of the condition now named canine infectious respiratory disease (CIRD). This name was given to distinguish the syndrome from the more familiar and milder condition of kennel cough, although the investigators readily acknowledged that the two conditions exist on a continuum of mild (kennel cough) to severe (CIRD) clinical disease.

Professor Brownlie's first task was to assemble a multidisciplinary team that allowed him to collect all relevant data from uninfected dogs, infected dogs and those that were infected and showing clinical signs. This required a team comprising clinicians, epidemiologists, pathologists, virologists and microbiologists. Over the first 3 years of the study, the team was able to highlight the importance of several microbial agents either new to science or not strongly associated with respiratory disease in dogs. In an analysis of a number of different agents, two, or possibly three, were demonstrated to have a significant association with the development of disease. ▶

Investigation of CIRD at Battersea Dogs & Cats Home *continued*

During the search for potential new agents, the team discovered a new canine respiratory coronavirus (CRCoV) (Erles *et al.*, 2003). This agent was shown to have a significant association both with the development of respiratory disease in longitudinal studies in groups of kennelled dogs and with regard to the dogs' subsequent serological responses (Erles and Brownlie, 2005). Unlike the canine enteric coronavirus (a Group 1 virus), CRCoV has a genomic sequence that clearly places it within the Group 2 viruses, and it has a strong tropism for the respiratory tract (Erles *et al.*, 2007).

Since the discovery of this virus, the researchers have established that it is widespread, with evidence of its existence in both Europe and North America (Priestnall *et al.*, 2006; 2007). It would be surprising, on the basis of this early data, if CRCoV were not prevalent worldwide. Thus, the association with disease and its potential worldwide epidemiology makes this new virus of considerable importance as a newly discovered pathogen in canine respiratory disease and as a candidate for a novel vaccine.

CRCoV has been shown to potentiate the effect of other infectious agents, thus increasing the severity of the disease. It affects the primary protection afforded by the innate immune response and disables the ciliary action of the respiratory epithelium in the upper airways. This, in turn, allows bacterial superinfection, often by bystander bacteria that are normally held in check by the innate immune response. In the studies outlined above, mycoplasmas were repeatedly recovered as microbial organisms able to take advantage of this primary viral infection (Chalker *et al.*, 2004). In a major analysis of more than 800 isolates of canine mycoplasmas isolated during these investigations (Chalker and Brownlie, 2004), the most frequent invading mycoplasma was found to be *Mycoplasma cynos*. In a few cases, the respiratory disease was peracute and sufficiently severe to be life-threatening. From these cases, the team recovered profuse cultures of streptococci. On typing, these isolates were not *Streptococcus canis*, as expected, but *Streptococcus equi* ssp. *zooepidemicus* (Chalker *et al.*, 2003) – an agent that has zoonotic potential.

Example of an assessment for a shelter with problematic canine infectious respiratory disease

- **Intake**
  - What is the make-up of the dog intake population? (Depending on the type of shelter, the intake may be a mixture of owned dogs from members of the public, 'walk-in' strays and strays that will have been housed in local authority kennels or similar.)
  - Are different groups housed separately?
  - Are there separate treatment blocks and rehoming areas?
  - Does the local authority keep medical records, and are these records shared with the shelter?
- **Metrics**
  - What is the size and density of the shelter dog population?
  - What is the throughput (number of dogs entering/leaving the shelter per day)?
  - What is the average length of stay?
- **Kennel design**
  - Make an assessment of the housing. What is the age/state of repair?
  - Are the flooring and surfaces easy to clean and disinfect?
  - Do the dogs have access to outside runs?
  - How are dogs separated within individual blocks?
  - Do they share exercise areas, etc.?
  - Are dogs kennelled individually or are they housed in pairs?
  - Do the kennels face each other?
  - Do the front of the kennels have bars or is there a solid surface, e.g. glass?
  - Is the ventilation adequate? Is there a strong disinfectant smell?
  - Is there effective temperature regulation (both in summer and winter) and comfortable humidity?
- **Husbandry**
  - Make an assessment of the effectiveness of the cleaning and disinfection regime.
  - What is the capacity of the laundry facilities?
  - Do the staff wear separate uniforms/footwear while working in their blocks?
  - Do all staff and volunteers have access to all areas?
  - Is there a constant stream of visitors to the blocks?
  - Look for potential disease vectors: food and water bowls, cleaning equipment, toys, etc.
  - Are there clinic facilities on site?
- **Management**
  - Get a sense of the stress levels in the kennels, particularly in the intake blocks. Try to visit at different times of the day, e.g. during the morning cleaning, feeding times, rest times, busy public visiting hours, etc.
  - Ask about working practices that may be relevant to the spread of disease, both directly and indirectly. Most shelters carry out some form of behavioural assessment, which will usually include observing how a dog behaves and interacts when in close proximity to another. Are these dogs from the same populations in terms of disease risk?
  - Have the staff and volunteers received any education on disease prevention?

It is important to build up a rapport with the shelter staff, and a level of trust, in order to fully engage them and build up a full picture of the working environment. Some kennels may be understaffed or have outdated facilities or unusual management practices, which can present considerable challenges for disease control. Staff may feel guilty about the state of their facilities; others may have worked at the shelter for many years and have established ways of working that may be difficult to change. It is easy to be critical in such instances, but to do so will only alienate the shelter staff and make the job harder.

Presentation and clinical signs

Depending on the dominant pathogen or mix of pathogens, and with the exception of canine distemper virus (CDV), the incubation period for CIRD is a few days. The signs are mostly common to all dogs and all age groups are susceptible. Clinical signs include:

- Cough: the dog will usually present with a cough, which may be harsh and hacking, often accompanied by retching (as in the traditional owner complaint of 'something stuck in the throat') or, equally, may be soft or sometimes barely noticeable. It may be spontaneous or prompted by exercise or pulling on the lead
- Submandibular lymphadenopathy
- Lethargy and inappetence may be present
- Mucous membranes may appear congested
- Pyrexia may present in the early stages and can be marked (up to 40/41°C is not unusual in some outbreaks)
- Serous or purulent nasal discharge (or may be haemorrhagic in the case of a haemolytic streptococcal infection)
- Conjunctivitis may be noted in some cases.

If the infection is confined to the upper respiratory tract and the dog is otherwise healthy, no other signs will be apparent and the dog should make an uneventful recovery (although the signs may be more marked in brachycephalic animals). The cough will usually last for 1–2 weeks but in some individuals it may persist for significantly longer.

If the infection spreads to the lower respiratory tract and progresses to a bronchopneumonia, then alterations in respiratory rate and effort will be observed. Dyspnoea and tachypnoea are likely and changes will be apparent on auscultation (wheezes, rales or decreased sounds depending on the pathology). If the dog is in shock, then the usual signs will prevail (tachycardia, pallor, slow capillary refill time, cool extremities, etc.) and, of course, if the dog has been inappetent or not drinking, there will also be signs of dehydration. In the most serious cases, weakness and collapse will follow.

There are two pathogens that provide a more distinct clinical picture: CDV and *Streptococcus* spp. (see Figures 14.1 and 14.2).

Canine distemper virus

The incubation period is approximately 10 days but may be greater than 4 weeks. The presentation and common clinical signs of distemper are:

- Dogs aged 3–6 months are most commonly affected (coincides with the fall in maternally derived antibody)

- Conjunctivitis, becoming purulent, with thick crusting around the eyes
- Productive cough
- Purulent rhinitis
- Pyrexia, lethargy and inappetence
- Diarrhoea may be present
- Hyperkeratosis of the nose and footpads 3–6 weeks after infection
- Dental enamel hypoplasia
- Neurological signs may develop around 4 weeks after infection and may include seizures, paresis, ataxia and muscle twitching.

Streptococcus

Streptococcus equi ssp. *zooepidemicus* is an important pathogen, as some strains can be extremely virulent and may produce a severe peracute haemorrhagic pneumonia. Dogs of any age may be susceptible; in the authors' experience, very nervous/stressed animals appear to be particularly at risk. Prompt and aggressive treatment is indicated but the mortality rate may still be high.

The presentation and common clinical signs are:

- Sudden onset (may present as sudden death)
- Cough frequently absent
- Marked lethargy, depression
- Shock
- Dyspnoea, tachypnoea
- Haemorrhage from the upper respiratory tract, in saliva or nasal discharge. Occasionally, where there is no cough, this may not be seen initially and may become apparent only if the dog dies or is euthanased.

Treatment

Mild cases, where the dog is bright and eating well, will not usually require any medication. Rest and provision of a calm environment are common-sense measures, and attempts to reduce airway irritation by using a harness instead of a neck collar when exercising the dog may be helpful in some individuals. Adequate ventilation and temperature control are important, as is attention to husbandry so that disinfectant fumes do not build up in the immediate environment and cause further airway irritation. Soft palatable foods (e.g. chicken, ham, sausages) are useful to tempt the dog to eat.

The use of non-steroidal anti-inflammatory drugs (NSAIDs) is controversial but may be indicated in cases with pyrexia. In the authors' experience, if NSAIDs are used in this way and at an early stage in the course of the disease, they can produce significant improvements to demeanour and encourage the patient to eat, without which an earlier decision to use antibiotics (unnecessarily) may have been made. The usual precautions apply when using NSAIDs.

Ideally, antibiotics should be used only when strictly necessary, as inappropriate usage contributes to antibiotic resistance. As bacteria and mycoplasmas are known pathogens in CIRD and secondary bacterial infections will frequently follow initial viral infection, antibiotics may be indicated if the clinician feels that the patient requires them. If the animal is clearly unwell, inappetent, pyrexic and/or has evidence of lower respiratory tract infection, then antibiotics are indicated, but a lot of cases fall into a 'grey area' where the clinician's intuition/pragmatism takes over. The sense that the very young, very old, brachycephalic or overly stressed patient requires antibiotic treatment at an earlier stage of the disease will come down to personal choice and experience. In the absence of culture and sensitivity testing, the standard choices would be co-amoxiclav or doxycycline for a minimum of 5 days, with fluoroquinolones being reserved for more serious infections.

There is no evidence that antitussives or mucolytics help to reduce the severity of clinical signs, nor have the authors witnessed an appreciable or consistent clinical improvement with the use of either of these types of treatment.

Supportive intravenous fluids are indicated in the event of dehydration or shock. In cases of dyspnoea due to pneumonia, oxygen must be provided, but careful thought should be given to the prognosis for recovery in these cases and the degree of welfare compromise. This is especially so in suspected cases of acute streptococcal pneumonia, where the prognosis can be guarded at best. Furthermore, these cases are expensive to treat in terms of drugs, consumables and staff time, and they also represent a real risk of cross-infection to other animals in the shelter. For all of these reasons, euthanasia should be strongly considered. In any case, these patients can deteriorate rapidly and should not be left unattended.

Prevention and approach to an outbreak

Infection is caused when a naive animal comes into contact with the respiratory secretions from an infected dog. This can happen in one of two ways:

- Direct contact with infected dogs, either through bodily contact or via aerosol spread from sneezing and coughing (Figure 14.3)
- Indirect spread via fomites, most commonly staff but also inanimate objects such as food/water bowls and toys.

It is, therefore, clear that prevention measures must focus on segregation of naive populations and isolation of infectious individuals. In addition, assuming that it is inevitable that some dogs will become infected, the aim should be to maintain as healthy and stress-free a population of dogs as possible to ensure minimal compromise of their collective immunity.

It is particularly important to remember that susceptibility to respiratory disease is very variable within the mixed population of a shelter environment and that particular pathogens or strains that may only cause mild disease in one individual may cause much more serious disease in another.

Whether it is a solitary outbreak or an endemic problem, the strategies for dealing with CIRD in a shelter will be similar. Some of these strategies represent the ideal solution, and may not be feasible for all shelters; it is important to identify a pragmatic approach that suits the individual shelter, based on the available resources. Some of the recommendations require considerable effort and commitment from the shelter staff and results may not be seen immediately, so realistic expectations should be set from the beginning.

Vaccination

Vaccination can only ever be partially effective in controlling CIRD due to the relatively large number of causal agents, not all of which have a vaccine, and the logistical difficulties of vaccinating a large and ever-changing population of dogs in order to achieve protection throughout their stay in the shelter.

Nevertheless, vaccination can still play an important part in respiratory disease control in the shelter. A list of available vaccines against canine infectious agents is provided in Chapter 11.

Isolation

One of the most important measures is to ensure that all staff know to immediately remove from the group they care for any animals showing signs of infection. Leaving these dogs *in situ* for even a short period of time will ensure that the disease spreads rapidly, increasing the number of cases and the build-up of environmental pathogens. Infected dogs should be housed in a separate area where they can be closely observed and where they can receive treatment if required (Figure 14.4). Furthermore, dogs that are recovering, or have recovered, from kennel cough and which may be ready for rehoming may still be infectious to others and should, therefore, still be housed separately in designated areas (see Chapter 9).

To do this clearly requires that some empty kennels are kept free in the 'infected' blocks at all times, so that there is no delay in separating out clinical cases from the uninfected population. Similarly, in an ideal situation, those in-contact animals should be monitored for a few days before other naive animals are introduced into the group,

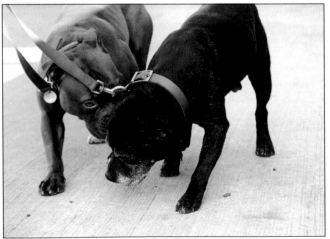

14.3 Direct contact between a naive dog and an infected dog can result in the transmission of disease.
(© Battersea Dogs and Cats Home)

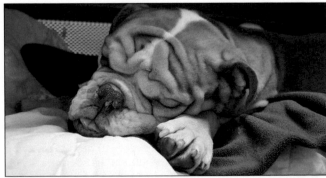

14.4 Infected animals should be isolated to prevent the spread of disease. They should be carefully observed and treatment administered as required.
(© Battersea Dogs and Cats Home)

to make sure that they have not contracted the disease and themselves become infectious. The biggest obstacle to this way of working is that most shelters run at full or close to full capacity and are under huge pressure to take in new dogs; yet, if respiratory disease is to be effectively managed, the shelter must be persuaded to leave sufficient kennel spaces in the isolation blocks to allow for movement of infected animals, and to manage their new intake accordingly. At times, when rates of rehoming are low, this can be particularly difficult to achieve, but the importance of this measure cannot be over-stressed.

Intake and animal grouping and overcrowding

The ability to house dogs in a way that helps in the effective control of respiratory disease will depend mainly on two factors:

- The level of occupancy, which in turn is influenced by animal throughput and length of stay in the shelter
- The kennel facilities, in particular the number of separate housing areas that can be used, as this dictates the extent to which different groups of dogs can be segregated.

What tends to happen is that, over time, the shelter population gradually becomes introduced to all the pathogens (and their varied strains) involved in CIRD as a result of infected individuals entering the shelter. These pathogens then become part of an ever-increasing reservoir of infection in the resident population that continues to infect new naive arrivals, and this perpetuates the problem.

With this in mind, if a significant proportion of the intake of a shelter is derived from local authority kennels or a similar source, then it will be advantageous to build good working relationships with those kennels. Providing advice on husbandry, disease and parasite control and, ideally, persuading the source kennel to vaccinate dogs on arrival, will all help to contribute to a healthier intake population with some immunity in place on arrival at the shelter.

Consideration should also be given to segregation of different groups of animals on arrival. For example, dogs from local authority kennels could be housed separately from those relinquished directly from their former owners' homes. Similarly, dogs that are identified as being potentially more vulnerable to infection (very nervous or stressed individuals; those in poor condition or ill health; pregnant or lactating bitches) might also benefit from being housed separately in quieter or calmer kennels, if available (see Chapter 10).

Animals should be housed singly wherever possible. Although certain individuals may gain some behavioural benefit by being paired up with another dog, the consequent increased risk of cross-infection should be acknowledged.

Whelping bitches should be housed separately. It is also advantageous to have designated housing for post-weaning puppies. If possible, housing these puppies in small groups of two to three per kennel will satisfy their requirements for company and social development, while minimizing the stress of competition for food and resources and the risk of bullying.

Fostering pregnant mothers and young puppies with experienced carers should also be explored. The puppies could be rehomed directly from the foster carer's home. If this is not feasible, they should spend as little time as possible back in the shelter before being rehomed.

Mixing

Many of the normal working practices of a shelter provide plenty of opportunities for dogs to mix – and to cross-infect one another if disease is present. Exercising, cleaning, behavioural assessments and viewing of dogs by members of the public should all be managed in such a way as to minimize contact between dogs or, where this cannot be avoided (e.g. in a dog-to-dog assessment), ensuring that the dogs that do have contact share the same infection status (i.e. both uninfected or both infected/recovered).

Length of stay

Given that the risk of acquiring infection increases with each day spent in the shelter, all efforts should be made to manage the 'journey' of the dog through the shelter as quickly and efficiently as possible. It is extremely important that the number of kennels and dogs on site reflects the rate of throughput. If there are many more kennels/dogs than are required to this end, then dogs will simply 'stagnate' while waiting for a new home and the risk of infection will increase correspondingly. See Chapter 7 for details of how to collect and use data on the length of stay and other metrics in optimizing the management of the shelter population.

Husbandry and disinfection

Staff should wear protective overalls, gloves and boots in the areas housing dogs with CIRD. Access should be restricted to the minimum, and any visitors should be provided with disposable overshoes, overalls and gloves. If these staff also work in other areas (e.g. if the shelter has insufficient staff to have dedicated workers in infected kennels), then they should work to the principle of going from 'clean' to 'infected' areas wherever possible (see Chapter 9).

Each block should have its own cleaning equipment. The standard husbandry protocol of cleaning surfaces of organic matter (faeces, urine, vomit, etc.) with detergent before disinfecting them should apply. Quaternary ammonium compound-based disinfectants will deal effectively with CIRD pathogens. Disinfectants should be used at the correct concentration, and minimum contact times as specified by the manufacturer should be observed. It is important not to use a higher concentration than recommended; although untrained staff may be tempted to do this, the fumes that this practice causes are irritant to airway mucous membranes and will aggravate and prolong clinical signs in dogs with CIRD (see QRG 9.1).

After the disinfectant has been rinsed off, the floor should be squeegeed and either left to air dry or, to speed up the drying process, be dried with towels. If the floor is left wet, this will increase the humidity in the block, favouring pathogen survival.

Cleaning and disinfection should include exercise runs, corridors and walkways outside the block. Grass or other natural surfaces are problematic in this respect.

Toys can make effective fomites and should ideally not be shared between dogs, but in any event they should be cleaned and disinfected after use (Figure 14.5). Likewise, grooming equipment can transfer infected saliva from dogs' coats and so must also be cleaned. Food and water bowls and utensils should be made of stainless steel (Figure 14.6); plastic is harder to clean and disinfect.

Bedding can be laundered daily, but it is more cost-effective to target only soiled bedding if the dog remains in the same kennel. This has the added advantage of leaving

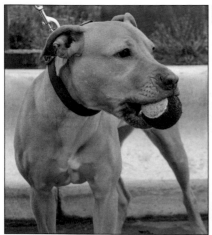

14.5 Toys, such as this ball, make effective fomites for disease transmission and should not be shared between dogs wherever possible. All toys should be cleaned and disinfected after use.
(© Battersea Dogs and Cats Home)

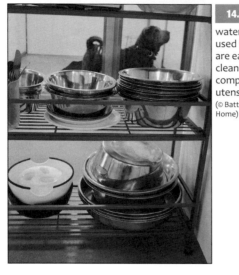

14.6 Stainless steel food and water bowls should be used in shelters as they are easier to effectively clean and disinfect compared with plastic utensils.
(© Battersea Dogs and Cats Home)

(unsoiled) bedding with the dog's scent on it, which will have a calming effect. Soiled bedding should be bagged up before collection and care should be taken not to allow cross-contamination with clean laundry.

Any vehicles used to transport animals should be cleaned and disinfected after each journey.

Sometimes, bowls of water are left in communal areas for dogs, especially on hot days, but these can be an effective source of cross-contamination. It may be simpler to provide disposable bowls on request (see Chapter 9 and QRG 9.1).

Stress

Measures to combat stress in the kennels will help to maintain the dogs' immunity and contribute to a healthier population. To this end, overcrowding should be avoided at all costs, and the blocks should be well ventilated and maintained at a comfortable temperature. The dogs should be exercised at least once a day and time should be spent socializing them both with other dogs (of the same infection status) and people, depending on their individual behavioural needs. Attention should be given to kennel enrichment and toys should be provided (see QRG 19.7). Radio/music may help to calm the dogs, but music and lights should be turned off at night. Particularly stressed or vocal animals will disrupt the whole block and efforts should be made to calm them or move them to a separate area.

It can be helpful to have consistency and continuity in staffing. Animals that would otherwise be wary of strangers will get to know their carers and become more relaxed. Similarly, the carers will become familiar with the dogs in their block and will be more readily able to detect early changes in the dogs' demeanour and health (see Chapter 19).

Facilities

These measures apply to existing facilities where changes can be made, but equally could be applied to the building of new purpose-built accommodation (see Chapter 10).

The ideal is to have multiple self-contained blocks with a small number of kennels in each block, as this provides the most flexible accommodation. Solid partitions between adjacent kennels and their runs (communal runs are best avoided) eliminate the possibility of physical contact and disease transmission by this route. If the kennels face each other and have open fronts, then a distance greater than 1 m between them is required to create an effective sneeze barrier. Alternatively, glass or plastic fronts to the kennels can be used. This has the slight disadvantage of lessening staff interaction with the dogs in the kennels, but may be preferable in blocks to which members of the public have access. It can be almost impossible to stop visitors putting their fingers through the bars of wire-fronted kennels to try to touch the dogs, no matter how much signage is employed advising them not to do this; this type of contact is a very effective way to spread disease from one kennel to another.

The individual kennels should provide adequate space for the breed/size mix of the shelter intake population and should be designed with ease of husbandry in mind, with cleanable surfaces, effective drainage, multiple water outlets throughout, good ventilation and temperature control. There should be adequate kitchen facilities and secure storage for food, utensils, bowls, cleaning equipment and uniforms/personal protective equipment, ensuring that rodent/bird access is prevented. The layout should allow for staff movement to flow from clean to infectious areas; in addition, well sited boot-cleaning stations will help to prevent cross-contamination of these areas.

It is helpful to have a small clinical examination area in the infectious/isolation blocks so that minor procedures can be carried out *in situ* without having to move a dog to another part of the shelter and risk spreading infection.

Ideally, ventilation should allow for a minimum of eight air changes per hour. The intake air should be fresh, as recirculation systems may reintroduce infection back into the air space. Humidity should stay below 50% if possible and the temperature should be maintained between 15 and 18°C; attention should be paid to preventing draughts in the kennel sleeping areas (see Chapter 10).

Segregation

One way to attempt to reduce cross-infection in a shelter is to introduce a simple colour-coding system to identify infected and non-infected animals (Figure 14.7), the staff responsible for them, and their kennel blocks, exercise areas and walkways. This can be especially helpful in urban shelters where space is at a premium and dogs are more likely to come into close contact with one another. The nature of respiratory disease control is such that it requires full engagement and compliance from all staff and volunteers (and visitors) if it is to be successful. By effectively making the disease status 'visible', a colour-coding system also reinforces the sense of personal responsibility of staff, making it clear to everyone when protocols are not being followed.

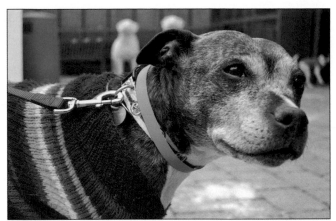

14.7 A simple colour-coding system can be used to identify infected and non-infected animals. In this case, the disposable green collar indicates that the animal is free from disease.
(© Battersea Dogs and Cats Home)

So, for example, green may be chosen to represent 'non-infected' and red to represent 'infected'. In this case, when dogs first arrive at the shelter, if they are free of clinical signs they are fitted with a green collar. If any dog starts to show clinical signs of infection, it is immediately fitted with a red collar, which remains on for the duration of the dog's stay until it is rehomed. When walked around the site, dogs would also have matching red or green leads for additional visibility.

The kennel blocks would then also be designated red (infected) and green (non-infected), as would any exercise areas. Having clearly marked red and green walkways around the shelter site will ensure that infected and non-infected dogs do not cross paths, which is important as it is very difficult to stop dogs sniffing one another when they meet and, in so doing, passing on infection.

In addition, staff may be defined with a coloured badge or armband depending on the blocks they are working in.

As members of the public can be effective disease vectors if they are able to handle the dogs or touch the dogs through the bars of their kennels, thought should be given to managing the flow of visitors from 'green' to 'red' dogs/kennels when viewing animals for rehoming.

As dogs may continue to shed pathogens after they have clinically recovered from CIRD, it makes sense to leave the red collar on a dog that has been infected until it is rehomed. While their infectious status will lessen with time, possibly to the point where they are no longer infectious, the extent to which this is the case will be largely unknown, and so they should still be kept apart from known non-infected 'green' dogs. 'Red' dogs that have recovered are more likely to be immune to further infection and are, therefore, less at risk from continuing to be housed with other 'red' dogs.

Training and education

All staff and volunteers should be educated about CIRD, preferably at induction or soon after. This should include non-operational staff who do not work directly with the animals (e.g. office staff), as their movements and actions can contribute to the spread of disease around the site.

Points to cover should include:

- The potential seriousness of the disease (the perception of 'kennel cough' outside of shelter establishments is usually that of a mild cough and uneventful recovery)

- The cost to the shelter (lengthened stays, cancelled procedures, effect on dogs' temperament, large financial burden)
- Overview of the disease, its complex nature and how it is transmitted, emphasizing vector transmission by both people and inanimate objects, especially toys
- How organisms that cause only mild disease in one dog may be potentially lethal to another
- The incubation period. This is an important point to convey to lay staff. Often, the organisms that cause CIRD may be spread by entirely innocent actions, such as fussing, cuddling or playing with a dog, and the nature of the incubation period means that the individual responsible is extremely unlikely to be able to correlate their actions with the resulting sick dog a few days later
- Carrier status/shedding of pathogens
- How increased length of stay increases the risk of dogs contracting CIRD
- Any control measures that have been put into place at the shelter.

In addition, the animal care assistants (and volunteers, if possible) should be given some basic animal health training. Staff and volunteers should be able to identify clinical signs of respiratory disease so that they can alert clinic staff or, if they are not immediately available, at least isolate the animals until they can be examined.

Visitors to the shelter should receive appropriate advice on disease spread, if possible. This could be done via posters on display, leaflets given out on arrival or a video at reception. Clear signage in the rehoming kennel blocks should alert visitors as to their responsibility to ensure that they do not cross-infect animals. In addition, the walkways around the kennel blocks could be arranged so as to direct visitors to view dogs in non-infectious kennels first.

Hand sanitizers should also be placed throughout the rehoming areas, with appropriate signage advising on correct use (see Chapter 24).

Data collection and audit

It is important to establish a reliable way of measuring and recording the incidence, prevalence and severity of respiratory disease in order to determine the magnitude of the problem, changing trends and response to any interventions. This can be done on a paper-based record-keeping system but will obviously be easier to achieve on a software system (see also Chapter 7).

A reliable set of criteria must first be established to define the severity of the disease. These could be based on clinical signs (presence of cough, nasal discharge, inappetence, pyrexia, chest complications, etc.) or treatment protocols (use of NSAIDs, antibiotics, fluids, etc.). This information must then be entered on to the record in a reliable fashion, whether using agreed terminology or, perhaps more easily, as a 'clinical score', so that the data can be extracted and put into a report format.

These data can be used to measure or identify:

- Incidence of disease (percentage of intake)
- Severity of disease
- Prevalence of disease on site at any given time
- Effect on length of stay
- Disease trends (e.g. seasonal)
- Risk factors (e.g. animal groupings, breed types, etc.)
- Success or failure of any interventions.

References and further reading

Chalker VJ, Brooks HW and Brownlie J (2003) The association of *Streptococcus equi* ssp. *zooepidemicus* with canine infectious respiratory disease. *Veterinary Microbiology* **95**, 149–156

Chalker VJ and Brownlie J (2004) Taxonomy of the canine Mollicutes by 16S rRNA gene and 16S/23S rRNA intergenic spacer region sequence comparison. *International Journal of Systemic and Evolutionary Microbiology* **54**, 537–542

Chalker VJ, Owen WA, Paterson C *et al.* (2004) Mycoplasmas associated with canine infectious respiratory disease. *Journal of Microbiology* **150**, 3491–3497

Chalker VJ, Toomey C, Opperman S *et al.* (2003) Respiratory disease in kennelled dogs: serological responses to *Bordetella bronchiseptica* lipopolysaccharide do not correlate with bacterial isolation or clinical respiratory symptoms. *Clinical and Diagnostic Laboratory Immunology* **10**, 352–356

Erles K and Brownlie J (2005) Investigation into the causes of canine infectious respiratory disease: antibody responses to canine respiratory coronavirus and canine herpesvirus in two kennelled dog populations. *Archives of Virology* **150**, 1493–1504

Erles K and Brownlie J (2008) Canine respiratory coronavirus: an emerging pathogen in the canine infectious respiratory disease complex. *Veterinary Clinics of North America: Small Animal Practice* **38**, 815–825

Erles K, Dubovi EJ, Brooks HW and Brownlie J (2004) Longitudinal study of viruses associated with canine infectious respiratory disease. *Journal of Clinical Microbiology* **42**, 4524–4529

Erles K, Shiu KB and Brownlie J (2007) Isolation and sequence analysis of canine respiratory coronavirus. *Virus Research* **124**, 78–87

Erles K, Toomey C, Brooks HW and Brownlie J (2003) Detection of a group 2 coronavirus in dogs with canine infectious respiratory disease. *Virology* **310**, 216–223

Mannering SA, McAuliffe L, Lawes JR, Erles K and Brownlie J (2009) Strain typing of *Mycoplasma cynos* isolates from dogs with respiratory disease. *Veterinary Microbiology* **135**, 292–296

Mitchell JA, Brooks H, Shiu KB, Brownlie J and Erles K (2009) Development of a quantitative real-time PCR for the detection of canine respiratory coronavirus. *Journal of Virological Methods* **155**, 136–142

Priestnall SL, Brownlie J, Dubovi EJ and Erles K (2006) Serological prevalence of canine respiratory coronavirus. *Veterinary Microbiology* **115**, 43–53

Priestnall S, Mitchell J, Walker CA, Erles K and Brownlie J (2013) New and emerging pathogens in canine infectious respiratory disease (CIRD): a review. *Veterinary Pathology* **51**, 492–504

Priestnall SL, Pratelli A, Brownlie J and Erles K (2007) Serological prevalence of canine respiratory coronavirus in Southern Italy and epidemiological relationship with canine enteric coronavirus. *Journal of Veterinary Diagnostic Investigation* **19**, 176–180

QRG 14.1: Rehoming a coughing dog
by Jenny Stavisky and Gemma Bourne

'Kennel cough' or canine infectious respiratory disease (CIRD) is commonly seen in shelter environments. This is likely to be due to close-quarters mixing of dogs – and their attendant pathogens – from multiple different sources. Although the syndrome is typically not life-threatening, it can be challenging to manage the treatment of both individual cases and outbreaks, while maintaining the movement of dogs through the rehoming process.

There are four main points where concerns occur:

- Care within the shelter
- When and whether to rehome
- Advising prospective owners
- Follow-up care after rehoming.

Care within the shelter

When an outbreak of CIRD occurs, it may be necessary to triage cases to determine which animals need veterinary attention in order to prioritize the available resources. As a general rule, animals that are immunocompromised or overtly unwell should always be seen. Otherwise fit and healthy dogs with a manageable cough may recover with rest and basic nursing care such as feeding soft food. However, it is wise to exercise caution and remember that not every coughing dog in a shelter will be suffering from an infectious disease. A thorough examination should always be carried out to ascertain whether the list of

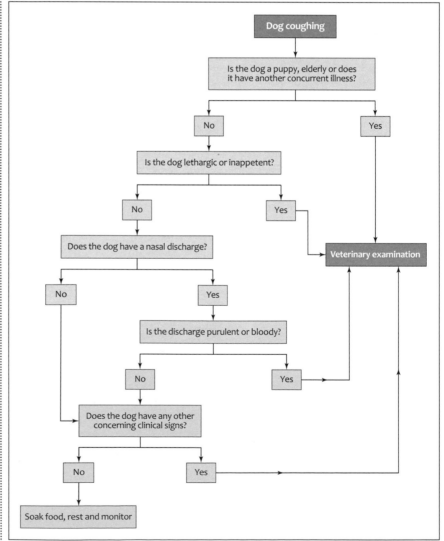

Flowchart suggesting a system for triage of coughing dogs.

QRG 14.1 *continued*

differential diagnoses should include other causes of cardiothoracic disease, such as heart failure, collapsing trachea or even pharyngeal foreign body.

When veterinary attention is required, it is not necessary to swab every dog for culture and sensitivity testing. Most dogs will respond to non-steroidal anti-inflammatory drugs and cough suppressants if required. Antimicrobial therapy may be justified in those that are pyrexic, systemically unwell or showing a discoloured nasal discharge. In order to choose appropriate antibiotics, it can be useful to keep a record identifying every coughing dog presented for treatment, the severity of signs and the treatment given. Over time, this can help to highlight successful and unsuccessful therapeutic options.

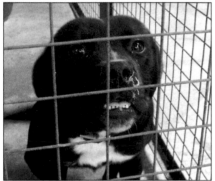

Purulent nasal discharge may be an indication to treat a coughing dog with antimicrobials.
(© Jenny Stavisky)

One of the biggest challenges when rehoming a coughing dog can be managing the risk of contagion against the need to prepare dogs for rehoming. If adoption is dependent on prior surgery (e.g. if the shelter has a policy that all dogs must be neutered prior to adoption), then consideration should be given as to whether an exception can be made so that the animal can return for the procedure at a later date. Often, the greater risk involved with surgery relates to spreading the disease to unaffected animals on the premises rather than to the coughing dog itself.

When and whether to rehome

Dogs in shelters will quite often be left with a residual cough following CIRD. It is likely that factors such as constant barking, which causes irritation to the trachea, can contribute

to this. Removing a dog from the shelter environment will often remove the stimulus to bark and thus allow a chronic cough to resolve. Therefore, it can sometimes be desirable to rehome a dog while it is still coughing. This can also break the cycle of reinfection in a high-challenge multi-pathogen stressful environment.

It may be helpful to have a standard recommendation regarding whether to rehome in such circumstances. Sensible limitations on rehoming would suggest that dogs that are systemically unwell or have a sustained pyrexia or concurrent disease should be kept at the shelter until their recovery is more advanced. However, factors such as the shelter's facilities, prospective owner's experience and the presence of other dogs in the prospective household can be used on a case-by-case basis to determine whether a particular dog would benefit more from being rehomed or held back. If appropriate, offering a repeat check at the shelter can encourage compliance with veterinary care and provide the new owner with support while the dog fully recovers.

Advising prospective owners

It is vital to obtain informed consent when considering rehoming a dog with any illness and to discuss potential issues with the prospective owners. Common concerns when rehoming a dog that has had kennel cough, or still has signs of the disease, centre on the risk that the dog poses to other dogs. Owners may also be apprehensive about what is involved in caring for a coughing dog, especially if they have not done so before, and some of them can find the process worrying and distressing. Additionally, the small but important risk of zoonotic infection must be taken into account.

The infectious period varies considerably both between different pathogens and from dog to dog. The table shows the infectious periods for organisms commonly implicated in kennel cough.

It is probably most noteworthy that *Bordetella bronchiseptica* has the potential to be shed for 12 weeks post infection. However, shedding does not necessarily correlate well with whether or not a dog is coughing. Therefore, decisions around the infectious hazard a shelter dog poses to other dogs or other species need to

be made on a pragmatic basis. If a dog is non-pyrexic, systemically well and showing no other signs of active infection, it is reasonable to consider rehoming the dog, with the informed consent of the new owner, particularly if there are no other susceptible pets or humans within the household. Sensible precautions might include ensuring that if there are any other dogs or cats in the household, they are suitably healthy and vaccinated, and that the new owner is fully aware of the risk of transmission to existing pets. It is also important that the low risk of zoonosis is discussed, with particular reference to susceptible individuals such as young children, pregnant women or immunosuppressed individuals. Advice should include the need to take sensible precautions, such as good hand hygiene following handling of affected dogs and avoiding allowing the dog to lick people's faces.

It is difficult to make firm recommendations about when to begin mixing the new dog with other dogs outside the home, but empirically a minimum period of 1–2 weeks of quarantine could be considered sensible.

Follow-up care after rehoming

Coughing is a frequent cause of concern post-adoption. Many owners struggle to take in information alongside the excitement of adopting their new pet and so it may be prudent to provide written information for owners to refer to. In cases where coughing is persistent, it may be wise to send dogs to their new home with medication, as this can go a long way towards offering owners reassurance. Inevitably, some owners may be concerned enough to seek veterinary attention. It will be necessary to decide whether this can be offered at the shelter. If not, is any support offered for private veterinary care? For dogs that appear clinically well at the point of rehoming, it is advisable to counsel owners that there can be no guarantees that the dog will not develop clinical signs once in its new home, but that this need not cause undue concern. It may be helpful to discuss kennel cough policies with local veterinary practices where new owners are likely to register their dogs. This can avoid conflicting advice being given or blame being mistakenly directed towards the shelter. ➡

QRG 14.1 *continued*

Organism	Incubation period	Asymptomatic carriage?	Other notes	Vaccine available?
Viruses				
Canine adenovirus-2 (CAV-2)	3–6 days	Yes	Closely related to CAV-1 (infectious canine hepatitis); vaccine offers cross-protection. Possibly also associated with enteritis	Live subcutaneous vaccine available
Canine herpesvirus (CHV)	6–10 days	Latent infection	Transplacental infection can cause abortion; infection may be fatal in puppies under 4 weeks	Subcutaneous subunit vaccine is normally used for pregnant bitches
Canine parainfluenza virus (CPiV)	2–10 days	No		Live subcutaneous and live intranasal vaccines available
Canine respiratory coronavirus (CRCoV)	2–7 days	Yes	Different from enteric coronavirus; respiratory coronavirus is not associated with diarrhoea	In development at the time of publication
Bacteria				
Bordetella bronchiseptica	2–14 days	Yes	Care must be taken with infected animals and when administering vaccines to avoid iatrogenic zoonotic infection. Cats are also susceptible	Live intranasal (UK); subcutaneous vaccines available elsewhere (e.g. Australia, New Zealand)
Streptococcus equi ssp. *zooepidemicus*	Not yet known	Reported, but rare – more evidence needed	Haemorrhagic pneumonia, high mortality. Sudden deaths may occur	No

Incubation period and vaccine availability for major causes of CIRD.

Information for new owners about kennel cough

Woofs-R-Us shelter.   4.3.2015

Dear Mr and Mrs Bloggs

This sheet is to provide some information regarding kennel cough.

Rex developed kennel cough during his stay with us. This is a condition which can affect any dog, but is especially common in dogs in rescue shelters and boarding kennels where lots of dogs are living in close contact. It is often caused by viruses, so we do not always treat it with antibiotics. Most dogs recover over a few days or weeks, and it is very rarely serious. However, there are some things to be aware of.

- Rex may be infectious to other dogs for a few days or weeks. To prevent him passing on the infection, a sensible precaution would be to keep him away from other dogs for 1–2 weeks after he has stopped coughing.
- If you have a dog at home, there is a chance it could become infected. We will have discussed this with you already. There is an intranasal (up the nose) vaccine, which helps to protect against some types of kennel cough, and although it does not guarantee immunity from infection we would recommend your dog has this vaccine before Rex comes home.
- Occasionally, some of the bacteria that cause kennel cough can be transmitted to cats. We will have discussed this with you already. There is an intranasal (up the nose) vaccine available for cats, and we would recommend that you discuss this with your vet before Rex comes home.
- Very rarely, some of the bacteria that cause kennel cough can be transmitted to people. This is extremely uncommon, but has been reported occasionally in people who are already suffering from health problems or particularly vulnerable. This includes anyone with immune suppression (e.g. those with HIV or on very high doses of steroids), transplant or chemotherapy patients, pregnant women and the very elderly or very young. If there is anyone of that description in your household, we would suggest delaying taking Rex home. Otherwise, sensible hygiene (do not let him lick your face, wash your hands after handling him) should eliminate any risk.

Rex may continue to cough occasionally for a few days or even weeks, as his throat may remain sensitive even after the infection has gone. You can help by avoiding pressure around his throat, e.g. walking him on a harness rather than a collar and lead.

Rex has been treated with some medication.

He is/is not going home with: ....

He does/does not need to be rechecked on: ....

It is likely that this problem will resolve quickly and that Rex will recover very soon. However, if you are worried about Rex, particularly if his cough gets worse or he seems lethargic or does not want to eat, please telephone us on 0115 111 1111.

Sample information sheet for new owners adopting a dog with kennel cough.

Chapter 15

Respiratory disease in the cat in the shelter environment

Rebecca Willby, Alan Radford and Maria Afonso

It is important for veterinary surgeons (veterinarians) to have a good understanding of feline infectious respiratory disease, since it represents a continual challenge in the shelter environment. The shelter population is particularly at risk because a number of factors compound to create an environment conducive to the acquisition and transmission of the pathogens responsible. Without knowledge of those factors, it is easy to focus on the treatment of individual cases without considering the population as a whole. Failing to recognize this 'bigger picture' can have serious consequences for the welfare of cats within the shelter, adversely affect staff morale and have negative financial consequences for the organization.

This chapter will focus mainly on infectious respiratory disease in the shelter cat. Most of the agents involved predominantly affect the upper respiratory tract; therefore, the term feline upper respiratory tract disease (FURTD) will be used when describing the disease complex.

Where appropriate, consideration will also be given to lower respiratory tract conditions and more unusual manifestations of respiratory infections such as virulent systemic feline calicivirus (VS-FCV).

The challenge of the shelter environment

The factors involved in the development and transmission of infectious respiratory disease can be grouped under two main headings, namely, those affecting the host and those affecting the shelter (Figure 15.1).

Many of these factors overlap; for example, concurrent health issues may negatively affect immunity. Prevention and control of FURTD demands a multifactorial approach. If the shelter has an excellent vaccination protocol but neglects the other factors listed in Figure 15.1, it will be harder to control disease. This chapter aims to arm the veterinary surgeon with the information required to formulate a rational approach to managing and preventing FURTD in the shelter environment.

Host factors	Shelter factors
• Host susceptibility • Immunity • Stress • Concurrent health issues • Carrier status	• Exposure to pathogens • Shelter design and traffic patterns • Presence of infected cats • Air quality • Hygiene and staff protocols • Stocking density and turnover

15.1 Factors involved in the development of feline respiratory tract infection.

History taking

Depending on the nature of the working relationship with the shelter, the veterinary surgeon may have a varying degree of knowledge of the disease burden of the shelter population at any particular time. It is vital for anyone involved in regular shelter medicine work to develop a good communication channel through which information is freely shared and updated. A veterinary surgeon performing regular frequent visits to a shelter will develop a deeper understanding of working practices and the 'normal' day-to-day challenges faced by the shelter staff. For those who are less acquainted with the normal practices and population dynamics, it will be crucially important to ask the right questions when consulted about a particular disease problem. The more involved a veterinary surgeon can be in advising and supporting the shelter, the more a proactive approach can be taken in the management of disease. For example, time taken with the shelter's management team to discuss and formulate hygiene and disinfection protocols and an outbreak management protocol will pay dividends.

The shelter veterinary surgeon may be asked to examine an individual cat affected by infectious respiratory disease, but, in such circumstances, the clinician should always be thinking of the rest of the population. Questions to cover during history taking can be grouped under three headings: the **population**, the **shelter** and the **individual**. Answers to these questions will help formulate a picture of FURTD in the particular shelter at that moment in time and provide a platform from which a management strategy can be developed (Figure 15.2).

Differential diagnosis

Figure 15.3 shows the main pathogens involved in FURTD with details of epidemiology, pathogenesis and diagnostic tests that can be used for each one.

Feline calicivirus

Feline calicivirus (FCV) is a small, non-enveloped, single-stranded ribonucleic acid (RNA) virus that infects domestic cats and other Felidae. As an RNA virus, FCV can evolve and adapt extremely quickly, leading to the emergence of a large number of different strains with varying antigenicity and pathogenicity. However, there is sufficient cross-reactivity between strains to group them all in a single serotype with some degree of cross-protection between them. Genetic diversity has led to the development of typing methods based on sequence analysis to differentiate FCV strains and to explore in depth the epidemiology of infection. Such methods have been used in shelters to explore the frequency of transmission events (Coyne *et al.*, 2007).

FCV can survive for up to 1 week in the environment, or possibly longer if the environment is damp. Fomite spread is, therefore, possible. Following infection, the majority of cats are believed to shed virus for approximately 30 days, significantly after the majority of clinical signs have resolved. Such clinically normal FCV-positive cats are termed carriers. Thereafter, a 75-day half-life has been described,

History taking	
The population	
What is the endemic or 'normal' level of infectious respiratory disease in the shelter? How does this compare with the number of cats currently showing clinical signs?	Disease surveillance data are useful to monitor trends (see section on Outbreak management later in this chapter). For example, recording and analysing the incidence (the number of new cases over a specific period of time) of cats showing signs of FURTD may be useful in detecting whether the current level of disease constitutes an outbreak (see also Chapter 7). The definition of an outbreak will vary from shelter to shelter depending on the population and the particular circumstances accompanying each. Shelters with low background levels of FURTD may decide to define an outbreak with a smaller number of new cases than a shelter with a higher background of disease
Is there concurrent respiratory disease in dogs in the shelter? What other diseases are concurrent within the shelter?	Some causes of FURTD are shared with dogs, notably *Bordetella bronchiseptica* Concurrent disease provides context to shelter biosecurity and may impact directly on FURTD through immunosuppression
The shelter	
Is disease present in one area of the shelter only, or are there clusters of affected cats in different areas?	The answer to this question could provide clues as to where the disease originated, whether it is confined to one area or whether it may have spread within the shelter
Is there a designated isolation area? If so, how is it decided that a cat should be moved there?	Properly designed and managed isolation facilities are crucial to minimizing the risk and impact of outbreaks
How are cats housed – in groups or individually?	Mixing of cats at housing, especially those from different origins, will inevitably increase opportunities for disease transmission
How is accommodation arranged? Can cats contact each other? Are there sneeze barriers? Is there at least 1.2 m of space between facing cages? What provision is there for ventilation and air flow?	The maximum distance of droplet transmission is not precisely known and depends on air flow, but it is generally considered that viral particles within droplets can travel distances of up to 1.2 m (Povey and Johnson, 1970). Poor ventilation allows accumulation of infective agents as well as dust and fumes, which can irritate the respiratory tract and thus can contribute to disease
What is the staff:animal ratio? Has this changed recently?	If the shelter has become short staffed there may be increased pressure on staff, with the result that husbandry and biosecurity are compromised
What is the routine staff movement pattern – e.g. do they routinely start work in one area and then move to another?	Tracking patterns of work may enable the veterinary practitioner to develop a picture of how disease may spread within the shelter
Are adequate hygiene and disinfection protocols in place and are they being adhered to? Have all staff received up-to-date training?	The details here are important. All disinfectants are not equally good, and they have to be used correctly. Any biosecurity can only be as strong as its weakest component
The individual	
What clinical signs are being displayed?	This is crucial in disease recognition and formulation of the case definition (see section on Outbreak management)
Are tests required to diagnose the likely cause of the clinical signs, or are they suggestive on their own?	Although not always necessary, a microbiological diagnosis can identify the possible cause of FURTD, inform treatment and management of outbreaks, as well as inform interventions to mitigate against future outbreaks
Could all the clinical signs be attributable to one agent, or could there be two or more possible pathogens?	In populations with high turnovers, mixed infections are not uncommon
What is the known history of each affected cat – e.g. was it found as a stray, has it been relinquished by an owner? If so, what is the vaccination history?	This can help to understand how cases of FURTD are getting into the shelter and being transmitted through the premises. Vaccination history can suggest a possible cause, and is also clearly important in deciding how to use vaccines in the shelter
What type of vaccine was used (modified live virus (MLV) *versus* killed)?	MLV preparations are generally considered to achieve a more rapid onset of protection (Möstl *et al.*, 2013). However, MLVs may occasionally revert to virulence and have, albeit rarely, been associated with disease
When did clinical signs start in relation to the date of admission?	Signs of FURTD within 1–2 days of admission are more likely to be due to infection before intake, whereas those occurring after 5 or more days are more likely to be due to either exposure within the shelter (Dinnage *et al.*, 2009), given that the incubation periods of the main feline respiratory agents are 1–6 days, or recrudescence of latent infection in carriers
What age and body condition are affected cats?	Cats in poor condition are perhaps less likely to have been vaccinated and may have underlying disease/infection. They may be immunosuppressed, making them more susceptible to acquiring infection
Is there concurrent disease?	This is helpful in identifying why certain individuals may have contracted disease and may help in decision-making regarding 'rehomeability'

15.2 Questions to ask when taking a history of feline upper respiratory tract disease (FURTD) in a shelter.

Pathogen	Incubation period	Pathogenesis	Diagnostic tests	Shedding	Carrier	Notes/relevant epidemiology
Viruses						
Feline calicivirus (FCV)	2–14 days	Replication in oral and respiratory tissues. Virus causes vesicles that rupture, forming mouth ulcers	Viral isolation (from oropharyngeal swabs in viral transport media) is gold standard RT-PCR	~30 days (most animals)	Yes; clinically normal	Multi-cat households have high prevalence. At least 10% of clinically normal cats arriving at shelter are likely to be shedding virus
Feline herpesvirus (FHV)	2–6 days (may be longer in cases where the cat is challenged by low levels of virus)	Replication mainly occurs in the nasal mucosa, nasopharynx and tonsils, causing multifocal epithelial necrosis. In severe cases, replication may lead to turbinate bone damage	PCR (higher sensitivity) or virus isolation from conjunctival, corneal or oropharyngeal swabs. Positive results should be interpreted along with present clinical signs	Up to 3 weeks	Yes; most animals should be suspected of being carriers	Following recovery from infection, virus becomes latent in ganglia. Recrudescence is common after periods of stress; minimizing stress is highly important to decrease viral shedding
Bacteria						
Bordetella bronchiseptica	3–6 days	Bacterium secretes specific proteins and toxins that allow it to colonize the ciliated epithelium of the respiratory tract, leading to failure of the mucociliary clearance mechanism. Upper respiratory tract more commonly affected but lower tract can also be colonized (bronchopneumonia)	PCR and bacterial culture of oropharyngeal swabs (transported in Amies charcoal medium or similar) or bronchoalveolar lavage	Up to 19 weeks	Yes; clinically healthy animals can be infective	Dogs with *B. bronchiseptica* respiratory disease are a risk for cats
Chlamydia felis	2–5 days	Obligate intracytoplasmic bacterium. Replicates in conjunctival epithelium	PCR (ocular swabs) Antibody detection in unvaccinated cats	~60 days (conjunctival shedding)	Persistent infections may develop	Most cases occur in young animals less than 1 year old
Mycoplasma felis	Unclear	Mycoplasmas reproduce well in environments such as mucosal membranes of respiratory tract	Culture and PCR (available from commercial diagnosis providers)	Unclear	Possible, but it is uncommon to isolate mycoplasmas from clinically healthy cats	Role in primary respiratory disease is not very clear. Role as a secondary pathogen is well described

15.3 Differential diagnosis of feline upper respiratory tract disease (FURTD): the main pathogens involved. PCR = polymerase chain reaction; RT-PCR = reverse-transcription PCR.

during which half of a given group of carriers will stop shedding. While this is almost certainly an oversimplification of the reality, it is a useful model to have in mind when seeing cats with FCV. It follows from such a model that only a small proportion of cats develop long-term and perhaps lifetime persistence of infection; it is these cats that are likely to play the biggest role in maintaining infection in the shelter population.

Because of the carrier state, clinically normal cats can often test positive for FCV. The likelihood of a cat testing positive is dependent on many factors, but in this context, the larger the group of cats, the higher the prevalence of infection can become, increasing from 10% in populations of cats living alone to well over 50% in some multi-cat households. The shelter veterinary surgeon needs to be aware that at least 10% of the clinically healthy cats arriving in the shelter are likely to be shedding FCV.

Mouth ulcers are the major and most consistent feature of FCV and can take more than 3 weeks to heal (Figure 15.4). Other clinical signs caused by FCV include an acute shifting lameness and conjunctivitis. Lower respiratory tract infections, including pneumonia, have been described but are not frequent.

FCV is also associated with the chronic gingivostomatitis complex, and veterinary surgeons should be aware that most cats with this challenging and stressful condition will be shedding FCV.

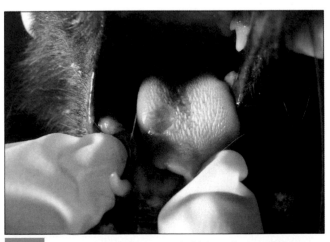

15.4 Cat with a lingual ulcer, typical of feline calicivirus infection.

The finding of oral ulcers in a cat with FURTD points to FCV involvement; however, lesions are not specific, and virus isolation or reverse transcription polymerase chain reaction (RT-PCR) on oropharyngeal (Figure 15.5), nasal or conjunctival swabs is required for definitive diagnosis. FCV-positive results should be interpreted carefully due to the existence of asymptomatic carriers; positive cats should be considered infectious, but the presence of virus does not necessarily mean it is the cause of any observed disease. Serology is not very useful for diagnosis, since the seroprevalence is high because of widespread vaccination and field infection of cats.

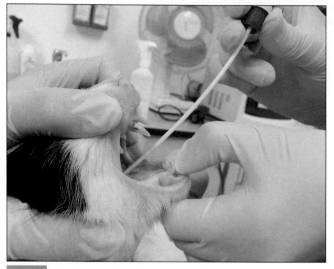

15.5 Oropharyngeal swab being taken from a cat.

Feline herpesvirus

Feline herpesvirus-1 (FHV-1) is an alphaherpesvirus with many similarities to herpes simplex virus (the cause of 'cold sores' in humans).

As a deoxyribonucleic acid (DNA) virus, FHV-1 isolates are generally similar with respect to pathogenicity and antigenicity, and are all considered to be in a single serotype. Following recovery of the cat from acute infection, FHV-1 sets up a lifelong infection, mainly in the trigeminal ganglia. This carrier state is characterized by periods of latency where no infectious virus is detectable, interspersed with episodes of virus shedding, where infectious virus is present in oronasal and ocular secretions, often in the absence of clinical signs (reactivation). In some cases, carriers show mild clinical signs while they are shedding (recrudescence), which may act as a useful indicator that such individuals are likely to be infectious to other cats. The switch from latency to active viral shedding may occur spontaneously but is most likely to occur following exposure to a stressor, for example after a change of housing (e.g. entering a rescue cattery) or kittening, or following corticosteroid treatment. Shedding does not occur immediately after the stress: there is a lag period of approximately 1 week, followed by a shedding episode of up to 2 weeks' duration. Thus, carrier cats are most likely to be infectious from 1 to 3 weeks after experiencing a stress.

FHV-1 infection generally causes a more severe upper respiratory tract disease than that seen following FCV infection, particularly in young susceptible animals. Initial signs include depression, marked sneezing, inappetence and pyrexia, followed by conjunctivitis and serous, becoming mucopurulent, ocular and nasal discharges (Figure 15.6). Excessive salivation and ptyalism and, in severe cases,

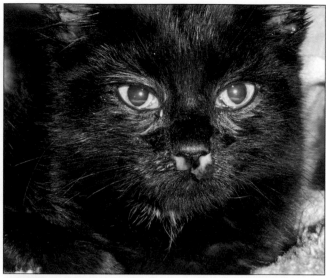

15.6 Cat with nasal and ocular discharges associated with feline herpesvirus infection.

dyspnoea and coughing may also occur. Oral ulceration is sometimes described, albeit less commonly than following FCV infection. Occasionally, pneumonia or generalized disease may also occur, particularly in young or debilitated animals. Other features of disease can include ulcerative or interstitial keratitis and, more rarely, skin ulcers and dermatitis, and nervous signs. Infection with FHV-1 is rarely fatal. However, in very young kittens or immunosuppressed cats the mortality rate may be higher due to secondary bacterial infections and, more rarely, generalized viral infection.

Clinical signs generally resolve within 10–20 days. However, in some cats the acute damage may have been severe enough to lead to permanent damage of the mucosae and turbinates, leaving affected cats prone to secondary bacterial infection and chronic rhinitis, sinusitis and/or conjunctivitis.

In terms of diagnosis (see Figure 15.3), positive results should be interpreted in the context of the clinical signs that are present.

Bordetella bronchiseptica

Bordetella bronchiseptica is an aerobic, Gram-negative coccobacillus. It is a well-known respiratory pathogen in many species, including dogs, pigs and rabbits; it also causes occasional opportunistic infections in humans and is considered a rare zoonosis, especially in immunocompromised individuals. As well as its role as a secondary pathogen, *B. bronchiseptica* can behave as a primary pathogen. It is likely that many factors may ultimately determine the outcome of infection, including environmental factors such as stress or overcrowding or, in some cases, preexisting viral infection.

Chlamydia felis

Chlamydia felis is an obligate intracytoplasmic bacterium. Following infection, the bacteria replicate in the conjunctival epithelium, leading to serous ocular discharge, chemosis, blepharospasm and hyperaemia: initial unilateral signs frequently become bilateral (Figure 15.7). Respiratory signs are usually very mild or non-existent. Infection commonly requires close contact between cats and ocular secretions are the main means of infection.

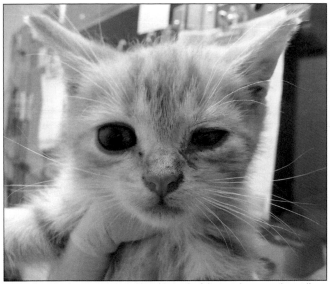

15.7 Ocular signs caused by *Chlamydia felis* may begin unilaterally, later progressing to become bilateral.

Mycoplasma felis

Mycoplasma species lack a cell wall; this has important implications for their susceptibility to antibacterial agents (see Treatment, below). Many species are considered to be commensal organisms associated with mammalian mucosal membranes. Several species have been isolated from domestic cats, in both colonies and households, and several studies suggest that some species may be more common in cats with respiratory disease than in healthy cats. While evidence for their role as a primary pathogen is perhaps still lacking, there is a general consensus that they can behave as secondary pathogens, exacerbating disease in co-infections. It may, therefore, be desirable to consider them as a complicating factor in any outbreak situation and to treat accordingly (Lee-Fowler, 2014).

Treatment

Overview

Treatment of FURTD cases in a shelter setting should be pragmatic to avoid excessive costs. If exercised badly, treatment measures can lead to prolonged stays and compromised welfare and, without good preventive measures in place, the risk of disease spread (see Chapter 3).

Decision-making in FURTD treatment

It is a good idea to have a set protocol for treatment of FURTD (e.g. detailing the clinical signs that will be an indication for starting antimicrobial therapy) with enough room for interpretation according to individual need, to ensure that cats are given appropriate treatment for the appropriate length of time with regular reviews of the treatment of individual cases. Shelters may decide under veterinary guidance to focus treatment on the cases that are most likely to recover fully and in a timely manner. It is not uncommon for FURTD to be the deciding factor in a euthanasia decision, especially if the cat has ▶

Decision-making in FURTD treatment *continued*

concurrent health issues. Ultimately, it is better all round to focus resources on prevention of FURTD rather than just treatment, although treatment will be an inevitable part of dealing with a cat shelter population.

As for all infectious diseases, treatment of FURTD has to take into account the cost of the treatment itself and the labour required to administer it. For example, it may be more cost-effective to use a treatment that needs only once-daily administration but is slightly more expensive than one that requires twice-daily dosing when staffing levels are stretched. In addition, the more treatment interventions a cat has, the higher the stress it is exposed to, which in turn can negatively affect the cat's wellbeing and recovery.

If a cat with FURTD is unable to eat enough to maintain at least its daily caloric requirements, it will be slow to recover (if at all), and during this time its welfare may be compromised. The mainstay of supportive therapy is ensuring adequate fluid, electrolyte and nutritional intake, although this can be a challenge. Many affected cats will not eat due to congestion causing a lack of sense of smell, or as a result of pain associated with oral ulcers. Severely affected FHV-1 and FCV cases can require fluid therapy and nutritional support for several days; the shelter may lack the financial resources for such cases to be hospitalized at a veterinary facility, especially if there are several cats affected at any one time.

Cats do not tolerate syringe feeding well, especially when they have nasal congestion, so any cat that is not eating at least a maintenance quantity of food for 3 days consecutively would ordinarily be an indication to have a feeding tube placed. In the shelter setting, however, such interventions are not often possible, and so reaching this stage may precipitate a decision to euthanase the individual on welfare and resource-sparing grounds

---

Fluid and nutritional support

Strong-smelling food that is highly palatable should be offered; warming the food will increase its flavour and smell. Appetite stimulants (e.g. mirtazapine) may be used in the short term. Fluid administration should take account of electrolyte losses through inappetence and secretions, as serum potassium may be depleted in such cats.

Steam inhalation

Placing affected cats in a steam-filled room may assist with decongestion (Gent, 2013), but this may not be practical in the shelter setting.

Analgesia and antipyretics

Pain can result from oral and nasal ulceration, as well as ocular inflammation. Pyrexia can be alleviated with the use of non-steroidal anti-inflammatory drugs in the well hydrated cat.

Topical ocular treatment

Specific treatment of ocular lesions associated with FHV-1 may be indicated. Treatments include the antiviral agents trifluridine, idoxuridine and ganciclovir (Thiry *et al.*, 2009).

Other indications for use of topical eye medications include treatment of secondary bacterial infections and providing lubrication to ease ocular discomfort. Chloramphenicol, administered as eye drops four times daily or ointment twice daily, is effective against a wide range of Gram-positive and Gram-negative organisms. Fusidic acid will treat Gram-positive infections. Fluoroquinolone, such as ofloxacin, should be reserved for those infections in which sensitivity to other antibiotics is limited (Gent, 2013). Systemic use of doxycycline is more effective at treating and eliminating *C. felis* infection than topical treatment (Sparkes *et al.*, 1999).

Topical corticosteroid or antibiotic/corticosteroid preparations are generally not indicated for routine treatment of conjunctivitis and should be reserved for chronic cases, especially where an immune-mediated process is suspected. They should not be used in suspected cases of FHV-1 due to the risk of recrudescence or aggravation of an existing FHV-1 infection (Gent, 2013).

Nursing and environment

Cats will benefit from having ocular and nasal discharges regularly cleaned away and being groomed. Minimizing stress will help to decrease the incidence of FURTD, so attention should be paid to minimal handling, reduction in environmental noise, having a predictable routine and providing hiding places for the cats.

Antibiotics

In some cases of FURTD, the use of topical or systemic antibiotics may be appropriate. Topical treatment in cases of ocular lesions is outlined above.

As well as exposure to primary bacterial pathogens, the compounding factors of FURTD and stress from being in a shelter environment can mean that affected cats have decreased resistance to secondary bacterial infections. In ensuring judicious use of antibiotics, a balance should be struck between ensuring that affected cats are treated as necessary, while minimizing the risk of promoting the development of antibiotic resistance. Therefore, establishing guidelines – for example, reserving antibiotic treatment for the most severely affected cats with purulent ocular or nasal discharges – may be prudent.

In the shelter setting it is often not practical to take swabs from every case for culture and sensitivity testing, and shelters may use antibiotics empirically in the first instance. However, there is an absolute need to use antimicrobials responsibly, to minimize the development of resistance. The Small Animal Medicine Society (SAMSoc)/BSAVA PROTECT guidelines are a valuable resource and can sensibly be included in antibiotic treatment policies for shelters (SAMSoc and BSAVA, 2011). Thus, antibiotics should primarily be reserved for cases of *M. felis*, *C. felis* or *B. bronchiseptica* infection; a good first-line antibiotic in such cases is doxycycline (10 mg/kg). Additionally, antibiotics should be used in cases where there is clear evidence of bacterial infection, such as bacterial rhinitis, chronic rhinitis and sinusitis. In such cases, a good empirical first choice is co-amoxiclav. Doxycycline can cause oesophageal ulceration and strictures; therefore, tablet administration should always be accompanied by syringing at least 5 ml of fluid. Tetracyclines can cause teeth staining of neonates when used in late pregnancy or the first few weeks of life. Though not well documented in animals, it is prudent to restrict use of tetracyclines in young cats; there is less of a concern of these effects with doxycycline than oxytetracycline (Ramsey, 2014).

Antivirals

There is a lack of published data supporting the efficacy of systemic antivirals for treatment of FURTD caused by FHV-1 (Thiry *et al.*, 2009), and the cost of these treatments often puts them beyond the realm of pragmatic usage in the shelter setting. Aciclovir has been widely used in human medicine, but has poor activity against FHV-1 *in vitro* (Gaskell *et al.*, 2007). Recently, famciclovir has been used in cats with FHV-1, but more field trials are required. Very few antivirals used in veterinary medicine have activity against RNA viruses such as FCV.

L-lysine

The rationale for using L-lysine is that it is an antagonist of arginine, which is essential for FHV-1 replication. Supplementation with L-lysine has been shown to have some activity against FHV-1 in experimentally induced infections, reducing the number of shedding episodes associated with reactivation of latent virus. It may, therefore, have an application in reducing the severity of disease at times of stress (Gaskell *et al.*, 2007).

Interferon

Although feline interferon omega has been shown to decrease viral replication *in vitro*, it has not been shown to make a significant clinical difference when used in cats with FCV or FHV-1 infection. Some authors advocate its use in the chronic gingivostomatitis complex (Southerden and Gorrel, 2007). With regard to FCV, there are no published data evidencing the benefit of human or feline recombinant interferon in the management of rhinitis associated with this virus (Reed and Gunn-Moore, 2012).

Treatment of specific conditions
Bacterial infections

Most isolates of feline *B. bronchiseptica* are susceptible to tetracyclines and the drug of choice is doxycycline (Egberink *et al.*, 2009). In cases of *C. felis*, doxycycline should be administered for 4 weeks to ensure complete resolution of infection (Dean *et al.*, 2005). Clinical signs improve rapidly once administration of doxycycline has begun (Dean *et al.*, 2005) but if treatment is administered for an insufficient duration, shedding may continue with the potential for recurrence. *M. felis* is also susceptible to tetracyclines and at least a 4-week course is recommended; some authors recommend 6 weeks' treatment for upper and lower respiratory tract infections caused by *M. felis* (Foster and Martin, 2011). As *M. felis* organisms lack a cell wall, beta-lactam antibiotics (e.g. penicillins) are ineffective (Lee-Fowler, 2014).

Lungworm

The feline lungworm *Aelurostrongylus abstrusus* can cause clinical signs of lower respiratory tract disease, including coughing and dyspnoea. Although cases are usually sporadic, they may be confused with other more common causes of feline respiratory tract disease, and so information is included here for completion. Feline lungworm can be difficult to diagnose, and, in any suspected case, it would be prudent to administer treatment. Imidacloprid/moxidectin and emodepside/praziquantel have proved effective, and both have the advantage of being easy to administer and being effective against a wide range of endoparasites.

Potential sequelae

Chronic stomatitis

The aetiology of this condition is uncertain, but affected cats will usually be shedding FCV. It is characterized by marked proliferative inflammation of the gingiva and oral mucosa. Resulting oral pain can cause inappetence, ptyalism and weight loss. Chronic stomatitis is usually very difficult to treat, and affected cats often need to have ongoing medical management and sometimes total tooth extraction.

Chronic rhinosinusitis

This condition is characterized by chronic mucoid or mucopurulent nasal discharge, which is often bilateral and accompanied by blood. Pathology includes turbinate erosion and mucosal inflammation. Cats with this chronic condition often require intermittent treatment for years to manage the clinical signs. In some cases there is a possible link with historical acute disease associated with FHV-1 infection.

With both chronic stomatitis and chronic rhinosinusitis, successful adoption may be a challenge, and consideration should be given to the ongoing welfare of the cat and the expectations of a potential adopter when deciding whether such an affected cat should be treated and rehomed or not.

Prevention

The stressful environment associated with large numbers of animals, often with a high stocking density and population turnover, within the sight, sound and smell of other animals, and with varying degrees of susceptibility to infectious disease, brings with it a high risk of infectious disease. Nevertheless, a well thought through preventive management programme, which should be broad-based enough to cover both infectious disease and cats' wellbeing as a whole, will help reduce the risk of infection.

Some of the key features of the main pathogens involved in FURTD that should be considered in prevention strategies are summarized in Figure 15.8.

Maintenance of general health

Shelters should have a system for prompt identification of medical needs, for example, a full health examination by a veterinary surgeon at or shortly after intake. In addition, prompt instigation of routine treatment with ecto- and endoparasiticides (see Chapter 11) will address parasitic burdens that may compromise a cat's immune system.

Vaccination

Vaccination strategies should be specifically tailored for shelters, where the considerations are different than for the individual privately owned cat. Vaccination is covered in depth in Chapter 11. Vaccination should take place as close as possible to the time of intake and should be limited to the diseases that are likely to be transmitted within the shelter. Vaccines against FHV-1 and FCV (and feline panleukopenia virus (FPV)) are considered core (Scherk et al., 2013). Consideration may be given to using these vaccines at an earlier age than is recommended for pet cats (i.e. off-licence use), especially where the shelter's management protocols mean that young susceptible kittens are at risk of infection.

Stress reduction

An animal's wellbeing encompasses both emotional and physical health (see Chapter 19). It is well recognized that stress can have immunosuppressive effects (Möstl et al., 2013), rendering a cat more susceptible to contracting infectious respiratory disease or inducing shedding and/or recrudescence in the case of FHV-1. Before shedding of infective virus, there is a lag phase of 4–11 days; the shedding period itself lasts 1–13 days. Hence, an FHV-1 carrier cat experiencing stress (such as that associated with entering a shelter) is likely to shed infectious virus over the following 3 weeks (Gaskell et al., 2007). Thus, incoming cats should ideally be quarantined for 3 weeks unless they are likely to be rehomed sooner (Figure 15.9). Where this is not possible, strict barrier nursing will help to contain the spread of potential pathogens (Möstl et al., 2013). Some researchers have argued that while quarantine is important for the control of other infectious diseases, such as FPV, its use purely to reduce risk to the healthy cat population from FURTD has limitations (Dinnage et al., 2009). This is because this study (and others) has shown that the length of stay in a shelter is strongly related to the risk of developing FURTD, with the daily incidence of disease increasing with each day a cat spends in a shelter. The reason for this is that a very high percentage of incoming cats are likely to be latent carriers of FHV-1, and others will acquire the infection during their stay. Therefore, unless other control measures are optimal, prolonging an animal's stay in a shelter by imposing a quarantine period may have limited impact on the incidence of FURTD. Strict hygiene precautions are necessary even when dealing with healthy cats, since so many of them shed pathogens associated with FURTD.

Adherence to a predictable daily routine will help to reduce chronic stress. Natural circadian rhythms should be supported by turning lights in the cattery off at night (Newbury et al., 2010). Good-quality food should be provided and dietary changes should be avoided unless indicated. Cleaning should be done in the least disruptive manner possible. Consideration should be given to spot cleaning where appropriate (for healthy cats or those with non-infectious disease (Steneroden, 2013); this refers to low-level cleaning of the pen during a cat's stay, with deep clean/disinfection needed only when the pen becomes heavily soiled or between occupants. The cat remains in the pen and cleaning is performed around it. Cats benefit from having somewhere to hide within the pen while spot cleaning is taking place. This procedure reduces handling and stress, and leaves the cat's scent on materials within the pen; it is also saves shelter staff/volunteers time.

It almost goes without saying that the best way to avoid stress is to rehome cats as quickly as possible. Many shelters choose to alert potential adopters to the risk of FURTD, and this would seem to be a prudent move.

Steps should be taken to avoid overcrowding. A well meaning, overambitious intake policy will only lead to breakdowns in hygiene and infection control if the shelter lacks the resources to cope with the numbers of animals.

Route of transmission	Lability	Susceptibility to disinfectants	Vaccine	Immunity	Zoonotic potential	Cross-species infection
Viruses						
Feline calicivirus (FCV)						
Direct cat-to-cat contact (and droplet over distances less than 1.5 m), indirect (fomite, ocular, nasal, oral secretions, possibly urine/faeces)	Can survive up to 28 days in the environment, even in dried state; longer in cold temperatures	Not reliably killed by quaternary ammonium compounds (QACs) or many alcohol hand sanitizers. Killed by bleach (5% sodium hypochlorite at a 1:32 dilution), potassium peroxymonosulfate (Virkon) or chlorine dioxide (Radford et al., 2009)	Modified live virus (MLV) intranasal; MLV and killed parenteral. Vaccination will help prevent disease but not infection. May not protect equally well against all strains, including those associated with virulent systemic FCV	Level of maternally derived antibody (MDA) generally higher and of longer duration than for FHV-1. Virus neutralizing antibodies are generally higher than for FHV-1 and correlate well with immunity to the same strain. Additionally, infection with one strain can significantly reduce the clinical signs associated with a different strain and oral shedding may be reduced	None known	Felidae. Similar viruses have been isolated from dogs but their significance is unknown
Feline herpesvirus-1 (FHV-1)						
Direct cat-to-cat contact (and droplet), indirect (fomite, ocular, nasal, oral secretions). Latent infection of kittens is possible following exposure to an infected queen even in the presence of MDA	Variable potential to remain viable outside the host, depending on environmental conditions (few hours at 37°C to months at <4°C). Relatively unstable as an aerosol	Glycoprotein lipid envelope, therefore readily destroyed by disinfectants	MLV intranasal; MLV and killed parenteral. Vaccination reduces disease and virus excretion upon infection, but not infection itself. MLV vaccines may cause clinical signs if aerosolized vaccine contacts mucosal surfaces therefore care should be taken to reconstitute the vaccine away from the cat	Level of maternally derived immunity is generally quite low. Some kittens do not have MDA beyond 6 weeks of age and most will have none by 10 weeks of age. Natural infection does not induce solid immunity (1–3 months duration only); therefore recovered cats should still be vaccinated. In general, immunity protects against infection but not disease	None known	Felidae only
Bacteria						
Bordetella bronchiseptica						
Direct cat-to-cat contact, fomites, aerosol, shed in oral and nasal secretions	May persist in the environment in fluids	Readily killed by routine disinfectants	MLV vaccine available in the UK. Not considered a core vaccine for shelter use. Consideration may be given to vaccinating high-density populations with a history of disease. Not effective in cats receiving antibiotics	Acquired immunity not long-lasting. Naturally acquired immunity protects against subclinical infection, but vaccination does not. Hence, both vaccinated and unvaccinated cats may become persistently infected carriers	Risk to immuno-compromised people or to those suffering from pre-existing respiratory disease	Dogs, cats, rabbits, pigs, humans

15.8 Key features of the main pathogens involved in FURTD. (continues)

(Data from Browning, 2004; Coyne et al., 2006; Gaskell et al., 2007; Gruffydd-Jones et al., 2009; Miller and Zawistowski, 2011; Advisory Board on Cat Diseases, 2014; International Cat Care; Koret Shelter Medicine Program)

Route of transmission	Lability	Susceptibility to disinfectants	Vaccine	Immunity	Zoonotic potential	Cross-species infection
Bacteria continued						
Chlamydia felis						
Direct cat-to-cat contact, most importantly via ocular secretions, fomites, aerosol. Kittens can be infected during parturition, as organisms are shed from the reproductive tract	Poor survival outside host	Reliably killed by QACs	MLV and killed parenteral. Not considered a core vaccine for shelter use. Consideration may be given to vaccinating high-density populations with a history of disease. Effective against development of disease but not infection. No reliable data comparing efficacy of killed *versus* MLV vaccine	Infected cats develop antibodies; kittens are protected for the first 1–2 months by MDA. Duration of immunity post vaccination unknown but thought to be <12 months	Has been known to cause chronic conjunctivitis in at least one immuno-compromised person (Browning, 2004)	Felidae only
Mycoplasma felis						
Normal commensals of conjunctiva and upper respiratory tract, therefore opportunistic secondary invaders? May be a primary pathogen in lower respiratory tract disease. Transmission route currently unclear	No information available	Reliably killed by QACs	None	Uncertain	Low risk but at least one case of septic arthritis in an immunosuppressed person documented (Greene, 2012)	Felidae only

15.8 (continued) Key features of the main pathogens involved in FURTD.

(Data from Browning, 2004; Coyne et al., 2006; Gaskell et al., 2007; Gruffydd-Jones et al., 2009; Miller and Zawistowski, 2011; Advisory Board on Cat Diseases, 2014; International Cat Care; Koret Shelter Medicine Program)

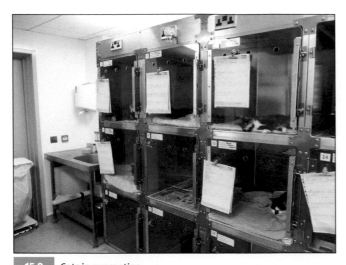

15.9 Cats in quarantine.

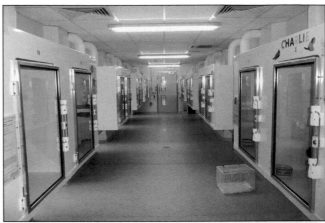

15.11 Cat accommodation block with an impervious, easy-to-clean floor.

Enrichment

Regular positive daily interactions with people (e.g. play, grooming, stroking) for socialized cats (but not for those fearful of humans) should be a daily part of shelter life. Such contact inevitably increases the risk of transmission of diseases between cats, and this risk must be considered. Precautions should be taken to minimize disease spread, for example, by the use of disposable gloves when touching cats, or by each member of staff interacting with only a consistent, small number of healthy cats. Placing food in puzzle toys or cardboard boxes is a good form of enrichment. Cats may also benefit from being able to see their surroundings (Figure 15.10). It is common for shelters to use feline facial pheromones to provide a sense of well-being, and this practice is recommended by some authors (Beck, 2013; see also QRG 19.8).

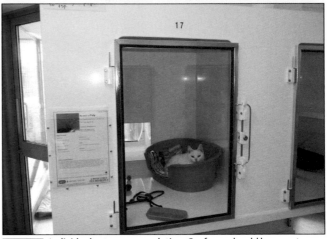

15.12 Individual cat accommodation. Surfaces should be easy to clean.

adequate to enable there to be 60 cm of triangulated distance between the litter tray, water and food bowls (Newbury *et al.*, 2010) (see also Chapter 10).

Cats showing signs of FURTD should be immediately isolated, preferably in a building separate from other accommodation areas, including the quarantine area (Figure 15.13). Sneeze barriers between pens can help reduce droplet transmission of pathogens (Figure 15.14).

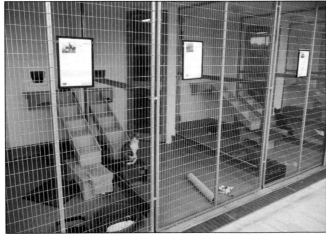

15.10 Cats may benefit from access to runs where they can see the outside environment.

Shelter design and accommodation

Consideration should be given to having separate housing for different groups of cats according to their disease susceptibility. Therefore, kittens should ideally be housed away from the adult population, and nursing queens would ideally be fostered with their kittens and not kept within the shelter for any longer than is necessary, due to the vulnerability of young kittens to infection. Ideally, surfaces in the cattery should be impervious and easy to clean (Figures 15.11 and 15.12), and pen sizes should be

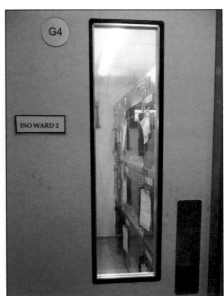

15.13 Shelters should be able to isolate cats showing signs of infectious disease in a separate accommodation area, away from other groups of cats.

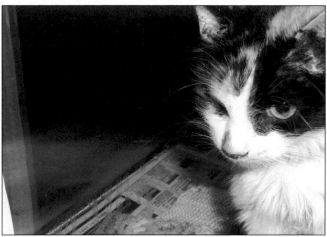

15.14 Sneeze barriers (e.g. made of glass or Perspex®) can help to reduce droplet transmission of pathogens.

Biosecurity

For more in-depth coverage of the various aspects of bio-security in shelters, see Chapter 9.

Traffic patterns and good husbandry practice

Daily feeding and cleaning should be conducted in an order such that the healthiest, most vulnerable groups are dealt with first, followed by those at lower risk of contracting infection, and proceeding finally to those known to be infected (Figure 15.15). Ideally, on any given day, staff working in the isolation area should not work in other feline accommodation areas. Where staffing is insufficient for this to be feasible, protective personal equipment (PPE) (gloves, aprons, overboots, etc.) should be changed when moving from one area to another.

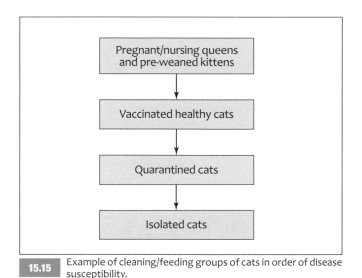

15.15 Example of cleaning/feeding groups of cats in order of disease susceptibility.

Staff hygiene and cleaning protocols

Use of PPE is one weapon in the armoury of disease transmission control. However, it acts only as a temporary physical barrier and does not eliminate infective organisms, and should not be relied upon as the sole method of transmission control.

The shelter should have a written cleaning and disinfection protocol, which all staff are familiar with and have been trained in.

Sections to include in a shelter cleaning and disinfection protocol

- Instructions regarding the use of PPE
- Directions for safe and correct mixing of chemicals (detergents, disinfectants), including dilution rates for given scenarios in accordance with manufacturers' recommendations
- Step-by-step instructions for cleaning and disinfection procedures, including recommended contact times
- Frequency of cleaning for different areas and equipment
- Instructions regarding disinfection of the cleaning equipment itself

Disinfection

It is important to remove all organic matter from surfaces with detergent before disinfecting them. FCV is particularly difficult to inactivate, so a disinfectant with manufacturer's claims to be effective against non-enveloped viruses should be used (with attention to the correct dilution and contact time) (see Figure 15.8 and QRG 9.1).

Separate cleaning equipment

Different areas should have separate cleaning equipment, ideally colour coded by area; a minimum requirement is separate equipment for the isolation facilities (see Chapter 9).

Barrier nursing

Hand hygiene is extremely important in any biosecurity programme (Figure 15.16). Staff should receive regular training in hand hygiene. Handwashing supplies should be kept topped up. Hands should be washed in between handling each cat and each litter tray. Alcohol gel sanitizers are useful but are no replacement for strict hand hygiene. The use of disposable gloves should be considered, especially with those cats likely to be most infectious.

Concurrent medications

Corticosteroid treatment may induce shedding of FHV-1 in approximately 70% of cats, so these medicines should be used judiciously in the shelter setting (Gaskell *et al.*, 2007).

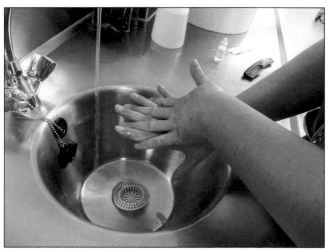

15.16 Hand hygiene is an essential part of any biosecurity programme.

Temperature and ventilation

The ambient temperature should be kept at between 15.5 and 26.6°C, but additional measures may need to be taken to provide extra warmth or cooling where indicated (Newbury et al., 2010). Good air quality is important in reducing pollutant gases, such as ammonia, airborne pathogens and heat. There should be a minimum of 10–12 air exchanges per hour (Möstl et al., 2013; see also Chapter 10).

Outbreak management

It is useful to have an outbreak management plan in place to provide guidelines for shelter veterinary surgeons and staff to help them effectively investigate and manage an outbreak of infectious disease.

Case definition

An important term to understand is 'case definition'. This is a set of epidemiological criteria enabling the clinician to decide whether or not an individual has the disease in question. The case definition can include confirmed and suspected cases, depending on how restrictive the clinician wants to make the criteria. So, for example, a cat may be judged to have FURTD if it has some or all of the following clinical signs: ocular or nasal discharge, sneezing with or without nasal congestion, coughing, dyspnoea, blepharospasm, lingual ulceration and keratitis. As these signs are strongly suggestive of FURTD, the case definition may not need to include a positive test result for one of the causative agents. However, if the veterinary surgeon was investigating a potential outbreak of a more unusual specific causative agent, such as VS-FCV, they may include only cases confirmed by diagnostic testing. The tighter the criteria for case definition, the higher the potential for missing mild cases. Conversely, the looser the criteria, the higher the likelihood of identifying all positive cases – but, at the same time, the higher the likelihood of identifying false-positive cases that are then treated in the same way as infected cases and isolated. This may have far-reaching consequences if the shelter has a policy of euthanasing cats with FURTD at times when resources are stretched or the shelter is at capacity.

Data collection and record-keeping

It can be useful to plot the number of animals affected in a population over time to produce an 'epidemic curve' (Figure 15.17) (see also Chapter 7 for more information on the use of shelter metrics in outbreaks of disease). Analyses of such data will indicate whether the level of infectious respiratory disease is changing. When managing a specific outbreak, a spreadsheet capturing data on 'who', 'what', 'where' and 'when' can be used alongside an epidemic curve and may potentially help to trace the source of infection and enable triggers for specific actions to control the outbreak. Obtaining a comprehensive history, for example, by asking the questions detailed in Figure 15.2, will guide the clinician as to the possible origin of the outbreak and its progression (see Chapter 7).

Communication

During an outbreak, shelter staff and volunteers should be updated daily on any new developments. This also has the advantage of enabling deployment of workers and task allocation on a daily basis. Consideration should be given to informing other interested parties of the potential or actual outbreak, including recent adopters and any other establishments where animals have been transferred to and from the shelter.

When to test

It may not be necessary to perform diagnostic tests to successfully contain and manage an outbreak of FURTD. Screening every cat within a shelter is clearly not pragmatic or cost-effective and will almost certainly detect carriers that may not be clinically relevant to the current outbreak. It would be prudent to consider diagnostic tests where symptoms deviate from the expected (e.g. there are lower respiratory tract signs, or signs suggestive of VS-FCV, such as ulcerative dermatitis and cutaneous oedema) or in situations where it is thought that a change in the vaccination plan is warranted – for example, whether or not to vaccinate against C. felis or B. bronchiseptica. Where antibacterial treatment is instigated, especially for large numbers of animals or for prolonged periods, this should be informed by diagnosing the infection and, when appropriate, assessing resistance of the pathogen to antibacterial agents.

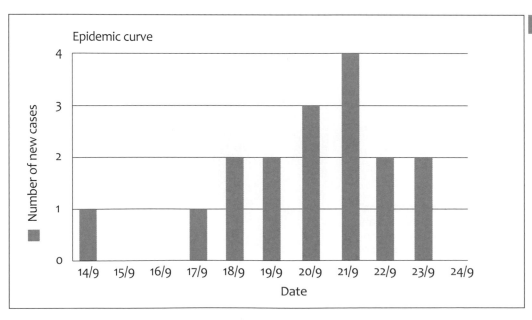

15.17 Example of an epidemic curve.

Control measures

Cats diagnosed or showing signs of FURTD should be isolated as soon as possible to protect the rest of the population from infection. The subpopulation the identified individual has come from will contain cats that may have been exposed and be at risk, depending on factors, such as biosecurity and vaccination, age and health status. If biosecurity is poor, the risk may extend to cats in other parts of the shelter too. An assessment needs to be conducted to identify cats that have been exposed to the disease and are, thus, at risk, and so that measures can be taken to monitor and, if possible, quarantine them until the risk has passed. In cases of FURTD, vaccination is no guarantee of protection, especially when the time between vaccination and exposure is as short as it often is in a rescue shelter. Therefore, it cannot be assumed that a vaccinated cat is 'safe' and does not need quarantining. It is important to remember also that vaccination does not prevent infection with either FHV-1 or FCV, and so vaccinated cats can still shed these viruses and be infectious.

Role of the incubation period in determining when a cat may be removed from quarantine

The duration of quarantine (the physical separation of animals that may have been exposed to a contagious disease but are not currently displaying clinical signs (Gingrich and Lappin, 2013)) needs to be balanced with, among other things, the risk of infection associated with prolonging a cat's stay in the shelter. If possible, cats that are quarantined should not be returned to the general population until the maximum incubation period for the disease has passed with no sign of infection; a period of 14 days will include the incubation period for FHV-1, FCV and *M. felis*. If necessary, shorter periods in quarantine of approximately 5–7 days would still capture a significant number of cases (see also Chapters 9 and 10 for more information on the use of quarantine).

Reintroduction of cats that have recovered from FURTD into the main population

Whether it is possible to reintroduce cats that have recovered from FURTD will depend on the biosecurity of the main population. Recovered cats will shed virus for variable amounts of time after infection, although most likely at lower levels than when they were showing clinical signs of FURTD. Attention to good hygiene measures is essential in preventing the spread of infectious agents in such circumstances.

New intake

New admissions to the shelter should be admitted into a 'clean' area separate from quarantined or isolated cats (Figure 15.18). If such a clean area cannot be created, consideration should be given to a temporary cessation of cat intakes until the outbreak has resolved. Clean areas should be clearly marked and staff should not move between clean and infected areas unless absolutely necessary, and then only after a change of PPE. Dedicated equipment should be provided for each area.

Vaccination as close as possible to the time of admission with an MLV vaccine becomes even more pertinent during an outbreak of FURTD. Consideration may be given to using an intranasal preparation, if available, because of the earlier onset of immunity these vaccines confer. In addition, the age at which kittens are first vaccinated may

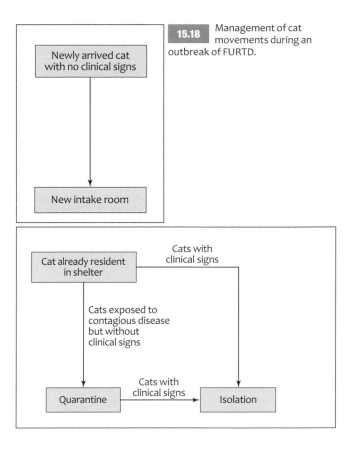

15.18 Management of cat movements during an outbreak of FURTD.

Newly arrived cat with no clinical signs → New intake room

Cat already resident in shelter → Cats with clinical signs → Isolation

Cats exposed to contagious disease but without clinical signs → Quarantine → Cats with clinical signs → Isolation

be reduced at such times to 4 weeks of age and the vaccine interval reduced to every 2 weeks (Möstl *et al.*, 2013) (note that this is off-licence vaccine use).

FCV-associated virulent systemic disease

VS-FCV disease was first described in the USA; more recent reports have described a similar syndrome in other countries, including the UK, Italy and Germany. The incubation period for VS-FCV can vary from 1 to 12 days. The pathogenesis of this clinical syndrome is not fully understood, but it is thought that it may include viral evolution and other factors, such as overcrowding of individuals and the endemic presence of FCV (Pesavento and Murphy, 2014). Infection with hypervirulent strains of FCV can lead to a febrile syndrome with high mortality. Clinical signs may include, but are not limited to, subcutaneous oedema, facial, mouth and skin ulcers, pneumonia, organ necrosis, lameness and jaundice. Disease is usually worse in adult cats than in kittens and can affect both vaccinated and unvaccinated animals. Any affected cats should be immediately isolated. VS-FCV is rare, but outbreaks can be difficult to manage so it may be necessary to seek expert advice.

References and further reading

Advisory Board on Cat Diseases (2014) *Bordetella bronchiseptica* infection. www.abcdcatsvets.org/wp-content/uploads/2015/06/ABCD_Fact_Sheet-Bordetella.pdf

Beck A (2013) Use of pheromones to reduce stress in sheltered cats. *Journal of Feline Medicine and Surgery* **15**, 829–830

Browning GF (2004) Is *Chlamydophila felis* a significant zoonotic pathogen? *Australian Veterinary Journal* **82**, 695–696

Coyne KP, Edwards D, Radford AD *et al.* (2007) Longitudinal molecular epidemiological analysis of feline calicivirus infection in an animal shelter: a model for investigating calicivirus transmission within high-density, high-turnover populations. *Journal of Clinical Microbiology* **45**, 3239–3244

Coyne KP, Jones BR, Kipar A *et al.* (2006) Lethal outbreak of disease associated with feline calicivirus infection in cats. *Veterinary Record* **158**, 544–550

Dean R, Harley R, Helps C *et al.* (2005) Use of quantitative real-time PCR to monitor the response of *Chlamydophila felis* infection to doxycycline treatment. *Journal of Clinical Microbiology* **43**, 1858–1864

Di Martino B, Di Rocco C, Ceci C and Marsilio F (2009) Characterization of a strain of feline calicivirus isolated from a dog faecal sample. *Veterinary Microbiology* **139**, 52–57

Dinnage JD, Scarlett JM and Richards JR (2009) Descriptive epidemiology of feline upper respiratory tract disease in an animal shelter. *Journal of Feline Medicine and Surgery* **11**, 816–825

Egberink H, Addie D, Belák S *et al.* (2009) *Bordetella bronchiseptica* infection in cats: ABCD guidelines on prevention and management. *Journal of Feline Medicine and Surgery* **11**, 610–614

Foster SF and Martin P (2011) Lower respiratory tract infections in cats: reaching beyond empirical therapy. *Journal of Feline Medicine and Surgery* **13**, 313–332

Gaskell R, Dawson S, Radford AD and Thiry E (2007) Feline herpesvirus. *Veterinary Research* **38**, 337–354

Gent G (2013) How to approach the red eye. *Companion* **November**, 14–19

Gingrich E and Lappin M (2013) Practical overview of common infectious disease agents. In: *Shelter Medicine for Veterinarians and Staff, 2nd edn*, ed. L Millar and S Zawistowski, pp. 297–328. Wiley-Blackwell, Ames

Greene C (2011) *Infectious Diseases of the Dog and Cat, 4th edn*. Elsevier Saunders, St Louis

Gruffydd-Jones T, Addie D, Belák S *et al.* (2009) *Chlamydophila felis* infection. ABCD guidelines on prevention and management. *Journal of Feline Medicine and Surgery* **11**, 605–609

Lee-Fowler T (2014) Feline respiratory disease: what is the role of *Mycoplasma* species? *Journal of Feline Medicine and Surgery* **16**, 563–571

Miller L and Zawistowski L (eds) (2013) *Shelter Medicine for Veterinarians and Staff, 2nd edn*. Wiley-Blackwell, Ames, Iowa

Möstl K, Egberink H, Addie A *et al.* (2013) Prevention of infectious diseases in cat shelters: ABCD guidelines. *Journal of Feline Medicine and Surgery* **15**, 546–554

Newbury S, Blinn MK, Bushby PA *et al.* (2010) Guidelines for standards of care in animal shelters. Association of Shelter Veterinarians. www.sheltervet.org/assets/docs/shelter-standards-oct2011-wforward.pdf

O'Quin J (2013) Outbreak management. In: *Shelter Medicine for Veterinarians and Staff, 2nd edn*, ed. L Miller and S Zawistowski, pp. 349–366. Wiley-Blackwell, Ames, Iowa

Pesavento PA and Murphy BG (2014) Common and emerging infectious disease in the animal shelter. *Veterinary Pathology* **51**, 478–491

Povey RC and Johnson RH (1970) Observations on the epidemiology and control of viral respiratory disease in cats. *Journal of Small Animal Practice* **11**, 485–494

Radford AD, Addie D, Belák S *et al.* (2009) Feline calicivirus infection: ABCD guidelines on prevention and management. *Journal of Feline Medicine and Surgery* **11**, 556–564

Ramsey I (2014) *BSAVA Small Animal Formulary, 8th edn*. BSAVA Publications, Gloucester

Reed N and Gunn-Moore D (2012) Nasopharyngeal disease in cats: 2. Specific conditions and their management. *Journal of Feline Medicine and Surgery* **14**, 317–326

SAMSoc and BSAVA (2011) Are you PROTECTing your antibacterials? Special edition. *Companion* **October**, 1–32

Scarlett JM (2009) Feline upper respiratory disease. In: *Infectious Disease Management in Animal Shelters*, ed. L Miller and K Hurley, pp. 125–146. Wiley-Blackwell, Ames, Iowa

Scherk MA, Ford RB, Gaskell RM *et al.* (2013) 2013 AAFP Feline Vaccination Advisory Panel Report. *Journal of Feline Medicine and Surgery* **15**, 785–808

Southerden P and Gorrel C (2007) Treatment of a case of refractory feline chronic gingivostomatitis with feline recombinant interferon omega. *Journal of Small Animal Practice* **48**, 104–106

Sparkes AH, Caney SMA, Sturgess CP and Gruffydd-Jones TJ (1999) The clinical efficacy of topical and systemic therapy for the treatment of feline ocular chlamydiosis. *Journal of Feline Medicine and Surgery* **1**, 31–35

Spindel M (2013) Strategies for management of infectious diseases in a shelter. In: *Shelter Medicine for Veterinarians and Staff, 2nd edn*, ed. L Miller and S Zawistowski, pp. 281–287. Wiley-Blackwell, Ames, Iowa

Steneroden K (2013) Sanitation. In: *Shelter Medicine for Veterinarians and Staff, 2nd edn*, ed. L Miller and S Zawistowski, pp. 37–48. Wiley-Blackwell, Ames, Iowa

Thiry E, Addie D, Belák S *et al.* (2009) Feline herpesvirus infection. ABCD guidelines on prevention and management. *Journal of Feline Medicine and Surgery* **11**, 547–555

Useful websites

Advisory Board on Cat Diseases:
www.abcdcatsvets.org

International Cat Care:
http://www.icatcare.org/

Koret Shelter Medicine Program:
http://www.sheltermedicine.com/

PROTECT website:
www.bsava.com/Resources/PROTECT/PROTECT.aspx

QRG 15.1: Rehoming a snotty cat
by Rebecca Elmore and Rachel Dean

Feline upper respiratory tract disease (FURTD), or 'cat 'flu', is endemic in shelter cat populations. Therefore, it can be assumed that any cat rehomed from a shelter may have had a clinical or subclinical infection with one of the causative agents. In clinical infections, the causative agent(s) is often undiagnosed due to cost and time constraints within the shelter. Therefore, it might be more appropriate to consider FURTD, or the 'snotty cat', in general terms:

* When and whether to rehome
* Advising prospective owners
* Follow-up care after rehoming.

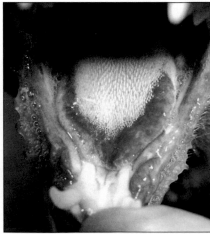
Lingual ulceration typical of FCV infection. FCV = feline calicivirus

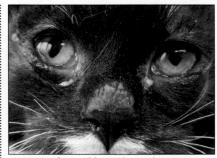
FURTD is often milder with FCV than FHV infection but the clinical signs are not pathognomonic. FCV = feline calicivirus; FHV = feline herpes virus.

QRG 15.1 *continued*

When and whether to rehome

It is a challenge to decide when to rehome a cat that is currently or has previously been 'snotty'. Most new adopters generally prefer to choose a healthy cat, so that they can bond with their new pet without the stress of administering medication and potentially having repeated veterinary appointments. However, cats with a current or prior history of FURTD pose an increased disease risk to the other cats at the shelter, and, therefore, expediting their rehoming can decrease the risk of transmission within the shelter. Additionally, space in the shelter is very often limited, so the sooner these cats can be offered for rehoming and adopted the better. When considering the welfare of the affected cat, the stress of changing environment to a new home may be offset to an extent by the benefits of leaving the shelter environment, although this will depend greatly on the individual.

Ideally, affected cats should be put up for adoption only once all severe clinical signs have gone and medication has been stopped, but this is not always practical, and, in some circumstances, rehoming cats with some clinical signs of FURTD may be appropriate. A shelter policy regarding the rehoming of cats with FURTD should depend on the veterinary and nursing care available at the shelter. However, in general, cats with severe clinical signs, anorexia and pyrexia should be withheld from rehoming until signs have largely resolved; this is particularly the case for young kittens.

As FURTD is commonly regarded as multifactorial, it is often unnecessary to perform diagnostic tests. However, if the causative agent has been identified, it may be possible to provide targeted treatment (see main chapter). If the pathogen is known, it is possible to give information about the possible disease progression, for example:

- Recurrence of keratitis and rhinitis with feline herpesvirus (FHV)
- Prolonged shedding of feline calicivirus (FCV)
- Treatment can be curative if given correctly for *Chlamydia felis*.

Even where definitive diagnosis is not practical, clinical signs can sometimes lead to a presumptive diagnosis, and this can help with management advice, for example:

- Oral ulceration can be associated with FCV
- Severe ocular signs with corneal lesions are often associated with FHV
- Conjunctivitis with no other signs may indicate *C. felis* or *Mycoplasma* spp.

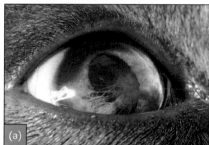
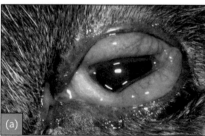

Clinical signs typical of FHV infection. (a) Anterior synechiae; (b) facial lesions.
(b, © Rachel Dean)

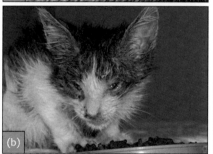
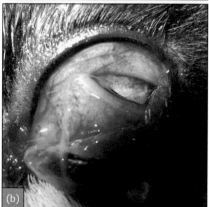

C. felis infection can cause (a) chemosis in the early stages and (b) chronic conjunctivitis that can last for months.
(a, © Rachel Dean)

Advising prospective owners

The advice given to new owners is vital to provide a smooth transition from the shelter to the home. It is equally important that veterinary surgeons (veterinarians) treating cats after rehoming have a good understanding of the challenges of managing cats in large numbers, so a 'blame culture' does not evolve.

It is essential to provide clear advice to prospective owners and obtain their informed consent when rehoming a FURTD-affected animal. Important points to explain include:

- Cats with clinical signs or a recent history of FURTD may be potentially infectious for long periods, or even lifelong
- Many cats without clinical signs of FURTD also carry infectious agents that can cause the disease
- Stress is a key factor that determines whether or not signs of disease are seen
- Signs may flare up again following rehoming, as this is a stressful event
- If there are other cats in the household, transmission of infection may occur
- However, other cats in the household may already be infected – and the stress of living with a new cat could trigger signs of FURTD in either or both animals.

Not all new owners will be experienced in treating cats, and so if the cat is rehomed while receiving treatment, it is important to ensure that the new owners will be able to administer all medication and that they will have the cat checked (if considered appropriate) at the end of the course. It is also important to provide the contact details of the veterinary surgeon who has treated the cat at the shelter, so clinical information can be exchanged with the veterinary practice where the cat is registered by the new owners. This should ensure continuity of care for the current episode of disease, as well as ensuring that future clinical decisions that might be affected by the cat's history of FURTD can be made appropriately (e.g. care with glucocorticoids in a potentially FHV-infected cat).

QRG 15.1 *continued*

Any cats owned by the prospective adopter must be fully vaccinated prior to the arrival of the new shelter cat. It must be explained to the new owner that vaccination does not prevent infection or development of a carrier state of any FURTD pathogen, but will reduce the severity and duration of the disease (see Chapters 8 and 11).

Follow-up care after rehoming

To veterinary staff and shelter workers, FURTD is an unwelcome but familiar part of life. To the prospective adopter, it can be a much more worrying experience. By preparing the new owner for dealing with their cat's recovery, the experience can be made much more positive. Shelters have various strategies for follow-up care, depending on the facilities available. These might range from a simple follow-up telephone call to a repeat consultation after rehoming, especially when animals are sent home on treatment. Advice sheets may be helpful, as the large amount of information given at rehoming makes it difficult for owners to retain it all.

In summary, although organizations struggle to minimize the extent of FURTD, it will inevitably occur in cat shelters. Due to the propensity for cats to have subclinical infections, which recrudesce under stress, it is inevitable that signs of FURTD will be seen in a proportion of cats around the time of rehoming. Each shelter will come up with a policy to suit its own facilities and needs. By gaining informed consent and preparing the new owner's expectations, the chances of a successful adoption can be maximized, even for cats showing some signs of FURTD.

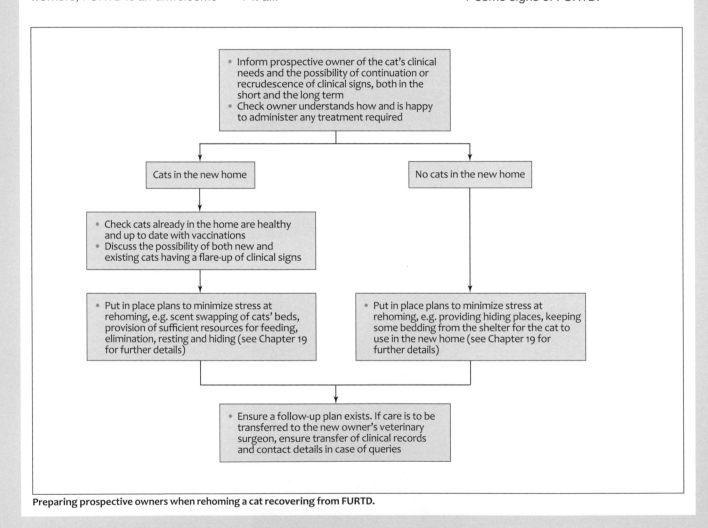

Preparing prospective owners when rehoming a cat recovering from FURTD.

Chapter 16

Skin diseases in shelter animals

Nathalie Dowgray and Steve Shaw

Skin disease is common in cats and dogs. The chronic nature and financial cost of managing dermatological conditions may result in animals with these diseases being more likely to be relinquished for rehoming, abandoned, or even being considered for euthanasia. Adverse comments about an alopecic animal or the difficulties in handling associated with ear disease leading to pain and aggressive behaviour may also add to this trend. However, many dermatological conditions are very amenable to diagnosis and effective treatment within the shelter without marked expense. Some larger shelters may have a small laboratory equipped with a usable microscope, which will further aid the speed of diagnosis and reduce costs. Prompt identification of infectious, contagious or zoonotic conditions (see QRG 16.1) is key to preventing spread within the shelter and to protect the shelter's public reputation. The identification of the disease will determine the prognosis, which, in turn, will indicate the treatment plan and the ongoing financial commitment, either for the shelter or the person who adopts the animal.

This chapter will describe dermatological problems of particular relevance in the shelter setting. Different organizations will have different policies with regard to treating and rehoming animals with a chronic condition. Charities that operate as 'no-kill' shelters or sanctuaries may invest more money in single animals and, in such a situation, decision-making for a veterinary surgeon (veterinarian) will be more similar to that with a private client. In contrast, organizations that operate as open-intake shelters are under pressure to accept animals and may not have the resources to commit to prolonged treatment courses for chronic conditions such as demodicosis or dermatophytosis, and identification of these conditions may result in euthanasia.

Procedures on admittance to the shelter

Procedures for animals being admitted into the shelter should include a thorough evaluation for skin disease. This is important to ensure not only that the animal receives appropriate ectoparasite treatment, but also that contagious diseases such as dermatophytosis are recognized to prevent outbreaks from occurring. The condition of the skin and fur will also give pointers to the general health of the animal. Where possible, the animal's veterinary and domestic history should be evaluated. In some circumstances, animals from the same source will have already been diagnosed with contagious disease or may have received prophylactic treatment, and knowledge of this history may affect how other animals are dealt with on admission.

The skin should be examined thoroughly under bright light. Shelter staff should be trained to recognize the significance of skin lesions and to bring them to veterinary attention. Educating lay staff can be achieved by having them spend time with the attending veterinary surgeon at the shelter during visits; this has proved to be a valuable way to educate people to ensure a consistent and effective approach. Findings should be recorded using written descriptions, lesion maps and, ideally, photographs. Describing the appearance and distribution of lesions adequately will ensure that all veterinary and ancillary staff will recognize improvement and deterioration over time, as well as directing the diagnosis. Any skin masses should be palpated and their size and location recorded; fine-needle aspirates or biopsy samples can be considered. Detailed discussion of dermal masses is outside the scope of this chapter, and readers are referred to the *BSAVA Manual of Canine and Feline Dermatology* for more information.

There are a number of simple clinical tests that can easily be performed at the initial veterinary examination. The wet paper test, coat brushings and Wood's lamp evaluation should be performed on all cases, although operators should understand the limitations of these techniques and appropriate quarantine procedures should be in place for new entrants. Skin scrapings, cytology and earwax examination should be performed as required, depending on the skin lesions that are present. The pinnal-pedal reflex and itch-scratch reflex may indicate pruritus. The most useful clinical tests are summarized in Figure 16.1.

As many ectoparasitic infestations cannot be ruled out on clinical examination alone, where possible, animals should be treated on arrival at the shelter and then regularly while in the shelter's care to reduce environmental contamination and transmission to other animals and to shelter workers. External parasites play a large role in dermatological diseases seen in many shelters, with fleas being the most common cause of problems. Authorized Veterinary Medicine – General Sales List (AVM-GSL) products that act quickly, such as nitenpyram, are well tolerated and can be given at the intake check to start the process of maintaining a flea-free shelter community.

Appropriate treatment for fleas should be the mainstay of the shelter's parasite prevention policy. If funds permit, treatments for other ectoparasites can be applied routinely, or alternatively on a case-by-case basis.

Test	Possible diagnoses	Technique
Wet paper test (WPT)	Fleas	Rub debris from the coat on to wetted paper and observe for the haemorrhagic colour of flea faeces. The WPT has poor sensitivity but is quick and cheap to perform
Coat brushings and microscopic examination	Fleas Lice *Cheyletiella* spp.	Use a comb to brush the coat; collect skin debris on folded paper and examine by eye or mounted in liquid paraffin for microscopy
Superficial skin scrapings	*Demodex* spp. (*D. canis, D. gatoi*)	Using a blunted scalpel blade, collect surface scale and crusts, and mount in liquid paraffin for microscopy
Deep skin scrapings	Scabies *Demodex* spp. (*D. canis, D cati, D. injai*)	Using a blunted scalpel blade, collect skin scales, scale and crusts, ensuring that there is capillary ooze, and mount in liquid paraffin for microscopy
Earwax examination	*Otodectes cynotis* *Demodex canis*	Mix the wax with liquid paraffin gently to avoid bubbles and mount in liquid paraffin for microscopy
Skin surface cytology	*Demodex* spp. Bacterial infection *Malassezia* infection	Using a glass slide, or (often better) clear adhesive tape, press hard on to the affected area. Stain with routine haematology stains
Pustule cytology	Bacterial infection Pemphigus foliaceus	Breach the pustule with a needle and then smear the pus carefully on to a slide. The presence of intracellular cocci is consistent with pyoderma. The presence of large numbers of acantholytic keratinocytes is typical of pemphigus foliaceus
Hair plucks	Trichography	Pluck hairs for microscopy to examine the ends of the hairs, to determine the presence or absence of trauma and to determine the stage of growth
	Demodex canis	Hair plucks for *Demodex* can be very useful for the feet, especially in chronic cases
	Dermatophytosis	Select broken hairs (possibly those shown to fluoresce under Wood's lamp illumination). Look for broken hair structure, hyphae and spores under microscopy
Wood's lamp	Dermatophytosis	Working in a darkened room, illuminate the affected area with a Wood's lamp that has been warmed up for sufficient time to be effective. Specific test (when properly conducted) for around 50% of *Microsporum canis* only
Scabies serology	Canine scabies	Submit serum for scabies-specific immunoglobulin G (IgG) serology. Sensitivity is high, specificity is reduced by cross-reactivity to house dust mites. Only useful 4–5 weeks after initial infection

16.1 Common clinical tests for the dermatology case.

Figures 16.2 and 16.3 list products commonly available in the UK and their uses. Some are AVM-GSL, while many others are classified as Prescription-Only Medicine – Veterinarian (POM-V) and need to be dispensed by a veterinary surgeon. Well thought out entry procedures, using a suitable product, will reduce the likelihood of flea infestation becoming established in the shelter. In shelters where animals stay for more than a brief period, further prophylactic treatment should be used as necessary (see Chapter 11).

Product	Fleas	Ear mites	Lice	Ticks	Demodex
Fipronil	Y	N	Y	Y	N
Imidacloprid	Y	N	N	N	N
Indoxacarb	Y	N	N	N	N
Selamectin	Y	Y	Y	N	N
Imidacloprid + moxidectin	Y	Y	N	N	N
Spinosad	Y	N	N	N	N
Nitenpyram	Y	N	N	N	N
Fipronil + (S)-methoprene + eprinomectin + praziquantel	Y	N	Y	Y	N
Selamectin + sarolaner	Y	Y	Y	N	?
Fluralaner	Y	(Y)	(Y)	Y	?

16.2 Common ectoparasite treatments for cats.

Product	Fleas	Sarcoptes	Lice	Ticks	Demodex
Amitraz	N	Y	N	Y	Y
Fipronil[a]	Y	N	Y	Y	N
Imidacloprid	Y	N	Y	N	N
Fluralaner[b]	Y	(Y)	Y	Y	(Y)
Afoxolaner[b]	Y	(Y)	Y	Y	(Y)
Sarolaner[b]	Y	Y	Y	Y	Y
Indoxacarb	Y	N	N	N	N
Selamectin	Y	Y	Y	N	N
Imidacloprid + moxidectin	Y	Y	Y	N	Y
Spinosad	Y	N	N	N	N
Nitenpyram	Y	N	N	N	N

16.3 Common ectoparasite treatments for dogs. [a] Fipronil may be useful in young puppies with scabies as it can be used at an early age. [b] Drugs in the isoxazoline group have been shown to be useful for a number of mite infections, including demodicosis and scabies. Those without marketing authorization at the time of writing are indicated by the use of brackets.

Fleas

The clinical signs of flea infestation vary depending on the number of fleas, the hypersensitivity response and the general condition of the animal. In dogs, cutaneous signs usually affect the caudal half of the animal, whereas in cats all four feline cutaneous reaction patterns (see the section on Allergy later in this chapter) can be seen. However, asymmetric lesions on the tail or caudal dorsum are more indicative of feline flea allergy than other allergic skin diseases. Heavy flea burdens can be fatal in young puppies and kittens, and fleas may transmit a variety of pathogens and parasites, including tapeworm (e.g. *Dipylidium caninum*) and *Bartonella* spp., in dogs and cats, as well as *Bartonella henselae*, a potential zoonosis causing 'cat scratch fever' in humans.

Treatment for fleas needs, in many circumstances, to encompass not only the animal but the environment. To provide a flea-free environment after infestation, all animals must be treated with a flea adulticide. The environment should be treated by cleaning and then application of an environmental insecticide (usually a permethrin combined with an insect growth regulator such as (*S*)-methoprene). Grass runs and other communal areas pose a particular problem in shelters; hence, it is advised that all animals are treated before entering these areas. More clinical areas are much easier to keep clean. Environmental considerations are also important where animals are fostered in domestic homes.

There are currently a large number of different products available for flea control (see Figures 16.2 and 16.3), and the individual circumstances and available funds will dictate the best product. Whatever the products used, the implementation of a strict flea treatment policy is essential for successful control (see Chapter 11).

Other common parasitic diseases

Sarcoptes scabiei, *Cheyletiella* spp., *Otodectes cynotis* and lice are contagious and commonly associated with pruritic disease. A novel *Demodex* species in cats (*D. gatoi*) is also contagious and may be associated with pruritus. The *Demodex* species *D. canis*, *D. injai* and *D. cati* are not contagious and pruritus is dependent on the degree of secondary infection.

Canine scabies

Scabies due to *Sarcoptes scabiei* var. *canis* is a common contagious disease of dogs and has the potential to be zoonotic. Infection is acquired from direct or indirect contact with affected animals. Due to the tunnelling nature of the mite, the primary lesion is a papule, with pruritus due to hypersensitivity following soon after. The ear margins, elbows and hocks are often affected, whereas it is rare to see disease affecting the plantar/palmar surface of the feet (Figure 16.4).

Diagnosis is made on the basis of clinical signs, finding eggs, faeces or mites on skin scrapings (Figure 16.5), or by serology. Treatment with topical selamectin, moxidectin/imidacloprid, amitraz and oral sarolaner is licensed in the UK for use in scabies. All four treatments are efficacious, but topical products must be applied carefully to ensure effectiveness. Following treatment, affected dogs can be mixed after 3–4 weeks, often after the second treatment when using spot-on treatments. Environmental treatment may be required in cooler climates. Secondary bacterial and yeast infection needs to be addressed.

Cheyletiellosis

Cheyletiella spp. may affect both dogs and cats, causing a powdery white scale in some dogs and miliary dermatitis

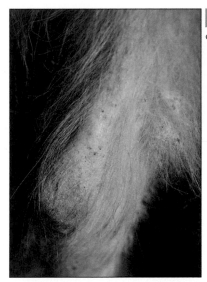

16.4 Alopecia, scale and papules in canine scabies.

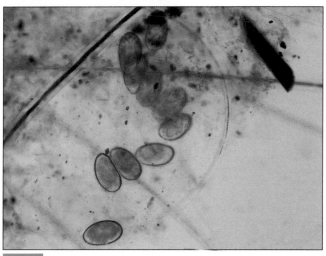

16.5 Eggs of *Sarcoptes scabiei* in a skin scraping preparation.

and other manifestations of pruritus in cats. Young animals are often affected. Pruritus is variable. Cheyletiellosis is a zoonosis, with small crusted papules commonly seen in people who have handled affected animals. There are currently no licensed medications to treat cheyletiellosis, and a variety of topical acaricides and insecticides are used. The authors favour selamectin in cats; a variety of products can be used in dogs, including selamectin, fipronil and moxidectin/imidacloprid combinations. It is likely that the isoxazoline group of ectoparasite treatments will also be effective in cheyletiellosis.

Lice

Felicola subrostratus (in cats) and *Trichodectes canis* and *Linognathus setosus* (in dogs) are infrequent causes of disease in the UK. Lice cause truncal pruritus, particularly affecting the head and shoulders (Figure 16.6). In cats, large numbers of lice frequently indicate another problem that interferes with grooming, and clinical evaluation for musculoskeletal and systemic disease, including testing for feline immunodeficiency virus (FIV) and feline leukaemia virus (FeLV), is indicated. *Linognathus* spp. may be associated with anaemia due to blood loss in severe infections. Many topical spot-on treatments are effective and such treatments may be included in the shelter's entry policy.

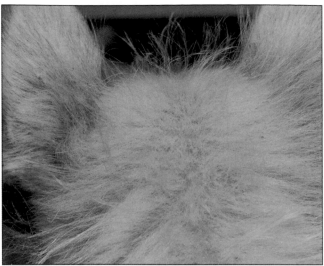

16.6 Alopecia and erythema around the head and neck of a dog due to lice.

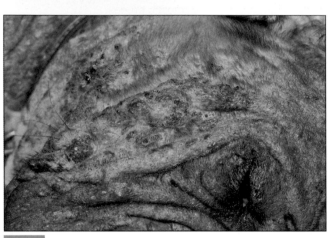

16.7 Comedones and pyoderma in a dog with demodicosis.

Otodectes cynotis

Otodectes cynotis is a common cause of otitis in young kittens and puppies. Typically, there is dark brown ear-wax and variable pruritus, and changes affecting the ears and surrounding skin. Diagnosis is often presumed when such wax is seen and there is a risk of misdiagnosis, but subclinical infestations may be difficult to recognize. Definitive diagnosis is made by demonstrating mites or eggs in wax or seeing mites on otoscopic examination. Many topical ear treatments are considered effective. Selamectin and moxidectin/imidacloprid are also highly effective and are essential in animals with ectopic infestations. The mite is highly contagious and can live off the animal for some time. Strict policies should be used to avoid introducing *O. cynotis* to animals grouped in the shelter (see Chapter 9).

16.8 Deep pyoderma due to demodicosis.

Canine demodicosis

Demodicosis due to *D. canis* is a significant problem in shelter dogs. The burden of treatment can be large in terms of veterinary costs and can also require considerable staffing to perform baths and other treatments. There are three common clinical syndromes associated with *D. canis*. The first, most common and least serious, is localized disease with a juvenile onset; alternatively, more generalized demodicosis can also occur in young animals, while a third group of animals develops demodicosis later in life. *D. canis* resides in the hair follicle causing a folliculitis resulting in the common features of bacterial infection and comedones (Figure 16.7). In some cases, the folliculitis extends to the underlying dermis, resulting in a deep pyoderma (Figure 16.8).

Common clinical syndromes

Localized juvenile-onset demodicosis

In localized juvenile-onset demodicosis (LJD), small patches of alopecia are seen with variable scale and come-done formation, often affecting the face, legs and chest. The disease represents an imbalance between host immunity and an initially low level of infection with this commensal organism, which is transferred from the mother in the early postnatal period. The disease is seen in growing puppies and will most often self-cure. In some animals, a stressful event or medical problem may induce the appearance of disease. Treatment of secondary infection, using shampoos and, if necessary, antibiotics, should be given, but treatment with an acaricide is not required. Local therapy of LJD will not prevent the development of the generalized form.

Generalized juvenile-onset demodicosis

Generalized juvenile-onset demodicosis (GJD) is a more severe form of LJD, with increased numbers of patches of lesioned skin (>10) or large areas of involvement. Pedal demodicosis may be seen in isolation from other disease, but, due to the very poor rate of self-cure, should be considered a form of GJD.

Adult-onset demodicosis

Adult-onset demodicosis (AOD) is clinically similar to GJD, but is seen in older animals where immunosuppression has led to a breakdown of the host–parasite relationship. Possible causes include unmonitored chronic administration of steroids, lymphoma and naturally occurring hyperadrenocorticism. In older dogs received at the shelter with signs of generalized demodicosis it can be difficult to know the onset of disease, and chronic GJD and AOD are often indistinguishable clinically.

Treatments

Antimicrobial therapy

Most cases of generalized demodicosis require antimicrobial treatment and, where the topical acaricide amitraz is being used, deep or extensive superficial pyoderma should be treated before this acaricide is applied. The performance of topical acaricides will be improved when topical antimicrobial treatments are used to clean and degrease the skin surface.

Acaricidal treatment

There are only a small number of available licensed treatments for canine demodicosis. Amitraz is a volatile liquid that is diluted in water to between 250 and 500 ppm and used as a dip. Long-haired dogs should be clipped and, in most cases, this reveals a greater area of disease than was previously appreciated. The skin should then be degreased. Traditionally, shampoos containing benzoyl peroxide were used for this purpose; although these shampoos act as an effective degreasing agent, they cause irritation in some cases, and an alternative shampoo containing chlorhexidine is recommended. The liquid should be applied with careful attention paid to the manufacturer's instructions regarding issues, such as adequate ventilation and the use of personal protective equipment (PPE) to ensure adequate protection for the operator. Where many baths are being performed at one site, the protection of staff becomes a major consideration, and an appropriate health and safety protocol must be implemented.

Moxidectin/imidacloprid spot-on is also licensed in the UK for use in demodicosis. An application is made every 1–4 weeks. In the authors' experience, this treatment is not as effective as amitraz, but the product is considerably easier to use. The skin should be clean, dry and lesion-free at the point of application, and bathing, with or without antibiotic treatment, will be needed to treat secondary bacterial or yeast infections. Bathing should be timed carefully so as not to remove the spot-on treatment.

Treatments without marketing authorization

In animals that have shown a poor response to the therapies described above, or where adverse events have been noted, ivermectin, milbemycin and moxidectin may be considered for use 'off-licence'.

Milbemycin is used at 1–2 mg/kg administered orally q24h. Ivermectin is not licensed for use in dogs, and in Collies may cause severe neurological signs and death. Such signs may also be seen in non-Collie breeds, and so the dose of this product is often titrated up to the recommended dose of 200–600 µg/kg orally q24h over at least 2 weeks, with careful observation during that time. Veterinary staff may be under considerable pressure to use ivermectin in cases of demodicosis in shelters, as it is inexpensive and readily available, but a licensed product should be used first (Mueller, 2004; Mueller *et al.*, 2012). Recently, the isoxazoline group of parasiticides has proved useful in the treatment of canine demodicosis, and reports in the literature support the use of fluralaner, afoxolaner and sarolaner, although at the time of writing none of these agents has marketing authorization.

Judging the response to treatment

Clinical appearance is a useful indicator of the progress being made when treating demodicosis, but does not replace the need for skin scrapings. Deep skin scrapings taken from multiple sites should be used to assess the dog before treatment and then repeated to assess the response to treatment. When many eggs or larvae are seen, treatment is likely to be required for some time, whereas seeing only dead adults is a sign of improvement. Treatment should not be stopped until two sets of skin scrapings taken 2–3 weeks apart are negative, and in cases where there has been chronic disease a longer period between negative scrapings may be required. Skin scrapings should be supplemented by hair plucks and by ear examination. For many severely affected cases, scrapings are not warranted before 6 weeks of treatment. A small group of dogs will never be completely cured, and chronic therapy, often at a reduced dose, is needed. Depending on the shelter's policy, euthanasia may be appropriate in these cases.

To perform adequate skin scrapings, many dogs need to be sedated; if medetomidine is used as the sedative agent, there may be a cumulative effect with the recent administration of amitraz, and a reduced dose of medetomidine may be needed. The initial frequency of scrapes is difficult to gauge and should be based on the clinical improvement. Even when there is rapid improvement, scrapes should still be performed to assess the presence of *Demodex*, as antimicrobial treatment can ameliorate many of the worst clinical signs.

Demodex injai

A small group of dogs with demodicosis are infested with *Demodex injai*; small terriers are predisposed (Figures 16.9 and 16.10). Affected animals commonly have very greasy skin and show marked pruritus, and often appear to be suffering from allergy. Comedones and hair loss are less common. The mites are usually found in deep skin

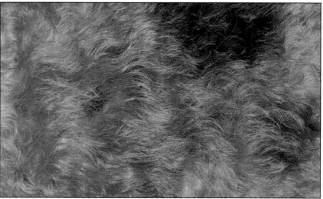

16.9 Grease, alopecia and erythema on the dorsum in *Demodex injai* infestation.

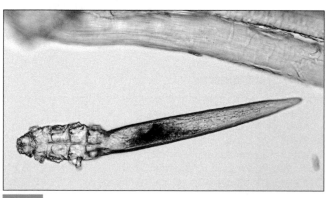

16.10 *Demodex injai.*

from the back, but other areas can be involved. When performing skin scrapings, the best results will be obtained by choosing areas where there is scale and hypotrichosis. Aggressive acaricide treatment is needed, as described above for *D. canis*.

Feline demodicosis

Feline demodicosis due to *Demodex cati* is a non-pruritic disease typified by alopecia and comedone formation. This disease is consistent with naturally occurring or iatrogenic immunosuppression, so evaluation for systemic disease, including FIV/FeLV testing, is advised.

Recently, *Demodex gatoi* has been reported in the UK. This short, surface-living mite causes alopecia and mild to severe pruritus. Unlike many other species, *D. gatoi* is contagious between cats; once it has been introduced to the shelter environment, considerable effort may be required to control its spread. The mite is difficult to find on skin scrapings, and cytology and faecal flotation tests are often more useful. *D. gatoi* is susceptible to treatment with topical lime sulphur, which should be applied weekly in the affected group.

Bacterial infections

Pyoderma in dogs and cats represents a group of secondary diseases, usually involving staphylococcal bacteria, with many different causes, including malnutrition, poor grooming, ectoparasites, allergy, and metabolic and hormonal disease (see the *BSAVA Manual of Canine and Feline Dermatology* for further information). Animals that have been in contact with hospital workers or other at-risk people, or that have been treated many times before, are at risk of carrying or being clinically affected by meticillin-resistant staphylococci, particularly meticillin-resistant *Staphylococcus aureus* or meticillin-resistant *Staphylococcus pseudintermedius*.

Common clinical syndromes

Intertrigo

Intertrigo, or folding of the skin due to conformation, obesity or disease, results in increased moisture and secondary bacterial infection on the surface. Large numbers of bacteria produce toxins, which cause inflammation and hair loss, and a sticky exudate on the skin surface results. Keeping the area as clean and dry as possible is the key to treatment. Superficial and subsequently deep pyoderma may result from inflammation and wetness in folded areas and then may extend to the surrounding skin in severe cases.

Superficial pyoderma

Superficial pyoderma is characterized by the presence of increased numbers of bacteria on the skin surface and most often involves the hair follicles. The basement membrane is not breached and a neutrophilic exudate is seen in which intracytoplasmic cocci are present. The neutrophilic exudate results in pustules, but these are short-lived, and the various signs of pyoderma that follow need to be recognized (Figure 16.11). In the dog, pyoderma may be recognized as pustules, crusted papules, multifocal

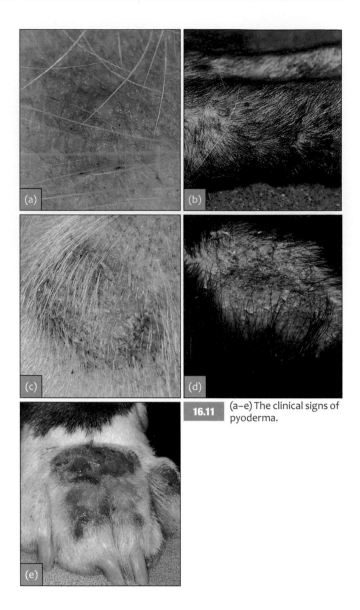

16.11 (a–e) The clinical signs of pyoderma.

alopecia, epidermal collarettes and macular hyperpigmentation. In the cat, crusted papules (miliary eczema) may be a sequel of bacterial infection. Superficial pyoderma is often pruritic.

Deep pyoderma

Deep pyoderma involves invasion of the dermis. On examination, the skin will feel thickened and there is often pain associated with the lesions (see Figure 16.11). Deep pyoderma is common in pedal demodicosis. In the cat, some eosinophilic granulomas are associated with infection, and some cases may resolve on appropriate antibiotic therapy (Figure 16.12).

Treatment

Treatment for bacterial infection should avoid the use of antibiotics if possible. For impetigo in puppies, surface pyoderma, such as intertrigo, and mild cases of superficial pyoderma, chlorhexidine-based shampoos will often successfully treat the infection. When antibiotics are needed for more severe superficial pyoderma or deep pyoderma, the period of treatment should be long enough to ensure clinical cure. This often requires antibiotic treatment for 1 week beyond the point of clinical cure in superficial

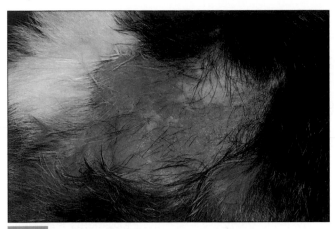

16.12 Eosinophilic plaque in a cat with deep pyoderma.

infections, and 2–3 weeks beyond clinical cure in deep pyoderma. In all cases, the veterinary surgeon should consider the underlying reason for the pyoderma in detail and address this accordingly to try to avoid a return of the infection.

Dermatophytosis (ringworm)

Dermatophytosis is the most common infectious and contagious skin disease in cats and commonly affects kittens and puppies. Dermatophytosis is a zoonosis; because of this, an outbreak can have a great impact on the reputation of the shelter (Newbury and Moriello, 2014).

Dermatophytosis is a non-fatal and usually self-limiting disease, but it is highly infectious and has zoonotic potential. It causes great concern among shelter staff, owing to the resources required to treat and adequately control the spread of infection when an outbreak occurs, as well as the fear that euthanasia of infected animals will be required as part of the control measures.

Dermatophytosis is common in cats; however, dogs, rabbits, guinea pigs and rodents can also be affected. *Microsporum canis* accounts for over 90% of cases of feline dermatophytosis, with other *Microsporum* spp., *Trichophyton* spp. and *Epidermophyton* spp. accounting for the remainder. Dermatophytes produce arthrospores that are highly resistant and can survive in the environment for up to 12 months. In a shelter setting, the aim is to identify and isolate any suspected cases of dermatophytosis on admission to the shelter, to prevent the possibility of spread of infection and an outbreak occurring.

M. canis is a zoophilic dermatophyte, which means that the reservoir and source of infection are animals. Dermatophytes may be cultured from the coats of normal (uninfected) animals in contact with infected animals, and subclinical infection can also occur; in both cases, animals that have been exposed but are not showing clinical signs can act a source of infection. Outdoor cats can be exposed to geophilic (soil-living) dermatophytes, and hunting cats/farm cats can be exposed to other zoophilic dermatophytes; however, these species are less often associated with outbreaks within shelters.

Predisposing factors for the development of disease are age (<2 years), immunosuppression, concurrent skin disease, nutritional deficiency and environmental factors such as high temperature and humidity. In animals infected with a dermatophyte, the hair shafts are weak and hair

containing arthrospores can easily transmit disease either directly or via fomites, such as in-contact cats, the hands and clothing of shelter staff and cleaning equipment. Healthy animals with healthy skin may not develop dermatophytosis when they come into contact with arthrospores, but in a shelter situation many of the animals are young, stressed, in a poor nutritional state and suffering from pre-existing skin trauma due to ectoparasites, so they are more vulnerable to infection. Older cats with suspected ringworm should be tested for FIV and FeLV.

Clinical signs

Clinical signs can vary greatly. Subclinically infected animals and fomite carriers may have no obvious clinical signs. Classically, dermatophytosis is seen as circular alopecia with crusting and hair breakage, commonly on the head and ears (Figure 16.13). However, in cats especially, dermatophytosis can resemble many different skin diseases, with relatively mild scaling and miliary dermatitis in mild cases and severe scale, alopecia and crusting over a wide area, complicated by secondary bacterial infection in immunocompromised animals.

Diagnosis is made on the basis of clinical signs, backed up by positive fluorescence in the Wood's lamp test, microscopy and positive culture. Historically, it was thought that only 50% of *M.canis* infections fluoresce with a Wood's lamp, but this is likely higher if a good technique is used. The lamp used should produce light with a wavelength of 365 nm. Mains-powered models are usually more effective than battery-powered lamps. The lamp should be warmed up for 5 minutes and the area of interest should then be illuminated in a darkened room for 3–5 minutes, as it can take time for the glowing hairs to become visible. Infected hairs glow bright green at the base and along the shaft, but not at the tips. Debris and topical medications can also fluoresce.

Ideally, all animals should be checked for ringworm at admission to the shelter. If this is not possible, then all animals with signs of skin disease noted on admission should be barrier nursed until these examinations can be performed. Microscopic examination of hair shafts can also be used as a rapid detection method; shafts are examined for hyphae and arthrospores (Figure 16.14). This method is not highly sensitive but is specific, although misinterpretation of debris can occur.

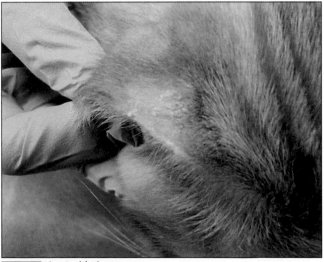

16.13 A cat with ringworm.
(© Cats Protection)

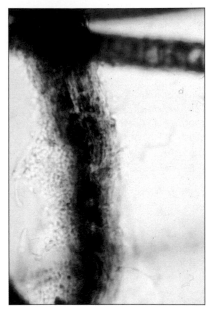

16.14 Microscopic appearance of *Microsporum canis* on an infected hair.

Culture is the gold standard for diagnosis of dermatophytosis. There are many media plates available for use in-house. Care in monitoring and recording results is required, and it is advisable to send the diagnostic samples to an accredited laboratory for definite identification of the dermatophyte. This may be more economical in the long run than relying only on in-house diagnostic methods. The sample should be collected by selecting fluorescent hairs identified on Wood's lamp examination and plucking these or, better, by collecting the sample using a toothbrush; a new toothbrush is vigorously brushed over the whole coat for 3–5 minutes, paying careful attention to the area around the toes and the head and ears. Skin lesions should be sampled last so as not to contaminate the rest of the coat. When using an in-house plate, gently push the toothbrush bristles into the centre of the plate first and then work outwards. If the sample is being sent away to a laboratory, place the toothbrush in a clean envelope and then package it for postage – do not seal it in in a plastic container with no oxygen.

Isolation and environmental contamination

Dermatophytes are spread via arthrospores. Spread can occur via direct or indirect contact or on fomites such as staff or equipment. Housing animals individually or in small groups of related animals will reduce the risk of an outbreak occurring. Any animal suspected of having ringworm should be isolated immediately, and any in-contact animals should be barrier nursed while awaiting the results of culture (see Chapter 9).

In shelters, reinfection from environmental contamination, and environmental contamination causing false-positives in subsequent cultures, cause considerable problems. The environment should ideally be cleaned daily with a 'hard clean' to remove hair and other debris from surfaces followed by a disinfectant that is active against ringworm (e.g. bleach at a 1:10 dilution). Many shelters have insufficient staff/volunteers to perform daily cleaning; in such situations, twice weekly cleaning is the minimum. Bedding for animals with ringworm should be disposable and replaced at each cleaning. The use of disposable food bowls and litter trays may be useful to reduce the risk of fomite transmission. Toys, water bowls and other potential fomites should be treated with disinfectant, thoroughly rinsed and returned to the same animal. Staff working in these areas should wear disposable PPE to reduce the risk of spreading disease to other animals.

Treatment

In the UK, the first line of treatment for cats with ringworm caused by *M. canis* is oral itraconazole using pulse therapy (7 days on and 7 days off for 3 treatment weeks, i.e. a total 5-week period) (Moriello, 2004; Carlotti *et al.*, 2010; Moriello and Verbrugge, 2013). If a cat or dog is infected with another dermatophyte, continuous therapy is often recommended. In such cases the pharmaceutical manufacturer should be consulted to get the most up-to-date treatment recommendations.

Systemic therapy will kill the arthrospores in the hair follicles but may not kill arthrospores located more superficially in the hair shafts. Topical therapy can be used to kill these arthrospores to aid in reducing environmental contamination and also to reduce false-positive cultures. Enilconazole or lime sulphur are recommended; topical treatment should be applied to a dry coat every 3–4 days. Enilconazole is licensed in the UK for use in dogs but not cats; a 1:50 dilution is advised in dogs but a 1:100 dilution has been reported for cats. There is a lime sulphur dip (marketed for the treatment of equids) available in the UK, and this should be applied at a 1:16 dilution. Under the prescribing cascade, enilconazole should be the first choice of topical treatment for dogs, but for cats lime sulphur may be a better first choice as it has a more rapid sporicidal activity. All topical treatments should be applied in a well ventilated area, and kittens/puppies and debilitated animals should be monitored for signs of hypothermia while the treatment is drying. Care should be taken to ensure that treated animals (and staff) do not ingest either topical preparation.

Clipping can cause micro-trauma to the skin, worsening the infection. It also poses a risk of introducing a large amount of infected hair into the environment, so clipping should not be routinely performed but can be considered if the coat is matted, the cat or dog has long hair, the lesions are diffuse and extensive, or soaking the coat is not easy. Small focal lesions can be trimmed using scissors, and infected whiskers should be trimmed or plucked if only a small number are infected.

An animal is considered free of infection when two consecutive negative cultures have been obtained. In general, these cultures should be taken at the end of itraconazole treatment and again the following week. As it takes 12–14 days to obtain a negative culture, even straightforward cases of ringworm require 8 weeks of isolation and barrier nursing. For veterinary surgeons working in a shelter treating large numbers of ringworm cases, there is an argument to start culturing weekly from the end of week 1 of treatment, especially if using a combination of systemic and topical treatment; the cost of an in-house culture plate is similar to the cost of keeping an animal in isolation for a day. Weekly cultures can also be used to measure the efficacy of the treatment. If weekly cultures are performed in this way, animals may be able to come out of isolation considerably earlier. This is important, as there are welfare issues associated with confining young animals in isolation, especially as it may limit their socialization. Some shelters require at least one of the negative cultures to be from an external laboratory. Depending on the size of the organization, discounted rates negotiated with external laboratories may mean that external cultures are the same price as or even cheaper than in-house culture.

Managing an outbreak

An outbreak of ringworm in a shelter occurs when there has been known transmission between animals kept in the shelter. The steps needed to control and treat an outbreak are shown in Figure 16.15.

1. Identify and isolate all animals with skin lesions.
2. Identify and barrier nurse all in-contact animals.
3. Perform a Wood's lamp examination and toothbrush sampling and culture on all animals.
4. Animals with skin lesions that are Wood's lamp positive should be started on itraconazole and topical treatment; for those that are not Wood's lamp positive, only topical treatment should be used.
5. In-contact animals should be started on topical treatment.
6. Stop intake of new animals.
7. Disinfect the environment.
8. Culture-negative animals can be returned to the disinfected environment.
9. Culture-positive animals should all be started on systemic and topical treatment and kept isolated until they produce two consecutive negative cultures; collect samples for culture weekly.

16.15 Steps to manage an outbreak of dermatophytosis.

Allergy

Chronic pruritic skin disease due to allergy is common in dogs and cats, and accounts for the most common dermatological presentations in these species. Animals may have been relinquished to the shelter due to signs of disease causing annoyance and embarrassment to the previous owners, or due to the long-term economic burden of treatment. Flea allergy requires consistent flea control measures, and these are discussed earlier in this chapter.

When presented with a pruritic animal in which there are signs of bacterial or yeast infection, these infections should be dealt with first; however, there may be a requirement to provide relief from severe pruritus, and this may delay diagnosis, a prognosis and, subsequently, rehoming. When animals are kept in the clean shelter environment for longer periods, the signs of atopic dermatitis may subside, only to reappear after rehoming when they encounter the allergens associated with domestic environments. This can be very frustrating for the new owner.

Clinical signs

The most important clinical sign in allergy in both dogs and cats is pruritus. As a complication, some anxious dogs will show increased pruritus, usually affecting the neck and shoulders. In animals that are more disturbed, a more localized area of linear alopecia and excoriation affecting one or both legs, sometimes resulting in acral lick dermatitis, may be seen. However, when pruritus is present, there is nearly always a non-psychological cause. Canine allergic pruritus is usually bilaterally symmetrical and affects the glabrous areas, face, feet and ears (Figures 16.16–16.18).

In cats, pruritus is often more difficult to observe, and one or more of the four cutaneous reaction patterns often indicates the presence of self-trauma. The reaction patterns are: symmetrical (barbered) alopecia; head and neck pruritus; eosinophilic dermatoses; and miliary eczema (Figures 16.19–16.21). Unfortunately, these reaction patterns are not pathognomonic for allergy.

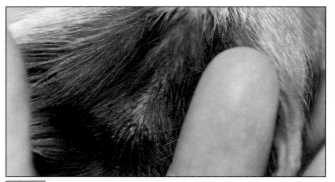

16.16 Pedal saliva staining due to allergic dermatitis in a dog.

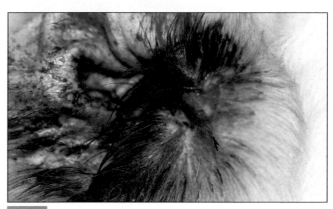

16.17 Severe *Malassezia* otitis in a dog with atopic dermatitis.

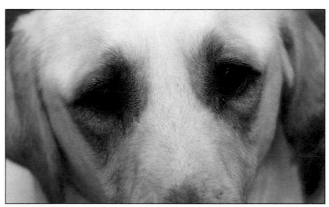

16.18 Periocular alopecia, erythema and staining in a dog with atopic dermatitis.

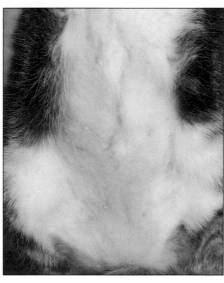

16.19 Barbered alopecia of the abdomen of a cat with flea allergy.

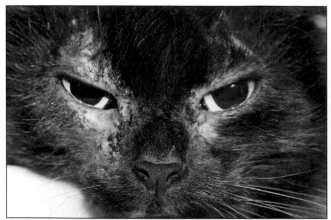

16.20 Signs of facial pruritus in a cat with non-flea hypersensitivity disease.

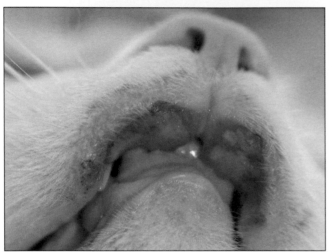

16.21 Eosinophilic granuloma ('rodent ulcer') affecting the lips of a cat.

Diagnosis

Allergic skin disease can be divided into three major groups: hypersensitivity to ectoparasites; cutaneous adverse food reaction (CAFR); and atopic dermatitis (allergy to house dust mites, pollens and moulds). There are no single diagnostic tests to determine that an animal has one of these allergies. Confusingly, these allergic diseases may coexist, and diagnosis is a process of elimination. Animals should first be free of ectoparasites and infectious (bacterial and yeast) dermatitis. For many cats that are fastidious and in which a food trial cannot be performed, a diagnosis of non-flea hypersensitivity disease (NFHD) is then appropriate if the signs continue. In most dogs, a food trial can be performed, which will allow distinction between CAFR and atopic dermatitis. It is not necessary to perform allergy testing unless immunotherapy is being considered, which is unlikely in shelter settings. Recently, updated criteria for atopic dermatitis and NFHD have been published (Olivry, 2010; Favrot et al., 2010, 2012).

Treatment

It is outside the scope of this chapter to describe the treatments for atopic dermatitis in detail, and only a brief overview is given. The minimum level of treatment to keep the patient comfortable should be used (see Chapter 3). For

some patients, this may be impossible either medically or financially, and euthanasia is appropriate; however, the effects of secondary infection can be so profound that an immediate decision regarding the prognosis before an attempt is made to improve the condition with appropriate treatment should be avoided (Olivry et al., 2010).

The reader is referred to dermatological texts (e.g. the BSAVA Manual of Canine and Feline Dermatology) for treatment options. These are similar to those provided to non-shelter pets, including allergen avoidance, infection control through initial antibiotic therapy in some instances and then shampoos and wipes, as well as drugs that modulate the immune response, such as glucocorticoids, ciclosporin and oclacitinib. Allergy testing and immunotherapy are more likely to be used only in chronic management, as are essential fatty acid supplements (see QRG 16.2) (Olivry et al., 2015).

Viral disease with cutaneous manifestations in the cat

Viral infections in the cat have been associated with skin disease. The viral agent of the common respiratory disease feline rhinotracheitis (feline alphaherpesvirus-1) is a frequent cause of respiratory disease in cats, and is commonly encountered in shelter cats. Although uncommon, oral and cutaneous ulcers may occur; ulcers may be found on the face (most commonly), feet and body. As with other herpesviruses, recrudescence may occur following apparent recovery, at times of stress. When there are clear respiratory signs, the diagnosis is more straightforward, but a skin biopsy sample is needed for definitive diagnosis.

Less commonly, feline calicivirus (FCV) may be associated with skin disease. FCV has been seen to cause pustular lesions at sites where the fur has been clipped, and in the recently described haemorrhagic form, distal limb oedema and ulcers affecting the nose, lips, pinna, periocular skin and distal limbs have been described (see Chapter 15).

FeLV and FIV infections have also been associated with skin disease. FeLV most commonly affects the skin via immunosuppression (Figure 16.22); chronic or recurrent

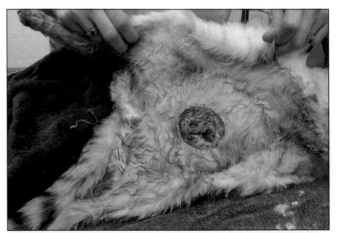

16.22 Non-healing wound in an FeLV-positive cat; the definitive cause was not identified. The haircoat on the ventral abdomen is stained by exudates. Cats with non-healing wounds should be tested for FIV and FeLV infections. Other differentials for non-healing wounds include atypical bacterial infections (e.g. Mycobacterium spp.), fungal infections, neoplasia, foreign bodies and corticosteroid therapy. FeLV = feline leukaemia virus; FIV = feline immunodeficiency virus.
(Reproduced from the BSAVA Manual of Feline Practice)

pyoderma, seborrhoea, exfoliative dermatitis and pruritus have been reported, as well as cutaneous horns and giant cell dermatosis. FIV may similarly manifest with cutaneous signs relating to immunosuppression, but it has also been reported to cause a generalized papulocrusting skin disease with alopecia and scaling, particularly affecting the head and legs. No treatment has been reported to be useful in these cases.

unexplained pruritus, erythema and scaling. Oral inflammation and ulceration are also common in CEL.

In older cats, hyperthyroidism, hyperadrenocorticism and diabetes mellitus will cause problems of recurrent infection and changes in the skin and coat quality, with scale being common. Smooth generalized alopecia is associated with thymoma, and exfoliative dermatitis is seen with pancreatic or hepatic carcinoma.

Leishmaniosis

Leishmaniosis is a growing problem in rescued dogs, and the increasing trend to rescue dogs from continental Europe and rehome them in the UK is bringing new burdens to shelter medicine (see QRG 16.3). Leishmaniosis is a sandfly vector-borne disease caused by *Leishmania* spp. such as *Leishmania infantum*. The disease is endemic around the Mediterranean and sporadic cases are reported in more temperate regions of Europe. Laboratory tests will often fail to determine the difference between exposure and disease, and this means that there is no simple way of screening potentially affected animals. The key history point will be that the dog has originated from southern Europe. A variety of cutaneous clinical signs may be seen, including scaling alopecia, nasal dermatitis, vasculitis and localized ulceration. In many cases there will be more systemic signs, such as uveitis, renal disease and anaemia. Treatment depends considerably on the location and severity of disease, and a detailed description is beyond the scope of this chapter (see QRG 16.1).

Miscellaneous skin diseases

In older dogs, endocrine diseases, such as diabetes mellitus, hyperadrenocorticism and hypothyroidism, should be considered as causes of otitis, pyoderma, *Malassezia* dermatitis and demodicosis. Cutaneous epitheliotropic lymphoma (CEL) should be considered as a cause of

References and further reading

Battersby I (2014) Using antibiotics responsibly in companion animals. *In Practice* **36**, 106–118

Carlotti DN, Guinot P, Meissonnier E and Germain PA (2010) Eradication of feline dermatophytosis in a shelter: a field study. *Veterinary Dermatology* **21**, 259–266

Favrot C, Steffan J, Seewald W and Picco F (2010) A prospective study on the clinical features of chronic canine atopic dermatitis and its diagnosis. *Veterinary Dermatology* **21**, 23–31

Favrot C, Steffan J, Seewald W *et al.* (2012) Establishment of diagnostic criteria for feline nonflea-induced hypersensitivity dermatitis. *Veterinary Dermatology* **23**, 45–50

Harvey A and Tasker S (2013) *BSAVA Manual of Feline Practice: A Foundation Manual*. BSAVA Publications, Gloucester

Jackson HA and Marsella R (2012) *BSAVA Manual of Canine and Feline Dermatology*. BSAVA Publications, Gloucester

Moriello KA (2004) Treatment of dermatophytosis in dogs and cats: review of published studies. *Veterinary Dermatology* **15**, 99–107

Moriello KA and Verbrugge M (2013) Changes in serum chemistry values in shelter cats treated with 21 consecutive days of oral itraconazole for dermatophytosis. *Veterinary Dermatology* **24**, 557–558

Mueller RS (2004) Treatment protocols for demodicosis: an evidence-based review. *Veterinary Dermatology* **15**, 75–89

Mueller RS, Bensignor E, Ferrer L *et al.* (2012) Treatment of demodicosis in dogs: 2011 clinical practice guidelines. *Veterinary Dermatology* **23**, 86–96

Newbury S and Moriello K (2014) Feline dermatophytosis: steps for investigation of a suspected shelter outbreak. *Journal of Feline Medicine and Surgery* **16**, 407–418

Olivry T (2010) New diagnostic criteria for canine atopic dermatitis. *Veterinary Dermatology* **21**, 123–126

Olivry T, DeBoer DJ, Favrot C *et al.* (2010) Treatment of canine atopic dermatitis: 2010 clinical practice guidelines from the International Task Force on Canine Atopic Dermatitis. *Veterinary Dermatology* **21**, 233–248

Olivry T (2015) Treatment of canine atopic dermatitis: 2015 updated guidelines from the International Committee on Allergic Diseases of Animals (ICADA). *BMC Veterinary Research* **11**, 210

Patel A, Forsythe P and Smith S (2008) *Small Animal Dermatology*. Saunders Elsevier, London

QRG 16.1: Zoonotic diseases in shelters
by Paula Boyden and Nathalie Dowgray

Background

Zoonotic diseases affect shelters on a number of levels. There is the risk of spread to shelter staff and other animals within the shelter, implications for rehoming and reputational risk to the shelter due to public health concerns. People who are immunosuppressed are at a greater risk of zoonotic disease, and this should be highlighted to staff and potential adopters.

Skin disease

For further information, see main text.

Ringworm (dermatophytosis)

Ringworm primarily affects puppies and kittens and can have a wide range of clinical presentations. Disease spread is *via* infected spores shed on the hair shafts. Staff should wear full disposable personal protective equipment (PPE) when

handling infected animals, and cases should be isolated. All animals should be treated and ideally two sequential negative cultures obtained before homing. Pens should be cleaned thoroughly between animals with a suitable disinfectant (5% and 1.84% sodium hypochlorite, 0.3% quaternary ammonium compounds, 3.2% lactic acid and 0.5% hydrogen peroxide have been all shown to be effective).

QRG 16.1 continued

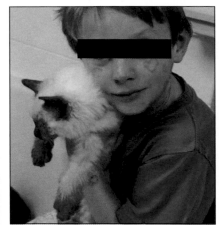

Child with ringworm caused by *Microsporum canis*.
(© Richard Malik)

Sarcoptic mange (scabies)

Sarcoptes scabiei mites have a preference for dogs but will cause skin disease in cats and humans. Lesions are intensely pruritic and are commonly found on the ear margins, elbows and hocks. As *S. scabiei* is a burrowing mite, diagnosis is made by examination of deep skin scrapes. Staff should wear disposable gloves, aprons and arm sleeves to reduce the risk of infection to themselves and indirect spread to other dogs. The mites can survive off a host for 21 days if environmental conditions are amenable but it is more common for them to survive only 2–3 days. Lesions on humans commonly develop on the hands and feet and are intensely pruritic. Affected dogs and all in-contact animals should be treated; a second treatment is advised after 4 weeks, before the dogs are mixed with other dogs. Washing bedding and drying it in the sun or a hot drying cycle should prevent repeat infection.

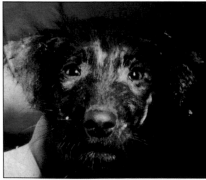

Classical distribution of *Sarcoptes scabiei* in the dog.

Cowpox

Rodents are the natural host for cowpox virus. Cats primarily develop solitary lesions but, occasionally, the virus can cause systemic disease. Cats should be tested for feline immunodeficiency virus/feline leukaemia virus, and usually recover with supportive care unless they are immunosuppressed. Staff should wear disposable gloves, aprons and arm sleeves when handling these cats. The environment should be cleaned with an oxidizing disinfectant or a quaternary ammonium product. Cats should be clear of lesions before rehoming. Most cases in humans cause mild exanthema on the face, arms or legs, but individuals who are immunosuppressed are at risk of severe smallpox-like disease, which can be fatal.

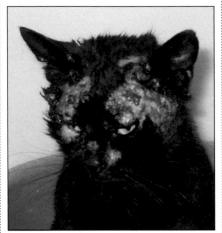

Severe cowpox in a cat.
(© Conor O'Halloran)

Mycobacteria

Infection with feline leprosy (caused primarily by *Mycobacterium lepraemurium* but also by other mycobacteria that cannot be grown in culture) and non-tuberculous (environmental) mycobacteria primarily presents as cutaneous or subcutaneous nodules. Cats with outdoor access are primarily at risk of infection. Zoonotic risk is low but is increased in immunosuppressed people. Gloves should be worn when handling affected cats, especially if they have draining lesions. Infection is by direct inoculation of the tissue, so the risk of transmission is low. Pens should be cleaned with a peroxidizing compound or sodium hypochlorite. Treatment is expensive and often prolonged, so this should be discussed with the shelter management before starting therapy.

Respiratory disease

For further information, see Chapters 14 and 15.

Mycobacteria

Tuberculosis complex (*Mycobacterium tuberculosis*, *M. bovis* and *M. microti*) and occasionally non-tuberculous mycobacteria can cause systemic disease, with visceral and respiratory disease being the common manifestations. Diagnosis can be difficult and is by suspicion on the basis of clinical signs, ruling out other causes and demonstration of the organism within tissue samples. The zoonotic risk is potentially increased with respiratory disease, but reported cases of transmission to humans are rare. It is important to recognize that transmission can also go from humans to animals, so animals coming to a shelter from a home where their owner had tuberculosis would be considered at higher risk. Other risk factors are animals living in rural communities and having outdoor access. Due to the poor prognosis of systemic disease, the cost and length of treatment and risk to staff, in a shelter situation euthanasia should be considered. M. bovis is a notifiable disease in companion animals in the UK.

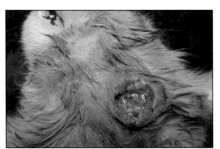

Cat with a skin lesion caused by *Mycobacterium microti*.

Bordetella bronchiseptica

This is a common cause of kennel cough in dogs. Although infection is often considered to be self-limiting, it can cause fatal bronchopneumonia in puppies. *Bordetella bronchiseptica* infection is less common in cats but can cause severe pneumonia. The pathogen can also cause pneumonia in immunosuppressed people, although it is different from *Bordetella pertussis*, the cause of whooping cough. Staff should wear aprons, gloves and arm sleeves when handling infected animals, which ➔

QRG 16.1 *continued*

should ideally be isolated from uninfected animals to reduce spread. This can be difficult with dogs. Dogs ideally should be treated with antibiotics only following diagnosis by culture and sensitivity testing; if this is not possible, then treatment should be given if they are systemically unwell. *B. bronchiseptica* does not survive well outside the host and is sensitive to most disinfectants. At adoption, the new owner should be informed that the animal may still be shedding (although this generally lasts for a period of weeks, it may on occasion be for several months) and advised to keep the dog away from any immunosuppressed people. Vaccination of puppies, in particular, is recommended.

Gastrointestinal disease

For further information, see Chapters 12 and 13.

Toxoplasmosis

This can be a cause of mild, self-limiting diarrhoea in cats. Systemic disease is seen in immunosuppressed cats or kittens with congenital toxoplasmosis. Spread to people from cats is via ingestion of oocysts shed in cat faeces. The risk to shelter staff is low, as long as they practise good hygiene when cleaning litter trays and handling the cats; use of basic PPE (gloves) is advised. Infection of previously unexposed women during pregnancy can cause birth defects in the fetus; this is why there is much concern about toxoplasmosis as a zoonosis. Most human infections are acquired from eating undercooked meat or coming into contact with cat faeces when gardening.

For prevention:

- Clean litter trays at least daily to reduce the number of sporulated oocysts (sporulation takes 1–5 days)
- Do not feed raw meat to shelter animals
- Advise adopters about good litter tray hygiene.

See also QRG 18.1.

Giardiasis

There are several assemblages (genotypes) of *Giardia*. While some are species specific, others are also common to humans, resulting in a zoonotic risk. *Giardia* is spread through the ingestion of infectious cysts, usually in contaminated food or water.

For prevention:

- Use good hygiene after handling animal faeces or cleaning contaminated areas
- Remove faeces to prevent ground water contamination
- Avoid pooling of water – ensure good drainage of exercise areas and allow pens to dry
- Clean pens with a peroxidizing compound, sodium hypochlorite or a quaternary ammonium product.

Giardia can be challenging to eliminate; oocysts will remain on the fur of dogs and cats, and may contribute to reinfection. While clinical cases should be treated, clinically well animals can also shed the pathogen. Treatment of clinically normal animals is controversial, as is repeated sampling for a negative result. Therefore, good hygiene is imperative at all times.

Cryptosporidiosis

Most up-to-date studies indicate that the host-adapted species of *Cryptosporidium* found in cats and dogs are not a cause of disease in humans.

Campylobacteriosis

A large number of isolates of *Campylobacter* spp. are found in cats and dogs both with and without diarrhoea – clinically normal animals can shed the pathogen. It is more prevalent in kennelled cats and dogs, with *Campylobacter jejuni* being the most common species. Animals fed raw meat diets are at higher risk of shedding isolates that may have public health significance. Transmission is via the faecal–oral route. Treatment with antibiotics is indicated only in animals with systemic disease. Good hygiene is advised when cleaning litter trays and removing dog faeces; gloves should be worn. Standard disinfection is suitable. Clinically well animals can be homed with advice given to the new owner on standard hygiene precautions. Repeat testing is not necessary if the diarrhoea has stopped.

Disease	Species affected	Route of infection	Diagnosis	Treatment
Toxoplasmosis	All species Cat is the definitive host	Ingestion of cysts	Paired serology	Clindamycin
Giardiasis	Variety of mammals, including dogs and cats. Some genotypes are species specific	Ingestion of infected oocysts. Thrive in moist environment	Faecal microscopy	Fenbendazole Metronidazole
Cryptosporidiosis	Reptiles, birds, mammals Species-specific: *C. canis* and *C. felis*	Faecal–oral: ingestion of oocysts	Faecal examination	Given current evidence indicates this is not zoonotic, symptomatic management should be tried first Azithromycin (little reported)
Campylobacteriosis	Cats and dogs. Higher prevalence in kennel environment	Asymptomatic carriers may be present Faecal–oral Transmission via contaminated food and water	Faecal culture	Multiple treatments are reported, including erythromycin
Salmonellosis	Mammals, including cats and dogs; birds, reptiles	Contaminated food, water, fomites	Faecal culture NB: Notifiable disease	Uncomplicated gastrointestinal signs: symptomatic treatment Antibiotics only if concurrent non-enteric signs are present

Enteric zoonoses.

QRG 16.1 *continued*

Salmonellosis

This is a notifiable disease in the UK and the diagnosing laboratory will contact the Animal and Plant Health Agency. Animals fed raw meat diets are at higher risk of shedding *Salmonella*. Treatment is indicated only if the animal is systemically unwell. The usual advice is to keep the animal quarantined until it is no longer shedding. Standard precautions with the use of good hygiene, disinfection and PPE are advised while the animal is in the shelter.

Other diseases

Leptospirosis

This bacterial infection can be transmitted by direct or indirect contact with infected urine. The pathogen has several different serovars (serotypes), many of which colonize the kidneys and are shed in the urine. The challenges associated with this disease are that many cases are chronic or subclinical (and therefore may not be recognized as such), there is no cross-protection between serovars, and vaccines will not necessarily prevent renal shedding of the bacteria. Leptospirosis is more frequently associated with dogs, although cats can be the incidental host for a number of serovars. With multiple animals in a shelter environment, consideration must be given to the handling of urine. Standard precautions with the use of good hygiene, disinfection and PPE are advised. Care must also be taken to avoid contamination of broken skin.

Bartonellosis

Bartonella spp. can be transmitted via infected flea faeces contaminating cats' claws and cause 'cat scratch disease'. Symptoms in humans are fever and lymphadenopathy, with more severe disease in immunosuppressed individuals.
  For prevention:

- Clean all scratches appropriately
- Apply flea control to all animals on entering the shelter
- Clean pens and bedding contaminated with flea faeces regularly.

Q fever

This is caused by *Coxiella burnetii*, a small bacterium. While sheep, cows and goats are the common reservoirs, cats can become infected via tick bites, ingestion of a contaminated carcase or aerosol exposure. Infection in cats will often be subclinical but fever, anorexia and lethargy can occur. Abortion can occur in pregnant animals but the organism has also been isolated during normal parturition. It is advised that shelter staff and veterinary surgeons (veterinarians) wear gloves and a facemask when assisting cats during labour and when cleaning up aborted or post-parturition material. Disease in humans can range from asymptomatic to mild self-limiting fever or myalgia, to severe pneumonia, hepatitis or abortion. On rare occasions, encephalitis, sepsis or myocarditis may develop and result in death. Shelters in rural areas where cats may be interacting with livestock before admission should be considered at higher risk.

Non-endemic diseases

For the purposes of this guide, non-endemic diseases are those that are not normally found within the UK. However, with the increased movement of dogs, in particular from other countries into the UK, consideration needs to be given to such diseases (see also QRG 16.3).

Leishmaniosis

Animals may present with scaling alopecia, nasal dermatitis and localized ulceration. They are likely to have a history of spending some time in southern Europe. Leishmaniosis can cause cutaneous or, less commonly, visceral disease in humans, although many infections are clinically silent. Spread is via infected sandflies and dogs act as a disease reservoir. At the time of writing, the sandfly vector is not established in the UK. There is no direct animal-to-human transmission.

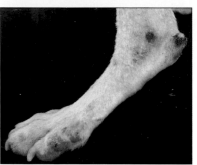

Cutaneous ulcers and exfoliative dermatitis in a dog infected with *Leishmania* spp.
(Courtesy of M Saridomihelakis and reproduced from the *BSAVA Manual of Canine and Feline Dermatology*).

Rabies

Currently, there is a very low risk of rabies in the UK, but due to changes in the Pet Travel Scheme (PETS) the risk has increased. Charities need to have good procedures in place to inform the appropriate authorities and isolate and test any animals that are suspected to have originated overseas but entered the country without the relevant documentation (pet passport) to confirm legal entry. Animals should not be rehomed until it has been confirmed they are not at risk of carrying rabies.

References and further reading

Jackson HA and Marsella R (2012) *BSAVA Manual of Canine and Feline Dermatology, 3rd edn*. BSAVA Publications, Gloucester

QRG 16.2: Dealing with the itchy dog: is it atopic dermatitis?

by Steve Shaw

QUICK REFERENCE GUIDES

Canine atopic dermatitis is a diagnosis of exclusion. In the context of shelter medicine, this can be time-consuming, although good practices at intake (as detailed elsewhere in this manual) may ensure that many problems have been eliminated. Errors and delays in the diagnosis can be minimized by considering whether the signs are typical and whether appropriate measures have been taken to rule out infections and infestations.

Key questions

Are the signs typical?

- Pruritus is the primary clinical sign and continues despite treatment of infection.
- Most often bilaterally symmetrical.
- Areas typically involved:
  - Face
  - Feet (plantar/palmar disease is common in canine atopic dermatitis)
  - Ventral abdomen and axillae
  - Perineum
  - Ears – otitis is common.
- Areas not typically involved:
  - Ear margins – consider scabies
  - Dorsal rump and tail head – consider flea infestation.
- Age of onset between 6 months and 3 years.

Have infections and infestations been ruled out?

- Demodicosis can be highly pruritic when only small numbers of mites are present (*Demodex canis*) and when apparently absent (*D. injai*). The areas involved are common to those seen with allergic dermatitis.
- Scabies may present as irritation with very few lesions.
- Fleas, lice and *Cheyletiella* may all cause pruritic disease resembling allergic dermatitis.
- *Malassezia* dermatitis may cause severe pruritus in some dogs.
- Superficial pyoderma is commonly pruritic.

Diagnosis

The process for diagnosis is shown in the flowchart below.

Treatment options

The minimum level of treatment to keep the patient comfortable should be used. For some patients, it may be impossible either medically or financially to provide relief from the clinical signs, in which case euthanasia may be appropriate. However, the effects of secondary infection can be so profound that, ideally, such decisions should be made only after appropriate antibacterial treatment (Olivry *et al.*, 2010 and Olivry *et al.*, 2015).

1 Allergen avoidance. Allergen avoidance may be useful in reducing clinical signs, but clinical experience would suggest that this is rarely a complete solution to the problem. Allergen exposure may be different in a shelter than a home; in some dogs, this may result in a significant improvement in their clinical signs while in kennels. This has to be borne in mind when rehoming an atopic dog, as the clinical signs may subsequently flare up.

2 Preventing secondary infection. Throughout the diagnosis and treatment of atopic dermatitis, patients should be evaluated using clinical examination and ear, skin surface and pustule cytology as required. When

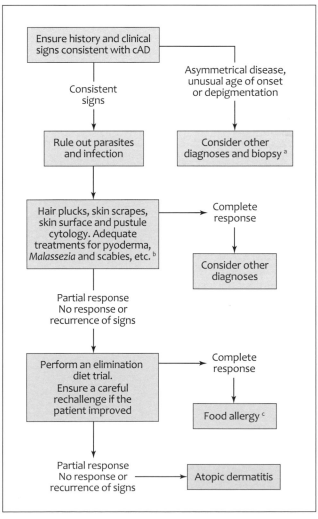

Diagnosis of canine atopic dermatitis (cAD).
[a] Biopsy is particularly important in older dogs, where epitheliotropic lymphoma may mimic atopic dermatitis.
[b] Use the information gathered during this part of the work-up to design appropriate long-term microbial control measures.
[c] Atopic dermatitis and food allergy may coexist.

QRG 16.2 *continued*

present, pyoderma should be treated aggressively, and further disease should be prevented through the use of shampoos, ear cleaners and good management of the underlying irritation.

3 **Glucocorticoids.** Oral steroids are often appropriate in treating atopic dermatitis. This class of medication is inexpensive, but can cause significant adverse effects if used inappropriately. In dogs, prednisolone is used for either a short course (in which a tapered reduction is not needed) or for longer periods, in which reduction to alternate-day administration and then a further graduated dose reduction should be used. Starting doses of 0.2–0.8 mg/kg orally q24h are appropriate in dogs. Side effects include polydipsia, polyuria and polyphagia (possibly leading to obesity), with muscle loss, fat redistribution, increased susceptibility to infection, depression and behavioural changes, urinary tract infection and intermittent digestive upsets. Nevertheless, this treatment provides good control of clinical signs in the majority of cases. Alternatively, for local areas, hydrocortisone aceponate is a potent steroid that is applied topically and has a reduced potential for adrenal suppression.

4 **Ciclosporin.** This offers good control of the signs of atopic dermatitis. In dogs, capsules or liquid are given at a dose of 5 mg/kg daily for around 1 month, and then the dose is titrated first to every other day and then, in many dogs, to twice weekly. Dogs that respond promptly in the first month are more likely to achieve the twice-weekly dose level. Ciclosporin has a relatively slow onset of action and pruritus may need to be controlled, using a short course of steroids, to ensure that the welfare of the patient is maintained. The clinical signs of canine atopic dermatitis are generally controlled by 21 days. Adverse effects of ciclosporin include intermittent vomiting, diarrhoea, hirsutism, viral papillomata and hyperplasia of the gums. Satisfactory control is seen the majority of cases. It is expensive to initiate therapy and, unless a marked dose reduction is achieved over time, ciclosporin may be outside the budget of many shelters.

5 **Oclacitinib.** This is approved to treat pruritus in dogs associated with allergic dermatitis, including atopic dermatitis. Around 60% of cases are controlled on maintenance therapy after 2 weeks. Oclacitinib acts quickly and effectively in many dogs, but this efficacy can be markedly reduced in cases with complicating otitis, pyoderma or *Malassezia dermatitis*. Haematology and biochemistry monitoring should be performed when oclacitinib is used long-term. Additional data regarding its use in chronic disease is as yet limited.

6 **Antihistamines.** A variety of antihistamines are used in dogs but they are unlicensed and have poor efficacy. There may be safety issues with more recent antihistamines in dogs. Antihistamines are most useful in cases where there is significant urticaria.

7 **Essential fatty acids.** A large variety of essential fatty acid supplements (EFAS) are available, containing evening primrose oil, cod liver oil and other oils, with widely varying dose rates recommended. Despite this variation, these products do seem to be helpful in improving coat and skin condition, and there is evidence in the literature of a steroid-sparing effect of EFAS. They have a very slow onset of action and few side effects, although softness of faeces and exacerbation of pancreatitis are possible. Shelter organizations should carefully consider the cost–benefit of these treatments, which, although useful, have only a limited effect on the level of acute pruritus and skin disease.

8 **Immunotherapy.** This is the only treatment that acts specifically at the level of antigen-specific responses to reduce clinical signs. It is not licensed in the UK for dogs. It is very slow to act, taking up to 9 months to have an effect, and as such the response is often best judged at 12 months to avoid seasonal variation in disease confusing the interpretation of the response. Although anaphylaxis is a potential side effect, in general, there are few side effects, with pruritus, urticaria and needle shyness being reported. In general, 50–60% of cases show benefit and around 20% of cases rely on immunotherapy as sole therapy. Many shelter organizations may not choose this option as allergy testing and immunotherapy are expensive and the treatment does not act quickly. This option might be deferred until after an animal is rehomed, at which point the dog's new owners may choose to pursue treatment.

References and further reading

Olivry T, DeBoer DJ, Favrot C *et al.* (2010) Treatment of canine atopic dermatitis: 2010 clinical practice guidelines from the International Task Force on Canine Atopic Dermatitis. *Veterinary Dermatology* **21**, 233–248

Olivry T, DeBoer DJ, Favrot C *et al.* (2015) Treatment of canine atopic dermatitis: 2015 updated guideline from the International Committee on Allergic Diseases of Animals (ICADA). *BMC Veterinary Research* **11**, 210

QRG 16.3: Exotic diseases in shelters

by Emily Newbury and Paula Boyden

Background

Exotic, or non-endemic, diseases can be defined as those that do not normally occur within a given geographical area. For the purposes of this quick reference guide, the area in question will be restricted to the UK and the Republic of Ireland. While both dogs and cats can be infected with the organisms discussed, patent infection is more likely to occur in dogs.

Relevance to the shelter environment

Following the expansion of the Pet Travel Scheme (PETS) and the relaxation of quarantine laws, more and more pets are crossing national borders. This increase in animal movements makes it more likely that any dog or cat relinquished to a shelter by an owner or collected as a stray may have travelled outside the UK. In addition, a number of puppies are imported each year for sale.

Given the potential for prolonged incubation or asymptomatic carriage of many vector-borne diseases, it is possible for a shelter to unwittingly accept an infected dog or cat. This has several serious implications:

- Certain organisms can lead to increased bleeding tendencies, a significant risk in a period when neutering may be carried out
- The presenting signs of unfamiliar exotic diseases could be incorrectly attributed to a more common cause and treated in a way that could further compromise the animal, e.g. the use of corticosteroids to treat dermatitis in dogs with unknown *Leishmania infantum* infection
- If an exotic disease is identified as the cause of clinical signs, it may be considered a pre-existing condition by insurance providers, leading to a marked financial burden both for the shelter and for potential adopters who wish to pursue treatment
- Some diseases have zoonotic potential (e.g. leishmaniosis, *Echinococcus multilocularis*)
- More than one disease could be present concurrently.

Management strategies

The first step in any management strategy is to consider the following questions:

- Does the shelter have a policy on accepting dogs or cats that have originated from or travelled overseas?
- Does the shelter know if it is accepting dogs or cats that have originated from/travelled overseas – are they asking the appropriate questions at relinquishment to gain this information?
- Will the veterinary surgeon (veterinarian) advise the shelter to accept dogs or cats with a known history of overseas travel?

> There are many factors that may influence whether a shelter feels able to accept animals that have travelled overseas. Veterinary advice about disease risk assessment and the financial and logistical implications of testing is crucial

Assessment of intake animals

Relinquished pets

Handover protocols

The best opportunity to obtain accurate information about an animal's origin and travel history is at or around the time of handover. If the topic is addressed prior to the admission of the dog or cat, it will be easier to ensure that all relevant documentation arrives with the animal.

> Key facts to ascertain when accepting relinquished animals:
> - Countries to which a dog or cat has travelled
> - Areas entered within those countries – disease risk can vary widely within a country
> - Approximate dates of travel – indicates the duration and frequency of exposure
> - Preventive measures utilized during travel (e.g. repellent collars, vaccines) – indicates the likelihood of infection.

Establish disease risks in the area of origin/exposure

In order to assess the risk of disease and to inform testing, the infectious organisms to which the animal may have been exposed must be identified. Specialist reference laboratories and websites (e.g. www.cvbd.org) both provide a useful starting point.

Testing protocols

Advice on the optimal testing protocols for each organism can be obtained from the veterinary practice's nominated reference laboratory. Briefly, testing may utilize a combination of serological testing to determine exposure and polymerase chain reaction (PCR) methods to detect antigen. These diseases are extremely rare in cats, so routine testing of cats with a history of travel is probably not indicated unless suggestive clinical signs are apparent.

Action to take in the event of a positive result: Although many of the exotic diseases discussed are treatable and hopefully curable, some are not. Protocols defining the criteria for treatment or euthanasia can be decided in advance or on a case-by-case basis. Having a protocol is preferable to ensure consistency and aid communication with staff.

Certain organisms present more of a challenge than others. Infection with *L. infantum* is generally lifelong and medication is likely to be required to maintain a state of 'remission'. It is also likely that an infected dog will require future monitoring tests and that its quality of life and longevity will be affected. There is also the theoretical risk of zoonotic transmission. Management of a *Leishmania*-positive dog can therefore be an expensive and involved process with an uncertain outcome. Access to appropriate medications may be more difficult in the UK than in countries with endemic disease.

QRG 16.3 *continued*

Disease (causative agent)	Vector	Common clinical signs	Asymptomatic carriage?	Diagnosis	Treatment	Human disease?	Risk to other dogs?
Anaplasmosis (e.g. *Anaplasma phagocytophilum*, *Anaplasma platys*)	Tick (mainly *Ixodes ricinus* for *A. phagocytophilum*, *Rhipicephalus sanguineus* and *Dermacentor* spp. for *A. platys*)	*A. phagocytophilum* – pyrexia, lethargy, thrombocytopenia, other cytopenias. *A. platys* – pyrexia, lethargy, bleeding tendencies due to platelet destruction	Yes? – chronic carriers?	Serological and PCR tests available (often combined, can be negative on PCR in chronic disease and negative on serology in early stages of disease prior to seroconversion). Blood smear may show *A. platys* but is insensitive	Doxycycline	Yes (via vector)	*Ixodes* ticks are present in the UK
Babesiosis (mainly *Babesia canis* in Europe[a])	Tick (*R. sanguineus* and *Dermacentor* spp.)	Pyrexia, haemolytic anaemia, haemoglobinuria, thrombocytopenia	Yes – chronic phase of infection	PCR and/or serology (latter less useful in acute disease). Blood smears from marginal ear vein stained with Giemsa may show piroplasms	Imidocarb	No	Vector carrying disease has been found in the UK
Ehrlichiosis (*Ehrlichia canis*[a])	Tick (*R. sanguineus*)	Three main stages of disease – acute, subclinical and chronic. Acute disease causes a wide range of clinical signs, including pyrexia, lethargy, lymphadenopathy, oculonasal discharge, anaemia and thrombocytopenia. Pancytopenia can occur in chronic disease due to bone marrow destruction	Yes – chronic phase of infection	Serological and PCR tests available (often combined, can be negative on PCR in chronic disease and negative on serology in early stages of disease prior to seroconversion). *E. canis* can sometimes be seen in blood, buffy coat and bone marrow smears in acute disease	Doxycycline	No	Vector not established in the UK but may complete life cycle indoors, e.g. in kennels
Heartworm (*Dirofilaria immitis*)	Mosquito	Congestive heart failure from adult worms inhabiting pulmonary artery	Yes – depending on many factors, e.g. prepatent phase, low worm burdens, use of preventive therapies	Usually combination of antigen testing and screening for microfilariae. Both will be negative in the prepatent phase (around 6 months). Shelter dogs with a history of potential heartworm exposure should be retested 6 months later. Clinical signs, radiography and echocardiography are also important	Prevention is preferable – macrocyclic lactones. Treatment will include both adulticidal and microfilaricidal drugs – see American Heartworm Society guidelines	Humans are considered incidental hosts	Vector not present in the UK (?)
Leishmaniosis (*Leishmania infantum*[a])	Sandfly (*Phlebotomus* spp.)	Complex of clinical signs. Dermatological signs prevalent with this species – alopecia, dermatitis ± cachexia, uveitis, anaemia and many other signs. Signs may wax and wane. Renal involvement is common. In endemic areas, a large proportion of infected dogs will be asymptomatic	Yes – prepatent phase, 'resistant' animals and asymptomatic carriers which may not show signs of disease for many years or even for life	Serological and PCR tests available (often combined, can be negative on PCR in chronic disease and negative on serology in early stages of disease prior to seroconversion). Also patient-side test kits available. Bone marrow and lymph node aspirates and biopsy samples of affected tissues, e.g. skin, conjunctiva, can also be used	Cure unlikely. Initial treatment (e.g. with miltefosine) followed by long-term management with allopurinol	Yes (via vector)	Vector not present in the UK

Common vector-borne diseases of dogs that are endemic in parts of Western Europe but considered exotic in the UK. [a] Other species are found worldwide.

QRG 16.3 *continued*

Alternatives to testing

If a shelter cannot fund pre-adoption testing for imported or travelled animals, there are other measures that can be taken. Information leaflets can be prepared for adopters, detailing the countries and areas visited by their new pet and the diseases that are present there. There are also some excellent leaflets for clients that contain information about the more common vector-borne diseases (e.g. *Taking your pets abroad*, BVA Animal Welfare Foundation www. bva-awf.org.uk/sites/bva-awf. org-UK/files/user/taking_your_pets_ abroad.pdf). Once informed, it is then up to that particular owner whether or not they wish to pursue testing.

Handling of passport documentation

If a dog or cat arrives with a pet passport, a decision must be made about whether or not to pass this documentation on to the eventual adopter. Factors to consider in this decision are:

- The shelter may be perceived by the adopter as 'validating' a passport. If a passport is deemed invalid during subsequent travel, some blame may be attributed to the shelter
- It is necessary to consider data protection if the passport contains any details that may facilitate identification of the previous owner.

Shelters are not in a position to provide advice about overseas travel. Adopters of all animals (whether travelled or not) should be encouraged to consult their own veterinary surgeon to discuss the implications and logistics of future travel with their pet.

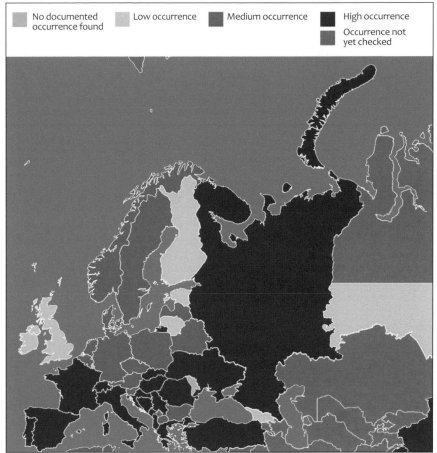

No documented occurrence found | Low occurrence | Medium occurrence | High occurrence | Occurrence not yet checked

Map of the distribution of canine vector-borne diseases in Europe.
(Courtesy of Bayer Healthcare, 13.10.2017)

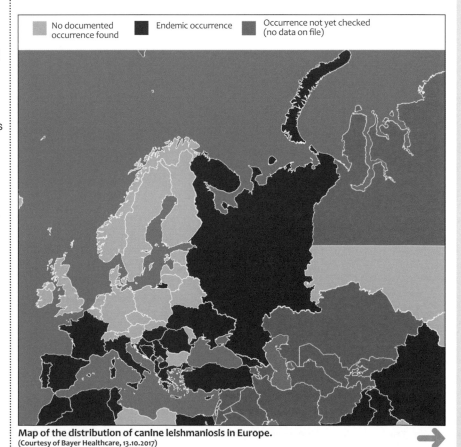

No documented occurrence found | Endemic occurrence | Occurrence not yet checked (no data on file)

Map of the distribution of canine leishmaniosis in Europe.
(Courtesy of Bayer Healthcare, 13.10.2017)

QRG 16.3 *continued*

Stray dogs and cats

Clues to previous foreign travel/origin may include:

* A microchip with a foreign country code. This is not proof, as microchips can be purchased online from international suppliers, but should be a consideration
  * European search engines, e.g. Europetnet (www.europetnet.com), might help to identify the origin of the dog or cat
  * If a dog or cat does have a foreign microchip but no traceable source, consideration should be given to whether that animal has entered the country legally and the implications of this, e.g. rabies serology
  * If there are concerns regarding potentially illegal import of an animal or notifiable disease, the relevant Government agency (at the time of writing, the Animal and Plant Health Agency (APHA)) should be contacted for advice in the first instance (see Chapter 21)
* Mutilations that are illegal in the UK, e.g. cropped ears or tail docking of non-traditionally docked breeds
* Rare breeds not commonly seen in the UK.

Rabies and *Echinococcus multilocularis*

Both of these diseases should be covered under PETS. However, it is possible that a shelter may encounter dogs or cats that are implanted with a foreign microchip but have no known history and cannot be traced. While the presence of a foreign microchip does not definitively identify the animal's country of origin, it raises questions. As such, it is advisable that all such animals are treated immediately against tapeworms (with praziquantel). This should be the case for **all** cats that have travelled overseas, as there is no mandatory requirement for this treatment within PETS. Consideration should be given to performing rabies serology to gain an indication of whether the animal has been vaccinated against rabies.

References and further reading

American Heartworm Society (2014) *Current Canine Guidelines for the Prevention, Diagnosis and Management of Heartworm (Dirofilaria immitis) Infection in Dogs*. American Heartworm Society, Wilmington. Available at: https://heartwormsociety.org/images/pdf/2014-AHS-Canine-Guidelines.pdf

Shaw SE and Day MJ (2005) *Arthropod-borne Infectious Diseases of the Dog and Cat*. Manson Publishing/CRC Press, Boca Raton

Useful websites

BVA Animal Welfare Foundation pet travel advice: www.bva-awf.org.uk/pet-care-advice/pet-travel

Companion Vector-Borne Diseases (Bayer Healthcare): www.cvbd.org

ESCCAP UK & Ireland: www.esccapuk.org.uk/professionals.php

Europetnet: www.europetnet.com

World Organisation for Animal Health rabies portal: www.oie.int/en/animal-health-in-the-world/rabies-portal/

Disease	Incubation period	Common clinical signs	Asymptomatic carriage?	Diagnosis	Treatment	Human disease?	Risk to other dogs?
Echinococcus multilocularis	4–8 weeks	No clinical signs in the dog or cat. The fox and the dog are definitive hosts. Cats are poor (and uncommon) hosts	Yes	Modified McMaster method or segment identification	Praziquantel – use in dogs every 4 weeks in endemic areas	Yes, through ingestion of eggs passed in the faeces of a definitive host (fox, dog). Asymptomatic incubation lasts 5–15 years. Result is alveolar echinococcosis with primary tumour-like lesion in the liver	Via ingestion of infected cysts from intermediate hosts (small rodents). *E. multilocularis* is not established in the UK
Rabies	Variable, can range from a few days to several months. Most cases present 2–12 weeks after infection	Variable, often a change in normal behaviour (unusually friendly or unprovoked biting), change in vocalization, excessive salivation due to inability to swallow	Yes	**Notifiable disease** – suspected cases **must** be reported to Animal and Plant Health Agency (APHA) as soon as possible. Virus isolation from samples of brain. If a dog has been bitten, euthanasia and early detection is required	None. Once clinical signs are present, the disease is invariably fatal within a week	Yes, through bites from an infected dog, or saliva on open wounds. The virus is extremely labile; therefore, immediate washing of a wound from an infected dog is imperative, in addition to post-exposure treatment	Via bites from an infected dog

Details of rabies and *Echinococcus multilocularis*, two non-vector-borne canine diseases that are endemic in parts of Western Europe but considered exotic in the UK.

Chapter 17

Managing feline immunodeficiency virus and feline leukaemia virus in the multi-cat/shelter environment

Beth Skillings, Tim Gruffydd-Jones and Victoria Crossley

Feline immunodeficiency virus (FIV) and feline leukaemia virus (FeLV) are retroviruses that are an important potential cause of disease in cats. Although commonly tested for together using combined tests, there are important differences between the two infectious agents, including risk factors for infection, testing methodology, prognosis and significance for infected individuals. An overview of the relevant characteristics and epidemiology of FIV and FeLV is given in Figures 17.1 and 17.2.

Despite these differences, FIV and FeLV are often considered together partly because combined tests are usually used to screen for these viruses using in-practice test kits but also owing to overlaps in their common clinical presentations. However, there are some clinical features that are more specific to each virus, which are outlined below.

Parameter	FIV	FeLV
Incubation	• Generally, months to years before cats may show signs associated with immunodeficiency • Some infected cats never develop clinical disease	• Months to years • Occasionally, very acute onset of signs (less common, often rapidly fatal)

Pathogenesis	• FIV is a lentivirus that targets T helper lymphocytes
	• Five subtypes (or clades) of the virus are known, but only subtype A is usually found in the UK
	• During the acute phase:
	  • Viral load peaks 2–3 months after infection and then subsides
	  • Signs of mild illness may be seen briefly, e.g. pyrexia, lethargy and lymphadenopathy
	• Typically, the acute phase is followed by an asymptomatic phase where viral load is stable, but T cell numbers decline over a period of years
	• This phase may ultimately lead to immunodeficiency, opportunistic infections, systemic disease and malignancies
	• Cats infected with FIV have low levels of antigen in their blood but persistent high levels of antibody
		• FeLV is a gammaretrovirus that replicates in leucocytes
		• Cats develop a significant plasma viral load early in infection
		• The p27 antigen is abundant in the plasma of infected cats and in infected cells
		• Infected cells transport virus to the thymus, spleen, lymph nodes and bone marrow
		• Migration to the salivary glands and mucosa leads to widespread excretion in body secretions
		• The most common outcomes of infection are:
		  • Persistent viraemia, where cats may develop FeLV-associated diseases
		  • Transient viraemia, where infection is regressive
		• Some cats seroconvert without ever showing detectable viraemia
		• Abortive and focal infections are possible but uncommon
		• Cats that overcome viraemia may be considered latently infected, but the risk of latent infection leading to shedding or FeLV-related disease is low

Diagnostic tests	• In-house screening kits based on detection of antibody by ELISA or rapid immunomigration are commonly used as the first-line test • Due to limitations of the in-practice screening tests, confirmatory testing using a different test method (e.g. PCR) at an external laboratory is recommended in many cases • Virus isolation may be regarded as the gold standard test but is not readily available • PCR tests are now available for direct detection of the virus	• In-house screening kits detect p27 antigen in blood samples • Positive results in healthy cats should usually be confirmed using a different test method at an external laboratory • Virus isolation, PCR for proviral DNA, immunochromatography and immunofluorescent antigen tests are available
Shedding and carrier status	• Viral shedding is continuous and lifelong • FIV is shed in saliva, nasal secretions, faeces and milk	• Transmission generally requires prolonged contact between cats • FeLV is shed in saliva, nasal secretions, faeces and milk

17.1 Characteristics of FIV and FeLV. ELISA = enzyme-linked immunosorbent assay; PCR = polymerase chain reaction.

Parameter	FIV	FeLV
Transmission	• In blood and saliva – usually via a bite from an infected cat • Transmission from mothers to kittens can occur *in utero*, at parturition and via milk, but the risk is considered low unless the acute stages of infection occur during pregnancy or lactation • The risk of transmission within a household may be influenced by the general health of the cats and how well the cats are socially adapted: 　◦ In a stable household the risk of infection is low 　◦ Risk is increased if fighting occurs, although transmission has occurred in closed multi-cat households where biting has not been observed • Virus is stable for only minutes in the environment	• Mainly in infected saliva, via mutual grooming; however, also possible by biting, close contact and sharing food bowls • Risk of infection is therefore high for susceptible, socially well adapted in-contact cats • Transmission also occurs across the placenta or in milk: 　◦ All kittens born to viraemic queens are expected to be viraemic 　◦ In latently infected queens, single kittens in a litter may become viraemic after birth if there is focal infection in a mammary gland, although this is rare • Virus is stable for minutes to hours in the environment
Disinfectant	• Quaternary ammonium compounds • Inorganic peroxygen compounds • Bleach	• Quaternary ammonium compounds • Inorganic peroxygen compounds • Bleach
Prevention	• No vaccine is available in the UK • FIV-positive cats should be housed separately from FIV-negative cats • Consideration should be given to rehoming (if appropriate) as indoor only	• FeLV vaccines are available and can be given optionally in a shelter environment • Vaccination from 8–9 weeks of age with second vaccination at 12 weeks • House cats in isolation pending confirmatory testing
Immunity	• Infection is lifelong	• Cats exposed to FeLV that seroconvert are protected from persistent viraemia • Duration of immunity is difficult to establish for FeLV vaccines. The European Advisory Board of Cat Diseases recommends booster vaccination every 2–3 years
Zoonosis	No	No
Cross-species transmission	No	No

17.2 Epidemiology of FIV and FeLV.

Feline immunodeficiency virus

A summary of the stages of infection of FIV is shown in Figure 17.3. Many infected cats do not show signs of infection owing to a long asymptomatic phase, but when signs are present they can be very variable. Some signs result directly from the virus, for example, neurological signs or diarrhoea. However, most clinical problems are secondary to immunosuppression and include chronic infections (e.g. chronic gingivostomatitis, chronic rhinitis), susceptibility to infectious agents that cats would normally be resistant to, or more serious consequences of clinical infections. Clinical signs depend on the body systems affected, but may include lymphadenopathy and weight loss. Evidence of clinical signs that affect multiple body systems increases the suspicion of immunosuppressive disease. FIV should be considered in the differential diagnosis for many sick cats.

1. Infection (usually occurs acutely, e.g. via a bite from an infected cat).
2. Virus is detectable approximately 2 weeks following infection. Antibodies are typically produced within 4–6 weeks of infection.
3. Viraemia peaks approximately 8–12 weeks post infection.
4. Decrease in plasma viral load associated with asymptomatic phase.
5. Signs of immunodeficiency may develop years later. Some infected cats never develop clinical disease.

17.3 Summary of the stages of FIV infection.

Feline leukaemia virus

A summary of the stages of infection of FeLV is shown in Figure 17.4. In the early stages of infection with FeLV, cats are unlikely to show significant clinical signs. However, the establishment of persistent viraemia usually results in either neoplastic disease, most often lymphosarcoma but occasionally leukaemia, or non-neoplastic disease, either

1. Infection (usually requires prolonged close contact with an infected cat).
2. Viraemia and significant proviral load develop within weeks; however, up to one-third of cats will seroconvert with no detectable antigenaemia.
3. Of those with detectable viraemia, a proportion will be only transiently infected (regressor cats) and will clear the infection within a short period. The chance of testing a transiently infected cat during this stage is low. The remainder will remain persistently infected and develop clinical signs.
4. A small proportion (5%) of cats will have detectable antigenaemia but no viraemia on testing (discordant cats). For the purposes of determining infection status, these cats are generally regarded as FeLV negative.

17.4 Summary of the stages of FeLV infection.

as a direct result of the virus or secondary to immunosuppression caused by the virus. Consequences of infection include anaemia, reproductive failure, uveitis, or features secondary to immunosuppression. FeLV should also be considered in the differential diagnosis for many sick cats.

Considerations for history and physical examination

The priority in history taking and clinical assessment with regard to FIV and FeLV is in assessing the likelihood of infection. The most important factor in determining the risk of infection is whether the cat is sick. Other factors that might be considered include: the background of how the cat was presented to the charity (e.g. relinquished by the owner, stray, from another charity, feral); how it was housed (indoor, outdoor); evidence of previous fighting, e.g. old healed bite wounds or abscesses (for FIV); the cat's vaccine history (for FeLV); information about any current or previous in-contact cats; and geographical location.

Epidemiology of infection

Proviruses

FeLV and FIV are retroviruses. This means that they insert DNA copies of their genetic material into the cat's own genome. The inserted material is called a provirus. In this way, every time an infected cat cell divides, the virus genome is also replicated using the cell's replication machinery. Some diagnostic tests are based on the specific detection of provirus rather than virus itself.

Transmission

FIV and FeLV are not viable in the environment, and direct contact is necessary for transmission (see Figure 17.2). FIV is typically transmitted by adversarial contact, such as bite wounds and fighting. FeLV is shed at high levels in all bodily secretions. Transmission most often occurs through transfer of saliva while cats in social groups are engaging in mutual grooming. Both FIV and FeLV can be passed on from queen to kittens, although this has been shown to be unusual for FIV. In a well managed rescue shelter with good husbandry and infectious disease control measures, transmission of FIV and FeLV should not be a problem if cats are housed individually or in small pre-established groups admitted from multi-cat households. Where group housing is utilized there is a risk of transmission within the shelter.

Many shelters have FeLV/FIV testing protocols based on the concern that, as there is often a long lag phase between infection and development of disease, cats may enter the shelter already infected with one of these viruses but appearing clinically normal. Therefore, if healthy cats in shelters are not tested, there is a risk of inadvertently rehoming an infected cat that goes on to develop disease some time later while in the new owner's care. In the period before overt signs of disease are shown, the cat will excrete virus and may infect other cats either within the same household or in the neighbourhood. As well as the obvious animal health implications of such a case, there is also the potential for reputational damage to the shelter. However, testing all cats has financial implications, and there can be concerns about unreliable results particularly when testing healthy cats (see below).

Prevalence

The prevalence of a disease describes the proportion of animals affected by the disease at any one time. For example, if five cats out of a colony of 20 have FeLV, the prevalence in that colony is 25% (5 ÷ 20 = 0.25). The current prevalence of FeLV and FIV in the healthy pet cat population of the UK is unknown but is considered to be low for FeLV (less than 1% and probably less than 0.1%), but higher for FIV (typically 3–5%). However, individual colonies and at-risk populations (e.g. in areas where neutering rates are low) may have endemic infections in which a significant proportion of cats are likely to be infected, so the prevalence of infection in different groups of cats is likely to vary considerably. As discussed further below, monitoring the prevalence of infection in the cat population(s) being tested is very helpful both when deciding on a population testing strategy and when considering how best to interpret test results.

Risk factors for infection

FIV

The prevalence of FIV is higher in sick cats than in healthy cats, but FIV-infected cats can be healthy at the time of diagnosis. For this reason, it can be difficult to determine whether FIV is the cause of clinical signs in a sick cat that is confirmed as positive when tested. It has been reported that cats in poor health, males, entire cats and stray cats are at increased risk of FIV (Levy *et al.*, 2006; Murray *et al.*, 2009). It is recommended that pregnant and lactating queens should also be tested as infection can be passed on to kittens (Figures 17.5 and 17.6). The proportion of kittens affected is variable depending on the queen's stage of infection, but is often quite low.

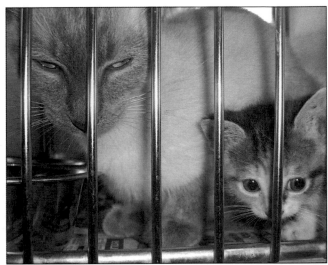

17.5 Testing pregnant queens or those with kittens for FIV or FeLV is a priority.
(© Rachel Dean)

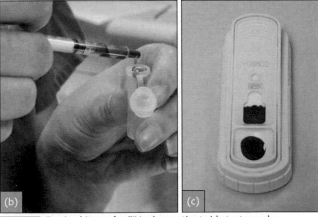

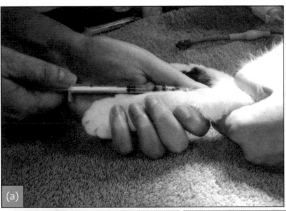

(a) (b) (c)

17.6 Testing kittens for FIV using patient-side tests can be unreliable. It is important to follow the manufacturer's instructions when undertaking tests as some require that serum or plasma is used rather than whole blood.
(© Cats Protection)

FeLV

Many clinical diseases may increase the index of suspicion that a cat may be infected with FeLV. Young cats, entire cats, those living in a high population density and in social groups are also at an increased risk of FeLV (Levy *et al.*, 2006). Again, it is recommended that pregnant and lactating cats should be prioritized for testing.

Testing for FIV and FeLV

When testing for any disease, it is important to consider the individual patient, the population from which the cat has come and the test to be used, as consideration of all these factors will help with the choice of test and the interpretation of the results. An understanding of the history, signalment and clinical signs of the patient will give the clinician an index of suspicion as to the likelihood that a cat may or may not be infected with FIV or FeLV. Knowing which type of population the cat has come from (e.g. feral colony, single indoor household, breeding group) will give an indication of how likely infection will be (i.e. the prevalence). It is important to recognize that no test is perfect

and knowing the likelihood of false-negatives and false-positives (i.e. the positive and negative predictive values which depend on the prevalence) is also vital when interpreting results. It is also important to know whether or not resources are available for confirmatory testing before deciding which cats to test. The epidemiological principles box below provides some basic epidemiological and diagnostic testing concepts that are useful when considering testing cats for FeLV/FIV, creating a testing strategy and interpreting test results.

Timing of testing

Testing cats at the earliest opportunity after they enter shelter care is recommended, as this ensures infected cats can be managed appropriately and helps to minimize the emotional attachment of shelter staff with cats that may be euthanased based on the policy of the shelter. It is theoretically possible that cats that have only just been exposed to infection might go through a stage before virus (FeLV) or antibody (FIV) is detectable in the blood, and will test (falsely) negative; however, this period is very short and is not generally regarded as a significant consideration unless there is reason to believe there has been very recent exposure.

Epidemiological principles to consider when deciding which cats to test

Diagnostic tests are not perfect and no diagnostic test is 100% reliable (see Chapter 8). False-positives and false-negatives occur in almost all diagnostic tests. The clinical examination is the first diagnostic investigation performed and all further test results should be interpreted in the light of the clinical findings.

* **True-positive** – test result is positive and cat DOES have the disease
* **False-positive** – test result is positive but cat DOES NOT have the disease
* **True-negative** – test result is negative and cat DOES NOT have the disease
* **False-negative** – test result is negative but cat DOES have the disease

Two terms that are often stated in relation to a test are **sensitivity**, the proportion of **affected** animals that test positive, and **specificity**, the proportion of **unaffected** animals that test negative.

However, the key considerations are the positive predictive value (PPV) and the negative predictive value (NPV), which are dependent on the prevalence of the disease in question.

* **Prevalence** – this is the number of animals with the disease at a particular point in time
* **Incidence** – this the number of new cases of a disease in a population during a given period of time

Positive and negative predictive values of a test are often more useful:

* **Positive predictive value** – this is the probability that an animal that tests positive *actually* has the disease
* **Negative predictive value** – this is the probability that an animal that tests negative **does not** have the disease

Another way of showing these principles is by using this table:

	Disease positive	Disease negative
Test positive	A	B
Test negative	C	D

True-positive = A	Sensitivity = A/A+C	Positive Predictive Value = A/A+B
False-positive = B	Specificity = D/B+D	Negative Predictive Value = D/C+D
True-negative = D	Prevalence = A+C/A+B+C+D	
False-negative = C		

When interpreting a result it is imperative to consider the patient in front of you: does the result make sense? Is it what you expected from your clinical examination?

The examples below show the impact of differences in disease prevalence and sensitivity and specificity of tests on test positive and negative predictive values. The figures used represent prevalence for FeLV (examples 1 and 2) and FIV (examples 3 and 4) in healthy and sick cats that may be encountered, however, actual prevalence will vary and risk factors for individual cats should be taken into account. The sensitivity and specificity for the tests are similar to those that might be expected for the performance of in-practice test kits for these diseases. When the disease prevalence is low (such as for FeLV in healthy cats), a high number of false-positives can occur even when test specificity is quite high, hence it is important that confirmatory tests are carried out. In contrast, the predictive values for FIV are generally high; even though the sensitivity is well below 100%, the NPV remains quite high because the number of true-negatives in the population is still comparatively large.

Example 1

In an FeLV test that is **100% sensitive** but only **98% specific**, if the **prevalence of FeLV is 1%** in every 100 tests, 1 cat that is disease positive will test positive (**red**). However, only 98% of the 99 cats that are disease free will test negative (n=97) (**blue**) and the remaining 2% (n=2) of non-infected cats will test falsely positive (**orange**). Therefore:

The **positive predictive value (PPV)** is:

$$\frac{\text{Number of true-positives}}{\text{Number of true-positives + number of false-positives}} \times 100$$

$$\frac{1}{1+2} \times 100 = 33.3\%$$

The **negative predictive value (NPV)** is:

$$\frac{\text{Number of true-negatives}}{\text{Number of true-negatives + number of false-negatives}} \times 100$$

$$\frac{97}{97+0} \times 100 = 100\%$$

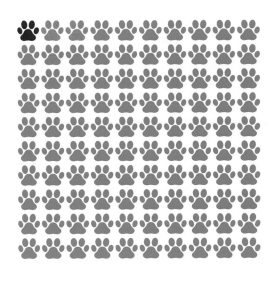

Example 2

In an FeLV test that is **100% sensitive** but only **98% specific**, if the **prevalence of FeLV is 8%** in every 100 tests, 8 cats that are disease positive will test positive (**red**). However, only 98% of the 92 cats that are disease free will test negative (n=90) (**blue**) and the remaining 2% (n=2) of non-infected cats will test falsely positive (**orange**). Therefore:

The **positive predictive value (PPV)** is:

$$\frac{\text{Number of true-positives}}{\text{Number of true-positives + number of false-positives}} \times 100$$

$$\frac{8}{8+2} \times 100 = 80\%$$

The **negative predictive value (NPV)** is:

$$\frac{\text{Number of true-negatives}}{\text{Number of true-negatives + number of false-negatives}} \times 100$$

$$\frac{90}{90+0} \times 100 = 100\%$$

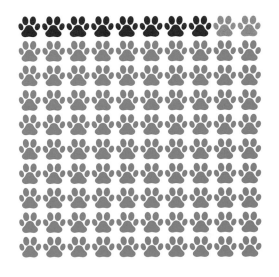

Example 3

In an FIV test that is **90% sensitive** and **100% specific**, if the **prevalence of FIV is 4%**, in every 100 tests only 90% of the 4 cats that are disease positive will test positive (i.e. 4/100 x 90 = 3.6, rounded up to 4, **red**). However, 100% of the 96 cats that are disease free will test negative (**blue**). Therefore:

The **positive predictive value (PPV)** is:

$$\frac{\text{Number of true-positives}}{\text{Number of true-positives + number of false-positives}} \times 100$$

$$\frac{4}{4+0} \times 100 = 100\%$$

The **negative predictive value (NPV)** is:

$$\frac{\text{Number of true-negatives}}{\text{Number of true-negatives + number of false-negatives}} \times 100$$

$$\frac{96}{96+0} \times 100 = 100\%$$

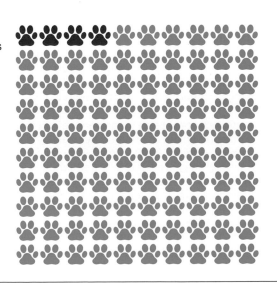

Example 4

In an FIV test that is **90% sensitive** and **100% specific**, if the **prevalence of FIV is 10%**, in every 100 tests, 9 of the 10 cats that are disease positive will test positive (**red**) and 1 will test falsely negative (**purple**). However, 100% of the 90 cats that are disease free will test truly negative (**blue**). Therefore:

The **positive predictive value (PPV)** is:

$$\frac{\text{Number of true-positives}}{\text{Number of true-positives + number of false-positives}} \times 100$$

$$\frac{9}{9 + 0} \times 100 = 100\%$$

The **negative predictive value (NPV)** is:

$$\frac{\text{Number of true-negatives}}{\text{Number of true-negatives + number of false-negatives}} \times 100$$

$$\frac{90}{90 + 1} \times 100 = 98.9\%$$

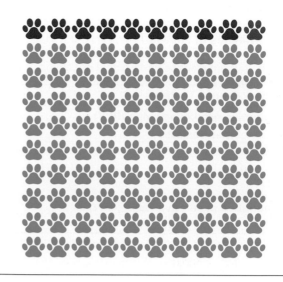

Tests available

In-practice patient-side tests

A number of tests for FeLV and FIV are available at the time of writing. Most commonly used are the patient-side tests. These are almost always combined tests for both viruses, which means that cats are likely to be tested for both even if they are considered high risk for only one or other infection. These tests work on the fundamental principle that an antibody will bind to its corresponding antigen. For FeLV, the test contains the antibody and will detect the FeLV viral antigen in the sample from the cat; whereas for FIV the test contains an antigen, which will bind to anti-FIV antibody if it is present in the sample. When these reactions occur, a colour change occurs on the test strip, giving a visible band or dot that indicates a positive result. Occasionally, molecules other than FeLV/FIV present in the sample will bind to the target antigen or antibody to give a false-positive result (Figure 17.7).

Potential errors with in-practice test kits are more likely when:

* The test is used at an incorrect temperature
* The test result is not read at the specified time (Figure 17.8)
* Whole blood rather than plasma or serum is used. False-positive results are considered to be more common when using whole blood. If whole blood is used initially and a positive result is obtained, it is recommended that the test be repeated using plasma or serum, or confirmed using an alternative method

The most commonly used screening tests in the UK are based on enzyme-linked immunosorbent assay (ELISA) or rapid immunomigration (RIM). Other in-practice test kits are available, but they are used less frequently. It is important to check how a test should be performed and interpreted according to manufacturer's instructions.

FIV: FIV tests are based on detecting antibodies to the viral core protein p24 or the transmembrane envelope protein gp40, which usually develop 4–6 weeks after infection. Positive results in (high-risk) cats over 20 weeks of age are generally reliable; however, false-negative results can occur,

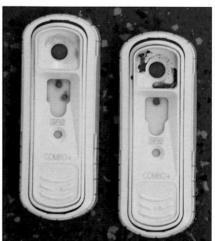

17.7 According to the manufacturer's instructions, the test on the left shows a positive result for FeLV. Positive test results can indicate infection or be a false-positive. The test on the right is negative for FIV and FeLV.
(© Rachel Dean)

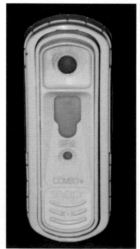

17.8 It is important to follow the instructions for patient-side tests. This test is not useful and needs to be repeated as the period between undertaking and reading the test was too long.
(© Rachel Dean)

and so a negative result in a cat with a high suspicion of infection should ideally be confirmed (see below). In-practice test results for kittens under 20 weeks of age can be complicated by the presence of maternally derived antibodies, and this type of test is not recommended in these cases (see Special considerations in screening programmes, below).

FeLV: Tests for FeLV are based on the detection of free p27 antigen and therefore results in kittens tested are not affected by maternally derived antibodies. There is a high likelihood of obtaining false-positive results with screening tests for FeLV when the prevalence is low (see Epidemiological principles to consider when deciding which cats to test, above). Therefore, positive results should ideally be confirmed at a reliable external reference laboratory, using an alternative confirmatory test methodology with higher specificity than the screening test. Exceptions to this could be sick cats (where false-positive results are less likely) and feral cats (see Special considerations in screening programmes, below).

Confirmatory external laboratory tests

Polymerase chain reaction (PCR) is the most common technique used by reference laboratories for confirmatory testing for FIV and FeLV, although other techniques may be used; practitioners are advised to contact the reference laboratory for up-to-date information on the tests used. PCR will detect provirus of the relevant virus in the sample. This is not yet available as a patient-side test but results from external laboratories are often available within a few days. PCR testing is more reliable than patient-side tests (see Chapter 8 for more information on PCR). Different types of test used for the diagnosis of FIV and FeLV are described in Figures 17.9 and 17.10.

FIV: Some infected cats fail to produce detectable antibody to FIV; this is a limitation for both in-practice and confirmatory antibody tests for FIV, such as immunofluorescence or Western blot. In cases with a high suspicion of FIV but negative results on antibody testing, retesting should be performed using a test based on the detection of the virus itself.

Type of test	Advantages and disadvantages of test
In-practice tests	*Tests for FIV are based on the detection of antibodies to the viral core protein p24 or the transmembrane envelope protein gp40, which usually develop 4–6 weeks after infection. Maternally derived antibodies in kittens can affect the results of these tests*
ELISA or RIM	• Quick results • Inexpensive • High specificity (99%), i.e. positive results are generally reliable (except in kittens) • Moderate sensitivity (80–98%), i.e. a negative result in a cat with a high relative risk of disease should ideally be confirmed by another test • Based on detection of antibodies, therefore maternally derived antibodies in kittens can lead to positive results but do not indicate active infection • Failure to mount a sufficient antibody response can lead to false-negative results
Confirmatory tests	*In cases with a high suspicion of FIV that give negative results on antibody testing, retesting using a test based on the detection of the virus itself rather than antibody may be considered. PCR tests are designed to detect specific subtypes of virus and, therefore, may not identify cats that are positive for a different subtype, e.g. cats that originate from a different country (see Chapter 8 for more detail on PCR)*
PCR for proviral DNA	• Generally sensitive and specific for particular subtypes of virus, but sensitivity and specificity are variable depending on the particular PCR test and the other subtypes (which may be seen in cats originating from other countries) for which the PCR was not designed • Particularly useful for confirmatory testing of kittens that test positive on screening, as PCR is not affected by maternally derived antibodies
Virus isolation	• Highly specific (100%), but not suitable for routine use and, therefore, not widely available
Western blot	• Based on antibody detection, which limits sensitivity in cats that do not mount a sufficient antibody response and limits use in kittens under 20 weeks of age. As this type of test detects antibodies rather than virus, it has similar disadvantages to in-practice tests

17.9 Advantages and disadvantages of tests for FIV. ELISA = enzyme-linked immunosorbent assay; PCR = polymerase chain reaction; RIM = rapid immunomigration.

Type of test	Advantages and disadvantages of test
In-practice tests	*Tests for FeLV are based on the detection of free p27 antigen and, therefore, results in kittens are not affected by maternally derived antibodies*
ELISA or RIM/ immuno-chromatography	• Quick results • Inexpensive • Highly sensitive (~100%). Negative results are, therefore, generally reliable in ruling out viraemia • Lower specificity (<98%). The low prevalence of FeLV within the population means that positive results on in-practice tests used in healthy cats have a high chance of being false-positives • Test is based on the detection of antigen and, therefore, is not affected by maternally derived antibodies in kittens
Confirmatory tests	*If a healthy cat tests FeLV positive, retesting using a confirmatory test is advised, as there is a high chance of the test result being a false-positive (see Epidemiological principles). If there is a high index of suspicion that FeLV may be a cause of clinical signs in a sick cat, confirmatory testing is also advised*
PCR for proviral DNA	• Highly sensitive and specific, but need to assess whether positive result indicates active viraemia • Positive results with low cycle threshold values are likely to be associated with regressive infection and are unlikely to be clinically significant
Virus isolation	• Highly specific (100%) but complex and time-consuming to perform • Virus isolation was the original confirmatory test for FeLV and is regarded as the gold standard for positive results. The main advantage of this test is that false-positives are not possible
Immunofluorescent assay	• Limited availability but reasonable sensitivity

17.10 Advantages and disadvantages of tests for FeLV. ELISA = enzyme-linked immunosorbent assay; PCR = polymerase chain reaction; RIM = rapid immunomigration.

PCR tests for FIV have been developed and are particularly useful for testing kittens, as they are based on the detection of part of the virus rather than detection of antibody to viral antigens. PCR tests are designed for detecting specific viral subtypes and, therefore, may not detects cats that are positive for a different subtype (e.g. cats that originate from a different country). Virus isolation is possible for FIV but is not practical for routine use.

FeLV: Virus isolation was the original confirmatory test for FeLV and is regarded as the gold standard for positive results. The main advantage of this method is that false-positives are not possible.

PCR tests that detect FeLV provirus are extremely sensitive. Very low levels of provirus are thought to represent residual infection in a cat that has previously encountered the virus, mounted an immune response and contained the infection. These low levels of provirus are not currently thought to be clinically significant. Interpretation of the results of these tests, therefore, requires consideration of the amount of provirus detected.

Discordant tests

Discordancy is a well recognized phenomenon where some cats persistently give positive results for FeLV on ELISA tests, but negative results on virus isolation. Generally, these cats are regarded as negative, that is, the ELISA results are regarded as a false-positive and the confirmatory tests are considered to give the true result.

To test, or not to test?

Whether and which cats should be tested for FeLV and FIV in rescue shelters is a challenging issue, and a number of different factors should be taken into account when making the decision. Shelters have a responsibility to balance the priorities of the health and welfare of the group of animals, the health and welfare of individual animals, and factors that may impact on potential new owners and in-contact animals, within the economic and environmental limitations of the organization.

In veterinary practice, the combined FeLV/FIV test is most commonly used for testing of an individual animal with suggestive clinical signs. However, within shelters, these tests are most commonly used as screening tests, to identify infected individuals (which may or may not have relevant clinical signs). This is an important distinction, as it affects the ways in which the test results may be interpreted and used.

The key issues in deciding whether and how shelter cats should be tested for FeLV and FIV are the likelihood of infection, future health implications for positive cats, whether confirmatory tests will be used to confirm results of screening tests and the concern of possible transmission to other cats following rehoming. Shelters often have limited budgets and, therefore, the use of FeLV/FIV testing must be balanced against the cost of housing, neutering, vaccination, microchipping and other healthcare measures. Testing can be expensive depending on the test used and whether it is undertaken at the patient's side or a sample is submitted to a commercial laboratory. Furthermore, the reliability and interpretation of patient-side test results can be complicated by a low prevalence of infection in some populations, which may also influence which cats require further confirmatory testing (see Epidemiological principles to consider when deciding which cats to test, above).

Designing a testing strategy

Shelters have the option to test all, none, or some of the cats admitted to their care for FIV and FeLV. Different screening strategies offer a range of benefits and drawbacks; these are outlined in Figures 17.11 and 17.12. No

Strategy	Advantages	Disadvantages	Comments
Test none	• Cheap • Avoids retaining cats for long periods while awaiting the results of confirmatory testing • On a population basis, investing in neutering rather than testing may represent a better overall use of resources and will actually reduce population infection rates more efficiently than test-and-remove strategies	• Infected but clinically healthy cats will be missed, resulting in increased potential for disease transmission to other cats and potential welfare compromise • Potential for reputational damage to the shelter	• This strategy may be appropriate for some trap-neuter-return programmes for feral cats or in settings with very limited resources
Test some (high-risk cats prioritized)	• Costs much less than a 'test all' strategy • By selecting high-risk cats, the prevalence of infection in the population tested is increased. This means that the positive predictive value of the test is increased (i.e. a positive test result is more likely to be correct)	• Risk of missing some clinically healthy but infected cats • Potential for adverse consequences as for a 'test none' strategy • Ideally, confirmatory testing of positive cats would still be carried out if finances allow, adding to the cost	• This strategy is common in UK shelters • Having a clear definition of what constitutes an 'at-risk' cat is key here and may vary depending on the intake of the shelter (e.g. does it take in a lot of stray entire males?)
Test all	• It will be very unlikely to miss an infected cat, therefore, there is very limited opportunity for an infected cat to be unknowingly rehomed • May prevent suffering in infected cats • New owners will be fully informed of the test status of their adopted cat • Minimizes any risk to the shelter's reputation that might arise from rehoming a positive cat	• Expensive • It will likely give rise to a high proportion of false-positives, especially where the prevalence of infection is low • Ideally, all positive cats should have a confirmatory test, adding to the expense and time in the shelter • If confirmatory tests are not carried out, cats may be labelled as positive for the rest of their lives (which may involve restrictions on their environment) or mistakenly euthanased	• This strategy may be appropriate for populations with a very high prevalence of infection • May be preferred by organizations that are very well resourced • Where disease prevalence is low in the tested population, this strategy represents a very inefficient use of resources

17.11 Advantages and disadvantages of different strategies for the use of patient-side screening tests for FIV and FeLV.

Strategy	Cat populations
Ideally test all as a minimum	• Sick cats (those that are either already sick when admitted to the shelter or become sick while in care) that show clinical signs of disease consistent with a retrovirus infection • Any cat before housing in a communal area
Recommended to test	• Pregnant and nursing queens • Entire adult males • All cats known to be in contact with cats that are FIV or FeLV positive (this includes all kittens of FIV-positive queens) • Feral cats (where finances are limited, it is recommended to test a proportion of a feral colony; if any test positive, all cats in the colony should then be tested) • Any cat before it undergoes extensive treatment or surgery
Others to consider testing if resources allow	• All stray cats • Orphan kittens • Kittens born to a queen whose FeLV/FIV status is unknown

17.12 Recommendations for which cats to test for FIV and FeLV.

single strategy forms a perfect solution, but by considering the priorities and resources of each organization the best fit can be selected. Understanding the epidemiological principles of positive and negative predictive values is critical in deciding which cats to test (see Epidemiological principles to consider when deciding which cats to test, above).

Once a cat is identified as positive, it is important for the shelter to have a clear policy as to whether rehoming or euthanasia is indicated. Whichever strategy is used, it is essential to ensure that potential adopters are properly informed about the organization's policy, preferably in writing.

Special considerations in screening programmes

Kittens

FIV tests based on the detection of antibody do not give a reliable indication of whether or not a kitten is infected until maternally derived antibodies have declined, which occurs by approximately 20 weeks of age. This is an important limitation when rescue centres wish to screen and rehome young kittens as soon as possible. When a queen is identified as FIV positive it is still worth considering testing the kittens if finances allow. This is because, although positive results for FIV on in-practice tests may be a result of maternally derived antibodies from an infected queen, a kitten with a negative result for FIV can be safely rehomed. If a young kitten tests positive for FIV antibody, this probably indicates that the queen is infected.

Kittens younger than 20 weeks of age that test positive for FIV initially should be retested using PCR or virus isolation from 8–10 weeks of age. If this is not possible, those that test positive for antibody to FIV should be considered as having an unknown FIV status and rehomed to indoor homes with no in-contact cats, depending on the shelter's FIV rehoming policy. The new owners should be advised that their kitten should be retested at 20 weeks of age. Alternatively, these kittens could be fostered or held in the shelter's care until they can be retested, but the implications in terms of animal welfare and practicalities (e.g. finances and demand on space and paid or voluntary workers) will need to be considered. A kitten that again tests positive at 20 weeks of age should be considered FIV positive.

FeLV screening tests are based on detection of antigen and are, therefore, not affected by maternally derived antibodies in kittens. However, similarly to healthy adult cats, false-positives will be common when testing kittens from populations where the prevalence of FeLV is low. Kittens born to FeLV-positive queens will invariably be infected and, therefore, kittens born to confirmed FeLV-positive queens may be regarded as positive without testing.

Cats recently in contact with FIV/FeLV-positive cats

Where a cat tests positive for FIV or FeLV (including confirmatory tests where appropriate), all recent in-contact cats (except nursing kittens of positive queens) should be separated from the positive cat and tested. The decision as to whether to keep recent in-contact cats that initially test negative in care, pending retesting before rehoming, should be carefully considered. The options for in-contact cats differ for FeLV and FIV. For either virus, in-contact cats may be euthanased, rehomed, or retained and retested after at least 1 month, depending on the policy of the shelter. It would be rare to retain a cat that has recently been in contact with an FIV-positive cat pending retesting (especially if the in-contact animal can be rehomed as the sole cat in a potentially indoor-only home until the results of retesting are known), but where centres feel that FIV retesting is necessary, it should be carried out 6 weeks after exposure. For cats in contact with a case of confirmed FeLV, it is more likely the cats will be retained pending retesting as persistently infected cats pose a high risk to others.

Feral cats

When dealing with feral cat colonies, the ways in which different test strategies will influence the management of the cats should be considered. There is no point in testing if the test results will make no difference to the way the cats are managed. In some cases, local carers of feral colonies will not allow positive cats to be euthanased or removed, in which case testing is of little value. However, on a smaller scale, decisions regarding testing may be influenced by the wishes of the carer/feeder and the health of the colony in question. Confirmatory testing of feral cats that test positive on in-practice tests is not justifiable, given the lower likelihood of false-positive results when using screening tests in this population. In addition, the need to confine feral cats while waiting for test results is generally considered detrimental to their welfare.

Practical application of test results

Shelters must decide on what actions to take for cats that test positive for FIV or FeLV. Rehoming, keeping in sanctuary care and euthanasia of these cats all carry ethical considerations. Euthanasia of an apparently healthy cat based on a screening test (with or without confirmatory testing) may be difficult for some shelter workers to accept, and may be considered an inappropriate strategy. Others will believe it is in the best interests of the wider owned and unowned cat population in terms of preventing disease transmission and avoiding welfare issues associated with confinement, while maximizing use of the shelter's resources in terms of money, workers and space to help more animals (see Chapters 2 and 3).

Cats testing positive for FIV

Healthy cats that test positive for FIV can have a normal life expectancy and, therefore, may be considered suitable for rehoming by some organizations. However, if FIV-positive cats are sick or considered not to have a good quality of life, euthanasia is recommended.

Most shelters neuter pregnant queens in view of the already large number of unwanted cats. For shelters that do not routinely adopt this policy, it may be useful to note that many kittens born to FIV-positive queens will not be infected. Transfer of infection to kittens is much more likely in a recently infected queen when levels of the virus are at their highest, but pregnancy during the longer (lower-risk) asymptomatic phase is more common. During lactation, the risk of transmission of the virus to the kittens is also low, and so, given the benefits of maternal contact on nutrition and behavioural development, early weaning and/or hand-rearing of kittens born to FIV-positive queens is not recommended.

Cats that test positive for FIV do not need to be housed in isolation facilities (standard disease control with individual housing should suffice) unless they are ill (for example, showing 'flu-like signs) and pose a potential risk to others through shedding of other pathogens. FIV-positive cats should be clearly identified in the shelter (Figure 17.13). Ideally, vaccination is recommended for any cat of uncertain vaccination history entering a shelter, but it is particularly important for FIV-positive cats.

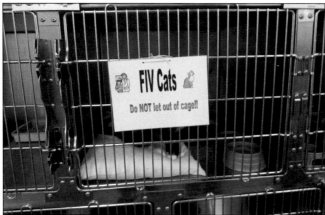

17.13 Clear identification of infected cats is important in shelter environments.
(© Rachel Dean)

Rehoming FIV-positive cats

FIV-positive cats that are rehomed should generally be rehomed as single cats, to avoid any risk of transfer to in-contact cats, and as indoor cats, to avoid the risk of transmission to cats in the neighbourhood. This also helps to protect the rehomed FIV-positive cat from exposure to infections from other cats, which may reduce the chance of progression of FIV-related disease. However, the risk of transmission to other cats within the same household is not clear, and some shelters choose to home FIV-positive cats in multi-cat households. This makes most sense if the cats go to a household where all of the existing cats are FIV positive. The risk posed by an FIV-positive cat to neighbouring cats is very variable and will depend on factors such as the location, the density of cats and how the cat responds to other cats – that is, whether or not it is aggressive. Some shelters may make a judgement that the risk posed by a new FIV-positive cat, particularly once neutered, is low, and be prepared to rehome such a cat to a household that will allow the cat outdoors. However, many shelters have a policy that FIV-positive cats that are not suited to living indoors pose a significant risk to others and should be euthanased even if they are healthy.

When cats that test positive for FIV are rehomed, the new owners must be made aware of the implications of having an FIV-positive cat, such as the potential for recurrent illness and increased cost of veterinary treatment (many insurance policies may exclude FIV-related conditions, such as gastrointestinal, skin and periodontal disease), and be willing and able to take on the extra responsibility (Figure 17.14).

Cats testing positive for FeLV

A cat that is FeLV positive on a screening test and is awaiting confirmatory test results should be housed in isolation, with food bowls, water bowls and litter trays cleaned separately and their use restricted to the same cat.

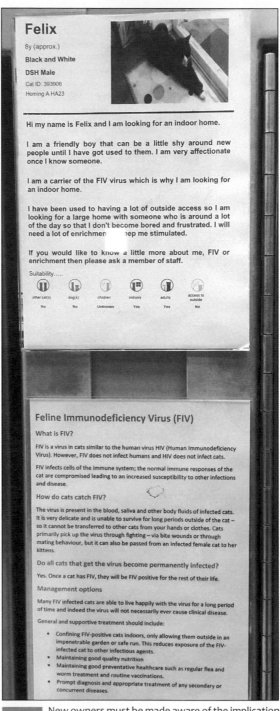

17.14 New owners must be made aware of the implications of having an FIV-positive cat.
(© Cats Protection)

If an apparently healthy cat (including a pregnant queen) tests positive for FeLV with the screening test and an external confirmatory test, it is not recommended to carry out any further testing. Euthanasia is advised for cats that test positive for FeLV where confirmed as appropriate, and for kittens of confirmed FeLV-positive queens, as these are invariably infected and have a poor prognosis. Eighty-five percent of cats that are persistently infected with FeLV are reported to die within 3 years of infection. FeLV-positive kittens usually die within 12 months. Most shelters euthanase sick and feral cats (the latter to avoid the welfare implications of confinement) that test positive, without conducting confirmatory testing.

Questions are sometimes raised as to whether positive FeLV results should be rechecked a few weeks later in case a cat has been in a transient phase of viraemia before an effective immune response has been mounted. However, this transient phase is very brief and the chance of testing cats during this phase is very small. Retesting is, therefore, generally regarded as unnecessary in view of the need to retain the cat for a longer period and the cost of retesting the cat, both of which have resource implications, as well as the effect on the morale of staff/volunteers caring for these cats.

Conclusion

There are many factors to consider in deciding whether or not to test a shelter cat for FeLV and FIV. Testing of all sick shelter cats is strongly recommended where possible, as there is an increased risk of such cats being positive and this will have serious implications for their future health.

Routine screening of healthy cats is more controversial. Detection of FeLV has very serious implications for any cat, whether sick or healthy. The outlook for a FeLV-positive cat is very poor even if it is healthy at the time of diagnosis. However, the prevalence of FeLV may be very low in healthy rescue cats, and therefore false-positive results are more likely than true-positive results. In an ideal world, routine screening of all cats would be backed up by a recognized confirmatory test; without this step, there are concerns that many of the cats that test positive are not genuinely infected and may be euthanased unnecessarily. However, the resources required for confirmatory testing may make this strategy impossible in some settings.

Screening for FIV is often considered more of a priority, as this virus is particularly common in certain populations of cats that may be encountered in rescue shelters. The main concern of a rescue centre is to avoid rehoming cats that are later found to be infected with FIV, with the resulting concerns to the adopter about health issues for the cat as well as concern about possible spread to other cats in the household or local area. However, many infected cats may remain healthy for a prolonged if not indefinite period, and some rescue centres will place the cats in selected homes when the adopter is aware of the potential implications.

It is recommended that when a cat is offered for rehoming, prospective owners are informed whether or not the cat has been tested for FeLV and FIV, the results of the tests performed and the implications of the results.

Top tips

- Testing every cat may not always be the best use of resources. Instead, ensure that the cats at most risk of infection are tested effectively
- Whether or not the resources are available to allow confirmatory testing to be carried out is key in determining a strategy for which cats to test
- Ideally, cats should be tested as soon as possible after entering shelter care
- From a welfare and economic perspective, if confirmatory testing is feasible, it may be preferable to obtain a sufficient blood sample at the time of performing the initial screening test, so that resampling is not required. Check with the individual laboratory as to the type and volume of sample preferred before taking the blood sample
- Interpret the test result in the light of the patient's clinical presentation and history, the sensitivity and specificity of the test, and the likely prevalence of disease in that population
- In kittens, anti-FIV antibody detected may be maternally derived rather than a result of infection
- Shelters must agree their own informed policies with regard to rehoming cats that test positive for FIV or FeLV
- Prognosis for FeLV-positive cats is poor for those that are persistently infected

References and further reading

Addie DD, Dennis JM, Toth S *et al.* (2000) Long-term impact on a closed household of pet cats of natural infection with feline coronavirus, feline leukaemia virus and feline immunodeficiency virus. *Veterinary Record* **146**, 419–424

Casey R and Bradshaw JWS (2008) The effects of additional socialisation for kittens in a rescue centre on their behaviour and suitability as a pet. *Applied Animal Behaviour Science* **114**, 196–205

Hosie MJ, Addie D, Belak S *et al.* (2009). Feline immunodeficiency. ABCD guidelines on prevention and management. *Journal of Feline Medicine and Surgery* **11(7)**, 575–584

Levy JK and Crawford PC (2004) Humane strategies for controlling feral cat populations. *Journal of the American Veterinary Medical Association* **225**, 1354–1360

Levy JK, Scott HM, Lachtara JL and Crawford PC (2006) Seroprevalence of feline leukaemiavirus and feline immunodeficiencey virus infection among cats in North America and risk factors for seropositivity. *Journal of American Medical Association* **228**, 371–376

Lutz H, Addie D, Belaket S *et al.* (2009). Feline leukaemia. ABCD guidelines on prevention and management. *Journal of Feline Medicine and Surgery* **11(7)**, 565–574

Möstl KH, Egberink H, Addie D *et al.* (2013). Prevention of infectious diseases in cat shelters: ABCD guidelines. *Journal of Feline Medicine and Surgery* **15(7)**, 546–554

Murray JK, Roberts MA, Skillings E, Morrow LD and Gruffydd-Jones TJ (2009) Risk factors for feline immunodeficiency virus antibody test status in Cats Protection adoption centres (2004). *Journal of Feline Medicine and Surgery* **11**, 467–473

O'Neil LL, Burkhard MJ and Hoover EA (1996). Frequent perinatal transmission of feline immunodeficiency virus by chronically infected cats. *Journal of Virology* **70(5)**, 2894–2901

Pinches MD, Helps CR, Gruffydd-Jones TJ *et al.* (2007). Diagnosis of feline leukaemia virus infection by semi-quantitative real-time polymerase chain reaction. *Journal of Feline Medicine and Surgery* **9(1)**, 8–13

Stavisky J, Dean RS and Molloy MH (2017) Prevalence of and risk factors for FIV and FeLV infection in two shelters in the United Kingdom (2011–2012) *Veterinary Record* **181**, 451

Managing feline coronavirus and feline infectious peritonitis in the multi-cat/shelter environment

Séverine Tasker and Nathalie Dowgray

Feline infectious peritonitis (FIP) is a serious and fatal disease that arises as a consequence of infection with feline coronavirus (FCoV). Although FCoV infection is very common in cats, particularly those housed in groups or at high density, FIP usually arises only sporadically (Pedersen, 2009), in a small percentage (~1–5%) of cats infected with FCoV.

Presentation and clinical signs

Epidemiology of FCoV infection and FIP

Features of FCoV infection

FCoVs are large enveloped ribonucleic acid (RNA) viruses. They are transmitted by the faecal–oral route, via ingestion of the virus in faeces and via sharing of litter trays. They are susceptible to many disinfectants (Figure 18.1), but they can survive for up to 7 weeks in dried faeces, so careful cleaning and disinfection of surfaces and materials in the shelter is important.

Kittens are usually protected from FCoV infection during early life, as they acquire maternally derived antibodies from the queen, which persist for 6–8 weeks. However, most kittens will then acquire FCoV infection from the queen or other in-contact cats, as soon as their maternally derived immunity wanes.

FCoV infection usually causes no clinical signs, although occasionally mild gastrointestinal signs (e.g. self-limiting diarrhoea) are seen. This is difficult to distinguish as a separate clinical entity from the transient diarrhoea that many cats experience on entering a shelter due to stress and dietary change (see Chapter 13). The possible outcomes of FCoV infection are shown in Figure 18.2.

Pathogenesis of FIP

FIP is believed to develop as a result of a virulent FCoV strain being present in the cat. Virulent strains are thought to arise through mutation of FCoVs during replication in infected cats (Kipar and Meli, 2014), which can occur weeks to months after the initial FCoV infection (Figure 18.2).

This theory of FIP pathogenesis, in which virulent FCoVs arise within individual cats rather than being transmitted horizontally between cats, is in line with the fact that the disease arises sporadically in FCoV-infected cats. It is thought that FIP-inducing FCoVs are probably less able to replicate within the intestinal tract and, thus, are not shed by infected cats. Hence, FIP outbreaks are very uncommon (see later, however, for further information on outbreaks).

Risk factors for FIP development

Most cats affected by FIP are young, typically 4 months to 2 years of age. Stress is believed to play a role in the development of FIP, with overcrowding, rehoming, neutering, changes in group hierarchy and vaccination all being potential triggers. Genetic lines may play a role; this may explain why certain pedigree breeds are predis-

Questions to ask	Comments
When did the cat enter the shelter? Was it healthy at the time?	This is important in determining whether FIP developed while the cat was in the shelter or before its admission
Where did the cat come from? Geographical location as well as source, e.g. foster home, relinquished by owner, stray?	May be useful in determining whether an FIP outbreak (fortunately, these are rare) is occurring, if a common source is identified for more than one case
Was the cat housed in a group or individually? If group-housed, are any of the other cats sick? Did the cat come in with any other cats, including siblings?	This will help decide whether any in-contact cats need monitoring for possible development of FIP
Has there been a source of stress, e.g. vaccination, neutering, regrouping or rehousing?	Identifying a source of stress and trying to prevent or reduce it may help prevent other cats from developing FIP
Are there enough litter trays for the cats? Are they regularly emptied? Are they cleaned and disinfected (including litter scoops) with an agent known to be effective against FCoV?	Aiming to reduce the faecal–oral transmission of FCoV by reducing the overall FCoV load present in a shelter may help to decrease the risk of FIP. Suitable disinfectants are bleach diluted 1:32, iodine compounds, oxidizing agents and alcohols. Cleaning of organic matter before disinfection is very important

18.1 Questions to ask when taking the history of suspected feline infectious peritonitis (FIP) in a shelter. FCoV = feline coronavirus.

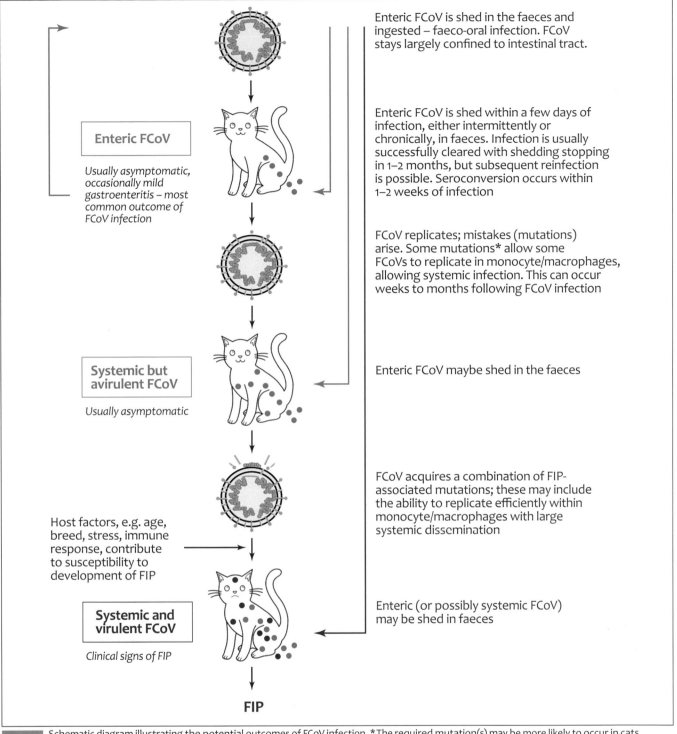

Enteric FCoV

Usually asymptomatic, occasionally mild gastroenteritis – most common outcome of FCoV infection

Systemic but avirulent FCoV

Usually asymptomatic

Host factors, e.g. age, breed, stress, immune response, contribute to susceptibility to development of FIP

Systemic and virulent FCoV

Clinical signs of FIP

Enteric FCoV is shed in the faeces and ingested – faeco-oral infection. FCoV stays largely confined to intestinal tract.

Enteric FCoV is shed within a few days of infection, either intermittently or chronically, in faeces. Infection is usually successfully cleared with shedding stopping in 1–2 months, but subsequent reinfection is possible. Seroconversion occurs within 1–2 weeks of infection

FCoV replicates; mistakes (mutations) arise. Some mutations* allow some FCoVs to replicate in monocyte/macrophages, allowing systemic infection. This can occur weeks to months following FCoV infection

Enteric FCoV maybe shed in the faeces

FCoV acquires a combination of FIP-associated mutations; these may include the ability to replicate efficiently within monocyte/macrophages with large systemic dissemination

Enteric (or possibly systemic FCoV) may be shed in faeces

FIP

18.2 Schematic diagram illustrating the potential outcomes of FCoV infection. *The required mutation(s) may be more likely to occur in cats carrying high FCoV loads; therefore, limiting the enviromental burden of FCoV and, thus, potentially, infection doses may be beneficial to help prevent FIP.
(Modified from Porter, 2014)

posed to FIP and why such predisposed breeds vary between different countries, although in the shelter environment the majority of cats that develop FIP will be non-pedigrees, in line with the profile of breeds taken in by the shelter. Littermates of kittens that have developed FIP are at a higher risk of developing the disease. Concurrent diseases or infections, such as feline leukaemia virus and feline immunodeficiency virus, may also predispose to FIP development.

Clinical signs of FIP

The clinical signs of FIP are traditionally divided into those associated with effusive or 'wet' FIP (in which widespread vasculitis leads to non-septic effusions) and those associated with non-effusive or 'dry' FIP (in which granulomatous reactions occur in localized tissues). In reality, there is marked overlap between the wet and dry manifestations of the disease.

Up to 80% of FIP cases present with effusions, the hallmark of wet FIP. Effusions occur most commonly in the abdomen but also in the pleural space and pericardial sac, causing bicavity or tricavity effusions. Cats affected with either the wet or the dry form of FIP can present with:

- Cyclical non-antibiotic-responsive fever
- Lethargy
- Reduced appetite
- Weight loss/failure to thrive
- Palpable abdominal masses due to omental and visceral adhesions, granulomas (e.g. on the kidneys (Figure 18.3) or in the liver) or mesenteric lymphadenopathy
- Jaundice is also relatively common
- Anterior and/or posterior uveitis can occur with both forms of the disease (Figure 18.4). The anterior chamber may show iritis, corneal oedema, aqueous flare, hyphaema, hypopyon and keratic precipitates, while retinal examination may reveal vessel engorgement, perivascular cuffing and/or subretinal fluid accumulation causing partial retinal detachment
- Neurological signs are reported in a small percentage (~10%) of cases and are typically associated with dry FIP. They are usually multifocal or diffuse, with

cerebellar ataxia, nystagmus and seizures most commonly reported. Hindlimb paresis, intention tremor, cranial and peripheral nerve deficits, hyperaesthesia, vestibular signs (head tilt) and behaviour changes are also seen.

As FIP is a progressive disease, the clinical signs change over time, so it is important to perform repeat clinical examinations to look for the development of signs (e.g. development of an effusion, uveitis) to aid diagnosis.

Diagnostic testing

Many young cats with FIP will present with a number of typical features of the disease, such as an abdominal effusion, pyrexia and uveitis. In such situations, the clinical picture may well result in FIP being the top differential diagnosis by far. In the shelter situation, it may be most cost-effective to consider euthanasia and post-mortem examination rather than embarking on diagnostic testing. Of the less invasive diagnostic tests available, demonstration of a reduced albumin:globulin (A:G) ratio in serum or in a sample of an effusion is probably most helpful in supporting a diagnosis of FIP. However, differential diagnoses (see later) should still be carefully considered before contemplating euthanasia and post-mortem examination without testing, and it may not be appropriate in cats showing less typical signs.

If the cat is euthanased, it is very important that a post-mortem examination is performed and, if at all possible, samples collected so that a diagnosis can be confirmed. Samples may not need to be collected or submitted for histopathology if gross post-mortem examination findings are very strongly suspicious of FIP. However, if there is any suspicion of another disease and/or other cats are showing clinical signs, it may be worth spending the money to get confirmation of at least the first case. Gross post-mortem examination does not require specialist skills and should be possible in all shelter situations (see Post-mortem examination in a shelter, below).

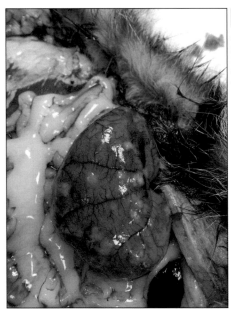

18.3 Appearance of granulomas on the kidney of a cat that was euthanased due to suspected dry FIP.

Blood tests

Serum biochemistry findings are usually most useful in aiding a diagnosis of FIP when funds limit diagnostic investigations.

Serum biochemistry

No serum biochemistry features are pathognomonic for FIP (Riemer *et al.*, 2016), but the following abnormalities are relatively common:

- Hyperproteinaemia (~60%) due to hyperglobulinaemia, usually with a low or low-normal serum albumin
- A:G ratio is low (<0.4 means FIP is very likely, >0.8 makes FIP very unlikely; reference range 0.45–1.2) (Sparkes *et al.*, 1991; Norris *et al.*, 2005; Tsai *et al.*, 2011)
- Hyperbilirubinaemia is often seen, especially in cases with effusion, often without marked elevations in liver enzymes
- α1-acid glycoprotein (AGP), an acute phase protein, is often markedly elevated in FIP (>1.5 g/l; reference range ≤0.48 g/l) (Duthie *et al.*, 1997, Giori *et al.*, 2011).

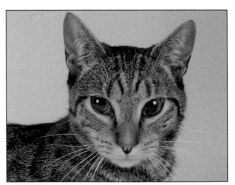

18.4 This 1-year-old male neutered Domestic Shorthaired Cat had a 2-week history of inappetence, lethargy and weight loss. Bilateral uveitis and renomegaly were found on clinical examination. Ultrasonography showed the presence of retroperitoneal and pericardial fluid. A diagnosis of FIP was confirmed on post-mortem examination.

Post-mortem examination in a shelter

All unexplained deaths or cases that have been euthanased with a high suspicion of infectious disease should have a gross post-mortem examination performed (Figure 18.5a). This is good practice and will take only a small amount of time. If gross post-mortem examination is highly suggestive of FIP, samples need not be sent for histopathology, saving the charity money. If there is a suspicion of FIP before euthanasia, it may be worth checking with research centres, such as those at Bristol and Glasgow Universities, to find out whether they are currently collecting samples for studies.

Preparation

Ideally, set up in an area of the practice or shelter that is quiet and where clinical work has finished. A tub table (if available) is very useful. Have a number of formalin pots for histology ready, some 5 or 10 ml syringes and some empty sample pots.

Post-mortem examination

Place the cat in dorsal recumbency (Figure 18.5b). Make a midline incision into the skin and retract the skin laterally (Figure 18.5c); an incision is then made into the abdomen (Figure 18.5de). Alternatively, the abdomen can be incised directly along with the skin with the initial midline incision. A syringe can be used to collect any abdominal fluid (Figure 18.5f). Investigate the abdomen, looking for any granulomatous lesions or plaques (Figure 18.5g). Look specifically at the mesenteric lymph nodes, liver, spleen, kidneys and intestinal surfaces. Also, examine the peritoneal lining of the abdominal wall and

diaphragm for plaques. Extend the incision up into the thoracic cavity (most cats' rib cages can be opened with scissors) (Figure 18.5h). Again, a syringe can be used to collect any fluid in the thoracic cavity. Inspect the lungs and mediastinal lymph nodes for granulomas, and the thoracic wall and diaphragm for plaques. The pericardium can also be examined for fluid.

Samples

If on gross examination typical fluid and/or granulomas are found that are consistent with FIP, a presumptive diagnosis of FIP can be made. In this case, it may be that no further testing is performed if the charity's funds are very limited. However, ideally, samples should be collected for histopathology to give a conclusive diagnosis. This is especially important for initial cases in a potential outbreak; later cases of suspected FIP in high-risk animals may require only a gross post-mortem examination. Samples do not always need to be submitted for analysis immediately; samples can be stored in formalin and some samples frozen (e.g. if mycobacterial infection is suspected) to send for analysis at a later date if further cases occur. Samples for histopathology are best taken from granulomas or plaques or enlarged lymph nodes, if present, first. Most laboratories charge the sample fee for up to four or five samples, so careful choice of tissues can maximize the information gained from histopathology. If no lesions are found but there is still a high suspicion of FIP, samples should be collected from the liver, spleen, mesenteric and mediastinal lymph nodes and small intestine.

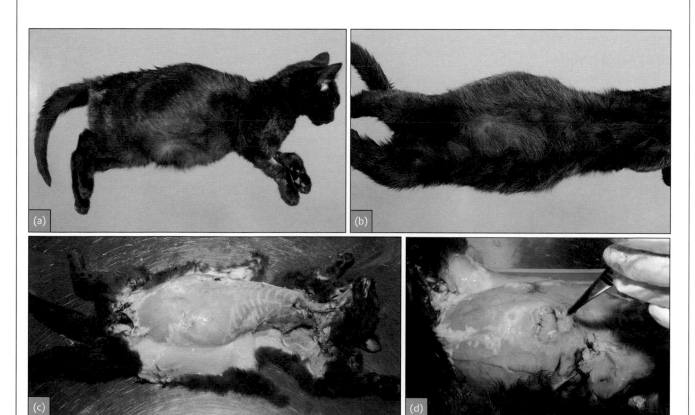

18.5 (a) This 16-week-old kitten has been euthanased due to suspected FIP; a marked abdominal effusion was present. (b) The kitten is placed on its back ready for post-mortem examination. Abdominal distension due to the effusion is evident. (c) A midline incision has been made into the skin and the skin has been retracted laterally to allow visualization of the chest and abdomen. An incision into the abdominal cavity has already been made in error here, resulting in some pale yellow abdominal effusion leaking out, as seen at the bottom of the photograph. (d) A small incision has been made into the abdominal cavity in the midline. (continues) ▶

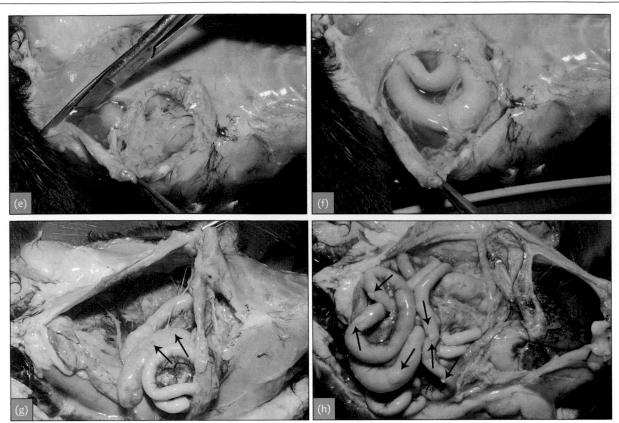

18.5 (continued) (e) Scissors are used to extend the midline incision cranially and caudally. (f) Visualization of the abdominal cavity shows a large amount of pale yellow abdominal effusion together with multiple whitish fibrin tags. A syringe can be used to collect fluid from the abdominal cavity. (g) Further opening of the abdominal cavity shows extensive fibrin tags to be present. Additionally, granulomatous lesions can be appreciated on a section of large intestine (arrowed). (h) Further evaluation of the abdominal cavity shows clear granulomas (arrowed) on the small intestine. The chest has also been opened, showing fibrinous deposits on the lung surface.

Routine haematology

Haematological changes are also non-specific for FIP and so may not be helpful, but if haematology is performed cases may show:

- Lymphopenia
- Neutrophilia
- Anaemia – mild to moderate normocytic normochromic.

Serology for FCoV antibodies

No serum FCoV antibody test can differentiate between antibodies associated with FIP and those associated with asymptomatic FCoV infection. Although cats with FIP tend to have higher FCoV antibody titres than healthy cats or cats without FIP, there is much overlap, so serology is of very limited value and often unhelpful. A negative titre may help to exclude FIP as a diagnosis, but this would be a very rare finding in a shelter situation as FCoV infection is so common; in addition, some FIP cases have negative titres due to the extensive binding of antibodies in antibody–antigen complexes. If the clinical signs and serum biochemistry and/or effusion analysis are supportive of a diagnosis of FIP, then the additional cost of serology is usually not justifiable.

Effusion analysis

Examination of effusion samples is very helpful in the diagnosis of FIP, so obtaining a sample of any effusion

present is particularly important in suspected cases and effusion analysis should be prioritized as a diagnostic test. FIP effusions are usually clear, viscous and straw-yellow in colour (Figure 18.6). They are protein-rich (frothy when shaken, with or without fibrin strands) with a total protein concentration of >35 g/l; protein levels in effusions can be cheaply evaluated in-house using a refractometer. The protein content of effusions comprises a predominance of globulins, with similar low A:G ratios

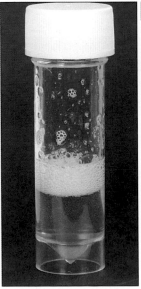

18.6 Typical yellow straw-like colour of FIP-associated effusion fluid. This sample has been shaken to reveal the frothy nature of the fluid. These fluids are typically high in protein (>35 g/l) with an albumin:globulin ratio of <0.4, and have poor cellularity (usually <5 x 10^9 cells/l).

(typically <0.4) and raised AGP concentrations to those in serum (see above). FIP effusions are poorly cellular (usually <5 x 10^9/l cells), consisting of non-degenerate neutrophils and macrophages. Thus, FIP effusions are classified as exudates based on their high protein concentration, but are more of a modified transudate based on their low cell counts. Immunological staining of FCoV antigen (see below) can also be performed on effusion samples.

Reverse-transcription polymerase chain reaction

Effusions, or tissue samples, can be submitted for reverse transcription polymerase chain reaction (RT-PCR) testing to amplify any FCoV RNA within them as an aid to the diagnosis of FIP, although the cost of testing will need to be balanced against the usefulness of the test results. No specific genetic sequences have been demonstrated for FCoVs associated with FIP, although genetic markers of systemic FCoV infection have been found (Porter *et al.*, 2014). Thus, positive RT-PCR results are not specific for FIP, although cats with FIP do have higher levels of FCoV in their tissues than cats without FIP (Porter *et al.*, 2014), so high levels in a tissue or effusion sample will be supportive of a diagnosis. Faecal RT-PCR is sometimes used to identify FCoV shedders to aid FCoV control in multi-cat households, but RT-PCR on faeces is not helpful in the diagnosis of FIP.

Cytological examination of samples

Fine-needle aspirates (FNAs) of tissues (e.g. liver, kidney or mesenteric lymph nodes) can be collected ante mortem (ultrasound guidance can be helpful for this procedure). Cytology usually reveals a mixed inflammatory pattern composed primarily of non-degenerate neutrophils and macrophages; these findings are not specific for FIP and are, thus, of limited diagnostic value, although they can help support the diagnosis of dry FIP. The costs involved in collecting samples may not be justifiable in the shelter situation.

Histopathological examination of tissues

Histopathology of samples of tissue (e.g. liver, kidney or mesenteric lymph nodes) collected ante mortem by ultrasound-guided percutaneous Tru-Cut biopsy, laparoscopy or laparotomy, or, more commonly, at post-mortem examination, can be evaluated for characteristic histopathological changes of FIP (pyogranulomatous parenchymal foci, perivascular mononuclear infiltrates, fibrinous polyserositis). Historically, this was the only method available for definitive diagnosis and is usually considered reliable alone to make a diagnosis.

FCoV antigen staining

Immunological staining of FCoV antigen can also be performed on samples taken for histopathology (tissues) or cytology (e.g. FNAs, effusions). Positive immunological staining in association with characteristic histopathological or cytopathological changes is widely regarded as the gold standard method of FIP diagnosis, and thus is an additional option for confirming the diagnosis, although additional costs are incurred. Unfortunately, negative FCoV antigen staining does not rule out FIP as a cause.

Differential diagnoses

As FIP cases present with a wide range and variety of clinical signs and clinical pathology changes, the list of differential diagnoses is long. However, the more clinical signs that are typically associated with FIP (e.g. unresponsive fever, jaundice, abdominal and/or pleural effusion, mesenteric lymphadenopathy, uveitis) seen together in a cat of appropriate signalment (age <2 years), the higher FIP should be on the differential diagnoses list. Important differential diagnoses to consider when dealing with a case of suspected FIP are listed in Figure 18.7.

Disease/condition	Possible distinguishing features from FIP ± course of action
Toxoplasmosis	**Transmission/epidemiology:** • Acquired via vertical transmission (young cats) or by hunting or eating raw meat (see QRG 18.1) **Signs:** • Cats may have hepatic, pulmonary, neurological, muscle and/or pancreatic involvement • Signs can include lethargy, anorexia, dyspnoea (pneumonia and/or pleural effusions can occur), jaundice, abdominal effusions, uveitis (especially posterior) and/or neurological signs **Testing:** • Clinical toxoplasmosis is less common than FIP and is not usually associated with the severe hyperglobulinaemia or reduced albumi:globulin ratio often seen with FIP • Serology (high IgM titre or rising IgG titres) may be helpful for diagnosis, or organisms may be found on sampling of lungs, lymph nodes **Treatment:** • If toxoplasmosis is suspected, trial treatment with clindamycin can be instigated to see if a positive response to treatment occurs
Lymphocytic cholangitis (LC)	**Epidemiology:** • Can also occur in young cats (Persians may be predisposed) **Signs:** • Often associated with jaundice, with some cats also having an abdominal (unicavity) effusion **Testing:** • The nature of the effusion is similar to that seen with FIP in terms of protein levels, although cell counts are usually higher • A marked hyperglobulinaemia can also be seen with LC • Unlike FIP, this disease is usually associated with marked increases in liver enzymes, especially cholestatic markers (ALP and GGT), and cats with LC are not usually as sick as those with FIP (e.g. they can be polyphagic rather than inappetant)

18.7 Important differential diagnoses to consider for feline infectious peritonitis (FIP), in approximately descending order of importance. ALP = alkaline phosphatase; FeLV = feline leukaemia virus; FIV = feline immunodeficiency virus; GGT = gamma-glutamyl transferase; Ig = immunoglobulin. (continues)

Disease/condition	Possible distinguishing features from FIP ± course of action
Neoplasia, e.g. lymphoma, abdominal carcinoma	**Epidemiology:** • Lymphoma can affect young cats **Signs:** • Lymphoma can involve multiple body organs, and, like FIP, it can result in lymphadenopathy and/or bicavity effusions • Cats are often systemically ill too **Testing:** • Sampling of affected tissues or effusions may yield a diagnosis of lymphoma on cytology rather than the mixed inflammatory cells typically seen on cytological sampling of FIP-affected tissues • Other neoplastic lesions, e.g. carcinomata, may be diagnosed on effusion cytology analysis
Pancreatitis	**Signs:** • May present with anorexia, jaundice and weight loss • Marked pyrexia is not usually a feature although pyrexia can occur in acute pancreatitis cases that are associated with severe pain and/or sepsis **Testing:** • A small amount of abdominal fluid (typically with a high protein and high cell count (non-degenerate neutrophils)) is sometimes present in acute cases • Diagnosed by ultrasonography of the pancreas and feline pancreatic lipase immunoreactivity measurement **Treatment:** • Trial treatment with anti-emetics and analgesics may be warranted
Retroviral infection	**Epidemiology:** • FeLV infection predominantly affects young cats, whereas FIV is an infection seen more commonly in older males **Signs:** • Both FeLV and FIV can be associated with pyrexia, lethargy, lymphadenopathy and uveitis **Testing:** • FIV infection can be associated with a marked hyperglobulinaemia. Retroviral testing may be performed upon entry to a shelter **Note: retrovirus-positive status may act as a risk factor for the development of FIP**
Mycobacterial infection including tuberculosis (TB)	**Epidemiology:** • Geographical variation in prevalence and usually associated with hunting history **Signs:** • Lymphadenopathy, respiratory signs and/or uveitis can be seen • Draining non-healing wounds may be seen • Affected cats may be relatively well despite their disease (pyrexia and inappetance are not common features) **Testing:** • It is not usually associated with the severe hyperglobulinaemia or reduced albumi:globulin ratio seen with FIP • Hypercalcaemia may occur • Cytology of affected lymph nodes or organs shows inflammatory changes (macrophages prominent) • Ziehl–Neelsen staining on cytology or biopsy samples may be positive • An interferon gamma test is now available to assist in the diagnosis of suspected feline TB cases, performed on blood, but is costly
Pyothorax	**Signs:** • Can be associated with pyrexia, and a pleural effusion is seen **Testing:** • Effusion analysis reveals very high cell counts due to marked neutrophilic inflammation with degenerate changes and possibly intracellular bacteria, although any previous antibiotic treatment may mean bacteria are not seen • Unicavity effusion
Septic peritonitis	**Signs:** • Can be associated with pyrexia, and an abdominal effusion is seen **Testing:** • Abdominal effusion analysis reveals very high cell counts due to marked neutrophilic inflammation with degenerate changes and possibly intracellular bacteria, although any previous antibiotic treatment may mean bacteria are not seen • Unicavity effusion
Congestive heart failure (CHF)	**Signs:** • Bicavity effusions in the pleural and peritoneal spaces are possible, although pleural effusions are more common with feline CHF, and abdominal effusions alone are rarely seen with feline CHF • The presence of a heart murmur, gallop sound or arrhythmia may increase index of suspicion for CHF • Jugular vein distension may be present with right-sided CHF • Pyrexia is not a feature **Testing:** • The fluid is a modified transudate with little protein, in contrast to the fluid seen with FIP • Echocardiography will confirm cardiac disease and CHF
Rabies	In countries where rabies is endemic, this must be considered as a differential diagnosis in unvaccinated cats presenting with neurological signs, especially acute behavioural changes and progressive paralysis

18.7 (continued) Important differential diagnoses to consider for feline infectious peritonitis (FIP), in approximately descending order of importance. ALP = alkaline phosphatase; FeLV = feline leukaemia virus; FIV = feline immunodeficiency virus; GGT = gamma-glutamyl transferase; Ig = immunoglobulin.

Treatment

Treatment for FIP is never curative, and treatment is unlikely to be undertaken in the shelter situation. Sometimes prednisolone (2–4 mg/kg/day orally, decreasing the dose) may delay the need for euthanasia by a few weeks or a few months, but in the authors' experience such a response is uncommon. Interferon has also been used, but this is most likely to be prohibitively expensive in a shelter situation and again is of limited value. If FIP is strongly suspected, or confirmed, euthanasia (with subsequent post-mortem examination) is usually indicated to minimize suffering.

Prognosis

FIP is considered to be fatal and all staff and volunteers should be made aware of the gravity of the disease.

Prevention

Considerations for housing, husbandry and the spread of FCoV

Communal *versus* individual housing

As FCoV is shed extensively in the faeces of infected cats, cats that are kept in groups in communal housing and share litter trays are more likely to become infected if a cat shedding the virus is introduced to the environment. This may not be a cause for concern, as most cats are often already infected with FCoV and the disease induced is usually mild (see Figure 18.2). However, if a particularly virulent strain of FCoV (see Suspected outbreaks of FIP, below) is introduced, then mortality rates associated with FIP can be very high (up to 50%). If the shelter uses communal housing, ideally only cats that have come from the same source should be kept together, as they are likely to have already been exposed to the same strains of FCoV; in addition, if they are an established social group, stress associated with communal housing will be reduced. If individual or small numbers of cats are being admitted into the shelter from different sources, communal housing is best avoided if at all possible. Housing cats individually will reduce their potential exposure to FCoV. More importantly, it will also reduce inter-cat aggression and stress, which can be a significant risk factor for the development of FIP.

Fomite and direct transmission of FCoV

In cats that are housed separately, fomite transmission is the biggest risk factor for the spread of FCoV (Figure 18.8). Cleaning procedures should be evaluated and amended as necessary so that used litter trays are disposed of promptly. It is not uncommon for cats (especially kittens) to escape from their pens during cleaning and have contact with another cat's faeces if litter trays have been left on the floor in corridor areas. The type of litter being used should also be considered, because if litter escapes from pens, it can act as a major fomite. Although larger litter is easier to identify and clean away, in litters of kittens with diarrhoea using torn up newspaper for a few days may help reduce the risk of fomite spread, as cats with diarrhoea may be likely to dig around in the litter more and flick it out of the

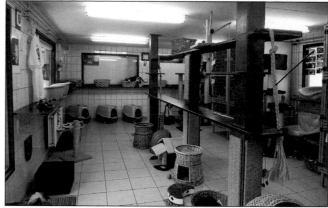

18.8 This communal space in a shelter cattery contains shared litter trays. In addition, direct contact is possible between the communally housed cats and the cats kept in pens. Both of these features are risk factors for the transmission of FCoV; in addition, communal housing can be more stressful for cats who are not accustomed to living with other cats.

tray. Litter trays should be kept in areas of the pen away from food bowls and any doors or gaps to reduce the risk of transmission. Cleaning protocols that allow regular removal of any escaped litter should be instigated.

People are another potential route of fomite transmission. Protocols should specify that all staff wear shoe covers, gloves and aprons when cleaning out cat pens, and to change these before entering the next pen (Figure 18.9), and steps should be taken to ensure that staff comply with these biosecurity measures.

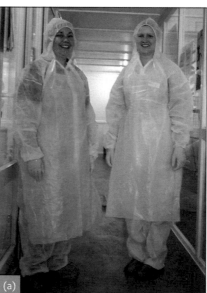
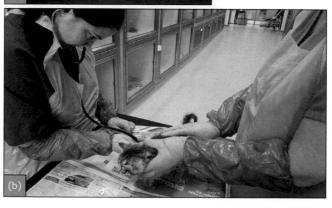

18.9 Barrier care in a shelter. Staff wearing (a) disposable overalls, aprons, gloves and overshoes for entering a cat pen and (b) disposable gloves, over-sleeves and aprons for clinical examinations. (© Cats Protection)

Direct contact should also be considered as a means of transmission. Pens that have open bars can allow cats (especially kittens) in adjacent pens to have direct contact with each other's paws; if this is the case, adjustments to the design or layout of the pens should be made to prevent contact.

Any movement of cats that occurs should be critically evaluated for its potential for FCoV transmission. A lot of movement that occurs in the first 14 days of arrival in the shelter is for veterinary care, for example, transporting cats for neutering and vaccination.

When examining cats, it is important for the veterinary surgeon (veterinarian) to reduce the risk of FCoV spread as far as possible. This includes ensuring that examination tables and hands are disinfected between each cat and/or the use of gloves, over-sleeves and protective aprons that are changed between cats or groups of cats (Figure 18.9b). Other considerations include evaluating how cats are transported and housed when visiting the veterinary surgery from the shelter for neutering. Shelter staff should be instructed to ensure that the vehicle used to transport cats is adequately cleaned. Cages/baskets should be covered to prevent direct contact between cats while in the vehicle. Staff in the veterinary clinic should be made aware that shelter cats represent a higher risk group for FIP than the average pet cat, and basic barrier nursing principles should be applied to shelter cats while in the clinic to help prevent the spread of any occult infectious agents to other cats. If the clinic has isolation space available, then using this to house shelter cats during their stay may be wise (see Chapter 9).

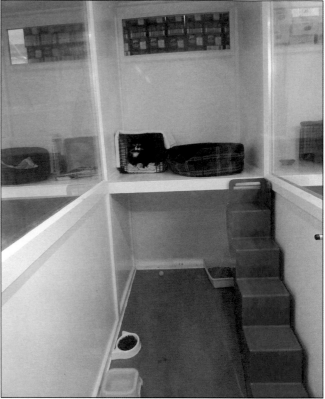

18.10 Example of an individual housing pen containing a cat basket in which the cat can hide.

Minimizing stress in the shelter

FIP usually develops within a few weeks to months (up to 18 months) after infection with FCoV, and stressors are often implicated in its development. These include changing housing/environment, neutering and vaccination. Trying to reduce stress within the shelter is, therefore, important not only for an individual cat's welfare but also to reduce the risk of FIP development. However, efforts to reduce stress have to be balanced against any potential negative effects of, for example, delaying neutering or vaccination.

Housing

- Cats should be housed individually or in established social groups only. It is important to note that pairs of cats are not automatically in the same social group; they may have coped in an environment where they had enough space to avoid each other (e.g. the previous owner's home), but in the confines of a pen conflict may occur.
- Cats should be provided with places to hide, e.g. Cat Hides, cardboard boxes, igloos, covered cat baskets (Figure 18.10) (see also QRG 19.8).
- Cats should be kept separately from dogs.

Neutering

Neutering is currently the only acceptable way of controlling the large population of stray and unwanted cats. All responsible shelters will arrange neutering of cats before rehoming. Transporting cats to the clinic for neutering, the time spent at the clinic and the procedure itself will inevitably cause some stress; however, applying good 'cat-friendly' principles in the veterinary clinic will help to reduce this stress (see *BSAVA Manual of Feline Practice*).

- Ensure that all cats are transported in covered baskets with appropriate bedding in them.
- Have a consulting room ready for the cats to be taken into, if a large number is being brought in at the same time, to minimize the time spent in the waiting room if there is not a separate cat waiting room. If large numbers of cats are brought to the clinic together on a regular basis, it may be wise to consider having a surgery day dedicated to shelter cat neutering.
- If a separate cat ward is not available, consider keeping the cats in their baskets in a quiet room until surgery.
- Staff at the shelter can be trained to do postoperative checks to minimize the need for the cats to return to the clinic.

Early neutering: Debate exists about whether early neutering increases the risk of FIP development. One of the authors has seen FIP developing before early neutering: FIP was detected in 9-week-old cats by the presence of an inflamed peritoneal membrane and a viscous abdominal effusion in female kittens, and scrotal enlargement due to a viscous effusion around the testes in male kittens (note that a small volume of clear low-protein fluid can be normal in kittens at the time of early neutering and it is important this is not confused with FIP). Other clinical signs of FIP then developed 3–14 days after neutering. It seems likely that FIP would have developed in these kittens regardless of neutering, although in other cats neutering may contribute to the risk of FIP developing. However, as neutering is a primary goal of most shelter charities and FIP is rare, this risk should not prevent charities from aiming to neuter all kittens before rehoming, as the benefits of doing so outweigh the drawbacks.

Vaccination against feline panleukopenia virus and 'cat 'flu'

Shelters are high-risk places for transmission of infectious disease, and the relative risk of a cat contracting feline panleukopenia virus (also known as feline parvovirus), or one of the agents responsible for cat 'flu, is higher than the risk of a cat developing FIP. Vaccination of all cats as soon as possible after entering the shelter is advisable to reduce the overall prevalence of these important infectious diseases in the shelter. While the act of vaccination may be considered a stressor that may increase the risk of a cat developing FIP, it is important to recognize that developing illness associated with cat 'flu, or a panleukopenia virus infection, is a greater stressor and may be associated with a higher risk of mortality.

Rehoming

Rehoming is a final stressor that could be a risk factor for FIP development in shelter cats. Like neutering and vaccination, this is a necessary stressor, as keeping cats in a shelter situation long term has negative welfare implications for the individual cats, as well as reducing the number of animals the shelter is able to help. The following can help to minimize the stress associated with rehoming:

- Keep cats in stable social groups when rehoming them
- Provide cats with their core needs (food, water, litter tray, bed and a place to hide) in a quiet part of the home and give them time to adjust to their new environment
- Perform any introductions to other cats or pets in the household slowly, once the new cat has had time to adjust; perform scent swapping for a period of time first. Information sheets regarding introductions can be given to new owners (see Useful websites).

Vaccination against FCoV

Currently no licensed FCoV vaccine exists in the UK. An intranasal vaccine is available in the USA, which is licensed for use after 16 weeks of age and is given as two doses 3–4 weeks apart. However, most cats are already infected with FCoV by 16 weeks of age, and reports showing efficacy of the vaccine in the field are lacking. Thus, FCoV vaccination is currently not recommended.

Management following confirmation of FIP in a shelter

The reality of FIP in the shelter situation is that the majority of cases will occur after cats have been rehomed, and the period before these cases arise can be quite lengthy. This means that veterinary investigations will be performed by the adopter's veterinary surgeon, and the amount of clinical information available can be variable. To facilitate communication, it is wise for the shelter to obtain contact details for the adopter's veterinary surgeon at the time of rehoming if this occurs during a period in which FIP is suspected in the shelter. The shelter veterinary surgeon and the adopter's veterinary surgeon can then get in touch to discuss any subsequent suspected FIP cases. Such communication can help to ensure that appropriate diagnostic testing and/or a post-mortem examination is carried out if FIP is suspected.

Following confirmation of a case of FIP in a shelter, it is important to consider the history, asking appropriate questions as necessary (see Figure 18.1). Shelter records should be evaluated to determine the source of the cat and whether other cats entered the shelter with it, as well as the age of the cat and how long it had been in its new home before it developed signs of FIP. If the cat entered the shelter individually, then the risk of any further cases is probably quite low if the cat was housed individually during its time in the shelter. If the cat was housed in communal housing then all other cats in the communal group have to be considered at risk of FIP. If the cat was part of a litter that were all adopted out recently, then there is a risk of further cases, as it can be assumed that all the cats in the litter were exposed to similar FCoVs and that they may have a similar genetic predisposition to FIP. However, the longer the period of time between adoption and FIP development, the less likely it is that further cases will develop. If the period from adoption of a cat to the development of signs of FIP is short, and littermates of the FIP case are still in the shelter's care, appropriate barrier nursing should be started and the littermates should potentially be held back from being rehomed until a period of time, after stressful procedures, such as neutering and vaccination has passed. Alternatively, they can be adopted out but with a disclosure (see Disclosure of FIP, below) made to the adopter that a littermate has died from FIP.

Disclosure of FIP

An FIP disclosure can be made in several ways when rehoming cats, but is best kept simple. Making a disclosure is important to help maintain the shelter and/or charity's reputation, as there is much misunderstanding in the veterinary world about FCoV and FIP. Thus, a disclosure can help prevent complaints and confusion in the event that a cat at slightly higher risk of FIP goes on to develop the disease. Cats that have been housed in the same area as cats with confirmed FIP should be rehomed with information documenting that they have possibly been exposed to a strain of FCoV associated with an increased incidence of FIP. Cats with littermates or other family members that have died of FIP should be rehomed with information documenting that they have probably been exposed to a strain of FCoV associated with an increased incidence of FIP and that a related cat has died of FIP, making them at a slightly increased risk for FIP development.

The following passages of text have been used by Cats Protection UK as disclosures when homing cats/kittens following an FIP outbreak (for further information see the link to the Cats Protection website at the end of this chapter):

- General FIP Disclosure: 'We have lost some kittens to feline infectious peritonitis (FIP), which can arise as a result of feline coronavirus (FCoV) infection. There is no test to determine which cats infected with FCoV will develop FIP. If your adopted cat shows any signs of ill health, please seek veterinary advice and let us know.'
- Specific FIP Disclosure: 'One or more of your adopted cat's kittens/littermates/queen has developed feline infectious peritonitis (FIP). It is likely that your adopted cat has been exposed to feline coronavirus (FCoV) and may potentially develop FIP, although only around 1–5% of cats infected by the virus go on to develop FIP. Unfortunately, there is no test to determine if this will occur. We advise that the cat is adopted with his/her littermates/queen only and not another cat, or to a home without resident cats'.

If the littermates of a confirmed case of FIP have already been adopted, a dilemma arises in whether to contact the adopters to inform them. If the adopters are not contacted and further cases occur, the reputation of the shelter could suffer. However, if the risk of FIP development is deemed to be low, informing the adopters could cause them unnecessary anxiety. The factors discussed above (whether the cat is related to an identified FIP case, whether it has had direct contact with a case or whether it was just kept in the same area as a case, for example) can help the shelter management make an informed decision as to the risk and whether adopters should be contacted. Before contacting the adopters, it is important to make sure that the person making contact has a good understanding of FIP and can either send or direct the adopter to good resources of information about the disease.

It is possible that an existing cat in a household develops FIP following the adoption of a cat from a shelter that has had a problem with FIP, although this scenario is likely to be uncommon. However, it is probably best for the veterinary surgeon to advise the shelter's rehoming staff that high-risk cats should be rehomed only as single cats or in their current established social group.

Suspected outbreaks of FIP

Occasionally, outbreaks of FIP are reported in which a larger proportion of FCoV-infected cats is affected (Barker *et al.*, 2013, Wang *et al.*, 2013); and when these arise, they often occur in shelter establishments. An outbreak is also considered likely when cases of FIP are reported in unrelated cats or cats from different sources that were in the shelter at the same time (see Example of an outbreak, below). Due to the lag period between exposure to virulent FCoV and the development of clinical signs of FIP, the presence of an outbreak may take some time to become apparent. Details of outbreaks of FIP that are reported suggest that sometimes virulent FIP-inducing FCoVs may replicate within the intestine of infected cats, resulting in shedding and potential transmission to other cats (see Figure 18.2). Alternatively, outbreaks of FIP could be explained by the existence in the environment of virulent FCoVs that have a particularly high potential to mutate to FIP-inducing viral strains in cats. Identification of particularly virulent FCoVs is not currently possible as the viral sequences associated with pathogenicity are not known (Porter *et al.*, 2014).

Possible approaches to managing an outbreak

The 'keep calm and carry on' approach

One accepts that FCoV infection is endemic in shelters and that the outbreak of FIP is simply 'bad luck'. This approach creates no additional work for the shelter, but it is likely that local groups and veterinary surgeons will become aware of the increased incidence of FIP in cats rehomed from the shelter, potentially damaging the shelter's reputation.

The thorough approach: separating cats by risk status

In this approach, high-risk and low-risk cats with respect to FCoV exposure are identified. Low-risk cats are often defined as cats that are housed in the same area as, but have had no direct contact with, FIP cases, so their risk of exposure is likely to be via fomites only. All low-risk cats can be rehomed as normal. High-risk cats are defined as cats with direct contact with FIP cases – for example, littermates, cats from the same original source or cats housed together in a group. All high-risk cats should be barrier nursed if still in the shelter, and have completed all likely stress-inducing procedures (e.g. vaccination, neutering), as well as a subsequent 4-week (if cats have been in the same area of the shelter as cats that have died of FIP) or 8-week (if cats belong to the same family group as cats that have died of FIP) period, before being rehomed. Rehoming of high-risk cats should be accompanied by a disclosure (see above) to the adopter. Rehoming to a home that already has another cat should be avoided, unless the resident cat is also at high risk of FIP. The disadvantage of this approach is that it goes against the recommendation of delaying stressful procedures to avoid the development

---

Example of an outbreak

Three litters of kittens and queens were admitted into a shelter from a single multi-cat source. After 4 weeks of care in the shelter, kittens from one of the litters showed signs of FIP at neutering, at 9 weeks of age. Ante-mortem testing was inconclusive. Euthanasia and post-mortem examination were performed 2 weeks later, and FIP was confirmed. The queen of the litter was adopted 2 days before the kittens were neutered, and was euthanased due to suspected FIP, based on clinical signs, approximately 3 weeks later. Several kittens from a fourth litter (from a different source) that was in the shelter at the same time as the three multi-cat household litters were euthanased due to FIP, approximately 4 weeks after adoption.

Full-barrier nursing was started in the shelter approximately 9 weeks after the three litters of kittens from the multi-cat source arrived at the shelter, which is when the initial exposure to a virulent FCoV strain is believed to have occurred. The multi-cat source was contacted at this time and confirmed that cases of suspected FIP were also occurring in the remaining cats in this source.

Overall, potentially 270 cats and kittens at the shelter were exposed to the virulent FCoV strain over the 9-week period before control measures were implemented. During this time, 19 cats died due to FIP, 9 in the shelter and 10 after adoption, giving a 7% mortality rate. Nine litters in total were affected, three of which were from the multi-cat source. A mortality rate of 40–50% was reported at the multi-cat source itself; this high rate was believed to be due to the overcrowding and stressful conditions in which the cats were kept. Post-mortem examination and subsequent research analysis of samples collected post mortem confirmed that the same strain of FCoV was present in cats at the shelter and at the multi-cat source.

This example shows the lag period between the initial cases of FIP and the recognition that an outbreak was occurring. The outbreak in this case was believed to have been caused by the introduction, from the multi-cat source, of a particularly virulent FCoV strain into the shelter, including the maternity wing, allowing exposure of young kittens.

of FIP in high-risk cats by reducing stress. It also requires a large amount of resources and blocks new cats from coming in to the shelter. It is likely to be most suitable for selective intake shelters rather than those with an open intake policy.

The cautious approach

As outlined above, cats are more likely to develop FIP following a stressful event. Rehoming high-risk cats into permanent homes or long-term foster care with concurrent spacing out of vaccination and delaying neutering for 3–6 months may reduce the likelihood of development of FIP. A full disclosure (see above) should be given to adopters in this situation and the cats should not be rehomed with any other cats (unless they are also at high risk). This approach concurs with the recommendation of delaying stressful procedures to avoid the development of FIP. The disadvantages are that if cats go on to develop FIP, the shelter's reputation could be damaged, and adopters of such cats may well experience emotional stress.

The pragmatic approach: euthanasia of high-risk cats

Euthanasia of all high-risk cats is the final option for managing an outbreak of FIP. This is a very hard decision to make as only a proportion of high-risk cats will go on to develop FIP, so euthanasia of cats that will never develop FIP would occur with this option. However, if the shelter's resources are limited, it is unable to keep cats for a holding period before adoption, as in the second of the options described above, and the risk to the shelter's reputation associated with the first and third options is too great, euthanasia of high-risk cats may be the best option. This option would be followed by thorough disinfection of pens where the high-risk cases had been kept, and would allow the shelter to reopen for intake again comparatively quickly.

Ten top tips about FCoV and FIP

- FCoV infection is extremely common in cats but FIP usually arises only sporadically.
- FCoV is shed in the faeces – good hygiene and disinfection can reduce the load of FCoV in shelters but elimination is likely to be impossible.
- FIP generally affects cats between 4 months and 2 years of age.
- There is often a history of recent stress.
- Cyclical non-responsive fever, lethargy, anorexia, weight loss and failure to thrive are typical signs – it is important to repeat clinical examinations, as the disease is progressive and new signs (e.g. effusions, uveitis) may appear.
- FCoV antibody tests provide information about exposure to FCoV, rather than a diagnosis of FIP; they do not differentiate between FIP-causing viral strains and asymptomatic infections.
- Serum biochemistry can be helpful, as cases can often show a reduced A:G ratio and hyperbilirubinaemia.
- If an effusion is present, however small, analysis of a sample will provide helpful information – effusions are typically highly proteinaceous (reduced A:G ratio) but poorly cellular. ▶

Ten top tips about FCoV and FIP *continued*

- FCoV antigen staining of effusion and/or histopathology samples in association with chracteristic cytology or histopathology change, is regarded as the gold standard for diagnosis.
- Gross post-mortem examinations (with or without analysis of collected samples) should be performed in any suspected cases.

References and further reading

Barker EN, Tasker S, Gruffydd-Jones TJ *et al.* (2013) Phylogenetic analysis of feline coronavirus strains in an epizootic outbreak of feline infectious peritonitis. *Journal of Veterinary Internal Medicine* **27**, 445–450

Duthie S, Eckersall PD, Addie DD, Lawrence CE and Jarrett O (1997) Value of alpha 1-acid glycoprotein in the diagnosis of feline infectious peritonitis. *Veterinary Record* **141**, 299–303

Giori L, Giordano A, Giudice C, Grieco V and Paltrinieri S (2011) Performances of different diagnostic tests for feline infectious peritonitis in challenging clinical cases. *Journal of Small Animal Practice* **52**, 152–157

Harvey A and Tasker S (2013) *BSAVA Manual of Feline Practice*. BSAVA Publications, Gloucester

Kipar A and Meli ML (2014) Feline infectious peritonitis: still an enigma? *Veterinary Pathology* **51**, 505–526

Norris JM, Bosward KL, White JD *et al.* (2005) Clinicopathological findings associated with feline infectious peritonitis in Sydney, Australia: 42 cases (1990-2002). *Australian Veterinary Journal* **83**, 666–673

Pedersen NC (2009) A review of feline infectious peritonitis virus infection: 1963-2008. *Journal of Feline Medicine and Surgery* **11**, 225–258

Porter E (2014) Virus and host determinants of feline coronavirus pathogenicity. PhD Thesis, University of Bristol

Porter E, Tasker S, Day MJ *et al.* (2014) Amino acid changes in the spike protein of feline coronavirus correlate with systemic spread of virus from the intestine and not with feline infectious peritonitis. *Veterinary Research* **45**, 19

Riemer F, Kuehner KA, Ritz S, Sauter-Louis C and Hartmann K (2016) Clinical and laboratory features of cats with feline infectious peritonitis – a retrospective study of 231 confirmed cases (2000-2010). *Journal of Feline Medicine and Surgery* **18**, 348-356.

Sparkes AH, Gruffydd-Jones TJ and Harbour DA (1991) Feline infectious peritonitis: a review of clinicopathological changes in 65 cases, and a critical assessment of their diagnostic value. *Veterinary Record* **129**, 209–212

Tsai HY, Chueh LL, Lin CN and Su BL (2011) Clinicopathological findings and disease staging of feline infectious peritonitis: 51 cases from 2003 to 2009 in Taiwan. *Journal of Feline Medicine and Surgery* **13**, 74–80

Wang YT, Su BL, Hsieh LE and Chueh LL (2013) An outbreak of feline infectious peritonitis in a Taiwanese shelter: epidemiologic and molecular evidence for horizontal transmission of a novel type II feline coronavirus. *Veterinary Research* **44**, 57

Useful websites

Cats Protection information for veterinary surgeons: www.cats.org.uk/cat-care/vets-info/ including information on FCoV and FIP and the text included in disclosures and pre-adoption FIP handout: www.cats.org.uk/uploads/documents/Feline_Coronavirus_and_Feline_Infectious_Peritonitis_0715-web.pdf

Cats Protection guide to FCoV and FIP: www.cats.org.uk/uploads/documents/cat-care-leaflets-2013/VG10_Feline_Coronavirus_(FCoV)_and_Feline_Infectious_Peritonitis_(FIP).pdf

International Cat Care information about FIP: www.icatcare.org/advice/cat-health/feline-infectious-peritonitis-fip

International Cat Care information about introducing a kitten: http://icatcare.org/advice/how-introduce-kitten-cat

International Cat Care information about introducing an adult cat: http://www.icatcare.org/advice/how-guides/how-introduce-new-adult-cat-your-cat

University of Glasgow School of Veterinary Medicine information about FIP: http://www.gla.ac.uk/schools/vet/cad/researchprojects/fip/fip.about/

Koret Shelter Medicine Program information about FIP/FCoV: www.sheltermedicine.com/library/resources/feline-infectious-peritonitis-feline-coronavirus-fip-fcov

QRG 18.1: Toxoplasmosis

by Sarah Caney

Knowledge of toxoplasmosis is relevant to rescue shelters in terms of understanding the disease that may be seen in infected cats, as well as the risk to people in contact with an infected cat and how to minimize this. Toxoplasmosis is the disease caused by infection with *Toxoplasma gondii*, a coccidian parasite.

T. gondii is present throughout the world and can affect most mammals, including cats and humans. Infection is common, although disease caused by *T. gondii* is rare. In general, around 50% of all cats are believed to have been infected with this organism at some point in their life; the prevalence of infection varies according to the cat's lifestyle.

Pregnant women who own cats commonly worry that the risk of exposure to *T. gondii* from their cat – and of harm to their unborn child – is high. These fears, often encouraged by midwives and other medical professionals, can lead to relinquishment of cats to a shelter. In reality, the risks of acquiring toxoplasmosis from a cat are extremely small, and simple hygiene measures can be taken to reduce these risks further, making it safe to care for a cat, even when pregnant. See also the section below on the risk of acquiring toxoplasmosis from a cat.

Life cycle

The life cycle of *T. gondii* is complex and involves two types of host, definitive and intermediate. Wild and domestic felids are the definitive host for *T. gondii*. Kittens can be infected *in utero* and by suckling their mother's milk, but this is uncommon. Most cats are infected by eating meat containing *T. gondii* cysts; this can include raw or inadequately cooked meat or, more commonly, prey species. A few days after a cat has been infected for the first time, it will start to shed millions of oocysts in its faeces. The oocysts are shed for only a short period of time, typically less than 18 days, before the cat's immune response stops oocyst production altogether. Although infected cats can start to shed oocysts again in the future, this is rare, and when it does occur it usually results in a much smaller number of

oocysts being shed. Even cats that are frequently re-exposed to *T. gondii* probably rarely shed large numbers of oocysts after their first infection. Experimental studies have shown that immunosuppressive drug therapy is rarely effective in triggering re-shedding. One study showed a higher rate of infection in stray cats compared with household cats; this may have implications for cats housed in a shelter (Savic-Jevdjenic *et al.*, 2006).

Other mammals, including humans and mice, are intermediate hosts of *T. gondii*. These hosts can become infected but do not produce oocysts. Oocysts passed in a cat's faeces are not immediately infectious to other animals, and must first go through a process called sporulation, which takes between 1 and 5 days, depending on the environmental conditions. A recent study indicated that sporulation in cat litter trays occurred within 2–3 days and that the resulting oocysts remained viable for 14 days (Dubey *et al.*, 2011). Once sporulated, oocysts are infectious to cats, humans and other intermediate hosts. Intermediate hosts become infected through ingestion of sporulated oocysts, and this infection results in the formation of tissue cysts (bradyzoites) in various tissues of the body. Tissue cysts remain in the host for life and are infectious to cats, humans and other intermediate hosts if ingested. Dogs (and perhaps other animals) can transport sporulated oocysts and spread these to other places if they ingest the oocysts and then pass them in their faeces, where they remain infectious.

Consequences of toxoplasmosis in humans

People who have been infected with *T. gondii* develop serum antibodies to the organism. The fetuses of pregnant women who have not been infected before pregnancy are vulnerable to *T. gondii*-induced disease if the mother is infected while pregnant. In around 20–50% of these women the fetus will be infected and may be miscarried or develop birth defects. The effects of infection are most severe when infection occurs

between months 2 and 6 of gestation. If a woman has been infected with *T. gondii* before she becomes pregnant (and, thus, has already developed antibodies) there is no risk of the infection being passed on to the fetus.

In most cases, people become infected via either ingestion of oocysts from the environment (e.g. through contact with soil containing sporulated oocysts when gardening or handling vegetables) or by eating inadequately cooked meat containing tissue cysts. In immunocompetent people, toxoplasmosis may be mild and pass undetected, or may cause symptoms such as fever and lymphadenopathy. Toxoplasmosis is most severe in certain 'high-risk' groups of individuals whose immunity is impaired. This group includes developing fetuses, babies, elderly people and immunosuppressed people. In this group, infection can be associated with severe illness, including encephalitis, miscarriage, stillbirth, birth defects, and other problems affecting the nervous system and eyes.

Clinical disease in cats with toxoplasmosis

Although infection with *T. gondii* rarely causes disease in cats, signs of illness can sometimes be seen. These include diarrhoea, inflammatory ocular, pancreatic, liver and neurological disease, in addition to more vague systemic signs of illness, such as anorexia and pyrexia. Congenital disease tends to be especially severe. Chronic clinical toxoplasmosis, associated with vague and recurrent signs of illness, is rare. Clinical toxoplasmosis associated with reactivation of latent disease has been suspected in a small number of cats receiving treatment with ciclosporin.

Detection of tachyzoites (the rapidly multiplying stage of *T. gondii*) in tissue biopsies or cytology samples (e.g. cerebrospinal fluid, bronchoalveolar lavage fluid) is diagnostic for toxoplasmosis. Diagnosis can also be made by measuring serum antibodies to *T. gondii* – IgM titres greater than 1:64 or a ➡

QRG 18.1 *continued*

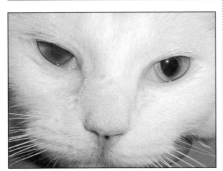

Uveitis can be a feature of clinical toxoplasmosis, as is the case in this Domestic Longhaired Cat.
(© Sarah Caney)

four-fold increase in IgG titres taken 2–4 weeks apart are generally indicative of recent or active infection. Clinical toxoplasmosis is suspected in cats with this antibody profile in addition to supportive clinical signs, exclusion of other possible differential diagnoses and a positive response to treatment for toxoplasmosis. Clindamycin (12.5–25 mg/kg q12h for 4 weeks) is the treatment of choice and a rapid response to treatment is often seen. Topical and/or systemic glucocorticoids are beneficial in cats affected by inflammatory ocular disease.

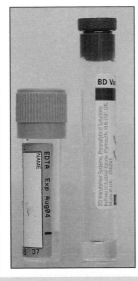

Detection of tachyzoites in cerebrospinal fluid is diagnostic for clinical toxoplasmosis.

Risks of acquiring toxoplasmosis from a cat

Research indicates that contact with cats does not increase the risk of *T. gondii* infection in humans. Studies have shown that it is rare to identify cats shedding oocysts in their faeces. Veterinary surgeons (veterinarians) working with cats are no more likely to be infected with *T. gondii* than the general population, including people who are not in contact with cats. Furthermore, contact with cats has no influence on the probability of people having antibodies to *T. gondii*, whereas consuming raw meat significantly increases the risk of acquiring the infection. Stroking a cat will not spread infection from cats to people – even when cats are shedding oocysts in their faeces, oocysts cannot be found on their coat. Studies in dogs have shown that oocysts do not sporulate on their fur, and it is likely that the same is true in cats. Cat ownership does not increase the risk of toxoplasmosis in people with acquired immune deficiency disorder (AIDS). Although people with AIDS are generally at an increased risk of clinical disease relating to *T. gondii* infection, this results from reactivation of a previous infection rather than the acquisition of a new infection from a cat or other sources. Furthermore, cats with feline immunodeficiency virus or feline leukaemia virus that are subsequently infected with *T. gondii* do not appear to shed oocysts for any longer, or in any greater numbers, than other cats. Therefore, the risk of infection from cats is very low, except for young children playing in soil contaminated with sporulated oocysts.

Although the risk of transmission of infection from a cat to its carer is very low, it can be reduced further by adopting the following recommendations for care of cats in shelters:

- People in 'high-risk' groups should not have contact with cat litter trays
- Empty litter trays daily
- Wear gloves when handling cat litter and wash hands thoroughly afterwards
- Use litter tray liners and periodically clean the litter tray with detergent and scalding water to kill oocysts
- Dispose of cat litter in sealed plastic bags
- Feed commercial cat food only
- Offer mains water to drink
- Wash hands after contact with a cat.

References and further reading

Dubey JP, Ferreira LR, Martins J and Jones JL (2011) Sporulation and survival of *Toxoplasma gondii* oocysts in different types of commercial cat litter. *Journal of Parasitology* **97**, 751–754

Savic-Jevdjenlc S, Vidic B, Grgic Z and Misic E (2006) Seroprevalence of *Toxoplasma gondii* antibodies in cats. In *Proceedings of the World Small Animal Veterinary Association Congress*

Chapter 19

Behaviour and stress management in the shelter environment

Rachel Casey and Nicky Trevorrow

Introduction

Behaviour is an essential consideration in a holistic approach to shelter medicine. Behavioural signs are key indicators of both physical and psychological health. Changes in behaviour are often the first indicators of disease, and help to identify cases requiring further veterinary care. Monitoring behavioural changes also provides shelter staff and veterinary surgeons (veterinarians) with a view on how animals are adapting to the centre, and enables them to adjust the animals' environments and management plans to aid their psychological wellbeing.

This chapter starts with a discussion of some of the main principles underlying the quality of life and behaviour of animals in the context of the shelter environment. This includes an introduction to stress and emotional states, the behavioural techniques often used in rehabilitation and how behaviours develop. The second part of the chapter focuses on the specific behavioural signs, issues and problems related to housing dogs and cats within shelters. It is beyond the scope of this text to provide detailed behaviour modification programmes, particularly as these need to be tailored to the specific needs of each individual case, but guidelines are provided on the main problems and the principles underlying prevention and resolution.

Stress

Definition of stress

The term 'stress' is used very widely, and has a number of different meanings in common parlance. It is often used to imply a negative situation or state, and the term is associated with compromised welfare. However, it is important to note that a stress response can be a good thing – and that it occurs equally as a result of positive and negative events. In fact, the stress response is associated with emotional arousal rather than valence (i.e. the degree of response to a stimulus, rather than whether it is positive or negative). With anticipation of something happening, or on a change of environment or context, it is adaptive for an animal to become more alert, aware of its surroundings and ready for activity. Anticipating a pleasurable experience induces a stress response in the same way that an unpleasant one does.

The stress response has central and peripheral components. The central component involves activation of pathways in the midbrain that lead to increased alertness and vigilance. Noradrenaline (norepinephrine) is one of the important neurotransmitters in these pathways: it is the main neurotransmitter within the locus coeruleus and pathways run from here to both the limbic and cortical regions. The peripheral component has different elements, but cumulatively they initiate the changes familiarly associated with the 'fight or flight' response. Sympathetic nervous system activation leads to increased heart rate, increased stroke volume, increased respiratory rate, pupil dilation, and vasodilation of blood vessels supplying the heart, lungs, skeletal muscles and brain. In addition, sympathetic stimulation of the adrenal medulla results in the production of adrenaline (epinephrine) and noradrenaline. Adrenaline stimulates glycolysis, and both hormones act to increase the heart rate and blood pressure, and also give rise to other sympathomimetic actions.

The stress response also includes activation of the hypothalamic–pituitary–adrenal axis, resulting in increased cortisol production from the adrenal cortex. Cortisol has a profound effect on glucose metabolism: blood glucose levels are increased to provide a supply of energy for muscular activity through the breakdown of carbohydrates, proteins and fats. Almost every cell in the body of an animal has receptors for cortisol, so changes in cortisol release can have wide-ranging effects on metabolic processes.

Although the stress response is highly adaptive, it has the function of enabling individuals to do something in response to external events. Where a behavioural response cannot occur, or where the behaviours shown do not resolve the situation, the stress response is prolonged and can become chronic. Chronic stress can have profound negative effects both physically and psychologically, and it is animals in this 'unresolved' state that are of greatest concern with regard to wellbeing.

The recognition and management of stress responses – particularly those associated with negative emotional states and those that are chronic, prolonged or repeated – are central considerations for all animals in shelters. Hence, the ability of shelter staff and veterinary teams to not only evaluate signs of stress, but also determine the emotional valence associated with behaviour changes, is fundamentally important.

Emotional states

The emotional state of an animal is a function of both emotional valence and arousal. Emotions can be considered to be either positive or negative – events are associated with a 'good' or a 'bad' feeling. This is adaptive, that is, biologically useful in an evolutionary sense – because it enables animals to associate events with different outcomes and alter their behaviour accordingly. If, for example, an animal associates a particular situation with a positive emotional state, it will do things to try to achieve that goal. Behaviours that are successful will become reinforced (i.e. more likely to be used again in the same circumstances). In other words, behaviours that 'work' to achieve a positive state are more likely to be repeated. In contrast, animals will show behaviours to avoid events associated with a negative emotional state. Behaviours that work to avoid these situations will also be reinforced, and are more likely to occur the next time the animal is in the same context.

The terms used to describe emotions in humans reflect both the valence and degree of arousal (e.g. 'panic' is a greater degree of arousal on the same axis of negative states as 'fearful', as is 'joyful' to 'cheerful' on the axis of positive states). The emotional states that have been the subject of the most discussion and research in shelter-housed animals are the negative states of fear and anxiety. However, the other negative emotional state that is important to consider is frustration, which arises when a behaviour that an animal anticipates will be successful at either achieving a positive goal or avoiding a negative event no longer succeeds.

- **Anxiety** is defined as the state when an animal anticipates a negative event or is not sure what might happen next or what the animal might do about it. It is a state of alertness and arousal that makes the animal ready for action to be able to best deal with whatever happens next. Most dogs and cats will be in a state of high anxiety when they first enter a rescue or rehoming centre environment, as they cannot predict what will happen next and are unable to control their environment at all. Unpredictability and perceived loss of control are the greatest causes of stress in both animals and humans, so entry to a shelter environment is a time when particular attention to animals' behavioural needs is important.
- A **fear response** is an immediate response to a stimulus that is perceived to be aversive. Unlike the whole-brain activation involved in anxious states, fear responses are thought to be rapid responses that pass through the phylogenically older parts of the brain. There is a brief period of emotional arousal leading to a behavioural response. Assuming this response is successful in resolving the perceived threat, the level of arousal then declines rapidly. Fear responses include behaviours such as climbing to a high shelf for a cat, or barking at someone approaching a kennel for a dog. Although some fears are thought to be innate, the majority of fear responses are learned through experience. For example, a dog might learn that an owner's angry facial expression and outstretched hand reliably predicts a bad outcome, and show a fear response to this specific collection of cues, such as running away and hiding under the table.
- **Frustration** is the emotion felt when an expected event does not occur. There are two broad causes of frustration. First, animals can be in a negative emotional state because they are not able to display species-specific behaviours. These are behaviours that animals are motivated to show because they were adaptive for survival in their evolutionary past. For example, many cats will show signs of frustration if

they are unable to show any predatory (or predatory-type play) behaviour over a prolonged period, and dogs may be frustrated by a prolonged lack of social contact. Second, individual animals can become frustrated if they are unable to utilize behaviours that they have previously learned are successful at achieving desired goals or avoiding perceived threats. For example, a dog that has learned that whining is successful at achieving the attention of its owner at home is likely to become frustrated if this behaviour no longer 'works' when it is in a kennel.

Recognition of stress

Recognizing the signs of stress is a very important aspect of managing animals in centres. Although some physiological and cognitive measures of stress are used in research contexts, behavioural indicators are most practicable for day-to-day monitoring of animals. This is because they are non-invasive, can be immediately reported, do not require any specialist equipment and change rapidly as the emotional state of the animal changes. The specific behavioural indicators of stress in dogs and cats are highlighted in the later sections of this chapter. However, it is important to note that, although behavioural signs are the most accessible measure of emotional state and stress, they can be difficult to recognize and interpret. This is partly because they can be very subtle, particularly in cats. For example, inactivity can be a sign of stress in cats, but shelter staff and other animal caregivers will often be more concerned about cats that show active signs, such as vocalization, than cats that are observed to be perfectly still in a pristine pen in the morning. Furthermore, several research papers have highlighted the relatively poor ability of people to recognize signs of negative emotional states in dogs (Tami and Gallagher, 2009).

Behavioural signs are also not directly correlated with individual emotional states. In other words, dogs or cats in similar emotional states may not necessarily show the same behavioural signs. One dog may respond to frustration at anticipating the loss of social contact by barking, and another by jumping up and grabbing a sleeve. To complicate things further, two dogs showing the same behaviour may do so as a result of different emotional states. Paw lifting (Figure 19.1), for example, can occur for appeasement,

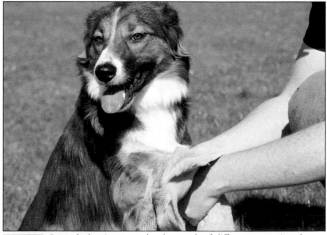

19.1 Some behaviours can be the result of different emotional states. For example, paw lifting by dogs can occur for appeasement, because of anxiety or to achieve attention. It is important for staff to pick up early signs of anxiety, particularly during handling, and change their approach accordingly.
(Courtesy of Daniel Thompson)

due to anxiety or even as a learned behaviour to achieve attention. This means that it is not possible to use individual behaviours as definitive indicators of emotional states. Rather, combinations of behavioural signs, and/or inter-preting signs in relation to other events or contexts, is key to gathering information about how individual animals are coping with their environment.

Using behavioural indicators to evaluate stress can, therefore, be complicated. To ensure that measurement is valid in terms of managing stress, there needs to be a clear process of assessment, documentation and review for each individual animal over time. It is also important to have staff training and development plans in place to make sure that all members of the team consistently recognize and appropriately interpret behavioural signs in the animals under their care.

Management and prevention of stress

Entering the rescue or rehoming centre environment is inevitably stressful for animals (Stephen and Ledger, 2006) because it is a novel environment with a range of new stimuli, and is associated with a loss of predictability and control. In most cases, indicators of stress decline over time after admission, as animals start to learn about the environment and predict what will happen when. However, the change in stress indicators over time varies consider-ably between individuals. Some retain high levels of stress over a prolonged period: they do not appear to adapt well to the environment because they find some aspects of it difficult to cope with. Others may appear to adapt more rapidly, but may then be more prone to signs of frustration as they try to show their normal behavioural repertoire. Interestingly, stress responses after admission to kennels decline faster in dogs that have experience of kennel environment, highlighting the importance of familiarity for an individual's responses (Hiby et al., 2006).

The key stages of stress management in rescue and rehoming centres are to:

- Recognize and record behavioural or physical signs of stress
- Determine the likely emotional state of stressed animals, in particular identifying anxiety, fear or frustration
- Consider what the specific cause or trigger of the stress response is for each individual animal
- Modify the environment or management routine to either avoid the situations identified as precipitating stress responses, or develop a modification programme to reduce the impact of those events for the animal
- Enable animals to show normal coping behaviours to reduce the impact of stressors
- Monitor how changes affect the signs identified, and review regularly to ensure that the animal is not exposed to chronic or repeated stress.

It is important to recognize that the causes of stress are different for each individual animal. Stress is some-times discussed as a generic concept in the kennel and cattery environment, with terms such as 'kennel stress' being used to describe how animals react to the environ-ment. A stress response for an individual animal, however, may be associated with different aspects of the environ-ment, including the close proximity of other animals, the approach of unfamiliar people, noise levels, unpredict-ability of routine, loss of expected outcomes to learned

behaviours or a combination of several factors. To put in place a suitable programme for each animal, the first stage is to identify the specific stressors and identify ways of reducing the impact of these through management or behaviour modification.

The other important factor in stress management and prevention is enabling animals to show behavioural responses that help to reduce their exposure (or per-ceived exposure) to stressors. This is important because it gives individuals some choice and, hence, control over their environment. These responses are sometimes called 'coping behaviours', and enabling these responses will help individuals to adapt to their environment. As dis-cussed earlier, the mechanisms of stress have the func-tion of enabling individuals to do something to resolve their situation. Enabling animals to perform appropriate coping behaviours, such as hiding, engaging in social interaction or chewing, will also reduce the risk that they will start to show abnormal or inappropriate responses when stressed. Allowing cats to hide in their pens by providing a box is a good example of enabling a normal coping response (Kry and Casey, 2007), which is discus-sed further later in this chapter.

Stress of confinement

Confinement in itself may be stressful for some animals, because it limits the opportunity for them to show coping responses or avoid stressors. The kennel or pen environ-ment can be adapted or enriched to reduce the impact of confinement, for example, by adding high shelves and hiding boxes for cats (see QRGs 19.7 and 19.8). However, if animals are very anxious in a confined environment despite the provision of enrichment – for example, because of anxiety about the presence of other animals or people – other options should be considered. Some centres have specialized temporary feral enclosures with cat-proof fencing, which provide feral cats the opportunity to main-tain a distance from people while a suitable relocation site is found. For dogs, having some facilities that enable them to avoid contact with other dogs or to maintain a distance from people apart from during controlled training sessions helps to manage animals that are very anxious. The option of fostering animals to non-kennel environments can also be a suitable alternative for some cases.

Confinement can also be a problem because it limits the opportunity for animals to show their full behavioural repertoire and can be a factor in the development of frus-tration. This may be particularly the case for animals that, for example, highly value human attention, which is limited by kennelling. The impact of housing in a confined area on frustration can be reduced with the imaginative use of enrichment and thoughtful management routines.

Behaviour problems

The majority of behaviours, whether desired or unwanted, develop through a process of learning. Each animal adapts to its environment in order to achieve things that it values and to avoid things that are unpleasant. As discussed earlier, this is essentially the function of emotional states – to drive animals to behave in a way that optimizes achiev-ing good things and avoiding bad things.

It is important to note that 'behaviour problems' are defined from a human perspective. They reflect those behaviours shown by animals that people find problem-atic, or that impact on their lives. Whether behaviours are a problem to owners does not necessarily equate with the extent to which they impact on the welfare of the animals themselves. For example, a dog that reacts to the anxiety of being left alone by chewing the kitchen units may be no more stressed than one that reacts by running from room to room, looking out of windows, whining, drooling or turning in circles. The first dog may be categorized as having 'separation anxiety' because of the damage caused and the impact on its owner's life; the latter may never be categorized as having a problem.

In dealing with problem behaviours in shelter animals, there are two key aims:

* To identify behavioural signs that indicate stress or inability to cope with the shelter environment
* To identify behavioural signs that may have developed in the domestic environment and need rehabilitation work for the animal to be suitable for rehoming.

Behavioural techniques

Prevention of problem behaviours

It is a common frustration for behaviourists that many of the problems they see in companion animals would have been preventable, had owners received the right advice when they first acquired their pet. Since behaviour problems are both common and preventable, it is important for animal welfare organizations to help reinforce the key messages to owners homing young or adult animals. It is also important to integrate the principles of good behaviour practice into the management of animals within shelters, to minimize the risk that the shelter environment contributes to the development of problems. The key aspects of practice for the prevention of problem behaviours are:

* Providing adequate opportunities for the socialization and habituation of young animals within shelters
* Ensuring that the environment and management of animals is designed to prevent the development of behaviours related to stress
* Providing owners homing puppies and kittens with appropriate advice on behavioural needs and training for their new pet
* Ensuring that adopters of older animals are aware of behavioural signs in their new pet and understand how to respond to changes in behaviour in different circumstances.

For dogs in particular, programmes of training or advice for owners of puppies and rescue dogs are important to ensure that they build a positive bond with their new pet and avoid the common pitfalls.

Socialization and habituation

Habituation is the process whereby a response gradually reduces with repeated presentation of the stimulus that elicits the response. Fear responses develop when animals are exposed to events or stimuli that they perceive as negative and salient, that is, above an individual threshold of tolerance (Grissom and Bhatnagar, 2009). In contrast, sensitization is the process whereby an animal's response increases on presentation of a stimulus (Davis, 1974). This is more likely to occur when the presented stimulus is of high intensity or low predictability to an individual (Gray, 1971).

Critical to whether an animal habituates or sensitizes to a stimulus is its judgement as to the degree of threat posed. This will vary with both the characteristics of the stimulus (e.g. salience, predictability) and the state of the individual animal at the time of stimulus presentation. Hence, controlling both these factors is very important to minimize the chance of an animal developing fear-associated behaviours. Gradual and careful habituation to new experiences is one of the key aspects of preventing behaviour problems in dogs and cats. This is particularly the case for their first experiences of new situations. If the first experience is a positive one, the animal will be less likely to subsequently develop a fear reaction in the same situation (Rooney et al., 2016). An example would be the first experience of visiting a veterinary practice or consulting room; by making this experience pleasant, with play and treats rather than doing any potentially aversive procedures, it is much easier to establish a positive perception of the environment.

The term 'socialization' is often used to describe the process of mixing animals with conspecifics, other animals or people. However, this term most appropriately refers to a specific sensitive period for development in the first weeks of life. The 'socialization period' is a period during which there is development and maturation of the senses before the young animal becomes more independent. In puppies, this is between approximately 4 and 16 weeks of age (Scott and Fuller, 1965), and in kittens it is between 2 and 7 weeks of age (Karsh and Turner, 1988), when the young animals become more independent. During this period there is enhanced synaptic plasticity, which results in exposure to environmental stimuli having a profound influence on later behaviour (Casey and Bradshaw, 2008). Ensuring that young animals have a positive experience of stimuli and situations they are likely to come across in their adult lives is commonly acknowledged to be beneficial in reducing the risk of fear-related behaviours in adult dogs (Appleby et al., 2002; Howell and Bennett, 2011) and cats (Casey and Bradshaw, 2008). In the past, it was considered that any exposure to new situations during this period would be beneficial for puppies and kittens. However, it is now clear that young kittens and puppies do experience fear from a young age, and it is essential to control exposure and the level of stimulus, increasing intensity gradually to avoid the risk of sensitization. For example, gradual habituation to an indoor crate, followed by an outdoor kennel environment, reduced physiological stress levels when search dogs entered military training kennels (Rooney et al., 2007). As the risk of sensitization is also increased in animals experiencing concurrent stress, the experience of young animals with respect to kennelling, handling and enrichment also needs to be considered when developing socialization programmes (see QRGs 19.3 and 19.4).

Desensitization and counter-conditioning, flooding and punishment

Desensitization and counter-conditioning

Desensitization is a term that is often confused with habituation. If an animal is feeling sensitized to a stimulus, then it needs to be desensitized to return to a normal emotional level. This is done by very gradually exposing the animal to a perceived threatening stimulus at a low level where the animal feels calm. Over time, the intensity and timing of exposure can be slowly increased. Counter-conditioning refers to changing the animal's perception from a negative association to a positive one, often using something appetitive such as a highly palatable treat.

In the shelter setting, a common situation is to have an animal that is anxious or fearful of the presence of or interaction with humans or other animals (e.g. dogs). When attempting desensitization, often the starting point is unknowingly set too high: for example, by walking a **stooge dog** past the kennel of a dog that is fearful of other dogs, as opposed to walking the stooge dog in another exercise area further away from the fearful dog. It is also important to have an appreciation for species-specific behaviour rather than taking an anthropomorphic perspective. As an example, many shelter workers are tempted to start by talking to and looking sympathetically at nervous cats, as these actions would tend to make another human feel better, whereas anxious cats would prefer to be completely ignored, with eye contact avoided.

Flooding

Flooding differs from desensitization in that the perceived threatening stimulus is presented to the animal at a high intensity without it having the ability to escape. If this is prolonged and the animal's normal coping mechanisms have proven unsuccessful, then the animal can enter a state of 'learned helplessness' where the animal appears to have calmed or learned, as it does not respond, and so shelter workers may think the behaviour problem has resolved. However, what has really happened is that the animal is 'shutting down' while still experiencing fear. This is one of the most significant and avoidable behavioural welfare issues facing shelter animals. For example, well meaning shelter staff may inadvertently use this technique to 'bring round' feral cats and kittens by exposing them to prolonged interaction until they stop hissing. As well as the welfare issues associated with this technique, the other problem is that the animal may become even more sensitized to the stimulus afterwards, and the original behaviour can return as flooding did not address the underlying cause.

Punishment

Punishment is an emotive word that often causes much confusion. In simple scientific terms, rewards and punishment happen throughout an animal's life to increase or decrease the likelihood of a behaviour occurring again; these are known as reinforcers and punishers, respectively. There are two types of each, shown in Figure 19.2.

Generally, when members of the public use the word 'punishment' they are referring to 'positive punishment', and they often may not realize that the term refers to anything the animal finds aversive, for example, shouting 'No!'

	Punishers = decrease a behaviour	Reinforcers = increase a behaviour
Positive = adding a stimulus	**Positive punishment** 'Give the bad thing' e.g. giving an electric shock	**Positive reinforcement** 'Give the good thing' e.g. providing a food reward
Negative = removing a stimulus	**Negative punishment** 'Take away the good thing' e.g. removing the animal's toys	**Negative reinforcement** 'Take away the bad thing' e.g. removing the pressure on a dog's neck when it stops pulling on a choke chain

19.2 Punishers and reinforcers.

There are numerous difficulties in using positive punishment, including:

- It is aversive and/or painful and, therefore, negatively impacts on the animal's welfare
- It does not address the underlying cause or emotional state
- The behaviour may worsen, or if the behaviour was inhibited by the punishment, it may reoccur later
- It can increase the animal's anxiety or fear in the context it is used and/or cause confusion about how to avoid the punishment
- The animal may form a different negative association from the one the owner/handler intended, including associations with other environmental factors that occurred at the same time, or fear of the owner/handler
- It may have dangerous health and safety implications for the owner/handler
- It can reduce the animal's ability to learn.

Qualified trainers and behaviourists recommend modern training methods that promote the use of positive reinforcement, which is not only effective but supports good animal welfare.

Psychopharmacology, pheromone therapy and complementary therapies

In some cases, the use of psychoactive medication can be valuable in conjunction with behaviour therapy. This is particularly the case where individual animals are so anxious that it is difficult to implement a behaviour modification plan and/or where chronic stress is having a negative impact on the animal's welfare. The decision-making process as to whether medication should be used in conjunction with behaviour modification, and the selection of agent(s) suitable for each case, can be complex and should involve collaborative working between the shelter veterinary and behaviour teams. Further information about the use of psychoactive medications is provided in the *BSAVA Manual of Canine and Feline Behavioural Medicine*.

There is insufficient scientific evidence that pheromone products are of benefit for reducing stress in cats or dogs in rehoming centres (Frank *et al.*, 2010), nor is there evidence of efficacy for any nutraceutical, herbal or homeopathic products.

Behaviour work in shelters

An emphasis on behavioural welfare is important at every stage of the process through a shelter, including the following areas:

- Preventing animals coming into the shelter, where possible, by providing advice to potential relinquishers
- Optimizing the welfare of animals when they are in the shelter
- Making the best matches of animals with owners to reduce the risk of return and promote long-term welfare.

Behaviour as a cause of relinquishment
Reasons for relinquishment

There is a significant number of cats and dogs in rescue organizations. One study estimated that 131,070 cats and 129,743 dogs entered the care of UK welfare organizations during 2009 (Clark *et al.*, 2012). There can sometimes be a perception by the general public that animal shelters are full of 'difficult' animals that come with 'baggage' or have been abused. While it will obviously vary depending on the organization's remit, many shelters deal with both stray and owned animals, many of which have been well loved and cared for. The main reasons for relinquishment are likely to vary between organizations, but behavioural issues are one of the most common reasons in dogs (Diesel *et al.*, 2010). By contrast, for cats, strays, owner's change of circumstances (including housing or financial difficulties) or unwanted litters are three of the principal causes of relinquishment. One study found that 7% of cats in UK shelters were relinquished for behavioural reasons (Casey *et al.*, 2009); this contrasts with 34% of dogs (Diesel *et al.*, 2010). It is likely that these figures underestimate the importance of undesired behaviour for relinquishment rates, as owners may consider other reasons more 'acceptable' or they may fear that a shelter may not take in animals with problem behaviours (DiGiacomo *et al.*, 1998). The impact of behavioural issues on the breakdown of pet–human bonds and relinquishment risk rates means that providing appropriate advice to members of the public, and training staff in giving this advice, are important roles for animal welfare charities.

Advice to owners to prevent animals coming into shelters

Providing appropriate advice when owners make contact with a shelter about relinquishing their pet can prevent the animal being given up for adoption, and this is an important aspect of shelter staff training (see below). However, it should be noted that many owners who have made the difficult decision to give up their pet are often 'at the end of their tether', feel that they have tried everything and are not necessarily receptive to receiving behavioural advice. In some cases, relinquishment may be the most appropriate option for the animal, for example, where the home environment or owner's situation is unsuitable. The veterinary surgeon has an important role in working with owners and shelter staff in determining the best environments to maximize the health and wellbeing of animals that can no longer remain in the home. Veterinary practice staff are also ideally placed to identify behavioural issues in companion animals before owners consider relinquishment. This includes preventive advice for puppy and kitten owners (see QRGs 19.3 and 19.4), asking owners questions during routine check-ups to identify behavioural problems sooner, and referring owners to suitably qualified trainers and behaviourists. In addition, veterinary practices can raise awareness among all pet owners about the help that is available, not only within the practice but also within the field of professional clinical behaviourists. Many owners may seek advice from inappropriate sources, and more are turning to the internet and social media for help with problems.

Optimizing the welfare of animals within shelters

It is also critical to integrate behavioural knowledge into management practices to optimize the welfare of animals once they have been admitted to a shelter. The overall aims of behavioural medicine within the shelter are shown in Figure 19.3. Achieving these aims involves an integration of several factors: ensuring adequate information is acquired at intake; ensuring the behaviour of each animal

---

Optimize the emotional welfare and quality of life of animals within and outside the organization's care by:

- Increasing positive emotional states through play, enrichment and social interaction appropriate for the species
- Promoting a normal behavioural repertoire, such as maintenance behaviours and appropriate use of space
- Reducing the risk of negative emotional states, such as anxiety, fear or frustration
- Avoiding stressful environments that may lead to reduced maintenance behaviours and stress-related illnesses.

Other potential benefits of enhancing animal welfare in shelters are:

- Reducing the length of time to rehoming and, therefore, increasing throughput in shelters
- Increasing the rates of adoption and retention in new homes
- Reducing the costs of animal care
- Increasing positive interaction between animals in care and staff, volunteers and visitors
  - May reduce relinquishment through provision of appropriate advice
  - Improves public perception of shelters
  - Makes animals more attractive to potential adopters
  - Improves staff and volunteer morale and satisfaction
- Consistent messaging across the organization.

19.3 Aims of a shelter behaviour programme.

is incorporated in health assessments; adapting management routines to the needs of each individual animal and enabling appropriate staff training in behavioural skills.

Training programme for staff and volunteers

Knowledge of animal behaviour, level of education and experience, and behavioural practices can vary widely among an organization's staff. As understanding the behaviour and welfare of animals in a shelter's care has a widespread impact on both staff and animals, it is crucial that training in this area is prioritized and consistent. Some shelters employ in-house qualified behaviourists who can provide training. Other shelters may outsource the training, and some shelters may have no access to a behavioural specialist. Knowledge from the behavioural field is constantly increasing and changing; keeping up to date and having the skills to evaluate new research and practice is, therefore, vital not only for animal welfare and the shelter behavioural programme, but also for motivating staff. While many animal caregivers wish to learn how to resolve behavioural problems, sufficient time must be taken to train shelter staff and volunteers by building a foundation of knowledge on basic ethology, behavioural development, socialization, facial expression and body language, environmental management and the welfare needs of animals. For more information about training and education programmes for staff and volunteers, see Chapter 24.

Intake history from owner

It is important to collect as much information as possible about an animal at the time it is relinquished to a shelter. Entering a shelter environment is a stressful experience for animals, and the information collected at intake can help minimize problems, for example, by identifying environments or routines that the animal is familiar with or particularly anxious about. Information obtained at relinquishment can also help with husbandry, provide a useful history for those animals that show a medical or behavioural problem while they are in the care of the shelter, and assist with matching the right animal to the right owner. Many charity staff and volunteers report that it can be very difficult to collect information, particularly if the owner is emotional, wants to sign the animal over quickly or does not provide honest responses when questioned. Compliance can be improved by making the process easier for owners and by educating them about the difference the information will make in helping the shelter to find the right home for their pet. It can help to have a comfortable private room, away from a busy reception area, to discuss the animal in more detail, where owners are more likely to feel that extra time is being taken to understand their animal.

Most owners struggle to think of specific details about their animal when asked broad questions such as 'Tell us more about your pet's interesting quirks'. Targeted questions are more likely to elicit informative responses. Areas that could be asked about include but are not limited to:

- Animal's details (e.g. name, age, breed)
- Medical history and details of the current veterinary practice, in order to gain access to medical records
- Reason for relinquishment
- Previous history, including where the pet was obtained, information on socialization, etc.
- Any insights into the animal's personality or temperament
- Reaction to handling and grooming
- Toileting habits
- Feeding regime and dietary preferences
- Preferences for exercise and play
- Information about species- and/or breed-specific behaviours (e.g. hunting behaviour in cats, or chasing behaviour in collies)
- Interactions and relationships with other animals and people (e.g. if the animal is anxious about contact with other animals/people)
- Home environment and routine
- Any behavioural problems.

The importance of history taking

An example of why history taking is so important is provided by the following case:

A cat was relinquished into a shelter by its owner. While in the shelter's care, the cat displayed inappropriate urination and defecation in its pen. The cat was initially examined by a veterinary surgeon to rule out medical problems, and then general behavioural measures, such as extra litter trays and different types of litter were tried. When these measures did not resolve the problem, a shelter worker telephoned the previous owner to ask for more information about the cat's toileting habits, only to be told that the owner used to provide the cat with an empty cardboard box with no litter as a litter tray. A cardboard box was given to the cat and its toileting problems resolved. The cat was then gradually trained to use an ordinary litter tray and was rehomed successfully. Had this information been collected at the point of intake, time, resources, expense and frustration could have been spared.

A cost-effective way of collecting information about animals that are to be relinquished is to e-mail a questionnaire to the owners for completion before the animals come into care. This method also has the advantages of reducing the time required for shelter workers to collect this information, and it can assist those managing the intake waiting list. It is also easier for the owners as they can take time to fill in the questionnaire, the information they need is more readily available in their home and they

are likely to be less emotional than they would be at the point of relinquishing their pet. Some shelters have an intake coordinator whose sole responsibility is to correspond with owners wishing to relinquish an animal, collect each animal's history and then manage the intake to achieve the optimum throughput. Knowledge about 'hot' pens or kennels (the ones from which animals seem to be rehomed more quickly than others, perhaps due to their position in the shelter), and the quiet pens/kennels that are best to allow nervous animals to settle in more easily, can help to manage intake of animals more effectively. Encouraging shelter staff to improve history taking at intake will assist shelter veterinary surgeons in clinical diagnosis of medical conditions, as well as optimizing the management of each individual while in the shelter.

Observations of behaviour

While it is acknowledged that animals will naturally behave differently in an unfamiliar, confined and often stressful environment, such as a shelter, it is still useful to monitor and record how the animal's behaviour changes over a period of time in the shelter. Different shelters take very different approaches to the assessment of behaviour, for example, observing responses over a number of days or following a standardized assessment protocol at a particular period of time after the initial assessment. However, there is currently little evidence that these assessments are reliable, and they have generally not been validated against the animal's behaviour post homing (Patronek and Bradley, 2016).

Undertaking behavioural assessment over a period of time after admission to a shelter is likely to be of value for the following reasons:

- Observation of behaviour changes over the period after admission enables assessment of how an individual animal is adapting to its new environment
- Different behavioural signs are likely to be better observed at different times, and this will reduce the risk of missing responses (i.e. false-negatives). For example, the response to separation in dogs is more likely to be valid if tested once the dogs have formed a bond with a caregiver in the shelter
- Single assessments may be subject to specific circumstances on the test day
- Repeated test protocols on the same day may cause stress and create 'false-positive' responses to later tests that day.

Keeping daily observational records of an animal's behaviour can aid communication within the shelter and reduce the incidence of bites and scratches. Staff and volunteers can be trained to record facial expressions, body language and the context, rather than trying to attribute an underlying cause or write vague descriptions such as 'nice boy'; training can also help them to appreciate the importance of taking time to complete the records accurately (see the BSAVA Manual of Canine and Feline Behavioural Medicine).

Behavioural aspects of homing and reducing returns to shelters
Matching the right animal to the right owner

Understandably, rehoming shelters have a vested interest in the animals' welfare both while in their care and once homed, and, therefore, shelters need to identify a suitable owner for each animal. The selection criteria often vary among shelters and sometimes there is not a consistent approach even within a single organization. Many shelters have policies and guidelines that detail their approach to rehoming animals (see Chapter 20). The chances of an appropriate match are increased by taking into account the information from the previous owner, the behavioural observations and animal training while in care, and matching these to the prospective adopter's lifestyle and preferences. The owner's level of satisfaction with their new pet is likely to be enhanced if their expectations have been carefully managed throughout the adoption process. Many owners expect the animal to settle into its new home within a period as short as 48 hours; if this does not happen, they may be disappointed or even take it personally, and perceive that the adoption is 'not working' rather than the animal is displaying normal behaviour. Veterinary staff can assist shelter workers by educating potential adopters about what to expect and ensuring that they give consistent messages at subsequent visits to the practice (e.g. for neutering). Successful rehoming where the animal remains in the new home and is not returned to the shelter is key.

Advice and ongoing support for new owners

Regardless of whether they have taken on a young or senior animal, or one with medical or behavioural problems, all adopters will need individually tailored advice about their new animal and ongoing support. It should also not be assumed that just because an owner has plenty of experience, this represents up-to-date knowledge. It is important to disclose both medical and behavioural information about the animal to the new owner and record the information given. Many charities use specific documents to record this information, which can help reduce the number of complaints and can be useful if legal action is taken against an organization.

It can be difficult to avoid overwhelming the owner with too much information. People generally do not absorb and retain verbal information particularly well, so a multimodal approach using written materials, visual and/or auditory aids (e.g. diagrams or videos) and interactive approaches with which the owner can engage (e.g. owner information evenings, online e-learning resources) can make a huge difference. Much like in veterinary practice, the owner's attention is easier to maintain when they are away from their animal. It is essential that the adoption experience is positive and interpersonal skills are vital to ensure that, should the adopter have any problems with their new pet, they feel happy to contact the shelter for help and advice.

Some of the most important areas in which to provide information and support to the new adopter are:

* How to settle an animal into the new home environment and what behaviour to expect
* How to gradually integrate the new animal with pets already living in the home
* Essential resources for the species and appropriate placement of resources within the home
* Contact details of the shelter and/or sources of behavioural advice
* Management of any medical or behavioural problems
* Understanding normal species-specific behaviour and body language
* The welfare needs of the species, including the adopter's duty of care under the Animal Welfare Act 2006 (see also Chapter 21)

* Recommended reading and resources about companion animal behaviour
* Basic training and where to go for more advice or training classes
* Preventive advice for common behavioural problems (e.g. litter tray management).

Behaviour of shelter cats

Understanding feline ethology and species needs

In order to meet the five welfare needs (see Chapter 21), it is important to appreciate how they relate to a particular species and the circumstances in which the animals are kept. For domesticated species, it is useful to consider animals with a shared ancestry, as these give insight into previous selective pressures that influenced the evolution of behavioural signs. Cats were domesticated relatively recently in evolutionary terms, and have been selectively bred for only approximately the past 200 years. This means that they have changed relatively little, in contrast to other species such as the dog. By understanding the behavioural characteristics of the African wildcat (*Felis silvestris lybica*), owners and shelter staff and volunteers can recognize the underlying influences on the domestic cat:

* Largely solitary, hunting independently
* Have large individual territories that have limited or no overlap with those of other wildcats
* Obligate carnivores that eat frequent small meals
* Hunting drive increases with hunger but is independent of satiety
* Use scent as an important medium for orientation and communication
* Have limited ability to show complex facial expressions
* Small predator that responds to threats predominantly through avoidance (running away, climbing up to a high place or hiding). Aggression is a defensive reaction to threat that occurs usually where avoidance is unsuccessful.

For more information about the origins and behaviour of the domestic cat, see the link to the Cats Protection website at the end of the chapter.

For those working in mixed-species environments, there can be a temptation for work with dogs to take precedence, especially as cats can often be viewed as independent and self-sufficient. In a shelter, it is easy to presume that the cats are not as stressed as the dogs because, at a glance, they may appear to be less active or sleeping, whereas kennelled dogs are often showing more obvious behaviours such as barking or jumping up at the kennel door. In addition, understanding of canine behaviour is more established than for feline behaviour, and misunderstandings of cats' needs are perhaps more common. It is certainly true that 'cats are not small dogs'.

Social behaviour

A particularly common misunderstanding of cats relates to their social needs. Cats are a unique species in that they can be highly social and benefit from contact with other cats, but can also be very stressed by being close to other cats (see QRG 19.2). It is interesting that, while some socially obligate animals, such as rabbits, are often still housed singly, cats are often kept in multi-cat households of two or more individuals. The success of these groups depends on the extent to which the individual cats are compatible and regard each other as part of the same social grouping. A cat may choose to be in the same social group as another cat, but this is very much on an individual basis. Furthermore, cats that are friendly with one cat may not necessarily be so with others. Cats that are in the same social group show social behaviours that are reciprocal between pairs of cats; this includes mutual grooming (allogrooming) and rubbing on each other, choosing to sleep together so that they are touching and approaching to greet one another with nose-to-nose sniffing and a 'tail up' posture. The absence of agonistic behaviours does not mean that cats are in the same social group, as many owners unfortunately assume. Cats that do not get on can cohabit by avoiding contact, for example, by 'time-sharing' key resources, including their owners.

The misapprehension that cats are happier living in groups can lead to cat lovers and shelter workers or volunteers adopting a number of cats that need homes. In some cases, these actions risk creating problems resulting from the high cat population densities within their homes. Veterinary staff can provide useful input by educating shelter staff and volunteers about cat ethology and highlighting any concerns about cat welfare or even hoarding (see QRG 23.1) with the relevant staff at the organization.

Although the presence of other cats in the same social group can be beneficial for their welfare, proximity to unfamiliar or incompatible cats is one of the most common causes of stress-related behaviours in cats. Being aware of the subtle signs of whether cats are in the same social group or not is, therefore, crucial in reducing stress levels. In shelters, the confined nature of the pens often means that stress or conflict between cats is more likely. The behaviours of cats that were carefully avoiding one another in the home – by, for example, time-sharing a resource or occupying different spaces – are easily missed by many owners and so not reported at relinquishment. Many owners request that their cats be rehomed together as, in the absence of witnessing hissing or fighting, they assume that their cats must get along with each other. Continual monitoring in the shelter is needed to help assess relationships between cats and determine whether pairs of cats may require being separated and will perhaps benefit from being rehomed separately.

The concept of 'dominance hierarchies' remains prevalent among cat owners and shelter workers, and many such people refer to one cat in a multi-cat household/group as being the 'top', 'boss' or 'alpha' cat over the others. The problem with dominance theory is how caregivers apply it to cats, such as by allowing cats to 'sort out who is the boss' during new introductions. People often consider aggressive encounters to be a necessary part of the process of integrating cats with each other, despite the reality of poor welfare that results from the conflict and stress experienced by the cats involved. Research over the past few decades has suggested that the concept of dominance is too simplistic for the complex social groupings found in species such as cats and dogs. There is now a consensus that dominance theory is flawed and out of date, and is, therefore, not applicable to either cats or dogs. Instead, it is more useful to look at interactions between each pair of cats to understand the quality of the relationship, with the knowledge that the response of each cat is influenced by its level of socialization, personality, motivation, previous experience of interactions with the other individual and any underlying medical conditions that can influence behaviour.

Cats' needs in a shelter environment

The confined shelter environment presents a set of challenges for cats, the most obvious being the space limitations and the loss of predictability and control over their environment. Cats are very attached to their home range and thrive on routine, familiarity and the ability to exercise choice. Given the unknown environment of the shelter, the unfamiliar smells and the close proximity to unfamiliar cats, it is common for cats to be stressed when first entering a shelter. While stress levels often decrease as individual cats adapt to their new environment, it is an important aspect of their care that signs of stress are monitored carefully over this period. Individual cats vary considerably in the rate at which they adapt to being in a shelter, and appropriate management techniques and enrichment choices need to be selected to ensure that levels of stress do not remain high for a prolonged period.

Facial expressions and body postures

With an ancestral species adapted to living largely solitary lives, cats lack the complex facial musculature to show a rich variety of expressions. Cats do have facial expressions, but they are much more subtle and can be harder to 'read' than those of species such as the dog. Cats are also very adept at hiding pain and stress as a self-preservation mechanism. The key to reading any species' facial expression and body posture is to look at all the signs as a whole and examine the context in which they are being shown. For example, a common sign of stress in cats is dilated pupils; however, they can also have dilated pupils in low light levels, when in pain or with increased levels of sympathetic activation, such as during play or hunting. Many of the signs of a stressed cat are extremely similar to those shown by a cat that is in pain.

A common complaint from shelter workers is that a cat has displayed aggressive behaviour that was 'without warning' or 'unprovoked'. Almost all cats will show a warning before displaying aggression; however, the difficulty can be that the cat's reactions are particularly quick, and so the warning sign can be easily missed by the worker while performing routine husbandry tasks. Key features to look at in the cat are summarized in Figures 19.4–19.8.

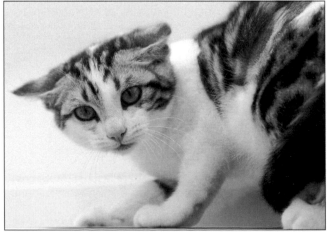

19.4 Flattened ears indicate that this cat is fearful and/or stressed. (© Cats Protection)

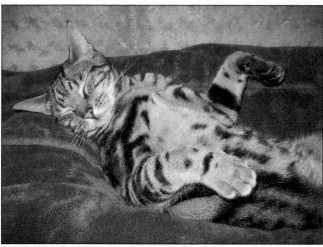

A relaxed cat sleeping on its back.
(© Cats Protection)

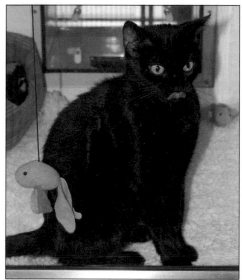

Lip licking where the tongue touches the nose, where it is not related to eating, may be a sign of stress or anxiety.
(© Cats Protection)

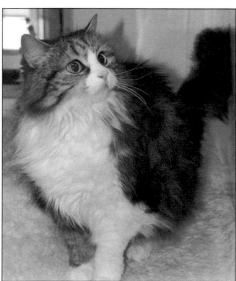

This cat is tense as indicated by the dilated pupils and the ears slightly turned out to the side. Context is important, e.g. the pupils were dilated due to the stress of the novel shelter environment rather than play.
(© Cats Protection)

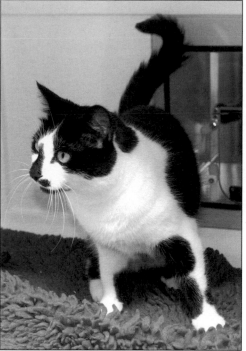

Constricted pupils combined with a raised tail that is curled at the tip usually indicate that the cat is relaxed and in greeting mode.
(© Cats Protection)

Behavioural aspects of cat accommodation

Pen design

Designing the cat pens in a shelter to maximize feline welfare should be paramount. Veterinary surgeons may be asked to provide input not only on the veterinary aspects, such as infectious disease control measures, but also on improving the psychological wellbeing of the cats housed in the pens (see Chapter 10). From a behavioural perspective, the key areas for pen design are:

- Provide the cat with choices so that it can feel more in control of its environment
- Provide elevated perches and places to hide to make the cat feel safe and reduce stress levels (Kry and Casey, 2007)
- House cats from different households away from each other (i.e. do not house communally)
- Avoid cats being able to see other cats by careful positioning of the pens in relation to one another and/or constructing the sides of the pen from a fully opaque (i.e. not frosted) material
- Take into account the likely locations for resources such as litter trays
- Have areas where the cat can choose to avoid and feel hidden from people (e.g. visiting members of the public)
- Provide an interesting and stimulating view (e.g. to an outside space).

Essential feline resources and appropriate placement

Even in the very limited and constricted area of a shelter pen, providing a cat with appropriate resources can make a positive difference to its welfare (Figure 19.9). The 'feline principles' of where cats generally prefer their resources

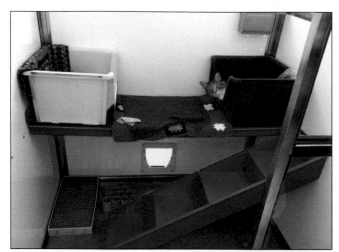

19.9 Even in the limited area of a shelter pen, providing a cat with appropriate resources and enrichment can make a difference to its welfare. This photograph shows half of a two-compartment pen; an outside run is accessible through the cat flap.
(© Cats Protection)

are as follows (although it should be borne in mind that every cat may have individual preferences):

- Litter tray somewhere private, accessible, away from other resources and not overlooked by other cats. Some cats prefer open litter trays, while others feel safer in a covered litter tray
- Food bowls positioned away from the water bowl, even if by only a short distance (several centimetres)
- Both food and water bowls positioned away from the litter tray
- Some cats find that plastic bowls taint the water and prefer to drink from metal or ceramic bowls; ideally these should be wide and shallow
- Scratching facilities should ideally be disposable. Many commercially-bought scratching posts, e.g. the sisal-based ones, are very difficult to disinfect fully and may act as a fomite for disease. Carpet tiles or corrugated cardboard can be obtained, often free of charge, and can be attached to the pen door (depending on its design) with a cable tie at the correct height to allow the individual cat to stretch fully while scratching
- The sleeping place may vary depending on the design of the pen; however, placing a bed or blanket in an elevated position will help the cat to feel safe. Operating a 'double bed' system by providing the cat with at least two blankets, and alternately removing one for washing to be replaced with a clean blanket, will provide scent continuity. If space allows, cats should be provided with at least two sleeping places so that they can display their natural behaviour of rotating sleeping locations
- Provide safe toys and feeding enrichment that can encourage self-directed play and mental stimulation; rotate the toys regularly to maintain their novelty.

Environmental enrichment

Providing suitable environmental enrichment is an essential part of the daily care and management of cats in the shelter environment. Enrichment needs to be relevant to the individual cat's needs, which may vary over time – for example, as cats adapt to being in the shelter environment. Hence, for cats newly arrived in the centre it is often more appropriate to provide a place to hide than to try to

initiate interactive play. Owing to the importance of infectious disease control, enrichment materials should be either disposable or easy to disinfect. Owners can also be educated about ideas for enrichment to improve the welfare of their cats (see also QRG 19.8).

Integration with other cats in the new home

Poor integration into the new home, especially with other resident cats, is one of the most common reasons for cats to be returned to a shelter after homing (Casey *et al.*, 2009). Unrealistic owner expectations and poor compliance with advice on integration may play a significant role in this occurrence.

An integration programme is the process of gradually introducing two animals to each other so that they may at least tolerate one another. Veterinary practice staff are ideally placed to help manage the owner's expectations and provide advice and support to owners regarding integration. The process of integration involves various stages; in general it should be viewed as a very gradual process, but each individual cat will vary in terms of how long each stage will take. Initially, the new cat needs to be kept in a separate 'sanctuary room', such as a spare bedroom, with all its resources, and be allowed to settle. Once the cat has adapted to this environment, a process of swapping the scent of the new cat and the other cat(s) in the household can begin. A clean cloth is rubbed over each cat to collect pheromones from its scent glands. The cloth bearing the scent of one cat is then placed in the territory of the other cat and vice versa. Once the cats are ignoring each other's scent, the next stage is to allow them to see one another briefly through a solid barrier, such as a glass door. The more stages that can be used the better, and some owners may be able to accommodate a mesh barrier for the next stage (Figure 19.10). The final stage is the cats meeting face to face; it can take weeks or even longer to reach this point.

The key points of integration are:

- It should be very gradual – at the cat's pace, rather than the owner's
- The scent transfer stage should constitute the longest part of the process; many owners either skip through this step or progress too quickly, so the provision of advice on this step is important
- Cats should always be given choice and control over their environment. Therefore, managing the integration

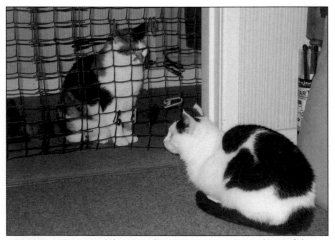

19.10 Using a mesh barrier when integrating cats can be useful as one later stage of the process.
(© Cats Protection)

process in small steps and providing hiding places and escape routes is preferable to, for example, trying to integrate the new cat while it is kept in a crate in the new owner's home

- It is easiest to monitor the cat's reaction to the scent cloth of another cat by placing the cloth in the middle of the room and observing whether the cat chooses to avoid the scent cloth or to sniff it and subsequently ignore it
- Ensure that the home has plenty of appropriately placed resources to reduce any competition
- Counter-conditioning the cats by using treats, attention or interactive play can help them to form positive associations to the presence of the other cat
- **The same principles apply when integrating a new cat with a dog.**

For more detailed information on integration, see the links to videos produced by Cats Protection at the end of the chapter.

Common behavioural problems and solutions

Preventing behaviour problems is key to a shelter behavioural programme. A large proportion of the available resources should be directed at preventing rather than addressing problems. Prevention strategies can be a part of many areas of the organization's work, including:

- Educating the public about cats' needs and the resources that are available to prevent behavioural problems developing and/or the owner–companion animal bond breaking down
- Advice given to owners to prevent potential relinquishment where appropriate
- Appropriate pen design from a feline behavioural welfare perspective
- Environmental management and enrichment programme.

The shelter environment presents a unique set of challenges and is generally not conducive to resolving behaviour problems. Cats may present with pre-existing problems, shelter-induced problems or a combination of the two. It is crucial to recognize where there could be a behavioural problem and how it might affect the ease with which a cat can be homed. Depending on the specific issue, some behavioural problems may naturally resolve while the cat is in in the shelter's care. For example, cats that have been inappropriately toileting in the house due to inadequate litter tray/latrine facilities or infrequent cleaning of litter trays may cease showing this behaviour with the provision of appropriate litter trays and substrate, and a regular cleaning regime by the shelter.

While a detailed account is beyond the remit of this chapter, the main behavioural concerns observed in a shelter environment, and initial measures to address them, are discussed in the following sections. For all changes in behaviour or behavioural problems observed, it is vital to rule out any medical reasons that could have caused the behaviour and identify the underlying cause.

Hiding and avoidance

This is one of the most prevalent and yet under-reported behaviours, as it does not directly impact on the staff or volunteers as much as aggressive behaviour towards people. All cats will experience some degree of stress when entering the shelter environment. Hiding is a desired response to stress, as it will help to reduce the cat's stress levels as well as being less of a health and safety risk for personnel. Providing hiding places with entry and exit holes will reduce the stress response and enable the cat to adapt more quickly. All cats should be given the choice to hide and climb to elevated perches. Identifying whether a cat is anxious or fearful of the new environment, the close proximity of other cats or dogs, or people can help shape the behavioural plan. Individual cats will adapt to the novel environment at different rates. Creating a sense of predictability, with a familiar caregiver, consistent routine and hands-off approach, will help the cat to settle in. Some cats may require a gradual desensitization programme. However, these cats should not be held back from being homed, as the desensitization technique does not generalize to other situations; the new owners may need to continue working with the cat once it has gone to its new home.

Inappropriate toileting

In the shelter environment, inappropriate toileting is a regular occurrence. History taking from the previous owner about each cat's toileting preferences is absolutely vital to help provide continuity; ideally, the relinquishing owner should be asked to provide a bag of the current type of litter used by the cat. This can be gradually changed over to the type of litter used at the shelter. If resources permit, it is helpful for the shelter to have several different types of litter and trays available. It is worth noting that most cats prefer soft, sand-sized litter; however, it may not be economical to use this type of litter routinely.

Considerate pen design can play a huge role in inappropriate toileting behaviour. Ensuring that cats cannot see other cats or dogs and are provided with private areas for litter tray placement will reduce the incidence of this behaviour. Placing an open, rectangular litter tray inside a cardboard box can provide privacy cost-effectively. Cut two holes in the sides of the box and have the top of the box open to help the cat to feel more hidden, prevent the accumulation of odour, and ease identifying when the tray needs cleaning.

Another consideration in the shelter environment is olfaction. Many commercially available animal disinfectants and some litter types are scented, often for human benefit, but unpleasant and off-putting for the cat. Using non-scented products will help not only in inappropriate toileting cases, but other 'problem' behaviours such as aggressive behaviour.

Aggression towards people

There are numerous underlying causes of aggressive behaviour in cats; those that are most commonly experienced in the shelter environment are discussed here. An appreciation of the underlying emotions experienced by the cat can help shelter staff and volunteers to empathize with it, rather than anthropomorphically labelling it as 'vindictive' or 'spiteful'.

Fear-based aggression: In the absence of successful avoidance behaviour, some cats feel they have no choice but to resort to aggressive behaviour in response to a real or perceived threat. Whereas cats that show hiding behaviour may be 'passive responders' to stress, cats that show aggressive responses may be considered 'active responders'. Environmental management to encourage the preferred coping strategies of hiding and climbing to elevated perches is vital. Once the cat's stress levels have reduced sufficiently so they do not impede learning, a desensitization programme may be appropriate.

Frustration-related aggression: Frustration is commonly experienced by cats in the shelter environment; depending on how it presents, it can often be misunderstood. Cats that have adapted to the initial stress of entering the shelter environment can be at risk of frustration as they continue to be confined with comparatively little stimulation. This is one of the many reasons why it is imperative for cats to be rehomed in the shortest time possible. Cats that show frustration-related aggressive behaviour can be alarming to shelter staff, who may perceive that the behaviour was 'unprovoked'. This perception can be further complicated if they feel that the cat is not showing a fear-based response but fail to understand the underlying motivation for the behaviour. In these circumstances, shelter staff may view the cat anthropomorphically, and the lack of understanding of the reason underlying the cat's behaviour can impede meeting its needs. Identifying the underlying cause and emotion will guide the measures required for the individual cat. Many cats that are showing frustration-related aggression can benefit from environmental management and enrichment programmes.

Inappropriate play behaviour: Cats that learned in kittenhood that biting fingers and toes was a stimulating way to interact with people can continue to show this behaviour into adulthood. These games often develop further with adult cats to include ambushing behaviour. Many owners fail to recognize this behaviour as a type of predatory play. With any potential health and safety risk, such as that associated with cat bites and scratches, protective clothing must be worn to prevent injury. A consistent approach to minimize contact with hands and feet without eliciting a predatory response and redirecting the behaviour on to appropriate stimuli, such as a fishing rod toy, can help.

Over-grooming

One of the ways in which stress can manifest is through over-grooming. If medical reasons for this behaviour have been ruled out, then environmental management, particularly avoiding having unfamiliar cats in the affected cat's line of sight, as well as enrichment and interactive play sessions can help to some degree. However, many cases caused by an underlying stress response to the shelter environment are resolved once the cat has been rehomed.

Withdrawal

Cats that have experienced prolonged stress in an impoverished environment may suffer from apathy and withdrawal. A change in behaviour is the most notable sign. More specifically, this can include sitting with hunched shoulders, being disengaged from human interaction, decreased appetite and a lack of interest in play and the surroundings. This lack of responsiveness is seldom recognized as an important welfare concern, yet it is more significant than aggressive behaviour, where the cat is displaying coping mechanisms. Cats displaying withdrawal behaviour require a calm, patient approach to encourage them to respond positively and elevate their emotional state.

Behaviour of shelter dogs

Understanding the behaviour of dogs is central to ensuring their welfare within the shelter environment. This understanding is needed both to enable management practices and housing that minimize stress, and also to rehabilitate dogs that have been relinquished with problem behaviours, to ensure they are adequately prepared for rehoming.

Ethology and species needs

Historically, much of the behaviour of dogs was interpreted quite simplistically in terms of 'hierarchy' or social structure. It was believed that dogs were motivated to achieve a higher 'status' relative to other dogs or people, and that this desire led them to show behaviours such as aggression in order to achieve control. However, following advancements in science and clinical behavioural practice, it is now known that the foundations on which this theory was based are incorrect. The majority of animal trainers and behaviourists have changed their practices as a result. There is also now greater knowledge about how the brain works and how animals learn, which has enabled a better understanding of why behaviours such as aggression develop in dogs. This section summarizes why 'dominance' is no longer regarded as a useful explanation for the behaviour of dogs; a fuller review of this topic is available in Bradshaw *et al.* (2009).

Dominance came to be used to describe dog behaviour through the interpretation of studies of the grey wolf, a closely related species to the domestic dog. Early studies of wolves were done on artificial groups of animals kept in captivity. These individuals were unable to get away from each other, and the social groupings were not the normal family groups that are found in the wild (Mech, 1999). The results of these studies suggested the existence of a rigid hierarchy in which particular individuals ('alphas') had priority access to resources and maintained the group structure through the display of aggression to others (Zimen, 1975). Since the wolf shares a common ancestor with the domestic dog, it was suggested that similar social groupings may exist in dogs, and that the formation of these groups is based on the 'desire' or 'drive' of each individual to be the 'leader' or 'alpha' of the group, with a hierarchical structure resulting from competitive success among individuals in the group. This interpretation of dog social behaviour became so well established that it was also used to interpret interactions between dogs and people, with the underlying assumption that dogs also regarded people as competitors in the struggle for social status. Dominance has been described as a motivation for behaviours as diverse as aggression, attention seeking, destruction and even failure to return on recall.

More recent research on natural wolf populations has suggested that groups are based on cooperative family units, in which one breeding pair produces puppies and older siblings assist with rearing them (Mech and Boitani, 2003). In these family groups there is no 'alpha' status achieved by strength or aggression (Mech, 2008), and there is no evidence that individual wolves have a lifelong 'dominant' characteristic (Packard, 2003). Aggressive behaviour is very rare in stable groups (Mech, 1999), and where it does occur, it is flexible, being based on individual circumstance rather than being predictable between particular pairs of animals. Since a dominance hierarchy in which social structure is based on competitive ability does not appear to occur naturally in wolves, the argument that this model should apply to dogs, as a close relative, is poor (Van Kerkhove, 2004).

Research has also highlighted that the social behaviour of the dog has changed considerably from its ancestral species since domestication (Miklósi, 2007), and observations of feral dogs suggest that their social structure is completely different from that of owned dogs (reviewed in Bradshaw *et al.*, 2009). For example, mating is unrestricted in feral dog groups (Pal *et al.*, 1999), and although appeasement behaviour occurs, it is seen both within family groups and between individuals belonging to different groups, suggesting that it has a general function of defusing conflict rather than being a specific 'submission' behaviour to maintain group hierarchical structures. In addition, groups of domestic dogs do not form social groupings that can be interpreted in terms of a dominance hierarchy. One study, described by Bradshaw *et al.* (2009), investigated the interactions within a group of 19 dogs housed together in a sanctuary environment. Recorded interactions between each pair of dogs within the group identified no evidence of an overall hierarchy. Rather, the interactions suggested that each pair of dogs had a learned pattern of behaviour with each other, which may or may not vary between different situations, but which could not be combined into any overall group structure.

Although discussions around dominance are often portrayed as an academic argument, it is important to realize that the way people interpret the behaviour of their dogs has a strong influence on the way they behave towards them. Dispelling the myths behind the dominance theory is, therefore, an important step in enhancing the welfare of the dogs in the care of shelters. If owners believe that a dog does something to 'achieve status' or 'be the boss', it naturally tends to lead them to use coercive training techniques. These techniques rely on inducing a negative emotional state (e.g. fear or anxiety) in a dog in order to inhibit a behaviour, which has the risk of inducing further undesired behaviour or having a negative effect on the dog's welfare.

The behaviour of dogs, as with all other mammals, is driven by emotional states – trying to achieve things that are found to be positive, and avoiding negative situations. Hence, a dog that is running away or showing aggression will be doing so to avoid a perceived threat. Similarly, a dog that is jumping up or barking at its owner may be doing so as it has learned that these behaviours 'work' to achieve social attention. Understanding the underlying reasons for behaviour in dogs helps to direct behavioural rehabilitation methods more appropriately. Modern approaches are based on using the principles of learning to alter behaviour – for example, by changing the emotional response of a dog to a particular event, or changing the consequence of a behaviour to alter the animal's motivation to show it. It is an important part of the work of animal welfare and veterinary organizations to reinforce modern interpretations of canine behaviour to avoid misconceptions being used to justify inappropriate, punishment-based methods of training.

Facial expressions and body postures

Although the social groupings of domestic dogs are quite different from those of their ancestral species, they do retain the characteristics of a highly social species from their evolutionary past. This means that dogs are highly adapted to both displaying and learning about even very subtle behavioural signs in others. It is adaptive for social species to be able to demonstrate their emotional state and recognize how others are responding, to enable cooperative living – and dogs are masters of this.

Dogs communicate with each other, and with humans, using a wide range of body language, facial expressions, tail and ear positions, and vocalizations. Recognizing these signs is an important way of monitoring how individual dogs are reacting to their environment (Figures 19.11–19.13).

It is particularly important for those who work with dogs to understand the subtler signs of anxiety, fear and frustration. Identifying these signs early on means that interventions can be put in place before more obvious, and potentially problematic, signs become apparent, such as aggression or other avoidance behaviours. Recognizing the initial subtle signs gives an early warning that a dog is worried about a specific situation. It is much easier to address this situation immediately than once an avoidance response is established. Staff training and clear protocols for shelter workers to help them recognize these signs can make an important difference to both the wellbeing of dogs and the ease of managing them.

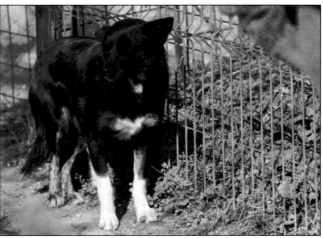

19.11 Turning away with eyes closed and a tense closed mouth are indicators of anxiety in this dog.
(Courtesy of Daniel Thompson)

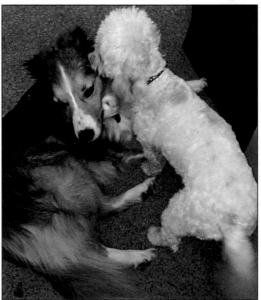

19.12 Dogs may show signs of anxiety in specific contexts or situations: here a dog is worried by close interaction with another dog.
(Courtesy of Daniel Thompson)

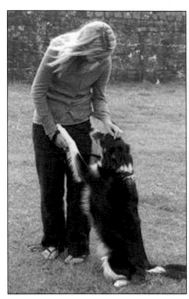

19.13 Dogs will learn behaviours which help them to cope with situations that cause them anxiety. In this case the dog is seeking attention from a handler.
(Courtesy of Bethany Loftus)

Resources, placement and pen design

Managing the behavioural wellbeing of dogs in shelters can be resource intensive. It requires staff resources for assessment and rehabilitation work, staff training to ensure consistent management of dogs, and the kennels and wider facilities to be designed in a way that enables optimal management of different behavioural presentations (see Chapter 10).

There are a number of beneficial aspects of shelter management and design that will improve a dog's welfare, and which organizations could implement depending on the resources available to them:

* Dedicated behavioural staff with appropriate knowledge and training skills can make a considerable difference in the ability of shelters to manage stress and rehabilitate dogs for rehoming
* A staff development and training process to ensure that all staff who handle dogs understand the body postures and facial expressions of dogs and know how to react to these different signs
* Pen design that at least ensures the basic needs of dogs, but ideally enables dogs to have some control over their environment, e.g. to move away from contact with people or get on to a raised area to see out
* Provision of enrichment, with the type, presentation and timing based on the needs of the individual dog (see below). Enrichment includes physical 'things' such as toys that dispense food on manipulation, but also social enrichment with people or other dogs
* Variability of kennel locations and access to enable easier maintenance of dogs that have fear or anxiety about specific situations. For example, where dogs are worried by the presence of other dogs, it is useful to have some kennels that dogs can enter and exit without passing other dogs in kennels. Having some kennels with easy direct access to exercise areas or compounds can be useful in the short term for dogs that are anxious about close handling
* Cleaning and management routines that reduce the stress for dogs. For example, for some dogs it may be appropriate to clean their kennels while they are out for exercise
* Adapting management routines to suit the requirements of individual dogs. For example, a dog that is fed last

and shows behavioural signs of frustration while waiting may benefit from being fed first
* Enabling sufficient exercise and physical activity to maintain health and reduce frustration
* Availability of quiet spaces or areas that enable quiet interaction with or training of nervous dogs away from the kennel environment.

Enrichment

Providing enrichment is an important aspect of managing stress for dogs in shelters. Enrichment is often considered generically as something that is of benefit to all dogs. It is also often thought of in terms of 'things', such as the provision of toys for all dogs. However, the enrichment needs of each dog will be unique and may also vary over time. For example, some dogs can benefit from enrichment that helps them show normal coping responses to stressors, such as barriers or high-sided beds that allow them to hide when they first arrive at the shelter. Anxious dogs also benefit from a predictable routine, having a limited number of handlers and being slowly introduced to new experiences. Other dogs may require enrichment that is focused more on preventing signs of frustration, for example, by providing a more varied routine and different experiences.

Social enrichment is an important part of reducing stress in kennels. Most dogs highly value human company, which is inevitably limited in a shelter environment. For dogs that are safe to handle and value human attention, a range of different types of contact and interaction may be beneficial, depending on the individual dog. These include spending time in the kennel with a handler, training sessions away from the kennel, walking on the lead, playing off lead and spending quiet time with a person without interaction (see QRG 19.7).

Common behavioural problems

An increasing number of dogs are relinquished to rehoming centres because of behavioural problems that their owners cannot tolerate. This means that a proportion of dogs within shelters will have issues arising from previous experiences, which impact on their wellbeing while they are in the shelter and can affect their likelihood of being successfully rehomed. In many cases these behaviours are apparent in the shelter, but in others the behavioural problem may be specific to the home environment and not be obvious while the dog is in kennels. Adequate assessment protocols are, therefore, important to ensure that such problems are identified, to enable the best matching of a dog to a new home and the implementation of any rehabilitation needed. The most common states leading to problematic behavioural signs being seen in the shelter environment are:

* Anxiety or fear about the approach of unfamiliar people, resulting in avoidance behaviours including aggression
* Anxiety or fear associated with handling or close contact, resulting in avoidance behaviours including aggression
* Anxiety or fear about contact with other dogs, resulting in avoidance behaviours including aggression
* Frustration associated with other dogs, for example, when they are passing the dog's kennel
* Frustration associated with the withdrawal of social attention or stopping of play, for example, when dogs are returned to kennels

- Anxiety or fear about being approached with resources, including toys and food, which may present as aggression
- Frustration based around limited opportunities for activity or mental stimulation
- Anxiety or fear about being separated from people.

The key to resolving these types of problem is often to concentrate on the underlying reason or motivation for the behaviour rather than try to change the behaviour that is observed. Where behavioural signs arise from anxiety or fear, the approach to rehabilitation may include identifying the specific contexts and cues that precipitate the behaviour and, where possible, avoiding exposure to these in the short term. This will enable subsequent desensitization and counter-conditioning if appropriate. With frustration-related behaviours, the options for rehabilitation can sometimes involve increasing the opportunity for the dog to show frustration-related behaviours, but may also require avoiding specific situations in the short term.

The development of a behaviour modification programme has to be specific to each dog and situation. Often there are multiple factors involved in each case, and so careful consideration is needed of the optimal approach and the order of treatment protocols to achieve the best outcomes. In some cases, medical conditions can affect behavioural signs, so close collaboration between the shelter veterinary surgeon and behavioural team is essential to ensure the welfare of dogs. The extent to which medical or physiological factors influence behaviour varies from case to case, from not at all (i.e. where the behaviour is entirely learned) to being the sole cause, with the behaviour being entirely unrelated to external events (Reisner, 1991). In most cases, a combination of learned and physical factors influences the development of behaviour – and it is an important skill of both the veterinary surgeon and behavioural practitioner to be able to interpret behavioural signs in the light of internal/physical factors. It is extremely important for veterinary surgeons to have a good understanding of how the various physiological and pathological conditions affecting their patients can impact on their behaviour, as well as knowledge of the influence of medication on behavioural signs. It is also important for behavioural practitioners to be able to interpret any elements of an animal's behavioural history that do not fit with expected patterns of learning, which may indicate a medical component to the problem. Failure to recognize that behavioural signs are associated with disease will affect the efficacy of treatment programmes and may also compromise the health and welfare of the animal.

References and further reading

Animal Behaviour and Training Council (2012) Socialisation of puppies to people. Animal Behaviour and Training Council, Carlisle. http://www.abtcouncil.org.uk/images/publicinfo/SOCIALISATION%20OF%20PUPPIES%20TO%20PEOPLE.pdf

Appleby DL, Bradshaw JWS and Casey RA (2002) Relationship between aggressive and avoidance behaviour by dogs and their experience in the first six months of life. *Veterinary Record* **150**, 434–438

Bradshaw JWS, Blackwell EJ and Casey RA (2009) Dominance in domestic dogs – useful construct or bad habit? *Journal of Veterinary Behaviour, Clinical Applications and Research* **4**, 109–144

Bräm M, Doherr MG, Lehmann D, Mills D and Steiger A (2008) Evaluating aggressive behavior in dogs: a comparison of 3 tests. *Journal of Veterinary Behavior* **3**, 152–160

Casey RA and Bradshaw JWS (2008) The effects of additional socialisation for kittens in a rescue centre on their behaviour and suitability as a pet. *Applied Animal Behaviour Science* **114**, 196–205

Casey R, Vandenbussche S, Bradshaw JWS and Roberts MA (2009) Reasons for relinquishment and return of domestic cats (*Felis silvestris catus*) to rescue shelters in the UK. *Anthrozoös* **22**, 347–358

Christensen E, Scarlett J, Campagna M and Houpt KA (2007) Aggressive behavior in adopted dogs that passed a temperament test. *Applied Animal Behaviour Science* **106**, 85–95

Clark C, Gruffydd-Jones T and Murray J (2012) Number of cats and dogs in UK welfare organisations. *Veterinary Record* **170**, 493–496

Davis M (1974) Sensitization of rat startle response by noise. *Journal of Comparative and Physiological Psychology* **87**, 571–581

Diederich C and Giffroy JM (2006) Behavioural testing in dogs: a review of methodology in search for standardization. *Applied Animal Behaviour Science* **97**, 51–72

Diesel G, Brodbelt D and Pfeiffer DU (2010) Characteristics of relinquished dogs and their owners at 14 rehoming centers in the United Kingdom. *Journal of Applied Animal Welfare Science* **13**, 15–30

DiGiacomo N, Arluke A and Patronek G (1998) Surrendering pets to shelters: the relinquisher's perspective. *Anthrozoös* **11**, 41–51

Frank D, Beauchamp G and Palestrini C (2010) Systematic review of the use of pheromones for treatment of undesirable behavior in cats and dogs. *Journal of the American Veterinary Medical Association* **236**, 1308–1316

Gray J (1971) *The Psychology of Fear and Stress*. McGraw-Hill, New York

Grissom N and Bhatnagar S (2009) Habituation to repeated stress: get used to it. *Neurobiology of Learning and Memory* **92**, 215–224

Hiby EF, Rooney NJ and Bradshaw JWS (2006) Behavioural and physiological responses of dogs entering re-homing kennels. *Physiology and Behavior* **89**, 385–391

Horowitz A (2009) Disambiguating the 'guilty look': salient prompts to a familiar dog behaviour. *Behavioural Processes* **81**, 447–452

Horowicz D and Mills D (2009) *BSAVA Manual of Canine and Feline Behavioural Medicine, 2nd edn*. BSAVA Publications, Gloucester

Howell TJ and Bennett PC (2011) Puppy power! Using social cognition research tasks to improve socialization practices for domestic dogs (*Canis familiaris*). *Journal of Veterinary Behavior: Clinical Applications and Research* **6**, 195–204

Karsh EB and Turner DC (1988) The human-cat relationship. In: *The Domestic Cat: The Biology of its Behaviour*, ed. DC Turner and P Bateson, pp. 159–177. Cambridge University Press, Cambridge

Kovary R (1999) Taming the dominant dog. *American Dog Trainers Network*. http://www.inch.com/~dogs/taming.html

Kry K and Casey R (2007) The effect of hiding enrichment on stress levels and behaviour of domestic cats (*Felis sylvestris catus*) in a shelter setting and the implications for adoption potential. *Animal Welfare* **16**, 375–383

Lindsay SR (2000) *Handbook of Applied Dog Behavior and Training. Vol. 1, Adaptation and Learning*. Iowa State University Press, Ames, Iowa

Mech LD (1999) Alpha status, dominance and division of labor in wolf packs. *Canadian Journal of Zoology* **77**, 1196–1203

Mech LD (2008) Whatever happened to the term 'alpha wolf'? *International Wolf* **18**, 4–8

Mech LD and Boitani L (2003) Wolf social ecology. In: *Wolves: Behavior, Ecology and Conservation*, ed. LD Mech and L Boitani, pp. 1–34. University of Chicago Press, Chicago

Miklósi Á (2007) Human-animal interactions and social cognition in dogs. In: *The Behavioural Biology of Dogs*, ed. P Jensen, pp. 205–222. CAB International, Wallingford

Packard JM (2003) Wolf behavior: reproductive, social and intelligent. In: *Wolves: Behavior, Ecology and Conservation*, ed. LD Mech and L Boitani, pp. 35–65. University of Chicago Press, Chicago

Pal SK, Ghosh B and Roy S (1999) Inter- and intra-sexual behaviour of free-ranging dogs (*Canis familiaris*). *Applied Animal Behaviour Science* **62**, 267–278.

Patronek GJ and Bradley J (2016) No better than flipping a coin: recognising canine evaluations in animal shelters. *Journal of Veterinary Behavior* **15**, 66–77

Reisner I (1991) The pathophysiologic basis of behaviour problems. *Veterinary Clinics of North America: Small Animal Practice* **21**, 207–224

Rooney NJ, Clark CCA and Casey RA (2016) Minimizing fear and anxiety in working dogs: a review. *Journal of Veterinary Behavior* **16**, 53–64

Rooney NJ, Gaines SA and Bradshaw JWS (2007) Behavioural and glucocorticoid responses of dogs (*Canis familiaris*) to kennelling: investigating mitigation of stress by prior habituation. *Physiology and Behavior* **92**, 847–854

Scott JP and Fuller JL (1965) *Genetics and the Social Behavior of the Dog*. University of Chicago Press, Chicago

Stephen JM and Ledger RA (2006) A longitudinal evaluation of urinary cortisol in kennelled dogs, *Canis familiaris*. *Physiology and Behavior* **87**, 911–916

Tami G and Gallagher A (2009) Description of the behaviour of domestic dogs (*Canis familiaris*) by experienced and inexperienced people. *Applied Animal Behaviour Science* **120**, 159–169

Trevorrow N (2012) Kitten socialisation. *The Cat Summer 2012*, 46–48. http://www.cats.org.uk/uploads/documents/The_Cat_Mag_extracts/Kitten_socialisation.pdf

Van Kerkhove W (2004) A fresh look at the wolf-pack theory of companion-animal dog social behaviour. *Journal of Applied Animal Medical Science* **7**, 279–285

Zimen E (1975) Social dynamics of the wolf pack. In: *The Wild Canids: Their Systematics, Behavioral Ecology and Evolution*, ed. MW Fox, pp. 336–368. Van Nostrand Reinhold Co., New York

Useful websites

The Animal Behaviour and Training Council:
www.abtcouncil.org.uk

Association of Pet Behaviour Counsellors:
www.apbc.org.uk

Association for the Study of Animal Behaviour, CCAB Accreditation:
www.asab.org/ccab

Bristol Veterinary School, Clinical Animal Behavioural Group:
www.bristol.ac.uk/vetscience/services/behaviour-clinic/dogbehaviouralsigns/
interpretingbehaviour.html

Cats Protection, E-learning:
www.cats.org.uk/learn/e-learning-ufo-care

Cats Protection, Cat behaviour:
www.cats.org.uk/cat-care/cat-behaviour-hub

Cats Protection, How to introduce cats:
http://bit.ly/catstocats

Cats Protection, How to introduce cats to dogs:
http://bit.ly/catstodogs

Cats Protection, Information leaflets:
www.cats.org.uk/cat-care/care-leaflets

Dogs Trust:
www.dogstrust.org.uk

Dogs Trust, Dog School:
www.dogstrustdogschool.org.uk

International Cat Care:
www.icatcare.org

PDSA Animal Wellbeing (PAW) Report:
www.pdsa.org.uk/get-involved/our-campaigns/pdsa-animal-wellbeing-report

UK Government, Code of Practice for the Welfare of Cats:
www.gov.uk/government/publications/code-of-practice-for-the-welfare-of-cats

QRG 19.1: Current thinking on dog behaviour
by Carri Westgarth

Humans are descended not from chimpanzees, but from a common ancestor of both species. DNA evidence shows that, in a similar manner, dogs are descended not from modern-day wolves, but from a common ancestor (although both dogs and wolves evolved much more recently than humans and chimpanzees). Comparison of the domestic dog and the wolf is helpful in understanding dog behaviour, but it has also been used to erroneously assume that dogs should be trained in particular ways regarding status, leadership and dominance. This QRG describes the basic principles underlying modern scientific opinion concerning dog behaviour and training.

Factors affecting canine behaviour

Certain genetic factors mean that dogs, which are canids, will behave to some degree like other canid species. There are both species- and breed-specific effects to consider, but also individual differences. For example, no two Labrador Retrievers will behave in exactly the same way, although they may have a liking for carrying objects around in their mouths. One trait that appears to have a strong genetic component is aggression.

The other factor that greatly affects a dog's behaviour is learning.

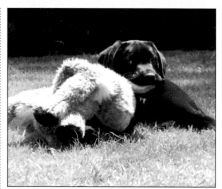

Labrador Retrievers may have a strong preference for holding things in their mouths, and this can be seen even early in life.

Although it is true that there are extra-sensitive periods for learning, such as the 'socialization period' in the first few weeks of life, learning continues throughout life. It is certainly possible to 'teach an old dog new tricks'.

Like wolves, dogs are behaviourally flexible and highly social animals. This means that they can adapt to living in many different environments, especially if they have experienced these during the first few weeks of life (see QRG 19.3). Dogs also have a need to be around others – be they dogs or humans – and use a variety of subtle methods of communication through body postures and facial signals. Unfortunately, people are not always good at noticing these subtle signals or reading them correctly.

History of the dominance theory

When modern-day wolves were first studied scientifically, it was easier to study unrelated wolves living together in captivity than small family groups living in the wild. As a result, more conflict and aggression was seen between individuals than occurs in free-living wolves. The idea that wolves compete with each other using aggression, with the highest-ranking wolf gaining priority access to resources, has now been superseded by the knowledge that a male and female pair naturally 'leads' the pack consisting of their offspring, rather like a family, and aggression is rarely seen. Unfortunately, the idea that to train a dog one needs to be 'dominant' over it, often using harsh methods to establish leadership, has permeated popular culture. Furthermore, scientific studies have shown that wolves and dogs are quite different in aspects of their behaviour.

To a behavioural scientist, 'dominance' is a term used to describe the outcome of repeated encounters between two individual animals. It is a term imposed by the observer to summarize the observed interactions between those individuals. It does not require that the animals have an awareness of this higher structure in order to decide how to behave next, although this is often assumed. ➡

QRG 19.1 *continued*

It certainly does not imply that they do things in order to strive for status as 'leader' or 'alpha'. Dominance therefore describes the product of interactions and not their cause.

However, in more everyday language, 'dominance' is often used in the sense of 'doing as told', and this is where the confusion in the use of the term may lie. Thus, a dog that tries to bite its owner may be regarded as being 'dominant' over the owner (as not many owners believe they have asked to be bitten). However, the root cause of any aggression is usually related to stress or fear. Likewise, when a dog does not 'do as it is told' this is usually because the dog either does not understand what is being asked of it or prefers to do something more rewarding.

The 'ladder of aggression'

Often, a dog is described as suddenly and unexpectedly becoming aggressive, but further investigation reveals that the signs were there but were not recognized. The more obvious behaviours associated with aggression, such as growling, snapping and biting, are preceded by more subtle signals that a dog is feeling stressed or under threat, which serve to try to appease the situation. The process of signals of stress/threat escalating to aggressive behaviour has been termed the 'ladder of aggression'.

These signals include licking the lips, yawning, lifting a paw, turning the head away, rolling over to expose the belly and walking away. Most dogs will try all of these behaviours before escalating to overt aggression (the exception being breeds that were bred to fight, which may not always show these signs as this would be a disadvantage). However, over time, dogs can learn that only growling, snapping and biting are successful in averting the threat, and may, therefore, escalate 'up the ladder' without displaying the intermediate behaviours.

Learning theory

If dog behaviour is not motivated by dominance, then what does motivate it? All animals, including humans, learn to respond to pleasant and unpleasant things in their

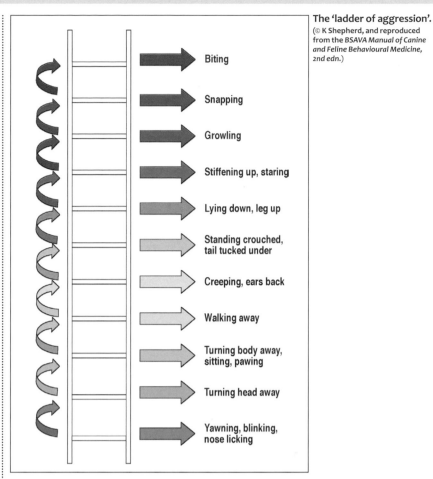

The 'ladder of aggression'.
(© K Shepherd, and reproduced from the BSAVA Manual of Canine and Feline Behavioural Medicine, 2nd edn.)

- Biting
- Snapping
- Growling
- Stiffening up, staring
- Lying down, leg up
- Standing crouched, tail tucked under
- Creeping, ears back
- Walking away
- Turning body away, sitting, pawing
- Turning head away
- Yawning, blinking, nose licking

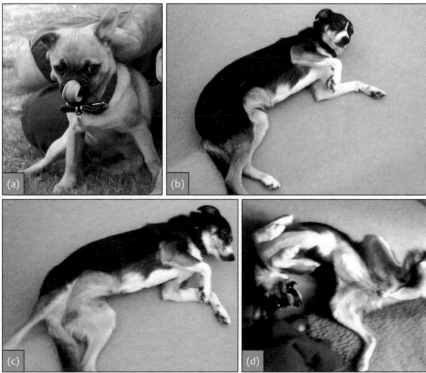

Some signs of stress/threat in the domestic dog. (a) Lip-licking/smacking is a sign of mild stress in a young dog interacting with a familiar, but not well known, person. The whites of the eyes can also be seen. (b) Rolling on the back to expose the chest as a sign of stress/appeasing signal in a Collie cross. Note also the flattened ear posture and raised front paw. (c) Extension of the signal to widen the back legs and expose the belly. Note also that the gaze is now averted away from the perceived threat. (d) The same dog in a relaxed rolling posture, used in a different context to instigate affection and play from the owner.
(b–d, © of Helen Taylor)

QRG 19.1 *continued*

environment. The concepts that have been developed to explain this are collectively termed 'learning theory'.

Classical conditioning

Classical conditioning is the term used to describe learning that involves simple associations. The classic example is that of 'Pavlov's dog', which learns to salivate when it hears a bell, because the sound of the bell always precedes the arrival of food.

Operant or instrumental conditioning

In contrast to classical conditioning, where an animal simply forms an association between two things in its mind, in operant (or instrumental) conditioning, the animal actually does something as part of the learning process.

Operant conditioning centres on the use of punishment, whereby unwanted behaviour subsequently decreases, and reinforcement (reward), whereby desired behaviour increases. Both punishment and reinforcement can be positive or negative. There is a misconception that these terms are used to describe training that is 'good' or 'bad'. In fact, 'positive' refers to something being **added** to the environment of the animal, whereas 'negative' describes the situation where something is **removed**.

For example:

- Positive reinforcement – something is added to make a behaviour increase, e.g. giving a treat every time a dog sits
- Negative reinforcement – something is taken away to make a behaviour increase, e.g. pressure from a collar and lead, head collar, harness or 'check' chain is removed every time the dog is walking on a loose leash
- Positive punishment – something is added to make a behaviour decrease, e.g. a spray from an anti-bark collar when the dog barks
- Negative punishment – something is taken away to make a behaviour decrease, e.g. withholding attention when a dog jumps up. A classic example of the use of

Parameter	Behaviour increases	Behaviour decreases
Something is added to the environment	Positive reinforcement	Positive punishment
Something is taken away from the environment	Negative reinforcement	Negative punishment

The four quadrants of operant conditioning.

negative punishment in humans is 'grounding' a teenager – i.e. taking away their freedom in order to decrease behaviours that are unwanted by their parents.

These four quadrants are used by all dog trainers to different degrees. Some trainers may claim to use only 'positive training', but this is a misunderstanding or simplification. A further complexity to consider is that in order to reinforce one behaviour, another corresponding (opposite) behaviour must be punished. For example, by rewarding a dog with a treat for sitting (positive reinforcement), the treat must be withheld when it is not sitting (negative punishment). To negatively reinforce a dog for not pulling on the lead, the dog must experience positive punishment when it is pulling.

Types of dog trainer

Different types of dog trainers are often portrayed as using rewards or 'positive' methods only *versus* using punishment. However, as outlined above, all trainers have to use more than one operant conditioning quadrant simultaneously.

The difference between trainers lies in two aspects:

- The degree of aversion that is deemed appropriate. For example, a head collar is generally deemed a less aversive or cruel way of training a dog than a check chain or pinch collar
- Which of the 'diagonals' in the operant conditioning model is the preferred approach to treating a behaviour problem?
  a. To positively punish unwanted behaviour and remove this punishment when the animal is behaving appropriately.
  b. To positively reinforce desired behaviour and ignore or interrupt and redirect unwanted behaviour.

Trainers also tend to subscribe to one or the other of the above theories relating to motivation for behaviour:

a. The dog is behaving due to dominance and being 'leader of the pack'
b. The dog is simply finding certain behaviours rewarding and avoiding unpleasant situations. Many problems are caused by the dog feeling fearful or anxious, even if over time the behaviour comes to look quite confident.

Although this is a simplified description, dog trainers tend to follow a strategy of either A or B when tackling behaviour problems. That is, 'Group A' trainers, who believe that dominance is the motivation of behaviour, tend to positively punish a dog's unwanted behaviour (e.g. using a rattle can, water spray, leash jerk or alpha roll (forcibly rolling the dog on to its back and restraining it in that position)); in contrast, 'Group B' trainers, who believe that learning theory explains behaviour, tend to apply a reward to a wanted behaviour instead (e.g. a food treat). This teaches the dog to perform a more acceptable behaviour, such as looking at the owner or sitting quietly, instead of barking and lunging at another dog.

To do this, a process called 'desensitization and counter-conditioning' is often used. Here, the dog is gradually desensitized to the presence of the fear-inducing stimulus at a distance, while being counter-conditioned to find the presence of that stimulus rewarding when it behaves in the desired manner. This has the effect of not only training the dog to do something different in that situation, but also changing the emotional state of the dog from negative to positive.

As noted above, there is controversy between groups of trainers and behaviourists over whether dogs are motivated by dominance or reward, and which types of methods should be used to train dogs. As a result, owners may receive conflicting advice from 'experts' and, thus, treat the dog inconsistently. Both types of trainers agree that this is a bad idea.

➡

QRG 19.1 *continued*

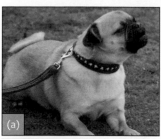

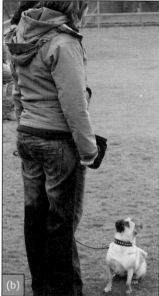

Tackling a problem behaviour of barking at other dogs during an agility training session by teaching the dog to quietly focus attention on the owner. (a) At first glance, the dog displaying the problem behaviour appears to be quite confident and excited. However, note the lowered body posture, backing away from the fearful stimuli and flattened ears. The problem worsens when the other dogs are running fast over the course, i.e. behaving in a more frightening manner; this provides further clues as to the cause of the problem barking being fear-based. (b) Training the dog to instead focus attention on the owner, and rewarding the calm behaviour (here, sitting is appropriate) with intermittent food treats. The dog is looking less fearful, sitting up with its ears pricked in anticipation. However, it is not as relaxed as ideal, as the left paw is slightly raised off the ground and one eye and the body are angled to quickly respond in the direction of the threat if required.

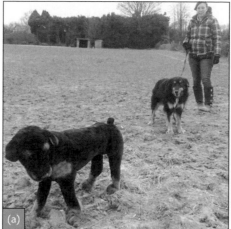

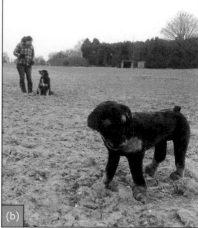

Demonstration of the desensitization and counter-conditioning process with a crossbreed dog. (a) The dog shows an anxious reaction even to a stuffed toy dog – note the tail under the body, back legs placed far back and ears back. (b) The stuffed dog (less frightening than a real moving dog) is used at a distance (less threatening than close up) to gently desensitize the dog to the presence of strange dogs. Note that the dog looks more relaxed, and is rewarded by the owner for focusing attention on her. Over time, the distance to the stuffed dog will be reduced, and real dogs will then be gradually introduced, again initially at a distance.
(© of Natalie Light)

Group B trainers believe that the methods used by Group A are dangerous because punishing a dog that is fearful causes escalation of aggression and because punishment is inherently cruel.

Group A trainers argue that Group B's methods are ineffective and their own training methods are, thus, justified, especially in cases of serious behaviour problems.

Both groups often see clients who have tried the other group's methods with their dogs and thought them to be ineffective or even to have made the problem worse.

Summary

There is controversy among dog trainers as to whether approaches should be based on the outdated theory of establishing dominance, or more modern theories of reward-based training to change unwanted behaviour into desired behaviour. The scientific evidence, organizations representing highly qualified behavioural counsellors and dog welfare charities all tend to support the latter approach.

References and further reading

Bradshaw J, Blackwell E and Casey R (2009) Dominance in domestic dogs—useful construct or bad habit? *Journal of Veterinary Behaviour: Clinical Applications and Research* **4**, 135–144

Bradshaw J (2012) *In Defence of Dogs*. Penguin Books, London

Donaldson J (1996) *The Culture Clash, 2nd edn*. James and Kenneth Publishers, Berkeley

Horowitz D and Mills D (2009) *BSAVA Manual of Canine and Feline Behavioural Medicine, 2nd edn*. BSAVA Publications, Gloucester

Pryor K (2002) *Don't Shoot the Dog! The New Art of Teaching and Training, 3rd edn*. Ringpress Books, Lydney

Useful websites

Welfare in Dog Training:
www.dogwelfarecampaign.org

QRG 19.2: Current thinking on cat behaviour

by Sarah Heath

Introduction

An understanding of feline communication and social systems is necessary to identify the emotional motivations involved in behaviours that result in cats being relinquished to shelters and which shelter staff report as being problematic. The emotional stability of cats is affected by genetics, early rearing and the limitations that the domestic environment places on normal feline behaviours. Ensuring that cats' environments meet their behavioural and environmental needs, and that humans have a better understanding of feline communication, are essential factors in improving the welfare of cats.

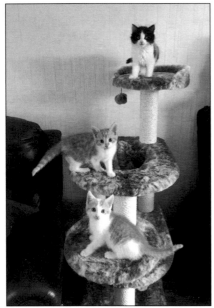

Three-dimensional space helps cats retain a sense of control, which is an important aspect of optimizing their emotional stability.

Principles of feline social behaviour

Cats are not an obligate social species, and much of their behaviour is the result of the fact that they are solitary survivors. They have a fundamental need to be in control, or to perceive that they are, and have very limited behaviours to facilitate cooperation with others. Avoidance is their preferred defence strategy in the face of stimuli that create a fear-anxiety emotional response, and they need to be able to evade or avoid sources of potential stress.

Social relationships do exist between cats and can be lasting in nature, but they are largely limited to relatives and, compared with those of socially obligate species, such as humans, they can be relatively fragile. Access to privacy and seclusion are considered to be positive features of the environment from a feline perspective.

Sociability

Research by Turner identified cats with differing levels of social interaction (Turner, 2013). Low-sociability cats tended to live on the periphery of social groupings, while those with a higher drive for social interaction would be found in the middle of the groupings. Mismatches between low-sociability cats and socially obligate humans, in terms of social interaction, can account for some of the misunderstanding between owners and their pets, and the misperceptions of those working with cats in a shelter or a veterinary context. When social contact does take place between cats it is characterized by low-intensity and high-frequency interactions, whereas human social interaction tends to be naturally high in intensity but low in frequency. Cats that initiate interactions will voluntarily spend more time in the company of people, and when they are given a sense of control within the interaction they are far more accepting of being handled. An understanding of this aspect of feline behaviour has resulted in the adoption of minimal handling techniques in both veterinary and shelter environments.

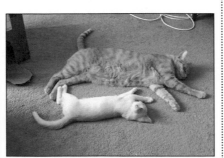

When social contact takes place between cats, it is characterized by low-intensity and high-frequency interactions.

Avoiding conflict

Since cats are not obligate social animals, they have a limited repertoire of appeasing behaviours. The consequence of this is that resolution of conflict is difficult for them. When cats are in a state of high emotional arousal, it takes considerable time for them to recover to a normal level of arousal. If avoidance of another cat (or a human) is not possible, and repulsion behaviours are shown, the resulting physical confrontation will often result in physical injuries to both cats – such as torn ears, puncture wounds or abscesses – or in significant injury to human handlers. It, therefore, makes sense for cats to avoid physical confrontation whenever possible and for humans to prioritize preventing confrontational interactions. Feline communication is designed to avoid unnecessary social encounters through body language and vocalization as well as indirect signals, such as urine marking. Ensuring that the environment enables cats to take avoiding action – for example, by providing places for them to hide – and to retain a sense of control is the most important factor in reducing the incidence of confrontational behaviours.

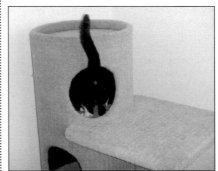

Cats need to have somewhere to hide to avoid conflict and other stressful situations.

Understanding feline social behaviour

Cats were once thought to be asocial and to come together only for breeding. Outside the breeding season, cats were considered to be solitary creatures. Groupings of cats were explained in terms of loose aggregations, 'like animals round a waterhole'. It is ➡

QRG 19.2 *continued*

now recognized that cats do display social behaviour and that their social groups are based on cooperation between related females. Social groups provide a communal den for kittens and allow for communal nursing and provisioning, as well as shared immunity (e.g. through shared maternally derived antibodies) and communal defence. In this type of social group, usually one adult tom breeds with the majority of queens in his territory, and other males are not well tolerated. Communication is vital in maintaining these social groupings, and affiliative behaviours, such as allorubbing and allogrooming, are of particular social significance. However, even when social relationships do exist in the feline world, they tend to be fragile and easily severed, due to the fact that survival is not a shared responsibility.

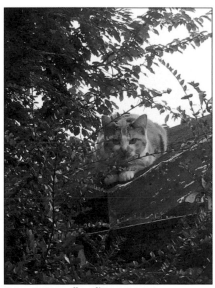

Cats are generally solitary creatures.

Keep it in the family

The most compatible combinations of cats are those that share genetic material, and taking on littermate siblings is considered to give the best chance of establishing a socially harmonious feline household. Forcing unrelated individuals to live in close proximity and to share essential resources can lead to chronic high levels of negative emotional arousal. The physiological effects of this will have physical consequences, and health conditions, such as feline idiopathic cystitis and infectious diseases, are commonly associated

with situations where cats are living in socially stressful environments. Relinquishment of cats to shelters is often related to unacceptable behaviours associated with social stress (e.g. urine spraying, destructive scratching as a form of marking), and if rehoming is to be successful, it is essential that adequate attention is paid to the social behaviour of cats and the potential for issues of social incompatibility in the new home.

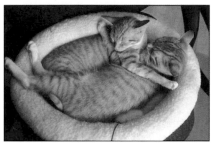

Social relationships between cats do exist, but they are largely limited to relatives.

Resource distribution

Maximizing feline harmony is not related just to the numbers of cats living in a household but also to the distribution of resources within the environment. Cats have a requirement for free and immediate access to resources at all times, and they do not possess the behavioural mechanisms for polite turn-taking. Restricted access to resources (e.g. food, water, litter trays, places to rest or hide) can result in frustration, and the presence of incompatible cats in the vicinity of life-sustaining resources can lead to activation of the fear-anxiety emotional system.

Feline feeding behaviour

Hunting and feeding are solitary activities within a feline context, and when it comes to the ultimate survival test – the acquisition of nutrition – the cat is on its own. Every aspect of the cat is designed for efficient hunting behaviour. The sensory system is tuned to receive olfactory, auditory and visual cues, and feline anatomy is perfectly suited to the hunting, capturing and dispatching of prey. Eating together is challenging for all cats, and in an ideal situation each cat would eat alone. If cats are housed in incompatible groupings, the offering of food in a communal area is very stressful and can result in both behavioural and physical consequences, including a predisposition to obesity.

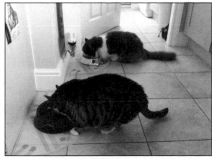

Cats are solitary feeders, and eating should occur when they are in a relaxed emotional state. Being fed together with other cats is challenging. The body posture and ear positions seen here indicate negative emotional arousal in both cats.

Activity and energy balance

In additional to the emotional effects on weight management, it is important to remember that cats will naturally spend 6–8 hours a day hunting. They carry out in the region of 100–150 hunting attacks per day but are successful in only about 10% of these. Their hunting forays involve many short bursts of energy expenditure and are fuelled by small but frequent meals throughout the day. The low success rate in hunting results in cats being very persistent in their behaviour and being undeterred by failure to succeed on the first attempt. When cats are fed from a bowl with easily digestible diets, the amount of energy expenditure to achieve adequate nutrition can be dramatically reduced. Therefore, using feeding systems that mimic natural predatory behaviour, such as puzzle feeders, can help to increase energy consumption, as well as improve mental stimulation and activate the positive emotional system of desire-seeking.

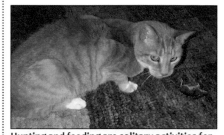

Hunting and feeding are solitary activities for cats.

Misdirected predatory behaviour

The motivation to hunt and the sensation of hunger are separately controlled, and,

QRG 19.2 *continued*

therefore, even a very well fed cat will still have the desire to hunt. When the desire-seeking emotional system is triggered, cats will respond with characteristic predatory behaviour, and if the opportunity to hunt real prey is denied, other targets will be used, such as moving ankles and hands of a human caregiver. This instinct must, therefore, be catered for through appropriate food-delivery systems and opportunities for play.

Environmental needs

As a result of the natural social behaviour of cats, there are some fundamental needs that the environment should fulfil. These are described in detail in the *AAFP and ISFM Feline Environmental Needs Guidelines* (Ellis *et al.*, 2013) and consist of the following five 'pillars':

- Provide a safe place
- Provide multiple and separate environmental resources: food, water, toileting areas, scratching areas, play areas, and resting or sleeping areas
- Provide opportunity for play and predatory behaviour
- Provide positive, consistent and predictable human–cat social interaction
- Provide an environment that respects the importance of the cat's sense of smell.

Summary

Understanding feline communication and the social behaviour that drives it can be hugely beneficial when interacting with cats in a shelter environment. Cats are social creatures, but their social behaviour differs greatly from that of people and dogs. They have a fundamental need to feel in control, and naturally live in small groups of related individuals, avoiding contact with other cats. It is,

therefore, understandable that cats can find it stressful to live in in proximity to unrelated cats. In addition, their social behaviour is based on low-intensity contact, and well intentioned human handling can be perceived as being restrictive and threatening. By paying attention to natural feline behaviours and modifying the environment accordingly, shelter workers can offer ethological solutions and manage feline shelter environments in a way that effectively minimizes the negative emotional impact on the resident cats.

References and further reading

Bradshaw JWS, Casey RA and Brown SL (2012) *The Behaviour of the Domestic Cat, 2nd edn*. CABI, Wallingford

Ellis SLH, Rodan I, Carney HC *et al.* (2013) ISFM and AAFP Feline Environmental Needs Guidelines. *Journal of Feline Medicine and Surgery* **15**, 219–230

Rodan I and Heath SE (eds) (2016) *Feline Behavioral Health and Welfare*. Elsevier, St Louis

Turner DC (2013) *The Domestic Cat: The Biology Of Its Behaviour, 3rd edn*. Cambridge University Press

QRG 19.3: Socialization of puppies

by Helen Zulch and Steve Goward

Evidence shows that a dog's early experiences may correlate with behaviour in later life. It is, therefore, important that those involved in raising puppies understand how to structure the environment and interactions that puppies experience to maximize the chance that their adult behaviour will be appropriate to the home in which they find themselves and promote their long-term welfare.

Although the focus of much puppy education is on socialization and habituation, dogs lose their homes, or even their lives, for behaviours that are related to emotions other than fear – for example, over-exuberance or lack of frustration tolerance. New owners frequently expect puppies to behave in a calm, controlled manner, but may have little knowledge of how to achieve this. For this reason, all interactions with puppies in a shelter should aim to foster behaviours that are appropriate to living in a family home. This should assist in reducing conflict with the eventual owners, which in turn minimizes the risk of

behaviour problems developing and maximizes the puppy's welfare.

This guide will describe a general approach to raising puppies, but it is important to remember that every puppy is an individual. There is evidence that a good predictor of longer-term behaviour is behaviour measured at the first exposure to a novel situation or stimulus, so shelter staff working with puppies should note individuals' reactions and tailor training and intervention programmes to account for them.

Teaching puppies what they need to learn

For most puppies, everyday life is a stream of new stimuli and experiences that they need to learn to cope with. In addition, there will be times in every dog's life when it experiences something unpleasant. Below are some suggestions for helping puppies to develop coping skills and resilience in a variety of common situations.

At all times when exposing puppies to new objects or social interactions, it is important to bear in mind two things:

- Watch the puppy's body language. If it appears anxious, 'back off' and take things more slowly. Never force or lure a puppy into a situation that worries it; instead, structure the situation differently to promote a positive association. This will mean that the puppy is less likely to escalate to aggressive responses (see QRG 19.1) when it is uncomfortable. Puppies vary in their responses to the types of situations described below; any puppies that become worried easily must be recognized, so that the pace and intensity of their exposure to stimuli can be managed very carefully to allow them to cope
- If the puppy becomes over-excited, encourage calm, considered interactions.

QRG 19.3 *continued*

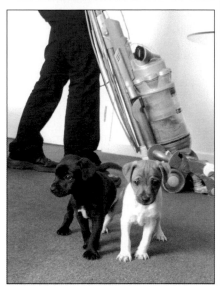

These puppies are not looking comfortable – note their tense posture, bodyweight distributed backwards and their tense and focused facial expressions. It is important to notice these signs and make sure that puppies are allowed to become comfortable in the environment in their own time (do not force them closer to objects) or, alternatively, to alter their environment in a way that helps them feel relaxed and able to explore.

Establishing the habit of calm interactions will reduce the risk of conflict with other dogs and people as the puppy grows up.

Environmental stimuli

- Before whelping, it is important to consider the dam's environment and to settle her into the whelping area and new routines before she gives birth.
- From the time the puppies are born (or before, if the dam also needs to become habituated), place a range of safe items in the whelping box, and change them every few days. Examples include:
  - Different textures on the floor – carpet tiles, different types of fabric, plastic shower mats, plastic garden mesh
  - Items that the puppies can interact with – cardboard boxes and tubes, plastic containers, soft toys, metal bowls, rubber or plastic food-dispensing toys or chew toys. Some of these items can be dangled into the whelping box from above
  - Different odours – different tit-bits of food for the dam.

- When the puppies are walking, introduce them to items that they can safely crawl over or through, such as plastic piping or crates (if these are slippery, glue carpeting on to them to provide safe footing).
- Play CDs of household and environmental sounds (a range of these CDs are available for habituating dogs) to the puppies intermittently, at low volumes to begin with. If the dam is fearful of noises, only play the CD at times when she is away from the puppies, but ensure that the puppies are feeling secure and relaxed at these times. Never pair the playing of the CD with any experience that distresses the puppies. Alternatively, create different noises in the environment for the puppies to hear – e.g. switching on a vacuum cleaner at a distance or tapping metal cutlery on a saucepan lid.
- Habituate the puppies to being alone by encouraging the dam to leave them for short periods – as short as a few seconds to begin with. Never force the dam to leave, but encourage her away using something she really likes, such as treats or a game.
- Once the puppies are a little older, introduce them to moving objects such as brooms and vacuum cleaners. This should only be carried out in an area with sufficient space for the puppies to move away if they choose. Ensure that the puppies are provided with other items (such as tasty chew treats) to minimize the risk of them chasing and grabbing the moving object. Attempts to chase and grab should be managed in a calm, neutral manner, by stopping

the object moving and distracting the puppies' attention to something more interesting.
- From around 5 weeks of age habituate puppies to wearing a collar or harness and lead. Initially, place a flat collar or harness on the puppies for short periods a few days before attaching the lead. The first lead should be light and should simply trail behind the puppy (be careful to ensure that it does not catch on anything in the environment). Puppies must not be dragged on the lead and should be gently distracted from grabbing or chewing it. Once habituated to the lead, the puppies can be lured with a food treat to follow the person holding the lead. Do not leave collars or harnesses on puppies when they are unattended.
- Once the puppies can be taken out of their kennel, ensure that when they are in new environments a safe hiding place is always available, equipped with blankets from the home kennel to give odour security. Never force puppies to leave this place of safety, but encourage them to join the other puppies, by using toys or games to show how much fun is available in the environment.
- If at all possible, take puppies for a ride in a vehicle in groups of about three, before a feeding time and with some of their familiar bedding in the travel crate. Journeys should initially be very short – less than 100 m to begin with – and gradually lengthened.
- If possible and appropriate, allow puppies to observe other species calmly from a distance, e.g. livestock and horses.

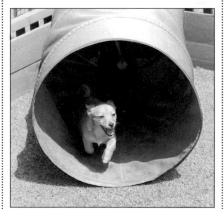

Providing puppies with objects to climb into, on to and through is important to help them develop confidence in their environment and with novelty.

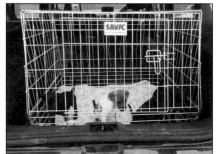

Taking puppies for short rides in a car is helpful in acclimatizing them.

QRG 19.3 *continued*

Social stimuli

- Immediately after birth, if the dam will allow it, puppies should be gently handled a few times a week (daily if possible). If the dam is protective, then this can be achieved while she is out on a walk, to avoid confrontation and prevent the puppies witnessing her reaction.
- Puppies should be gently lifted from their littermates and dam, cradled in a hand and gently stroked. If possible, puppies should be handled by a range of people rather than a single handler.
- After 3 weeks of age, having different people visit the puppies is advisable so that they get used to a range of people beyond their handler(s). If possible, include people wearing spectacles, men with beards, people wearing hats or high-visibility jackets, etc., and also children.
- All interactions should be on the puppies' terms. Ensure that the space is large enough for them to approach or retreat at will and do not force them to interact, but encourage them by providing toys and food treats.
- This socialization time is an excellent opportunity for the puppies to begin learning good manners. Everyone who interacts with them should apply the same set of 'rules'; for example:
  - Puppies should be encouraged to sit for attention (using a food lure held over their heads)
  - If a puppy grabs the person's hands, feet or clothing, the person must become totally still until the puppy stops and then substitute an appropriate toy. If the puppy shows no sign of stopping, its attention should be calmly redirected to something else.
- All people interacting with the puppies at any time can encourage them to sit for things that they want. This does not need to be on a verbal cue; puppies can simply learn the action of sitting as a default behaviour for getting what they want. Set the puppies up for success by giving rewards for desired behaviour; do not wait for a puppy to do something 'wrong' and then punish it.

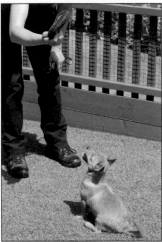

It is easy to teach puppies to sit for things that they want – in this case a toy – as long as everyone who interacts with them consistently expects this behaviour.

- Socialization with other dogs is also important. After 5 weeks of age, older, fully vaccinated and healthy dogs that are known to be calm, gentle and friendly towards puppies can be introduced to the puppies, if such dogs are available and the shelter's biosecurity protocols allow. The dam can be present or absent depending on her response to other dogs in this situation. No puppy should be forced to interact with a new dog, and there needs to be adequate space for the puppies to retreat and approach at will. Keep interactions short to begin with.
- To avoid puppies expecting to be able to interact with every other dog they meet – and, therefore, risk frustration problems developing later in life – it is valuable to put them in situations where they can see another dog but not reach it. Reward calm watching of another dog from behind a barrier such as a fence or, once the puppies tolerate a harness and lead, when restrained by a lead.

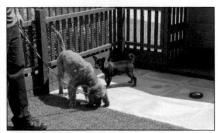

This puppy is being allowed to choose to interact with a relaxed adult dog. Note the space in which the interaction is taking place; the puppy can choose its proximity to the adult dog and can move away any time it wishes to.

Handling

Tolerance of handling will be introduced through the early interactions with people described above. This then needs to be built upon.

- Ideally, all puppies should be handled several times a week. Start at a time of the day when the puppies are likely to be calm and gently stroke them all over. Over time, stroking can evolve into gently lifting the pinnae, putting gentle pressure on the feet to splay the toes, lifting their tails, slipping fingers into their mouths, etc.

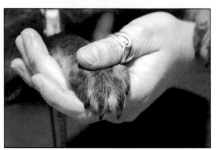

Ensuring that puppies are comfortable with having all parts of their body handled is very important. Feet, ears, mouths and tails are frequently more sensitive areas for puppies, so pay particular attention to ensuring they will accept handling of these areas in a relaxed manner.

- Keep all movements slow and calm to encourage reciprocal behaviour in the puppy. If the puppy tries to avoid being handled, note this and implement a programme of counter-conditioning in which touch is followed by a tiny tasty food treat. First, start with parts of the body that the puppy tolerates being touched (to establish the idea in the puppy's mind) and then move to the areas the puppy dislikes being touched. Give food rewards immediately after the interaction, not during it, so that the food serves as a learning tool rather than simply a distraction.
- If the puppy wriggles because it considers the interaction playful, first encourage calm behaviour by using food treats to encourage it to lie calmly on or next to the handler. Once the puppy learns that the only way to get the treat is to lie still, handling can be added to the situation – the puppy lies still, the handler touches the puppy, the puppy gets a treat.

→

QRG 19.3 continued

- Once the puppies are showing positive responses to being handled all over their bodies, additional actions can be added – a small piece of dry food or a treat can be popped into the mouth to simulate giving a pill; puppies can be groomed; puppies can be handled on a stable, secure raised surface and gently restrained to mimic a veterinary examination.
- It is ideal for the puppies to learn to accept handling from a range of different people.

Toilet training

Soiling in the house is usually expected of new puppies; however, the way new owners deal with soiling varies and often involves punishment. Encouraging puppies in the shelter to eliminate in appropriate areas can help them to develop habits that will be easier for the new owners to cope with.

Conclusion

These principles of encouraging and rewarding desired behaviours, while giving puppies the time to develop at their own rate will ensure that each puppy has the best possible chance to live successfully with its new owners in the community.

References and further reading

Appleby DL, Bradshaw JW and Casey RA (2002) Relationship between aggressive and avoidance behaviour by dogs and their experience in the first six months of life. *Veterinary Record* **150**, 434–438

Bailey G (2008) *The Perfect Puppy, revised edn.* Hamlyn, London

Seksel K, Mazurski EJ and Taylor A (1999) Puppy socialisation programs: short and long term behavioural effects. *Applied Animal Behaviour Science* **62**, 335–349

Serpell J and Jagoe JA (1995) Early experience and the development of behaviour. In: *The Domestic Dog: Its Evolution, Behaviour and Interactions with People*, ed. J Serpell, pp. 79–102. Cambridge University Press, Cambridge

Zulch H and Mills D (2012) *Life Skills for Puppies: Laying the Foundation for a Loving, Lasting Relationship*. Hubble and Hattie, Dorchester

Useful websites

The Puppy Socialisation Plan: www.thepuppyplan.com

QRG 19.4: Socialization of kittens
by Nicky Trevorrow

Preparing kittens to cope with the challenges they will face in their new home is one of the most important areas of cat welfare in the shelter environment. The responsibility for giving such kittens every chance of being lifelong happy and healthy cats lies predominantly with shelters. Shelters are frequently presented with pregnant queens, which are both experiencing stress and due to give birth, or with young kittens that require socialization. As the shelter environment is often so markedly different from a home, special attention needs to be given to successfully rear well adjusted kittens. Although the term 'socialization' may sometimes be used by shelter workers to refer to any interaction with kittens and adult cats, the process of 'kitten socialization' as discussed in this guide refers only to kittens during the socialization period. This distinction is important in order to appreciate the different forms of learning that occur in cats and apply appropriate behavioural techniques accordingly.

The kitten socialization period

The kitten socialization period refers to the important window of time when kittens are most receptive to learning appropriate social responses towards conspecifics and other species they may come into contact with. Studies have shown that this sensitive period, previously referred to as the 'critical period', is most significant during the ages of 2–7 weeks (Karsh and Turner, 1998). During this period, a kitten's brain undertakes huge growth as it develops new nerve pathways. During this time, it is vital that positive experiences are regularly repeated so that activated synapses are retained (Greenough *et al.*, 1999). Negative experiences, or lack of exposure to stimuli they will be exposed to later in life, can have a long-term impact on a cat's welfare. The overall result is that kitten socialization has a huge influence on behaviour into adulthood.

Getting used to people

Sociability towards humans is not an innate behaviour in cats and needs to be learned. Getting kittens used to a variety of social interactions with people can help them adapt to life as a domestic pet. Introducing gentle handling practices that involve touching the body in a way similar to a health check in veterinary practice is a great way of getting kittens used to being examined and having vulnerable areas, such as the feet, handled. Studies have shown that the sociability of kittens towards humans is influenced by the number of different people they meet, as well as by genetic factors (see below), personality and previous experience. The biggest impact can be achieved by introducing kittens to a variety of people, including, for example, men, women, children, older people and veterinary surgeons (veterinarians). This may present a challenge if rescue workers are predominantly female – an adverse reaction towards men may inadvertently reinforce the misconception by cat owners that their rescue cat 'may have been abused by men in the past', when in fact this reaction may simply be due to the cat not having been adequately acclimatized to men during the socialization period.

Habituation to the environment

The process whereby kittens learn to filter out non-harmful stimuli in their environment is known as habituation or 'social referencing'. As well as introducing the kittens to different social situations, it is crucial to expose them to a variety of →

QRG 19.4 *continued*

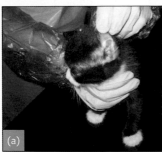

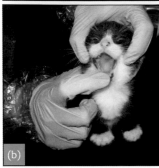

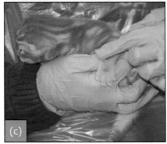

Get kittens used to health checks and having vulnerable areas such as their (a) ears, (b) mouths and (c) feet touched.
(© Cats Protection)

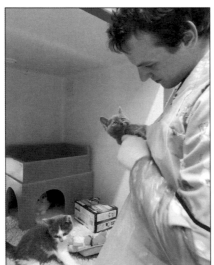

Regular, positive social interaction can improve the sociability of kittens towards men.
(© Cats Protection)

normal domestic sensory information. In the shelter setting, some of the domestic household sounds can be replaced by using a socialization CD (see Useful resources for more

information). These CDs feature a variety of noises, including a vacuum cleaner, fireworks, a baby crying and even gunshot sounds; while the latter may seem confusing, the idea is that kittens may learn to generalize sounds, so that if a dropped pan makes a loud clang on the floor, the kitten will still show a startle response but will recover more quickly, rather than hiding for lengthy periods.

Why is kitten socialization important?

The overarching reason for socializing kittens is to improve their welfare so that they can cope with novelty and the challenges of living in a household. These include any social or inanimate stimuli that kittens encounter after the socialization period, which may be approached more hesitantly as the onset of hazard avoidance or a fear response develops. This is often by 6 weeks of age, although some kittens appear to show a fear response even younger. It is worth noting that while socialization is important, other factors affect a cat's sociability. Genetics plays an important role. McCune (1995) found that kittens fathered by bold or friendly cats were themselves more likely to be friendly towards people. Conversely, fearful tom cats were more likely to sire fearful kittens.

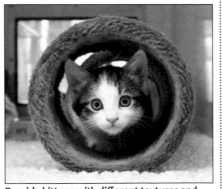

Provide kittens with different textures and tunnels to explore.
(© Cats Protection)

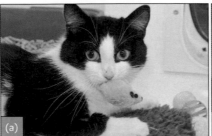

Give kittens different kinds of toys for self-directed play, such as (a) toy mice and (b) balls – these ones contain a bell to add interest.
(© Cats Protection)

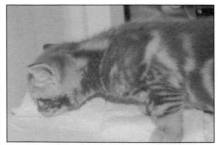

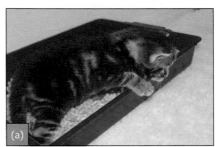

Providing kittens with the scent of a healthy, friendly, vaccinated dog can help get them used to dogs even if they have never met one.
(© Cats Protection)

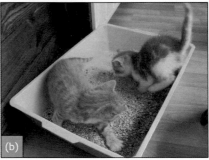

(a–b) Give kittens different types of litter to help them be more adaptable later in life.
(© Cats Protection)

Feral kittens

Different organizations may have different policies and approaches to dealing with feral kittens. The most important consideration is that of the animal's welfare and acting accordingly in its best interests. Some organizations may choose to socialize feral kittens found during the socialization period if sufficient resources and facilities are available.

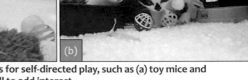

QRG 19.4 continued

This may vary on a case-by-case basis depending on the circumstances, such as whether a queen is present or not, the presence of other nursing queens in a colony, health and temperament of the kittens, availability of local veterinary surgeons practising kitten neutering (see Chapter 6 for information regarding early neutering), and whether the kittens can be returned to their natural environment. Generally, socializing feral kittens is more resource-intensive than socializing pet kittens. In addition, genetic effects from the feral fathers, which could produce more fearful kittens, mean that despite socialization efforts, the kittens could remain fearful towards people. It could be argued that where kitten neutering is available, it would be best to trap, neuter and return feral kittens to the site of capture. The Cats Protection Kitten Neutering Database lists local veterinary surgeons practising kitten neutering.

Infectious disease control considerations

Kittens are especially vulnerable to infectious diseases, and so special considerations are needed to reduce the risk. It is important for shelter staff and volunteers to understand the basics of disease transmission and accidentally acting as a fomite (see Chapter 9 for more detail). Wearing disposable personal protective equipment, such as plastic aprons, shoe covers and gloves, as well as consistently using an antibacterial skin disinfectant before and after socialization sessions, are vital to reduce disease transmission. Staff and volunteers should work with only one litter during a socialization session to reduce the risk of spreading disease between litters.

The shelter design and flow can also impact greatly on the health of the kittens. Having a separate maternity/nursery section away from high-risk areas, such as isolation or admission facilities in a shelter, as well as not mixing litters from different sources, can make a huge

difference. Where facilities allow, it may be beneficial to have individual litters fostered out to dedicated queen and kitten fosterers to prevent a large number of kittens from different sources with unknown disease risk and carrier status being kept in close proximity.

Kitten socialization can in itself be an important measure in reducing the risk of disease by reducing the kitten's stress levels. Stress impacts negatively on the immune system, so socialization may help them, from a disease reduction perspective, in the longer term.

Kitten socialization chart

Cats Protection has a structured kitten socialization programme developed by Dr Rachel Casey to address these challenges and prepare kittens with a variety of experiences that they may encounter later in life. The programme was originally part of a study, which suggested that kittens that had received additional structured handling and other positive experiences were less fearful, and their owners felt more emotional

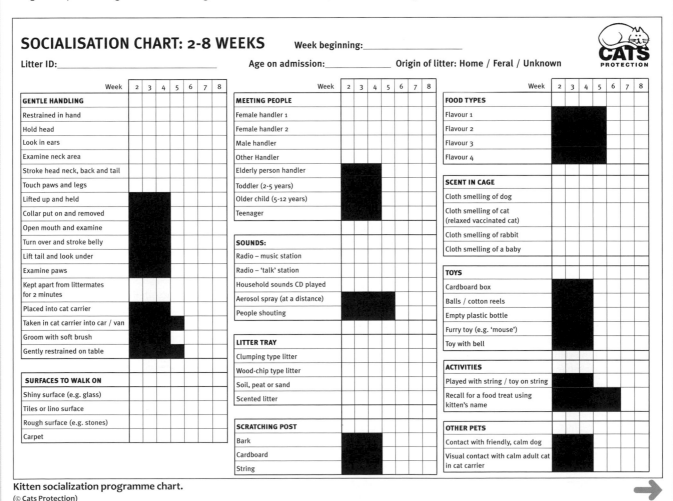

Kitten socialization programme chart.
(© Cats Protection)

QRG 19.4 *continued*

support from them, compared with kittens that received only ad hoc handling during cleaning (Casey and Bradshaw, 2008). Socialization is therefore likely to be an important factor in the retention of cats within homes.

References and further reading

Casey R and Bradshaw JWS (2008) The effects of additional socialisation for kittens in a rescue centre on their behaviour and suitability as a pet. *Applied Animal Behaviour Science* **114**, 196–205

Greenough W, Cohen N and Jaraska J (1999) New neurons in old brains: learning to survive? *Nature Neuroscience* **2**, 203–205

Karsh EB and Turner DC (1988) The human-cat relationship. In: *The Domestic Cat: The Biology of its Behaviour*, ed. DC Turner and P Bateson, pp. 159–177. Cambridge University Press, Cambridge

McCune S (1995) The impact of paternity and early socialisation on the development of cats' behaviour to people and novel objects. *Applied Animal Behaviour Science* **45**, 109–124

Useful resources

'Sounds Sociable' socialization CD: www.dogstrust.org.uk/help-advice/dog-behaviour-health/sound-therapy-for-pets

Cats Protection Kitten Neutering Database: www.cats.org.uk/what-we-do/neutering/enr/menu-early-neutering

QRG 19.5: Dealing with the aggressive dog
by Sarah Heath

Aggressive canine behaviour can be a serious concern in the shelter context, in terms of both the immediate safety of staff and the potential for rehoming the individual dogs concerned. If the dogs are to be handled safely and the staff are to implement suitable techniques to modify these behaviours, with a view to finding the dogs potential new homes, it is important to understand the underlying motivations for the behaviours being displayed. Inaccurate assessment of motivation can lead to miscommunication and avoidable escalation of aggressive behavioural responses.

- **Positive/negative emotional motivation:** the emotional systems that influence the willingness of the animal to put effort into achieving certain goals (motivation). Positive motivations are associated with achieving beneficial goals by gaining access to desired outcomes, such as the ability to reproduce (lust), the ability to care for others (care), the ability to gain access to vital survival resources (desire-seeking) and the ability to learn through play with other members of the species (social play). Negative motivations are associated with achieving beneficial goals by avoiding potentially undesirable outcomes, such as the ability to protect yourself and your resources from potential threat (fear-anxiety), the ability to protect yourself/recover from physical harm (pain), the

ability to achieve a presently unachievable outcome (frustration) and the ability to reconnect with sources of nurturing (panic-grief).

- **Behavioural responses to negative emotion**
  - Repulsion: a behavioural response which is designed to increase space and decrease contact between the individual and a perceived threat by using behaviours which lead the potential threat to effect that change, for example the threat stops interacting or moves away.
  - Avoidance: a behavioural response which is designed to increase space and decrease contact between the individual and a perceived threat by using behaviours which enable the individual to effect that change, for example the individual stops interacting or moves away.
  - Inhibition: a behavioural response which is designed to increase the availability of information about a perceived threat or situation of uncertainty by using behaviours which enable the individual to gather information about the threat or situation without engaging with it.
  - Appeasement: a behavioural response which is designed to increase the availability of information about a perceived threat or situation of uncertainty by using behaviours which enable the

individual to gather information about the threat or situation through engaging with it and offering information in return.

- **Passive interaction:** social interaction that is low in intensity, in terms of verbal and physical contact, in order to reduce the rate of emotional inflow that is generated by it.
- **Aggression:** overt, often harmful, social interaction with the aim of increasing space and decreasing contact between the individuals and with the potential of inflicting physical and emotional damage to one another.

Identification of motivation

Emotional motivation is most accurately determined by interpreting the dog's body language and vocalization. Education of shelter staff about this is essential. The majority of aggressive responses displayed by dogs in the shelter environment are defensive in nature and are designed to protect the individual dog from a perceived danger or threat. An understanding of the dog's perception is therefore essential to put the aggressive response into context and to formulate an appropriate human response. The aim is to prevent miscommunication, which can unintentionally escalate the perception of threat as it will serve only to intensify defensive motivation and lead to increasingly aggressive behavioural responses.

→

QRG 19.5 *continued*

Underlying emotions

The most common emotional motivations for defensively motivated aggressive behaviours in dogs are:

- Anxiety – the anticipation of a negative outcome
- Fear – a negative emotional response to a specific stimulus (e.g. a person or another dog)
- Frustration – the inability to achieve an expected or desired outcome.

Taking a thorough dog's history can help to identify potential triggers for negative emotional states. However, in the shelter environment information about the genetics of the individual dog, its physical and social environment when it was less than 8 weeks of age and its subsequent experiences before entering the shelter are likely to be unavailable. Observing the body language of the dog, combined with collecting information about the situation(s) in which aggressive responses are triggered, is necessary to accurately identify the emotional motivations involved (much of the information in the flow diagram in QRG 19.6 is also applicable to the so-called aggressive dog).

Body language signals

A combination of lowered body posture, tucked tail and retracted ears will alert the majority of shelter staff to extremes of negative emotional state in a dog. However, body language is dynamic and alterations are often both transient and subtle. The most accurate assessments will therefore be made over a number of observations, and will combine information about the dog's eyes, ears, tail and overall body posture. When the dog is giving aggressive or repulsion responses, it is not uncommon for offensive motivations to be attributed and the defensive nature of the behaviour to be less readily apparent. The result is that shelter staff often attribute more importance to repulsion responses. However, understanding that dogs can have a variety of alternative behavioural responses to negative emotions is equally important, both from a welfare perspective and from the point of view of risk assessment.

Looking at the individual features rather than the overall impression, can help to identify the more subtle signs of defensive motivation. When negative emotions result in behavioural responses of active avoidance it can be much easier to identify the fact that the dog is apprehensive or fearful. Passive avoidance and the behavioural response of inhibition are frequently overlooked but when these responses are seen in the shelter environment, it is important to remember that a change of context to a domestic home can trigger a change in behavioural response. If that change involves selection of repulsion, an animal that was considered to be 'fine' in the shelter may be dangerous in the new home. This highlights the need to be vigilant and to notice and act on signs of inhibition and avoidance with the same priority as signs of repulsion. Appeasement behaviours, through which the dog is offering and collecting information, are commonly misinterpreted as

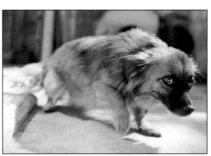

Lowered body posture, retracted ears and fixed staring 'whale' eyes are indicative of an extreme negative emotional state. The raised front paw is an additional sign of uncertainty.

friendly or submissive gesturing. Rolling onto the back is a common method of dissipating scent information but other appeasement behaviours, such as dribbling urine to release scent signals or licking faces to gather scent information, are also misinterpreted as signs of excitement.

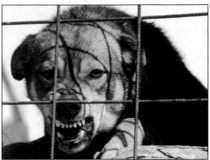

When negative emotions lead to aggressive behavioural responses it can be common for an offensive motivation to be attributed to the behaviour.

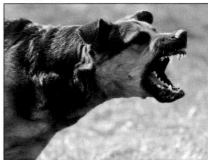

An overt display of teeth can lead to such concentration on watching the dog's mouth that people overlook other body language signalling and information from the body posture and tail position may be missed altogether. It is very important to observe the whole animal in order to determine the emotional motivation for the behaviour.

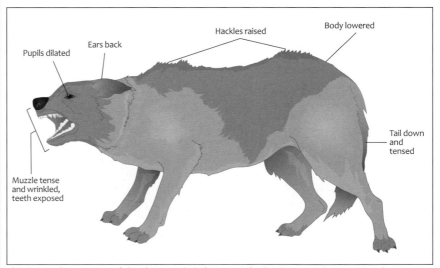

Pupils dilated · Ears back · Hackles raised · Body lowered · Muzzle tense and wrinkled, teeth exposed · Tail down and tensed

This image shows some of the characteristic features of a dog in a negative emotional state leading to defensive behaviour or repulsion. Note the lowered body posture with front end slightly lowered compared to the rear end leading to a perception of increased size. Also note the tucked tail, raised hackles, ears drawn back on the head, tense muzzle, corners of mouth drawn back and teeth exposed.

QRG 19.5 *continued*

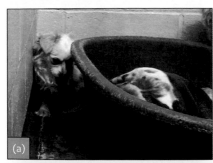

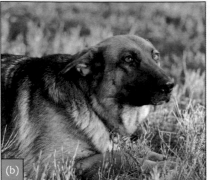

(a) When a dog is physically moving away at speed or simply retreating, it is often easier for people to identify the fact that the animal is in a negative emotional state. Active responses are often more obvious to people and they are more likely to consider that the dog needs help. (b) This dog is visually focused and is showing body language consistent with negative emotion. There is no attempt to approach the person and the dog is showing a combination of avoidance (keeping distance from the person) and inhibition (passively gathering information about the person) at this stage. The responses are very passive in nature and illustrate the fact that avoidance does not necessarily involve physical movement. This illustrates the need to be aware of subtle signals of negative emotion.

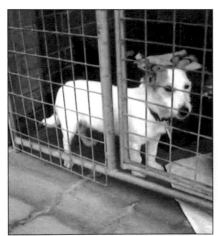

When dogs select inhibition as a behavioural response to negative emotion they may be overlooked in the shelter environment and assumed to be coping well.

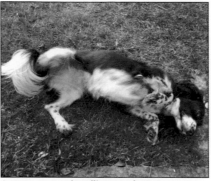

Appeasement signalling may be misinterpreted as friendly behaviour and the way in which people respond to these behaviours can unintentionally lead to an increase in anxiety. Misinterpretation of appeasement as submission can lead to perpetuation of the outdated theory of dominance and result in misguided justification of inappropriate training and handling methods.

Role of frustration

When aggressive behavioural responses are motivated by fear and anxiety and are related to a perception of threat, the behaviour can be further complicated by the effects of frustration. In a shelter environment, such factors can exacerbate frustration leading to intensification and acceleration of the aggressive response. Examples include restraining individual dogs on leads or housing them in accommodation with direct visual access to potential threats, such as when other dogs are walked past the front of the kennels.

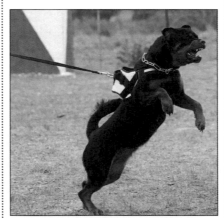

When a dog is thwarted from dealing with a perceived threat, for example due to being restrained on a lead, frustration can lead to acceleration and intensification of the response.

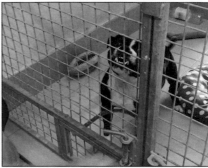

Confinement in accommodation, which allows direct visual access to potential threat, can lead to frustration.

Risk assessment

Although the emotional motivation for the majority of aggressive signalling in the shelter context is negative and the behaviour is defensive in nature, these dogs can still pose a safety risk both to humans and other dogs. Safety must always be a priority, and appropriate management of 'aggressive' dogs in a shelter environment is paramount. If the ultimate goal of the shelter is the rehoming of dogs in their care, then accurate assessment, observation and record keeping of aggressive behavioural responses are essential. Risk assessments should be carried out not only for the immediate and short term, in terms of housing the dog safely at the shelter, but also in the medium to long term, in terms of the potential to successfully rehome the dog without undue risk to the new owners, the public and other dogs. The welfare of the dog must always be a prime concern. Where the ability to reform defensively motivated aggressive responses is hampered by factors, such as the learned component of the behaviour, the restrictions of the physical layout of the shelter and limited resources, decisions will need to be made as to whether rehoming is a responsible approach or whether euthanasia should be considered. The overriding deciding factors for such decisions should be the welfare of the dog and the potential for risk.

Management within the shelter environment

In order to minimize risk and maximize welfare, it is important to appropriately manage dogs that are displaying aggressive behavioural responses while they are housed in a shelter environment. ➡

Identifying the potential triggers is the first step; following this, the aim is to minimize exposure to these triggers as much as possible. In particular, it is important to avoid exposure in contexts that favour the development of frustration. It can be helpful to house dogs with fear and anxiety in kennels that are not constantly in view of other dogs, a situation that allows for visual intrusion and perception of threat. It is also helpful to minimize walking fearful and aggressive individuals past the kennels of other dogs and to avoid situations in which these individuals are on the lead in the immediate vicinity of other dogs. Minimizing frustration in interactions with humans is also a priority. Any interaction that could be misinterpreted by a dog as a threat or confrontation (such as shouting at the dog or using intervention devices such as water pistols or rattle cans which are designed to suppress the behavioural response) should be avoided. Since the aggressive behaviour is defensively motivated, any attempt to use confrontation to suppress that behaviour runs the risk of increasing the dog's negative perception while suppressing its outward expression of that perception, and is extremely dangerous.

Approaching and handling dogs with aggressive behavioural responses

Working with dogs showing aggressive behavioural responses in a shelter environment can begin only once there is an element of trust between the dog and the handler. Passive interaction can be very beneficial in establishing trust. It is essential to avoid the use of confrontation, since this will serve only to increase negative emotions and favour the perception of threat. If immediate interaction is necessary, for example, in order to provide veterinary attention, the use of appropriate medication to achieve adequate sedation and, ideally, limit the dog's memory of the intervention should be considered. Medication that can be administered with minimal need for handling and

restraint, orally or by a single injection, is preferable. In order to minimize the duration of recovery, the use of reversible agents should also be considered.

If dogs with aggressive behavioural responses are to be handled effectively without the use of medication, it is essential to keep their emotional arousal level to a minimum to ensure that they have adequate emotional capacity to deal with the interaction. Reducing stimuli (e.g. visual and auditory) that could increase arousal is a first step, and housing these dogs in quiet secluded kennels rather than in the middle of a busy block is beneficial. The use of the pheromone product Adaptil to increase the dog's perception of the environment as safe is considered useful by some. The diffuser device for this product can be used to introduce the scent signal to the dog's environment with minimum disruption and without the need for physical handling. When it is necessary to move a dog that displays aggressive behavioural responses but direct handling is not essential, it is better to adopt a passive approach and use strategic placement of food trails to encourage the dog to move by creating a positive emotional response. When using food in this way, the pieces of food need to be extremely small and the delivery entirely passive; the food is placed on the floor, not offered from the hand. If it is possible to safely attach a houseline to a fixed collar on the dog, this can be used to guide the dog into compliance with the move, and removes the need for any attempt to grab at the dog's collar or use physical force to move the dog. The use of muzzles is obviously beneficial, but in order to use them effectively it is important to introduce them gradually and in association with positive experience. Basket-style muzzles should be used so that the dog can still express its emotional state by lip curling and baring its teeth. When possible, the muzzle training process should lead to the dog placing its head into the muzzle, rather than the muzzle being placed on to the dog's head. Obviously, this may not always be achievable in a shelter, and if a muzzle must be used without prior training it should be passively applied and used for the minimum time possible.

Low-restraint handling is always the aim, but in situations where time is limited, handling is necessary and medication is not considered to be appropriate, the use of restraint equipment may need to be considered. Slip leads that can be attached to the dog with minimal need for physical interaction, or dog catchers that enable the handler to remain at a safe distance, may have a place in such situations. However, these should always be used in the least threatening way and for the minimum duration of time possible.

Reforming aggressive behaviour with a view to rehoming

Keeping a dog safe within a shelter environment is very different from maintaining safety in a new home and, as previously discussed, the shelter has a responsibility to carry out a realistic risk assessment before considering rehoming a dog that is displaying behavioural responses related to negative emotional states. Aggressive responses may be the most obvious but all responses need to be given equal consideration. Ideally, behavioural modification work will be carried out before rehoming, but this can be achieved only with suitably qualified and experienced staff or by enlisting the assistance of a suitable external behaviourist. Implementing behavioural modification may be limited in the shelter context by the physical environment and by limited resources of staff and time. Interim housing in the form of a foster home may offer the opportunity to implement behavioural modification programmes in a home environment before making a final decision about the suitability of a dog for rehoming, but foster carers will require adequate training and support to carry out this role. At all times, the safety of people and other dogs, as well as the welfare of the individual dog concerned, must be paramount.

References and further reading

Bradshaw J (2011) *In Defence of Dogs: Why Dogs Need Our Understanding*. Penguin, London

Yin S (2009) *Low Stress Handling Restraint and Behavior Modification of Dogs and Cats: Techniques for Developing Patients Who Love Their Visits*. CattleDog Publishing, Davis

QRG 19.6: Dealing with the hard-to-handle cat
by Sarah Ellis and Vicky Halls

What does a 'hard to handle' cat look like?

Cats that are likely to be hard to handle or need careful handling due to feelings of fear, anxiety and/or frustration commonly show a number of behaviours, summarized below and in the flow chart.

Common behaviours related to fear and anxiety

- If real or potential danger is distant or inescapable:
  - Hiding response – cats often only need their head or eyes out of sight to feel they are hidden

- Freezing response – keeping still and often trying to make the body appear smaller while remaining highly vigilant.
- If real or potential danger is close but avoidable:
  - Flee response – cat attempts to run away.
- If real or potential danger is close and inescapable and there is no perceived hiding place:
  - Fight response – aggression involving biting and/or swiping.

Common behaviours related to frustration

- Aggression – biting and/or swiping, either as a direct result of

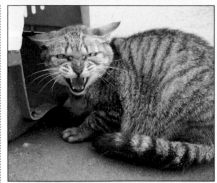

A cat displaying aggressive body language due to frustration (note pupil size).
(© Daniela Ramos)

being restrained/handled or redirected to a staff member in close proximity to the cat.
- Struggling.

Research into how to differentiate between a fearful, anxious or a frustrated cat on the basis of its body language and vocalizations is in its infancy, although a number of body postures/body language and vocalizations have been identified as generally occurring when a cat is experiencing one or more negative emotions. A cat can switch rapidly between such negative emotions and can even experience more than one emotion at the same time; for example, some cats can feel fearful due to an approaching handler but at the point of handling, feel frustrated by the restraint and the subsequent inability to escape.

Common body postures and body language involved in negative emotions

- Body: obvious signs of tension or hunching, limbs and tail pressed tightly to body, shaking, flattening.
- Ears: partially or completely flattened (more commonly associated with fear and anxiety), rotated sideways or backwards (more commonly associated with frustration).
- Fur and skin: piloerection (hair raised along the back and on the tail), skin rippling.
- Eyes: with fear and anxiety, pupils are often partially to fully dilated; eyes can vary from being wide open to pressed shut →

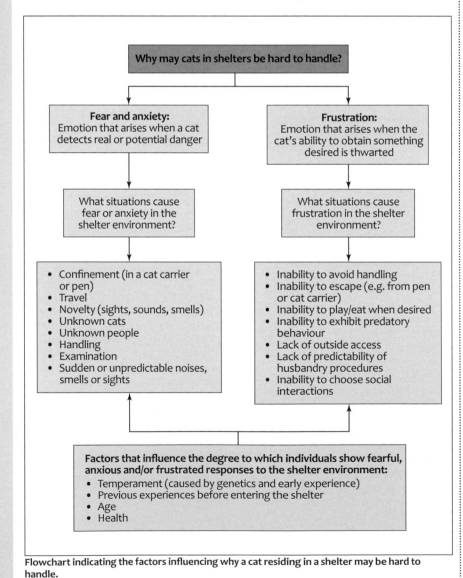

Why may cats in shelters be hard to handle?

Fear and anxiety:
Emotion that arises when a cat detects real or potential danger

Frustration:
Emotion that arises when the cat's ability to obtain something desired is thwarted

What situations cause fear or anxiety in the shelter environment?

What situations cause frustration in the shelter environment?

- Confinement (in a cat carrier or pen)
- Travel
- Novelty (sights, sounds, smells)
- Unknown cats
- Unknown people
- Handling
- Examination
- Sudden or unpredictable noises, smells or sights

- Inability to avoid handling
- Inability to escape (e.g. from pen or cat carrier)
- Inability to play/eat when desired
- Inability to exhibit predatory behaviour
- Lack of outside access
- Lack of predictability of husbandry procedures
- Inability to choose social interactions

Factors that influence the degree to which individuals show fearful, anxious and/or frustrated responses to the shelter environment:
- Temperament (caused by genetics and early experience)
- Previous experiences before entering the shelter
- Age
- Health

Flowchart indicating the factors influencing why a cat residing in a shelter may be hard to handle.

QRG 19.6 *continued*

(if the cat is motionless and appears hunched). Creasing can often be seen in the corner of the eyes when they are pressed shut. Both blinking and half-blinking have been shown to be associated with fear. With frustration, pupils may be dilated but can also be normal size (often dependent on cat's arousal levels); eyes can be open or protectively half-closed (if frustration linked to inability to escape from a threat).

- Tail: tucked close or under the body, swishing.
- Head: sharply turning towards the handler, always oriented towards the handler, pressed firmly into the chest with the nose facing the floor; rotating the head in circular movements (often witnessed when the cat is searching for an escape route).
- Mouth: nose-licking and tongue showing are both associated with frustration.

Common vocalizations that accompany negative emotions

- Hissing (particularly when frustrated).
- Growling.
- Repetitive miaowing.
- Silent.

Managing fearful, anxious and frustrated cats

Proper assessment

Recognizing behavioural signs of fear, anxiety and frustration will help identify those cats that are most likely to demonstrate aggressive behaviour during handling. In addition, obtaining as much background information on the cat will help assess how difficult it may be to handle in the shelter environment.

Questions that need to be asked include:

- For unowned cats:
  - What is the cat's origin?
  - Is it known or believed to be a feral or unsocialized cat?
  - Is it a stray?
  - Will it accept human contact?
  - How was it brought into the shelter (e.g. in a box/carrier, by car, sedated)?

- For owned cats:
  - How does the cat normally behave at the veterinary surgery, boarding cattery, around other cats, in confined spaces, such as the cat carrier or a pen?
  - What has proved helpful in the past, if the cat has been fearful or frustrated in other situations?
  - What preferences does the cat have in terms of food, bedding, toys, litter tray?
  - Does the cat like to be handled and, if so, how (e.g. picked up, stroked, where on the body, how often)?

A stay in a shelter environment involves a number of procedures that are likely to increase fear, anxiety or frustration in a cat. By taking appropriate steps as listed below, fear, anxiety and frustration can be minimized during each procedure, making handling of the cat easier when it is required.

Travelling to the shelter

- Choose an appropriate arrival time, e.g. when there is little activity and the waiting time will be minimal.
- Ensure the cat has been accustomed to a cat carrier before being transported.
- The cat carrier should have a top opening for ease of access or should be able to split in half.
- Transport the cat with items that carry a familiar scent placed in the carrier, e.g. something from the cat's previous environment or owner.
- Cover the carrier with a blanket or towel (ideally one that has a familiar scent).

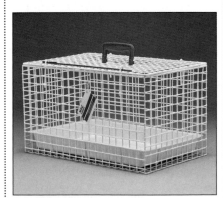

Cat carrier with a top opening.
(© MDC Exports)

Placing the cat in a shelter pen

- Move the cat from the carrier to the pen as quickly as possible, with minimal waiting time.
- Select a pen at waist level rather than either above eye or ground level, to facilitate easy access and comfortable and safe handling.
- Place the carrier directly into the pen and allow the cat to leave the carrier voluntarily (where this is not possible, see 'Examination and medical procedures' for how to remove a cat from a carrier).
- Provide hiding places in the pen, such as cardboard boxes, the carrier or an igloo bed.
- House cats away from dogs, not facing other cats, and in an area without harsh lighting and loud noises (e.g. telephones, doorbells, fans, air conditioning).
- Manage odours by cleaning and rinsing surfaces, washing hands between handling different cats and ensuring appropriate room ventilation, if possible. Challenging smells may cause anxiety (e.g. air fresheners, disinfectants, surgical spirit, deodorants, perfume, protective clothing or unfamiliar uniforms).
- Utilize recorded background information on the cat to provide it with familiar resources.

Approaching the penned cat

- Before opening the pen, ensure that the environment is secure, with no opportunities for the cat to escape.
- Angle yourself so that your side is facing the cat, thus avoiding confrontational behaviour such as direct eye contact and approach.
- Move slowly and deliberately, always speaking in a calm, quiet voice.
- Minimize hand gestures and ensure that hand approaches are initially no higher than the cat's nose height, thereby avoiding the hand looming over the cat.

Placement in a cat carrier for transportation within the shelter

- Always transport cats from the pen to other parts of the shelter in a carrier to reduce handling.
- Utilize a carrier with a removable top half.

QRG 19.6 *continued*

- Give the cat the opportunity to enter the cat carrier voluntarily. If the cat will not enter voluntarily, assess its body language and utilize background information about the cat to decide the best course of action.
- For cats showing limited signs of fear, anxiety or frustration, lift the cat smoothly and confidently, supporting its body with two hands, to move the cat from the pen to the carrier without distress. If cat is showing more intense signs of fear, anxiety or frustration, or these signs escalate on approaching the cat, or if the opening to the pen is small, hold a towel up, place it over the cat and then lift the cat into the carrier with the cat engulfed in the towel, using a gentle but firm 'scooping' action. Two towels doubled up to provide extra thickness can be used to protect the handler if the cat is showing particularly intense signs of fear, anxiety or frustration.
- Ideally these towels should smell familiar to the cat, e.g. used as bedding.

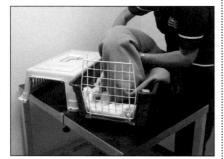

Covering a cat with a towel to place it in a carrier for transportation.
(© Vicky Halls)

Examination and medical procedures

- Always examine cats in a secure environment out of sight of other animals. If a procedure will be painful or surgery is planned, chemical restraint is necessary (see below). For all other procedures and examinations, the equipment needed should be prepared in advance to avoid unnecessary delays.
- Ideally, examine the cat while it is in the base of the carrier, to give the cat a perceived hiding place and enhance security.
- Always start with the least invasive procedure.

- Handle the cat as gently as possible and guard against using restrictive or heavy holding techniques as a result of handler fear, anxiety or frustration.
- The use of minimal restraint is often more acceptable for the hard-to-handle cat, so it is preferable to try this first before electing to use additional equipment or techniques.
- Treat each cat as an individual (assessing its body language and becoming familiar with background information about the cat) and continually adapt behaviour according to the cat's response to handling. Care should be taken when holding any part of the body to ensure that the cat is not being placed into an unnatural or uncomfortable posture.

Techniques and available equipment

Any handling equipment and aids should be used only when minimal restraint has not proved effective, and never chosen over sensitive handling and appropriate preparation. Cats may have a varying response to different pieces of equipment, so each cat should be monitored and alternatives used depending on the response. All equipment should be cleaned and disinfected between uses.

Food treats

Offering high-value food treats can be beneficial during handling. If the treats are not eaten, do not try to encourage the cat to eat them – simply offer them during each handling session. Over repeated exposures the cat may become comfortable enough to eat them, thereby developing a more positive association with being handled and/ or the individual handler.

Towel

This is the equipment of choice for particularly fearful or anxious cats. They can be removed from the carrier using a towel, as described above for placement in the carrier. They can then be kept calm by holding the towel at either side of their head, with the handler's arms supporting the cat's body. This allows the cat to be examined by lifting the towel from behind while the head is still covered,

thus preventing the cat bolting forward in an attempt to escape. Some cats may try to back out of the towel and resist having their head covered; it may be more comfortable for these individuals if the towel is wrapped around the body, leaving the head exposed. This technique should not be used to stop a cat from struggling if it becomes distressed; chemical restraint will be necessary in such cases. Staff should be well practised in the various techniques of using a towel for restraint and stress reduction.

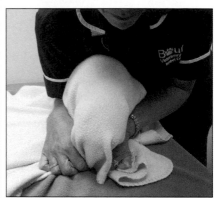

A towel held either side of a cat's head, with the arms supporting the cat's body, prevents it escaping forwards.
(© Vicky Halls)

Gloves

Various styles of gloves can be used, from strong leather gardening gloves to reinforced gauntlets. These may prevent injury to the handler but they hinder delicate or specific manipulation of the cat, may carry odours that further distress the cat and are difficult to disinfect.

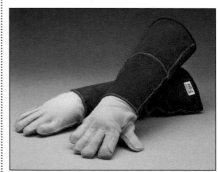

Elbow-length reinforced leather gauntlets.
(© MDC Exports)

Protective sleeves

These are elbow-length lightweight sleeves that also cover the main part of the hand, with a cut-out for the thumb, designed for use by operators of cutting machinery. Anecdotally, these appear to be

QRG 19.6 *continued*

fairly resistant to scratches and may be useful for handlers who are fearful of being injured by a cat, as the added security that these sleeves afford the user may be sufficient to enable gentler handling, which will appear less threatening to the cat.

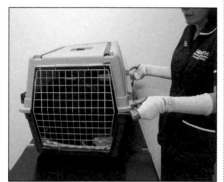

Protective sleeves may provide nervous handlers with some additional security against scratches and enable them to handle frightened or frustrated cats more confidently.
(© Vicky Halls)

Cage restrainer

A cage restrainer ('crush cage') is a top-opening wire carrier with a sliding internal panel that enables the cat to be restrained against one side of the cage for the purposes of administering an injection with the minimum of distress for the cat and handler. Such equipment is only recommended for feral cats that are generally unhandleable.

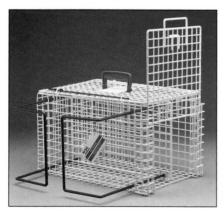

A cage restrainer showing the sliding internal panel.
(© MDC Exports)

Dropover carrier

This is a wire carrier with a removable sliding floor. The cat is contained by 'dropping' the carrier over it, and the floor is slid into place once the cat is secured. This type of carrier can also have a restraining panel that acts as a cage restrainer, so that an injection

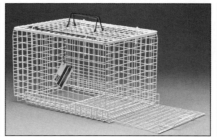

A drop-over carrier with a removable sliding floor.
(© MDC Exports)

can be administered. Such equipment is only recommended for feral cats that are unhandleable.

Chemical restraint

If a cat shows signs of fear, anxiety or frustration, possibly manifesting in aggression, then chemical restraint may be considered if the consensus is that the procedure would take longer and be more stressful without it. If a procedure will be painful or surgery is planned, then chemical restraint is appropriate. Agents that are administered via the intramuscular or subcutaneous routes are recommended, as they require minimal restraint or can be administered while the cat is in a cage restrainer (see above). Choosing agents whose actions can be reversed, would also be preferable.

Other handling equipment

Cat muzzle

A 'cat muzzle' is a fabric or leather device that is secured to cover the cat's face and eyes and, in some cases, to physically prevent the cat from biting. A muzzle should be used only if it calms the cat once fitted, and to facilitate a procedure. The cat should be monitored closely during use of a muzzle to ensure the device is not hampering breathing, and it should be removed immediately after the procedure has been carried out.

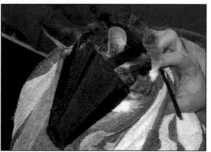

A cat being restrained with the use of a cat muzzle.
(Reproduced from the *BSAVA Textbook of Veterinary Nursing, 5th edition*)

Cat bag

This is a heavy-duty fabric bag that contains a cat while still allowing access to parts of the body for injections or venepuncture. Care should be taken to ensure the bag is not too tight, thereby restricting breathing, or too loose, as the animal would not be restrained sufficiently for the procedure to be carried out. A carefully placed towel wrap is likely to be a more comfortable alternative.

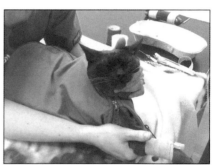

A cat being restrained for a procedure using a 'cat bag'.
(© Vicky Halls)

Other techniques and products are available (eg, nets, tight-fitting vests) and advertised as aiding handling and, in many cases, minimizing stress, based on immobilization of the cat. However, there is a lack of substantive scientific research to support the utility of such items; moreover, due to the biology and behaviour of the cat, it can be hypothesized that such items would be experienced negatively by the cat as a result of the restricted movement, inability to escape and lack of control. For this reason, use of such equipment is not advocated by some veterinary surgeons and behaviourists.

References and further reading

Bennett V, Gourkow, N, and Mills DS (2017). Facial correlates of emotional behaviour in the domestic cat (*Felis catus*). *Behavioural Processes*.

Cooper B, Mullineaux E and Turner L (2011) *BSAVA Textbook of Veterinary Nursing, 5th edn.* BSAVA Publications, Gloucester

Rodan I, Sundahl E, Carney H, Gagnon AC, Heath S, Landsberg G, Seksel K and Yin S (2011). AAFP and ISFM feline-friendly handling guidelines. *Journal of feline medicine and surgery* **13(5)**, pp. 364–375.

QRG 19.7: Environmental enrichment for dogs in shelters

by Steve Goward

Enriching an animal's environment is not a new concept and has been taken very seriously in zoos and wildlife parks across the world. However, domestic animals have received less attention in this regard, and it is quite common to visit an animal shelter in the UK and find little or no enrichment provided to the occupants. The research on enriching an animal's environment suggests that appropriate enrichment increases welfare and enhances quality of life. Enrichment of the environment in which animals are kept should be part of any shelter establishment's management routine. When adding any items to an animals' environment it is important to consider the health and safety of both the animal and people caring for them. A good understanding of the principles of infectious disease, transmission and biosecurity in shelters is essential to ensure protocols are put in place to reduce the risk of injury or disease via material used in enrichment (see Chapters 8 and 9). When devising a shelter's enrichment plan there are several considerations to ensure the wellbeing of the dogs in your care. Having segregated areas for dogs that are at different stages of their visit is essential, such as new arrivals, dogs in isolation due to infectious disease (e.g. kennel cough) and dogs that are at higher risk (e.g. puppies or older immune suppressed dogs).

What is environmental enrichment?

Environmental enrichment can be split into two main categories: **animate** and **inanimate**.

Animate enrichment essentially means other living animals to which the dog can develop an attachment – essentially, other dogs and other species, including humans. Inanimate enrichment simply describes items that can be added to the animal's environment for the animal to interact with or use and, in so doing, gain enrichment.

Dogs are a social species, and, therefore, it should come as no surprise that finding an appropriate partner for dogs in kennels can provide social interaction that is one of the most enriching parts of the dog's day. However, if a poor choice is made, this may well create negative experiences rather than enhance the dogs' welfare. Pairing dogs and/or mixing them in appropriate groups can enrich their lives with relatively little time input from the human caregiver, but must be done with extreme care to avoid fear, aggression and disease transmission.

Handling and exercise

How shelter staff and veterinary surgeons interact with the dogs in their care will have a direct impact on the dogs' quality of life and welfare. Ensuring appropriate handling by all staff and volunteers in all situations will enhance the positive interactions experienced by the dogs while in the care of a shelter. Whether the dog is being taken for a walk or restrained for veterinary examination, the use of equipment that is likely to cause pain or discomfort should be avoided.

Just a few minutes of positive reward-based training (see QRG 19.1) can create trust and enhance welfare, as well as have an impact on the ease of management and likelihood of adoption of the dogs in the care of the shelter. Appropriate exercise with other dogs or with the human caregiver, whether doing agility training or playing with a toy, has the bonus of removing the dog from the kennel area and allowing it to spend time with a social group. Socially isolated dogs are much more likely to suffer from poor welfare and associated conditions such as stereotypy and obsessive-compulsive behaviours.

A good volunteer programme can be a great way of increasing the amount of time dogs spend with people and opens up further potential for training and rehabilitation programmes once the volunteers themselves have received appropriate training. Volunteers can also help to build sensory enrichments (see below) and make activity toys, as well as spending social time with the dogs.

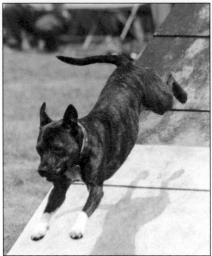

Learning agility gives dogs opportunities to grow in confidence and build a relationship with their handler.
(© Dogs Trust)

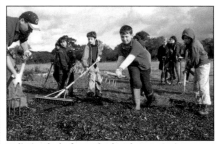

Enlisting help from the local community – whether from colleges, businesses or individuals – can free up shelter staff to concentrate on the dogs' daily activities. Here, a children's volunteer helps a group of children to prepare an enrichment area.
(© Dogs Trust)

It is important not just to consider the species being catered for, but also to think about various breed traits and remember that all dogs are individuals. Therefore, when a shelter is developing an enrichment policy it is preferable to include a wide variety of options, as some dogs will not be enriched by jumping over hurdles or fetching a toy and may find other activities or resources more enriching.

The general environment that surrounds dogs in kennels should be considered as it may be possible to enrich the immediate vicinity by adding creative planting or barriers, which can help to reduce the volume of noise and obscure some of the movement that goes on around a busy shelter, thus helping to →

reduce stress, or with a change of routine, such as a cleaning and feeding regime that caters for dogs' individual preferences. The shelter's design and layout may often contribute to the noise levels and therefore directly impact on the dog's stress levels (see Chapter 10).

Sensory enrichment

For dogs that enjoy exploring novel environments, there are a number of enrichment options that can be considered. A sensory garden does not have to be big or expensive to create. When planning a sensory garden, it is important to research and find safe (non-toxic) plants that have a variety of odours, and also prepare for the fact that male dogs are likely to scent mark the area.

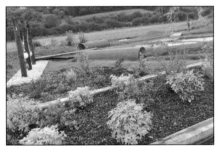

Providing items that enable dogs to engage their different senses can be a valuable form of enrichment, as in this sensory garden.
(© Dogs Trust)

Raised planting beds or large pots can be used to keep the plants out of harm's way. Scent trails strategically placed along the route of a walk can add interest to an otherwise monotonous daily activity. These can be made using metal bird feeders, plastic bottles or similar containers with holes in the sides, filled with a variety of plants, herbs, straw from a stable or a cloth scented with an essential oil, and spread out along the walk. The containers should be moved and changed frequently, as it is the novelty that drives the dogs' interest.

Along the same walking path there could be areas of varying substrate, such as sand, bark chippings (a type safe for dogs), pebbles and grass. Having points along the walk where there are signs describing tasks to be completed by the handler and dog creates opportunities to teach the dog basic commands including 'sit', 'down' or 'give paw'; this can help to build the dog's confidence and improve its

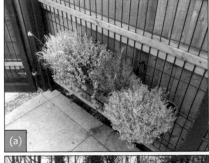

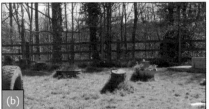

(a) Plant pots or (b) other containers filled with herbs, horsehair or other interesting-smelling items can add interest to exercise.
(© Jenny Stavisky)

adoption potential. Any opportunity to expose the dog to positive training interactions will have a beneficial impact on its welfare.

If there are trees along the walking path, items (e.g. wooden poles with holes cut out) can be attached to them that could hold food treats or toys for the dog to find while exploring. Having areas of interest along a walking route is particularly useful because the handler can allow the dog to explore, which is a very natural behaviour that is rarely catered for in dog shelters.

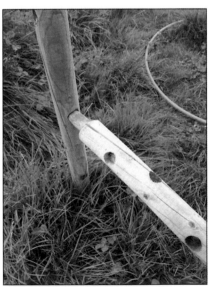

Opportunities to express investigative behaviours can have a positive effect on a dog's welfare. In this example, treats can be placed in holes drilled into a wooden post mounted at a height that dogs can easily explore.
(© Dogs Trust)

Play and social interaction

A place for dogs to play and socialize gives an excellent opportunity to enrich the shelter. This area can be used to promote the dogs for adoption as well as offering them a novel and stimulating space to interact with. Playgrounds do not need to be full of expensive agility equipment and can be put together on the smallest of budgets. Raised platforms, jumps, walkways and other areas for dogs to explore and interact with can develop their confidence and allow them to move away from other dogs in a group situation. Areas to dig in, such as a ball pool or sand pit containing hidden toys or treats for the dog to find, can be very rewarding for some dogs. As with anything that is added to a dog's environment, we must be sure that the materials used are safe and as easy to clean as possible. The use of plastics and rubber that could be ingested requires the dogs to be monitored in areas where the risk of chewing and ingesting materials is higher.

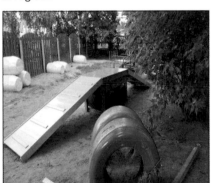

A raised area can facilitate social interactions by providing places for dogs to escape.
(© Dogs Trust)

Feeding enrichment

Food activity toys and puzzle feeders can be a great way to extend the time dogs spend finding and consuming their daily feed allowance. However, some caution is required with food activity toys, as some dogs find them frustrating and their stress levels can increase if the puzzle is too difficult to solve. For shelters on a tight budget, there are many inexpensive ways to make activity toys and games for the dogs to engage with in their search for food. For example, a puzzle feeder can be made from an old muffin tin or a cardboard tray from a coffee shop with food or treats placed

QRG 19.7 *continued*

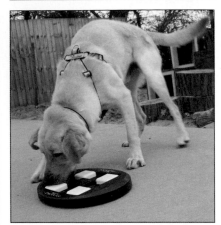

Feeding enrichment can be provided using either proprietary devices or cheaper homemade versions.
(© Dogs Trust)

in some of the indentations, with either tennis balls or balls of newspaper covering the food. An empty water bottle with the lid taken off and a few biscuits or treats inside can make a fun activity toy. Cardboard tubes can be filled with shredded or scrunched-up newspaper with treats mixed in; food items can be simply placed under some flower pots in various locations for the dog to find. When using food activity toys or puzzle feeders, it is important to monitor the dogs to ensure they do not damage or ingest the toys.

Even the number of feeds per day and their presentation can make a difference to the welfare of dogs in kennels. Understanding that dogs often enjoy seeking food items and are opportunistic feeders who may spend time looking for and consuming food items, should guide shelter staff towards being more imaginative about how food is provided. Scatter feeding in the kennel or in an enclosed exercise area, playing 'hide and seek' with portions of the food, or providing a scent trail for the dog to track to find the bulk of the food at the end of the trail are all good ways of providing enrichment with food. Caution is required when feeding more than one dog to avoid creating conflict or if an individual has exhibited possessive behaviour with food.

Housing enrichment

Items that may improve the individual dog's welfare can also be placed within the kennel. These include

furniture, such as a sofa or chair, or indoor crates with blankets draped over them, to provide the dog with an alternative sleeping spot or an area to retreat to when anxious. When housing dogs in groups, it is advisable to provide multiple areas for them to rest and drink. Increasing the provision of resources within the kennel will reduce the likelihood of resource-guarding problems developing.

In individual kennels, toys are often discarded or left half chewed and then just lie around looking untidy. However, the research on toys indicates that, although they can be effective as a tool for both enrichment and improving adoption rates (Wells and Hepper, 2000), the most likely age for sustained interaction is with puppies. The key to using toys effectively is the novelty factor, as this encourages dogs to interact with them. Having a routine that regularly allows for toys in the dogs' environment to be changed will create this novelty (DeLuca and Kranda, 1992; Kaulfuß and Mills, 2008). Considerations for disease prevention and spread must be made when devising a toy rota system and the toys need to be in good condition and easily cleaned with an appropriate cleaning solution. The research (Wells and Hepper, 1992; 2000) shows that even if a dog is not playing with a toy in its kennel, it is more likely to be chosen by an adopter than a dog sitting in a barren kennel. Preference testing toys to find out which types the dog enjoys playing with, can also help to encourage play and interaction with people. With a good shelter design

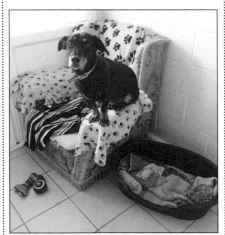

Household furniture can provide comfortable enrichment within a kennel, and donations of old armchairs and sofas are frequently easy to obtain.
(© Dogs Trust)

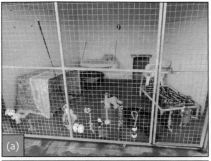

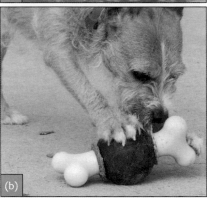

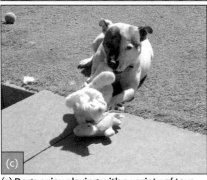

(a) Dogs enjoy playing with a variety of toys. (b) Encouraging play behaviour can help a dog to get noticed by adopters, as well as providing great photograph opportunities for advertising it. (c) Toys can also provide an important outlet for natural behaviours such as chewing.
(a–b, © Dogs Trust; c, © Jenny Stavisky)

(see Chapter 10), the dogs will be kept in separate areas dependent on vaccination/illness/disease status and it is wise to have separate toys for each of these areas to reduce the risk of contamination.

It may not be necessary, or possible, to carry out all of these activities and ideas every day, and not every intervention will be suitable for all dogs. However, by having a large portfolio of ideas and resources to enrich the lives of dogs in kennels, shelter staff are more likely to be able to enhance the lives of the dogs in their care. As with all new items and environments, it is important to monitor dogs to ensure no harm befalls them while engaging with environmental enrichment activities.

→

QRG 19.7 *continued*

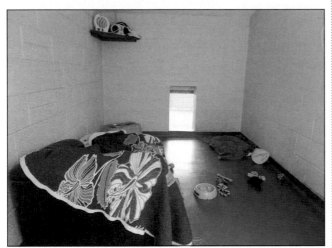

This kennel contains a donated sofa, puzzle feeder, toys, fan and radio to provide several different kinds of enrichment.
(© Jenny Stavisky)

References and further reading

DeLuca AM and Kranda KC (1992) Environmental enrichment in a large animal facility. *Laboratory Animals* **21**, 38–44

Kaulfuß P and Mills DS (2008) Neophilia in domestic dogs (*Canis familiaris*) and its implication for studies of dog cognition. *Animal Cognition* **11**, 553–556

Nicassio-Hiskey N and Alia Mitchell C (2013) *Beyond Squeaky Toys: Innovative Ideas for Eliminating Problem Behaviors and Enriching the Lives of Dogs and Cats*. Smart Pets Press, Lafayette

Pullen AJ, Merrill RJN and Bradshaw JWS (2010) Preferences for toy types and presentations in kennel housed dogs. *Applied Animal Behaviour Science* **125**, 151–156

Taylor KD and Mills DS (2007) The effect of the kennel environment on canine welfare: a critical review of experimental studies. *Animal Welfare* **16**, 435–447

Wells DL (2004) A review of environmental enrichment for kennelled dogs, *Canis familiaris*. *Applied Animal Behaviour Science* **85**, 307–317

Wells DL and Hepper PG (1992) The behaviour of dogs in a rescue shelter. *Animal Welfare* **1**, 171–186

Wells DL and Hepper PG (2000) The influence of environmental change on the behaviour of sheltered dogs. *Applied Animal Behaviour Science* **68(2)**, 151–162

Young RJ (2003) *Environmental Enrichment for Captive Animals*. Blackwell Publishing, Oxford

QRG 19.8: Environmental enrichment for cats in shelters

by Nicky Trevorrow

What is environmental enrichment?

Environmental enrichment refers to the meeting of species-specific needs through the creation of a suitable and stimulating environment. There are many different components to consider when designing an environmental enrichment programme. Rather than simply 'enriching' an environment, which may be too easily considered as adding an 'optional extra', environmental enrichment should be at the forefront of considerations as a normal and routine part of the cat's environment. It is perhaps more appropriate to use the term 'environmental needs' to emphasize its importance to a cat's overall wellbeing, in line with the duty of care of owners/carers to meet cats' welfare needs under the Animal Welfare Act 2006 (or relevant legislation in other jurisdictions; see Chapter 21).

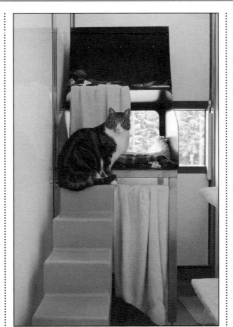

This bespoke cat bed unit with inbuilt heating in the raised sleep area provides opportunities for climbing and resting in a private elevated area.
(© Battersea Dogs and Cats Home)

Who is it for?

Many people may consider environmental enrichment as necessary for cats in the shelter environment that are hard to rehome, have been in the shelter for a long time or are perceived by the staff and volunteers as obviously not coping with the shelter environment. However, enrichment should in fact be provided and tailored for each individual cat in the shelter regardless of its situation. Providing environmental enrichment is also incredibly rewarding and therefore 'enriching' for the staff and volunteers working in the shelter.

This also applies to veterinary staff, who are ideally placed to advise their clients and those working in shelter environments. Many of the concepts discussed here can be applied or modified to suit cats in a variety of settings, from veterinary practice to boarding catteries. Incorporating discussions about environmental enrichment into clinical examinations has a huge impact on the health and welfare of cats, whether under the care of an owner or shelter, and the huge educational value cannot be underestimated.

QRG 19.8 *continued*

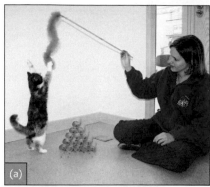

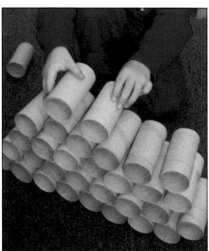

(a) Interactive play sessions are an important part of the cat's daily care routine. (b) Fishing rod toys can be homemade cheaply. Always store safely out of the cat's reach after the play session.
(© Cats Protection)

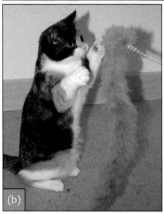

Children can get involved in making enrichment for shelter cats, which helps educate the next generation about animal care and welfare.
(© Cats Protection)

Why use environmental enrichment?

All animals have a need to perform certain species-specific behaviours. By providing outlets for their natural behaviour, caregivers are able to improve an animal's overall mood state and mental health and welfare. The shelter environment is particularly challenging for cats as it is an unfamiliar environment containing a number of potential stressors over which they have little control. Modifying the shelter environment to be more 'cat friendly' can help cats by:

- Enabling normal coping strategies to help them adapt to their situation
- Promoting normal 'maintenance' behaviours such as eating, drinking, toileting and grooming
- Increasing play behaviours
- Providing mental stimulation and, in some cases, problem-solving opportunities
- Encouraging physical exercise
- Preventing or managing behavioural problems
- Reducing the length of time to rehoming, increasing adoption rates and retention by adopters
- Promoting positive emotions and mood states.

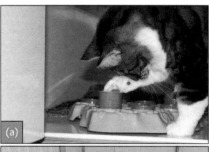

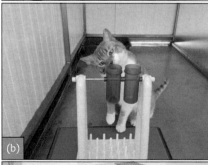

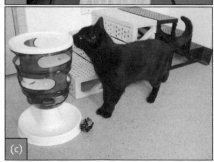

(a) AïKiou Stimulo feeding bowl and intelligence toy. (b) Trixie Cat Activity Turn Around. (c) CatIt Design Senses Food Maze.
(© Cats Protection)

Enrichment principles

Cats have a natural behavioural repertoire inherent to being a cat and this comes from their relatively recent domestication from a solitary and independent hunter. To gain an understanding of cats' environmental needs, it is important to take into account the behaviour of the African wildcat, *Felis silvestris lybica*, which shares its ancestry with today's domestic cat. More information about the origins of the domestic cat can be found at www.cats.org.uk/learn/e-learning-ufo.

Feline enrichment principles

- While some ideas for enrichment can be taken or modified from other species, enrichment does need to be appropriate for cats as a species.
- It needs to be tailored for the individual cat, as every cat is different.
- The enrichment should be suitable for the cat's current situation, life stage, physical and physiological health, mobility, level of socialization and emotional state. For example, cats that are newly admitted and scared are unlikely to want to play, but will benefit from having a safe place to hide.
- The items should be useful to the cat and not provided simply because they appeal to humans, e.g. teddy bears.
- Enrichment does not need to be expensive or time-consuming.

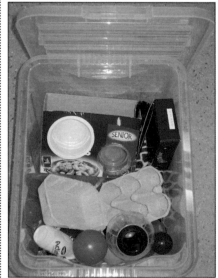

A collection of disposable items that can be used to create enrichment.
(© Cats Protection)

QRG 19.8 *continued*

- Interactive play sessions should ideally be short and frequent to replicate feline natural behaviour, moving toys in a way that simulates different prey species' movements (e.g. mice, birds).
- Items in the shelter need to be easy to disinfect or disposable to reduce the risk of transmission of infectious disease.
- Toys and feeding enrichment items need to be rotated to maintain novelty.
- Show cats how to use feeding enrichment items to prevent frustration (unless there is a human health and safety risk, such as a cat showing aggressive behaviour; for these cats, start with extremely simple feeding enrichment such as a scatter feed or dry food placed in an open egg box).
- Feeding enrichment can gradually increase in complexity – at the individual cat's pace.
- Enrichment is limited only by the caregiver's imagination.

Types of enrichment

The various types of enrichment aim to meet cats' needs through physical, sensory, social, occupational and nutritional aspects of their environment. Ultimately, it must not be forgotten that the best enrichment for a shelter cat is a permanent home, ideally one with appropriate resource placement. It is important to

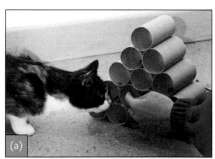
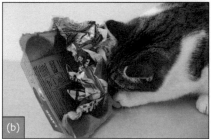

(a) Show the cat how to use a toilet roll pyramid to avoid frustration. (b) Dry food hidden in paper and placed in a cardboard egg box.
(© Cats Protection)

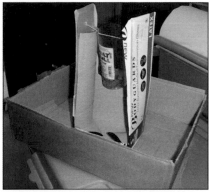

A homemade version of a puzzle feeder.
(© Cats Protection)

concentrate efforts to ensure a quick turnaround and minimize the time cats spend in the rescue environment.

The enrichment ideas listed below are separated out into the different stages of the cat's journey through a shelter.

Before relinquishment

- A cloth with scent from the owner's environment and/or the owner can be handed in with the cat to provide scent continuity.
- A blanket to cover the cat basket will help the cat feel more secure.
- The cat basket should be placed on a high surface, such as on the reception desk, when admitting the cat, to help it feel more secure than if placed on the floor.
- Find out information about the cat as an individual to enable a more tailored approach to the cat's care and facilitate matching the cat to the right owner.

On arrival in the shelter

- Provide places to hide, such as: an igloo-style bed; a proprietary product such as the Hide, Perch & Go box™ devised by the British Columbia Society for the Prevention of Cruelty to Animals, or the Feline Fort® developed by Cats Protection; or suitably sized cardboard boxes with two holes cut into the sides – the two holes are crucial so that the cat has an entry and exit point, providing potential escape routes if needed.
- Create more territory in the limited space available in the pen by making use of three-dimensional space and incorporating elevated perches, including some that only

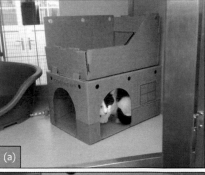
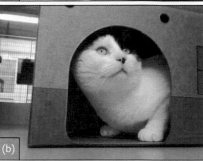
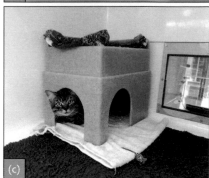

(a–b) Hide, Perch & Go box™ devised by the British Columbia Society for the Prevention of Cruelty to Animals. (c) Feline Fort® Hide developed by Cats Protection.
(© Cats Protection)

hold one cat, and corner shelves so that cats cannot be approached from behind, to help them feel safer.
- Have a predictable routine with the same, familiar caregiver where possible.
- Full opacity between pens is vital so that cats cannot see other cats in the shelter. If this is not possible, frosted materials are better than completely clear glass between pens; however, cats may still react to seeing the outlines or shadows of other cats.
- Synthetic facial pheromones, such as Feliway®, can help a cat feel more comfortable in its environment.
- Ensure that the cat's essential resources are appropriately placed.

QRG 19.8 *continued*

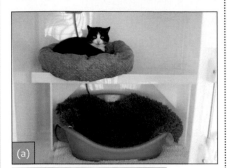

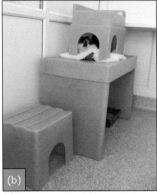

(a) It is easy to enrich an existing pen design by adding a shelving insert. (b) A Feline Fort® developed by Cats Protection, consisting of three modular pieces.
(© Cats Protection)

While at the shelter

- Continue with the items listed in 'On arrival in the shelter' during the cat's stay.
- Provide interactive play sessions with fishing rod toys for cats that have settled in and whose stress levels have reduced.
- Quality time with the caregiver interacting with the cat as part of the normal daily routine will help to lower stress and provide social contact.
- If possible, provide an interesting view outside the pen by placing bird feeders nearby, planting a buddleia (butterfly bush) to attract butterflies or bamboo for

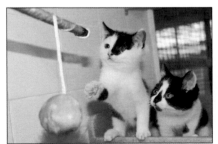

Both kittens and adult cats will benefit from an interactive game. Store safely out of the cat's reach when not in use.
(© Cats Protection)

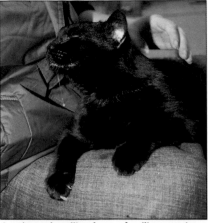

Consistent handling from a familiar caregiver.
(© Cats Protection)

movement and rustling noises, or hang CDs or other reflective items nearby. Be aware that while most cats will find these stimulating, some cats may find them frustrating.
- Provide suitable safe toys for self-directed play, and rotate (while observing good biosecurity) to maintain novelty.
- Introduce feeding enrichment, which can be commercially available or homemade items.

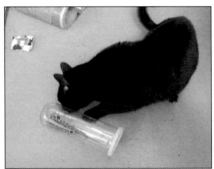

Another homemade version of a puzzle feeder.
(© Cats Protection)

- Provide disposable scratching facilities, such as carpet tile samples or corrugated cardboard that offers the choice of both vertical and horizontal surfaces and allows the cat to leave visual and scent marks.
- Provide sensory enrichment, such as quality catnip or cat mint, cloths that have been rubbed on to a healthy rabbit to collect its scent, or feathers from wild birds.
- Be mindful of the importance of scent to cats by using a 'scent-free' disinfectant.
- Use a 'double bed' system where the cat is given two blankets and only one is washed and replaced

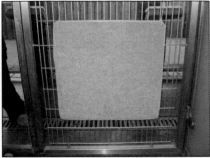

A carpet tile secured to the run door using cable ties provides a cheap scratching facility.
(© Cats Protection)

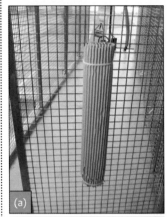

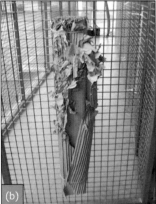

(a) A corrugated cardboard scratch post attached to the run with cable ties. (b) Simply dispose and replace once it is too worn.
(© Cats Protection)

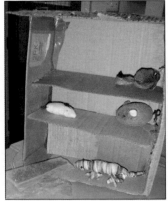

Catnip toys provide sensory enrichment.
(© Cats Protection)

QRG 19.8 *continued*

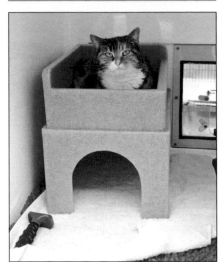

Feline Fort® Hide developed by Cats Protection.
(© Cats Protection)

with a clean blanket at a time. This provides scent continuity of the cat's own scent so that the environment will smell more familiar to the cat.
- Use a spot-cleaning protocol for areas with lower risk of infectious disease to maintain the cat's own scent.

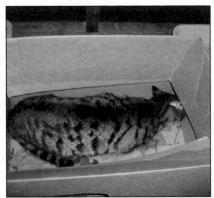

Cardboard box with dry food scattered among dry leaves.
(© Cats Protection)

- Provide different textures for the cat to sit on or investigate, such as cardboard, carpet tiles, soft blankets or bark.
- Some cats like to play with water – a clean litter tray half filled with water with a few ping pong balls floating on top can be provided.
- Laser pens and DVDs designed for cats featuring prey species and catching based games on tablet devices seem to interest cats, but again be aware that they may cause frustration as the cat cannot catch the stimulus. If these items are used, then the games need to end by providing a physical toy that the cat can catch and 'kill'.

Homing

- New owners can provide a cloth from home to start familiarizing the cat with the scent of the new home.
- A cardboard box from the pen can be homed with the cat for scent continuity and to provide a familiar hiding place.

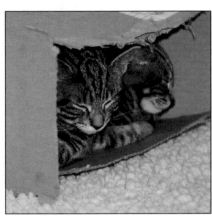

All cats need to be given a hiding place.
(© Cats Protection)

- A scent cloth from the cat's pen will also provide scent continuity.
- Advise the new owners about essential resources and appropriate placement in the home and general cats' needs – this is especially important for indoor-only cats.

Chapter 20

Charities, their policies and staff

Maggie Roberts and Wendy Adams

Charity structure

Most animal shelters and rehoming organizations are charities. In the UK, the majority are 'registered' charities. In order to become a registered charity, an organization must fulfil the criteria set out in the Charities Act 2006 and, crucially, must be 'for public benefit'. Importantly, while the 'advancement of animal welfare' is considered to be charitable, it is not considered charitable to 'offer sanctuary to fit and healthy animals' by the Charity Commission. Each country has its own regulations controlling the formation and actions of charities; for example, in the USA there are 'non-profit' state laws and a few national charities are controlled under federal law. There are no consistent regulations on charities across Europe, with each country having control over their governance. This can create difficulties for organizations that are working in more than one country, and it is important to be aware of the relevant legislation in each one.

There are several options for the legal structure of an individual charity. The specific structure will depend on a number of factors, including the size of the organization, whether or not it has paid employees, its annual turnover and whether it is incorporated. By law, a UK charity must apply to be registered with the Charity Commission if it is a charitable incorporated organization or if it has an annual income of more than £5000, although there are certain exceptions to this requirement.

A detailed discussion of charity law is outside the scope of this chapter, but further information can be obtained from the Charity Commission for England and Wales, the Scottish Charity Regulator or the Charity Commission for Northern Ireland. Regardless of the specific structure adopted, there are several requirements common to all charities (see also Chapter 21 for more details about the legislation governing animal charities in the UK).

Governing document

A charity must have a governing document. Essentially, this is a set of rules setting out what the charity was set up to do and the way it should be run. The governing document should include certain key rules for the charity. All trustees must have a copy of the governing document. The Charity Commissions for England and Wales and for Northern Ireland and the Scottish Charity Regulator provide guidance on writing a governing document.

Minimum requirements for the governing document of a charity

* The charitable objects (i.e. the purpose of the charity)
* Its 'powers', or what it can (and cannot) do in order to meet its objects, such as borrowing money
* Who runs it and who can become a member
* How and when meetings are held
* How trustees are appointed
* Rules about paying trustees, managing investments and holding property
* Whether trustees can change the governing document, including its objects ('amendment provisions')
* How to close the charity ('dissolution provisions')
* Other rules may be specified in addition to these

Trustees

All charities must have trustees, who are the equivalent of the board of directors in a commercial company. Trustees have considerable legal responsibilities in respect of the charity and, in the event of mismanagement, can be personally liable (see also Chapter 21). A charity should aim to appoint trustees who collectively have a breadth of skills and experience; veterinary surgeons (veterinarians) are often asked to act as trustees for charities, which may or may not be directly involved with animal welfare.

A veterinary surgeon acting as a trustee will have the same responsibilities to the charity as any other trustee, in addition to providing professional advice and support. A veterinary trustee may be required to advise or even arbitrate in the event that there is a conflict or disagreement between the charity and another veterinary surgeon.

Veterinary trustees can be very useful to an animal charity, as they have the knowledge and expertise to provide guidance on a range of veterinary and animal welfare matters. They must also be mindful of their responsibilities as a trustee and bear in mind that it is the trustees who lead the charity and decide how it is run. Trustees should take an active interest in their charity; indeed, a 'hands-off' approach may be in danger of becoming 'neglect'.

Purpose of the charity

The 'advancement of animal welfare', as defined in UK law, includes any purpose directed towards the prevention or suppression of cruelty to animals, or the prevention or relief of suffering by animals. Examples of the types of charities and charitable purposes falling within this description include:

* Those promoting kindness and/or preventing cruelty to animals
* Those offering advice and education on animal welfare matters
* The provision of veterinary care and treatment
* The care and rehoming of animals that are abandoned, mistreated or lost
* Feral animal control, e.g. via trap/catch-neuter-return programmes
* Some research and grant-awarding bodies linked to animal welfare
* Those promoting and strengthening the human–animal bond.

Many charities include more than one of these in their charitable objects (i.e. the formally set out purposes of the organization).

Shelters

There are currently no specific licensing requirements for animal rescue centres; however, they may need to be licensed or registered as a boarding establishment or even as a pet vending establishment, both of which are covered by specific legislation and are regulated by Trading Standards. All establishments where animals are kept are covered by the Animal Welfare Act 2006, although regulation and enforcement can be sporadic, and inspection may take place only in response to a complaint. This is often to the detriment of animal welfare, particularly in the case of very small 'rescues', which in some cases verge on animal hoarding (see QRG 23.1). Some of these smaller charities also blur the lines of what is considered charitable, and may in fact simply be keeping homeless but healthy animals or, at least, animals that start out healthy (Figure 20.1).

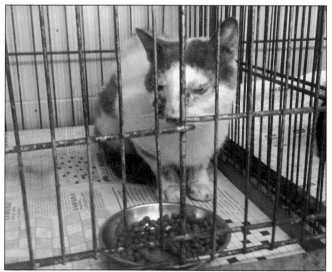

20.1 This cat's welfare has been compromised by being taken into the care of a no-kill organization with limited resources.
(© Cats Protection)

Veterinary care in the shelter

Where veterinary care for an animal rescue centre is provided on site by employed staff, the shelter needs to be registered and inspected as practice premises, regardless of whether veterinary services are offered to the public. If veterinary medicines are delivered and stored on site, then this part of the centre will be inspected by the Veterinary Medicines Directorate to ensure compliance with current legislation regarding the supply, use and disposal of veterinary medicinal products (VMPs), even if the veterinary work is carried out by veterinary surgeons from an external practice. This is not the case if the shelter is a client of a veterinary practice where services are provided off site only (or even with some on-site visits), as long as the only VMPs on site are prophylactic treatments such as parasiticides that have been prescribed by the attending veterinary surgeon (rather than being stored on site before prescription) and there is no delivery of pharmaceutical products to the site.

Veterinary care to the general public

Charities that provide veterinary care direct to the public in charity clinics (as opposed to those offering monetary contributions towards veterinary care carried out elsewhere, e.g. at a private veterinary practice) need to be registered as practice premises in the same way as any other veterinary practice. Veterinary care must be provided only by veterinary surgeons who are on the register of the Royal College of Veterinary Surgeons (RCVS), in accordance with the Veterinary Surgeons Act 1966. The range of services offered should be clearly set out and this information must include how emergency treatment can be accessed, particularly outside the times when the clinic normally operates.

Policies

Clearly defined policies are essential in any well managed charity to ensure transparency and consistency. This is particularly important in animal charities, where there may be many varied and strongly held views around animal welfare. Clear policies mean that staff, volunteers, supporters and donors are aware of the charity's position on fundamental issues and how its funds are being used. It is helpful to explain why decisions on polices have been made, particularly in relation to controversial issues. This assists in managing expectations and individuals can then make an informed choice as to whether they want to be associated with, or donate to, the organization.

The general ethos of the charity will often inform its policy-making. If the charity has a utilitarian ethos, aiming to help as many animals as possible with the resources available, its policies are likely to look different from those of an organization with a stance directed more towards 'animal rights', where the rights of the individual animal are considered most important (see Chapter 2 and QRG 5.2). However, the overarching principle for any such charity should be that animal welfare comes first, and it is important that human emotions and publicity-seeking do not override this fundamental point.

It is important for the charity to be open about its policies, even if they are contentious, and it can be helpful to summarize them in publications or on the organization's website.

Areas where it is important to have a defined policy

This chapter is not designed to dictate policy to any organization and the list that follows is not exhaustive. However, the list is provided to assist the many veterinary surgeons who may become involved in animal welfare policy development. Other policies, such as those on health and safety, are relevant but beyond the scope of this manual.

Euthanasia

A euthanasia policy is probably the most essential and contentious policy for any animal welfare organization. It is often viewed as straightforward by lay people but in reality it is much more complex. The euthanasia policy is inevitably linked to the intake policy; it will affect which type of supporters align themselves to the organization and may affect fundraising, as well as the welfare of the animals (see Chapter 2). Various possible euthanasia policy options are as follows.

Total non-euthanasia ('no-kill')

It is unrealistic – and might be considered unethical – to have a policy whereby no animals are euthanased in any circumstances. In practical terms, this could be achieved only if intake was highly selective and only animals that had been thoroughly assessed and deemed 'fit to rehome' were admitted. This may lead to poor welfare or animals being confined for excessive periods of time. A 'no-kill' policy may appeal to some supporters and could be used positively for fundraising. However, this may be at the price of animal welfare, as any animals with physical or mental conditions that cannot be resolved adequately may be left to live in pain or distress. Realistically, this is not feasible in the sanctuary situation, where animals receive lifelong care, without contravening the Animal Welfare Acts 2006 (in the UK) or equivalent legislation in other jurisdictions.

Euthanasia on veterinary advice only/no healthy animal is euthanased

Many animal lovers are appalled by the idea of healthy animals being euthanased, but understand that if an animal is suffering, euthanasia should be an option on welfare grounds. This approach should avoid animals with poor quality of life being kept alive and suffering. What may become challenging, though, is how 'healthy' is defined. Is, for example, an animal that is physically well but has severe behavioural problems 'healthy'? Using the phrase 'on veterinary advice' in the policy enables the veterinary surgeon to make a professional judgement on a case-by-case basis. This may be clear cut with completely healthy or very sick animals. With advances in veterinary medicine, there are many conditions that can be successfully treated or managed, but this may not always be feasible in the shelter setting.

This option can result in healthy animals being confined for extensive lengths of time, which may have a negative impact on their welfare. Intake will necessarily be limited to when space becomes available through rehoming or euthanasia. It may be necessary for the policy to highlight certain medical conditions that may warrant euthanasia due, for example, to severity, threat to other animals, availability of isolation facilities, zoonotic potential, cost of treatment, or likelihood of the animal being rehomed.

Euthanasia based on time spent in the facility

In some shelters, animals may be euthanased if they are not rehomed within a certain time period or due to pressure of space. If there is an open intake policy, animals may have to be euthanased to make room for more. The alternative is overcrowding and the inevitable outbreak of infectious disease, which may well depopulate a centre in what most people would consider a less humane way. This euthanasia policy may be unpopular with supporters and staff, but does increase the turnover of animals and, thus, the number of animals that can be helped, and avoids long-term confinement of individuals.

Euthanasia of animals that are sick but could be treated

Sometimes euthanasia is used as a form of disease control. For example, in cases of 'cat 'flu' or ringworm, attempts could be made to treat a sick individual but the highly infectious nature of the disease puts many other animals at risk; in a situation where the shelter does not have the facilities or resources to isolate and treat such cases, euthanasia is opted for. This may come under the umbrella of euthanasia on veterinary advice.

Sanctuary or rehoming?

The outcome for animals that come into the care of a shelter may be rehoming or staying in residence permanently, especially if deemed 'unhomeable' (e.g. disabled animals, feral cats or farm species). Providing lifelong sanctuary restricts the number of animals that can be assisted and may not achieve the maximum welfare for the resources available or meet the objectives of the organization. The needs of the animals may not be met, especially if there are many animals being cared for and space and funds are limited. If there is reluctance to euthanase animals, this could result in animals living with poor quality of life; some people would argue that if an animal is not fit to be rehomed, euthanasia should be considered. Keeping healthy animals in a sanctuary is not considered a charitable activity by the Charity Commission and related bodies, and care must be taken to avoid public funds being used to pay for what are, in effect, people's pets.

Which species?

The policy on which species will be admitted should be based on the available facilities, expertise and funding. Exotic species are particularly prone to husbandry-related problems due to the keepers' ignorance, and specialist knowledge is needed to care for these more uncommon pets. There may be certain types of animals that are not accepted due to their size, temperament or legal status. Breeds of dog banned under the Dangerous Dogs Act 1991 cannot usually be rehomed and so are rarely accepted by most organizations. Wolf or wildcat hybrids may be more difficult to keep or rehome safely, unless an adopter with suitable expertise can be found, and a Dangerous Wild Animals licence may be required depending on the generation cross (see Chapter 21). If the charitable objects state that only specific species are helped, the charity's funds cannot be spent on other species.

Intake

There is a close link between the intake and euthanasia policies. Each shelter will have a maximum capacity; overcrowding of animals results in many negative welfare outcomes and should be avoided. Many charities have found that 'bigger is not necessarily better', and a small centre with a high turnover of animals is often the most effective model in terms of the number of animals rehomed, disease control and the welfare of the individuals in care. There are far more animals in need than the capacity of UK shelters (see Chapters 4 and 6), so the intake policy may include issues such as whether to have a waiting list and how intake is prioritized (e.g. do strays have priority over animals that their owners wish to relinquish?). Some shelters may opt to have a contract with the local authority for taking stray dogs for the statutory holding period for a prearranged fee, in which case these dogs may take priority over those being relinquished by owners. It may be helpful to provide other support for animals on the waiting list for intake, such as assisting owners with getting their animals neutered or finding alternatives to relinquishment.

There may be limits or quotas on the intake of animals with significant health or behavioural problems, because of their welfare in the shelter and likelihood of being rehomed. Likewise, in order to maximize rehoming, it may be necessary to consider limiting the number of certain breeds of dog that may be commonly relinquished or over-bred (e.g. bull breeds), or types or colours – for example, black and black-and-white cats (Figure 20.2) take significantly longer to rehome than those of other, 'more desirable' colours. As younger animals tend to be rehomed more readily than older ones, there may be a selective approach to the age of animals taken in. Some centres have developed 'traffic light' systems to assess the likelihood of an animal being rehomed promptly, to ensure that precious pen/kennel space is not blocked by hard-to-home animals.

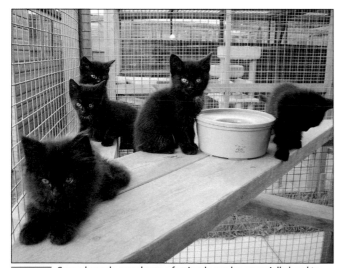

20.2 Some breeds or colours of animals can be especially hard to rehome; there are many reasons for this, including oversupply and/or superstition. It can be prudent to avoid having a high proportion of similar animals available for rehoming.
(© Cats Protection)

Legally or illegally imported animals

Some organizations actively promote the 'rescue' and importation of animals into other countries, including the UK, for rehoming. Factors to be considered in pursuing this strategy are the cost, the stress of transportation and the potential difficulties animals may experience in adjusting to the unfamiliar environment. Thousands of unwanted animals are euthanased annually in the UK,

and adding to the burden of 'unwanted' animals could be considered irresponsible. Imported animals may be carrying exotic or zoonotic diseases, which can be a significant problem both for the individual and for the naive UK population that may be more seriously affected by such an infection (see QRG 16.2). If imported animals are accepted they should be screened for exotic diseases, ideally before travel.

Increasingly, charities are faced with strays with foreign microchips implanted or animals that have been found in suspicious circumstances, such as in a foreign lorry. If a suspected illegal entry is found, Trading Standards should be contacted, but, as they may not give decisive direction, it is also important for the shelter to have a policy to ensure the safety of staff and adopters in such circumstances; this may include the requirement for rabies vaccination (see Chapter 21). Putting animals through quarantine or treating them so they are compliant with travel regulations under the Pet Travel Scheme (PETS) is expensive, so may not be the best use of the charity's funds. Depending on which countries animals are being moved from and to, they may need microchipping, rabies vaccination, rabies antibody testing, specific parasite control, screening tests and veterinary certification. The additional cost of transportation and (in some cases) quarantine can mean spending several thousand pounds on one animal that could instead be used locally to help a greater number of animals.

Relinquishment/strays

There are many reasons for relinquishment of an animal, including the health or circumstances of the owner, and perceived problems with the animal, such as chronic illness or behavioural problems.

It is a sensible precaution to have official paperwork completed for every animal admitted to the shelter. Owners relinquishing their pets can sign over ownership, enabling the rehoming process to begin immediately, and may be requested to have the animal health checked and vaccinated and/or pay a fee to the shelter to cover the cost of such veterinary care. As much information about the animal should be gathered as possible, including its medical history, to aid in its management and the process of matching it with a new owner. With a stray animal, it is useful to know where and when it was found, and to record the finder's details.

In some cases, where there are alternatives to relinquishment, education or support to the owner may be offered, for instance, when pregnant women have been made fearful about toxoplasmosis and initially approach the shelter seeking to relinquish their cat.

With stray dogs, there is legislation that dictates the length of time they must be held before rehoming or euthanasia. This is not the case with cats, as they are deemed property in law and, therefore, remain the property of the original owner, so each charity must decide what seems to be a reasonable holding period and how much treatment or preventive care is undertaken and at what stage. Most charities hold cats for a period before offering them for rehoming. Keeping detailed records is useful, especially if euthanasing an animal that may have an owner. Notes should be taken of the efforts made to locate the owner, such as the use of a paper collar before the animal is taken into the shelter, and advertising it as having been found. Every animal should be thoroughly scanned for a microchip on entry.

Veterinary care

Assessment on entry

A veterinary health check is advisable at or soon after admission. Some centres use an initial assessment by a member of staff to pick up urgent issues, followed by the veterinary assessment within the first few days. Observation records should be kept to monitor animals' demeanour, eating, toileting etc. A behavioural assessment is also important. Animals are often initially stressed, so it is worth giving them time to adjust and/or conducting multiple assessments. It is important to bear in mind that animals rarely behave the same way in the shelter as in a home environment.

Disclosure of health status

For the sake of transparency and the charity's reputation, it is important that potential adopters are made aware of any previous or ongoing health problems the animal has, what treatment (including preventive treatment) it has received and whether it is likely that there will be any recurrent problems. Sometimes a period of free insurance is offered to adopters, and it should be explained that any previous or ongoing conditions will not be covered by this insurance. The information can be provided as a copy of the medical record or a summary of this in lay terms. It can be helpful to have a disclaimer for adopters to sign to acknowledge that they have read the history and understand that it is not a guarantee that the animal is disease free.

Preventative care

The policy on what preventive regime is followed will be dictated by the shelter's financial resources, the local prevalence of infectious diseases and parasites, the health status of the animals coming into care and whether animals are kept singly or in groups (see Chapter 11). Most responsible animal charities would consider a veterinary health check, neutering, vaccination and parasite control to be the minimum requirement. Microchipping is compulsory for dogs but chipping and a limited period of free insurance may also be part of the 'package' and can be used to promote rehoming of a rescue animal.

Neutering

It is widely accepted by the majority of shelters that animals in their care should be neutered. However, a neutering policy is needed to provide clarity on the following issues:

- Minimum age of neutering
- Are all animals neutered before rehoming? If not, why not (e.g. age, stage of the oestrus cycle in a bitch, etc.)?
- Does the charity pay for animals to be neutered at a private practice after rehoming or returned to the shelter for neutering?
- Are pregnant animals neutered and, if so, at what stage of gestation?
- What happens if it is not clear whether an animal is already neutered – are the adopters advised to watch the animal closely for behavioural signs, or is the animal investigated via shaving to look for a scar, blood tests or exploratory surgery?
- What happens if an animal is rehomed as neutered but then gives birth? Does the charity pay for exploratory surgery and/or pay for the cost of the litter?

- Is there a policy regarding the procedure itself, e.g. flank or midline approach for ovariohysterectomy, choice of suture material, etc.?
- Are animals identified as neutered by, for example, microchipping or ear-tipping? (see Chapters 5 and 6).

Screening for disease

The shelter's policy on screening for specific diseases will depend on the local prevalence, infectivity, mortality and zoonotic potential of the disease, the risk factors in the individual animal and the accuracy of the available test(s). Transparency on which common diseases have and have not been tested for is crucial. Adopters' expectations can sometimes be unrealistic, as it is not financially viable to screen for every disease for which there is a test; however, in some circumstances it may be possible to offer specific testing, if the adopter is prepared to contribute towards the cost. Potential adopters should be informed of the test results and given guidance on their implications (see Chapter 8).

Realistically, there is no point in screening for diseases if the results are not acted upon. Will animals that test positive be euthanased, treated or rehomed with special conditions or ongoing support? If repeat testing is ideal (e.g. with healthy cats that test positive for feline leukaemia virus), are the animals held and retested or are the initial results acted upon? With several of the currently available in-house testing kits, confirmation of results by an external laboratory may be considered, especially if the outcome may be euthanasia. The decision will often depend on the charity's funds and capacity for holding animals, and whether the individual tolerates confinement.

Control of specific diseases

Most disease issues will be dealt with via protocols or guidelines rather than policies, as each case or outbreak will be different. Examples include outbreaks of parvovirus in dogs (see Chapter 12) or upper respiratory tract disease in cats (see Chapter 15). There may be some diseases where specific policies are needed, especially for infectious diseases with zoonotic potential (see QRG 16.1), such as *Mycobacterium* species or meticillin-resistant *Staphylococcus aureus* infection, or those that will make finding a home more challenging, such as diabetes mellitus. The choice is often whether to treat and rehome or euthanase the animal. Any suspected notifiable disease, such as rabies or *Mycobacterium bovis* infection, must be reported in the routine manner.

How far to pursue treatment

This is a difficult policy to make. It may be better dealt with as guidance rather than a rigid policy, as each case is different but some issues are clearer cut (see Chapter 3). Some conditions may not be treated at all and the animals may be euthanased; for example, most organizations would not rehome an animal with a mycobacterial infection due to its zoonotic potential, the difficulty, duration and cost of both diagnosis of the species of mycobacterium and treatment, the welfare implications of confining the animal for several months and the fact that the animal may never be clear of infection. There may be a maximum budget that is available to spend on each animal, or a policy whereby special permission must be sought to spend beyond this amount. The prognosis and potential for rehoming are crucial considerations. Certain drugs or treatments may not be sanctioned for use due to their cost or limited efficacy (e.g. chemotherapy, interferons). Where there are cost-effective alternatives to 'gold standard' medicine that achieve good welfare outcomes, their use may be encouraged – for example, amputation rather than extensive orthopaedic surgery in an animal with a complex limb fracture.

Dental treatment

Dental treatment can be an area of controversy. If there is significant dental pathology, therapeutic treatment is essential on welfare grounds, but where only a prophylactic descale and polish is warranted, consideration needs to be given to cost and the added stress of a non-essential anaesthetic. Once the level of dental care given is established, it is helpful to state this on homing paperwork to enable professional communication with the adopter's veterinary surgeon.

Treatment of geriatric animals

Special consideration needs to be given to how much treatment and monitoring is provided for geriatric animals, particularly in view of the chronic nature of the common diseases of this population. The prognosis, life expectancy and likelihood of rehoming need to be considered. It can be helpful to use standard systems, such as the International Renal Interest Society (IRIS) staging for renal disease to help guide policy development (see also QRGs 3.1 and 3.2).

Payment for treatment of ongoing conditions

Charities should decide whether they will pay for the treatment of ongoing conditions after adoption and, if so, in what circumstances. This can help with rehoming more challenging cases, such as animals with diabetes, but also runs the risk that the charity will make financial commitments that may be difficult to honour. Any arrangements should be clarified in writing, including what will and will not be paid for, whether prior authorization is necessary and whether a specific veterinary practice should be used.

Behaviour/aggression/feral animals

Any behavioural issues should be declared to potential adopters, with provision of adequate advice and support. Some behavioural problems resolve once the animal is settled in a home environment. Rehoming animals that show aggressive behaviour must be done with great care, as extremely negative publicity arises from an incident; alternatives, such as euthanasia, may be appropriate for such animals (see Figure 20.3 and Chapter 19).

Feral or street animals will not adjust to a normal home environment or confinement, so for such animals it is always advisable to have a policy of trap/catch-neuter-return to the original site. Re-siting can work but is challenging and less than ideal in welfare terms. The policy should include insisting on some form of marking, such as ear-tipping, to identify neutered animals. If funds allow, vaccination, parasite control and minor treatments may also be considered (see Chapter 5).

Rehoming

Shelters need to find suitable permanent homes for animals, but there are various ways to achieve this.

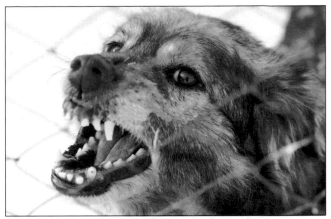

20.3 Homing an aggressive dog must be done with great care. (Stock image from www.dreamstime.com)

Information needs to be gathered from both the original and prospective owners to enable good matching of the animal to a new owner and to meet that owner's expectations. Often this is done via questionnaires and interviews, and the internet is a useful tool to aid matching. Home visits can be controversial; some shelters feel that they are essential, and others consider them to be a barrier. Anecdotally, there is no evidence that home checks result in more successful rehoming, and they can deter some adopters who see them as intrusive. If people are refused an animal, they tend to obtain one from another source (e.g. another shelter, or commercially), so it is often better to rehome a suitable animal to them and provide plenty of guidance and information.

Most rehoming policies are based around risks such as accidents or escape; they should not discriminate against adopters on the grounds of race, religion, sexual orientation, etc. Common policies consider issues of location, especially proximity to busy roads, the age of resident children and outdoor access. Often there is no evidence to back up homing policies, and on the whole, common sense and good matching of pet and adopter are the best tools.

It is important to provide information and advice when rehoming animals, even to experienced owners; this may be in the form of verbal advice or written material. Integration of the pet into the household is particularly important, especially if there are other pets already resident. Follow-up calls to check how the pet is settling into its new home and provide further advice, if necessary, may also be useful.

'Home-to-home' rehoming schemes

Some organizations will rehome animals directly from the relinquishing owner's home to the new owner. This has the advantage of not taking up valuable space in the shelter, being less stressful for the pet and reducing the risk of infectious disease. There can also be disadvantages, such as staff not being able to assess the health or temperament of the animal adequately and, therefore, match the pet and the new owner, or the relinquisher refusing to hand over the pet to someone they do not like or think unsuitable.

There are several different models that can be used, which vary in how much the shelter is involved with the procedures to get the animal ready for rehoming and matching and/or vetting prospective adopters. Any charity involved in this type of scheme should be clear in its policy about the level of involvement – and, therefore, responsibility – it has. The most common models are:

- Matching agency – owners and potential adopters are simply put in contact with each other and then make all the arrangements for seeing and handing over the animal themselves. This then is not the responsibility of the shelter, even if things go wrong; normally the shelter's paperwork is not used, and there is no fee or only a small donation is requested
- Full health check and preventive care, as for animals homed from a shelter's rehoming centre – the animal goes through the standard pre-homing procedures, such as the health check, neutering, vaccination and behavioural assessments, which are usually paid for by the shelter. Conventional matching procedures are followed and the animal is rehomed as an 'official' adoption with full paperwork and all that entails. Sometimes the rehoming itself takes place at the shelter so the new owner does not meet the original one.

There are many variations and hybrids of these models; whichever is chosen, it is important to be clear with the new owner how much responsibility the shelter has for the rehoming, particularly if problems arise.

Fees/donations

Most charities ask for a financial contribution when animals are adopted or relinquished, or when veterinary treatment is provided. This can be in the form of a voluntary donation to help the charity continue with its work; it cannot be classed as a donation for the animal or the treatment itself, as this should be freely given without the charity receiving anything in return. In the UK, Gift Aid can be claimed on genuine donations. If a fee is charged for adoption, the animals are classified as second-hand goods; this classification is based on case law after Gables Farm Dogs and Cats Home went to a Value Added Tax (VAT) tribunal in 2008. Some supporters are uncomfortable with this view, but in the UK this means that the 'sale' of animals from a shelter is zero-rated for VAT, and this allows the VAT to be reclaimed on purchases made to prepare the animal for rehoming. The fees policy may also include exceptions, for instance, reduced rates for disabled or elderly people, or different prices for different animals (see Chapter 21 for further information).

Paperwork and records

Good record-keeping facilitates animal management and is also useful for monitoring, audit and research purposes (see Chapter 7). Increasingly, records are computerized, which aids reporting, especially for organizations that have more than one site. The exact nature of what information is recorded and how long it is retained should be clearly defined. Records containing personal information must be kept in compliance with the General Data Protection Regulation (Regulation (EU) 2016/679).

Payment of private veterinary fees

Shelters may be asked to cover the cost of veterinary fees for owned animals. This may be outside the objectives of the organization; however, it is worth having a list of local charities that do this, to be able to give some assistance to enquirers. Assistance with veterinary fees may be provided in specific circumstances, such as for owners on a very low income or where the only other alternative is relinquishment of the animal. As this can be financially draining, it is important to have controls in place, such as a maximum contribution per case and/or a strict budget that is adhered to.

Ethical policy

Many charities have an ethical policy that states the types of companies, organizations or industries the charity will (or will not) be associated with. This usually covers accepting donations, investments, corporate partnerships and research projects (see below). As many companies, particularly larger ones, are owned by other multinational conglomerates, the policy should include whether parent or associate companies are included in any restrictions. Having an ethical policy helps to achieve clarity on associations with other organizations, especially if supporters question certain decisions that have been made.

Research projects

As shelters have significant numbers of animals, they can be in demand for involvement in research projects. This can be controversial; shelters are a good source of epidemiological information, but there may be negative repercussions if staff or supporters perceive that animals are being 'experimented' upon. Research projects should be ethically approved by a recognized body and within the law. In addition, some research requires a licence under the Animals (Scientific Procedures) Act 1986. The types of research that may be undertaken (e.g. observational or invasive) and how proposed projects are assessed should be clarified, particularly from an ethical, animal welfare and practical point of view. If a shelter does decide to become involved with a project, a written agreement with the researcher(s) is important, especially in respect of confidentiality and the ownership and control of data arising from the research.

Clinical services

Some charities offer subsidized or free veterinary treatment for animals owned by members of the public. Here, clear policies are equally important for the benefit of both clients and staff. These should set out the services offered, which pet owners are eligible to receive treatment (usually on grounds of low income or receipt of certain state benefits), which species and breeds will be treated, limits to the numbers of animals owned by one person that may be registered, the geographical area covered by the service, how out-of-hours emergencies will be covered and any other specific restrictions. Overriding this policy is the requirement to provide first aid treatment for any animal presented in an emergency. The details of these policies may be set out in a Scope of Service document, and all clinical staff should fully understand and adhere to its contents to ensure that the charity's funds are used responsibly. The scope of service should be evidence-based, but not be so restrictive as to interfere with an individual veterinary surgeon's clinical judgement.

It is also good practice to set out these policies clearly in the form of a client agreement, and to take time with each client at the point of registration to go through this agreement with them and have them sign a copy confirming that they understand the terms and conditions for receipt of veterinary care. This should reduce (although is unlikely to eliminate) conflict when a client presents an animal in circumstances that fall outside the agreement. The client agreement may include other conditions such as client behaviour and making regular payments, and should also make reference to the consequences of abusing the service, for example, banning a client from the premises for aggressive behaviour.

Targets and key performance indicators

Targets and key performance indicators can be useful in monitoring the success of a shelter in achieving its objectives; however, they should be used with caution. It is very easy to become target-driven, and to lose sight of the welfare of the animals being cared for (see Chapter 7 for further details of the use of shelter metrics).

If a charity becomes too focused on targets, there may be unintended consequences. For example, the average length of stay of animals in an adoption centre may become an issue. If a small minority of animals in the care of a charity are kennelled for such long periods of time that their welfare is considered to be compromised, the charity's response may be to make 'length of stay' a key performance indicator and to set a target maximum. The result of trying to reduce the length of stay and keep within the target maximum may be an increase in the number (and proportion) of animals that are euthanased.

When introducing key performance indicators and targets, it is important to be clear about their purpose and their limitations. Key performance indicators are a useful management tool insofar as they can be used to compare the performance of different sites (for a multi-site organization) or the year-on-year performance of a single site. They can highlight specific issues quickly and enable prompt intervention, and are also very useful for benchmarking against the performance of other comparable charities and the sector as a whole (Figure 20.4).

Targets can be positive if they are used as a 'carrot' and not a 'stick'; indeed, a bit of healthy competition can improve the overall morale and performance of staff and volunteers. However, there is a danger that they can be perceived by workers in a very negative way, especially if unrealistic targets are set. When setting targets, it is important to consult with the frontline staff, because they know their rehoming centre or scheme better than anyone and should know what is realistically achievable. It is also sensible not to set a target that is hugely different from current performance unless something substantial has changed to make the target feasible, for example, the opening of a new kennel block.

The list of useful key performance indicators set out in Figure 20.4 is by no means exhaustive, and the types of data that are reported as key performance indicators, which are used for internal research, may change depending on circumstances. For example, looking at intake, it may be of interest periodically to look at the reasons why people relinquish their animals to a shelter, but the key performance indicator may simply be the proportion of animals relinquished compared with those from other sources.

It is crucial that the charity does not lose sight of the underlying principle of animal welfare. For example, some people may have the view that a euthanasia rate of 0% is a desirable target; however, this may lead to serious compromise of animal welfare by, for example, prolonging suffering in a sick animal or causing overcrowding. Conversely, while some people may not consider euthanasia to be a welfare issue, since a dead animal can no longer have compromised welfare, some colleagues, volunteers, supporters and the general public may take a different view if the euthanasia rate is high.

People working with charities

The kind of people involved with an animal welfare charity can influence the ethos of that charity. Generally, they will all care about animals, but increasingly fewer have a background in animal welfare or even with animals (except possibly as pet owners), particularly at management level in larger organizations. With some (particularly larger) organizations' emphasis on being more 'business-like', and a trend towards emulating the commercial sector, it is easy to lose sight of animal welfare. There is also a danger that senior managers who have never worked 'at the coalface' may lack an understanding of the real challenges faced by the staff and volunteers working directly with the animals on a daily basis. At the other extreme, some people may have a 'rose-tinted' perspective and want to save every animal – again, at the expense of welfare in some cases. It is better to educate supporters and staff about these issues rather than to keep them happy to the detriment of animal welfare.

Veterinary professionals and charities

Charities can range from small local shelters, often run by a small group of volunteers with a shared passion, to large national organizations employing hundreds of staff, including veterinary professionals. Just as there is a wide spectrum of scale and structure for animal welfare charities, so there is a corresponding range in the level of involvement of veterinary professionals, from seeing the occasional welfare case in a general practice through to being directly employed as a full-time veterinary surgeon or nurse (Figure 20.5). The relationship may be paid or unpaid, and may be formal or on an ad-hoc basis. The responsibilities of the veterinary surgeon/team will depend on the nature of the relationship between them and the charity (see Chapter 22).

Whatever the level of involvement of the veterinary professional, there is often a need to balance professional responsibilities with the needs of the charity. A pragmatic

- Number of animals taken into the care of the charity and their source
  - Total intake
  - Stray and abandoned animals
  - Relinquished by owner
    - Reasons for relinquishment
  - Transfer from dog warden/local authority kennels
  - Transfer from other charity
  - Seized by authorities (welfare cases)
  - Transfer from another site within the same charity
- Number of animals rehomed
- Average length of stay
  - Total length of stay
  - Time to prepare for rehoming
  - Time to adoption once made available for rehoming
- Animals returned to the charity (unsuccessful rehoming)
  - Reasons for return
  - Time between rehoming and return
- Euthanasia figures
  - Total number euthanased
  - Proportion of intake euthanased
  - Reasons for euthanasia
- Neutering figures
  - Breakdown by species, sex, age
- Vaccination figures
  - Breakdown by species
- Number of cases of specific diseases (usually infectious)

20.4 Examples of useful key performance indicators (KPIs) that can inform and support management decisions in an animal shelter. Care must be taken not to base management decisions solely on KPIs, but to use them in the context of the bigger picture.

Unpaid (voluntary and *pro bono* work)
• Trustee
• Clinical
• In a shelter
• In a veterinary clinic
• Specific projects (e.g. trap-neuter-return programme)
• Advisory
• Training
• Providing occasional care for welfare cases and wildlife casualties
Paid
• Employed directly by a charity
• As a clinician
• Management role, advising on welfare, policy, education material, training, etc.
• Contracted to a charity
• The practice or individual has a contract to supply specific services to a charity such as:
– Neutering/routine veterinary care
– Out of hours
– Arrangement to see all welfare cases
– Seeing client-owned animals on behalf of a charity under a specific, contracted scheme (e.g. PetAid Practices)
• Accepting neutering vouchers
• Occasional work when an individual case is brought in
• Working with other agencies, e.g. the police

20.5 There are many ways in which veterinary professionals can be involved with charities. A veterinary surgeon may work for more than one charity, and have different relationships with each individual charity. For example, a practice may be contracted to do all the preventive work for one shelter, but to provide emergency treatment for another.

approach is required, but professional responsibilities and adherence to the RCVS Code of Professional Conduct must trump the charity's needs where there is a direct conflict, or the veterinary surgeon may be at risk of a complaint to the RCVS and, subsequently, its disciplinary process. It is prudent to have suitable professional indemnity insurance, even if the relationship with the charity is only advisory, in the event of a complaint either from the charity or from a member of the public.

Charities directly employing veterinary surgeons

The management structure should reflect the way in which veterinary professionals are used by the charity. Any charity that directly employs veterinary surgeons who provide clinical services should appoint a senior veterinary surgeon at director (or equivalent) status, as set out in the Guidance Notes to the RCVS Code of Professional Conduct for Veterinary Surgeons (updated August 2016). This appointee has overall responsibility for professional matters within the organization. The RCVS has no power to enforce this with the charity; however, where a charity does not comply, veterinary trustees may be held accountable in the event of a complaint regarding a charity policy that impinges on professional conduct – for example, a policy whereby veterinary treatment may be withheld or refused in certain circumstances, such as if an animal is

of a specific breed or has been bred for financial gain. The presence of a veterinary surgeon on the senior management team protects both the charity and any other veterinary surgeons directly employed by the charity. In charities where there is no veterinary director, there is often a tendency for employed veterinary surgeons to practise defensive medicine because they do not have a senior colleague to support their decisions. This can be costly for the charity, insofar as Schedule 3 procedures are not delegated to veterinary nurses, and unnecessary diagnostic tests are likely to be performed because the veterinary surgeon is concerned that the charity's management will not have the necessary knowledge or professional standing to support them. There can also be emotional pressure placed on the veterinary surgeon by staff or volunteers to pursue expensive or futile treatment of an animal because they have formed a deep emotional attachment to it.

Charities as clients

Where the charity is a client of a private veterinary practice, the practice should have a clear understanding of the charity's policies and, likewise, the charity should have an understanding of the responsibilities of the veterinary surgeon both to the charity and in terms of professional standards. To this end, a written agreement setting out the mutual expectations, agreed and signed by both parties, can be helpful. Such a service level agreement should include what services will be provided by the practice, where and when they will be provided, what provision there will be for emergencies and a fee structure (see Chapter 22).

References and further reading

Moynihan A (2015) *The Good Trustee Guide, 6th edn*. National Council of Voluntary Organisations, London

Useful websites

National Council of Voluntary Organisations: www.ncvo.org.uk/

Charity Commission for England and Wales: www.gov.uk/government/organisations/charity-commission

Scottish Charity Regulator: www.oscr.org.uk/

Charity Commission for Northern Ireland: www.charitycommissionni.org.uk/

Charity Governance Code: www.charitygovernancecode.org/en/

RCVS Code of Professional Conduct for Veterinary Surgeons: www.rcvs.org.uk/advice-and-guidance/code-of-professional-conduct-for-veterinary-surgeons/

Animal & Plant Health Agency (Pet Travel Scheme guidance): http://ahvla.defra.gov.uk/External_OV_Instructions/Export_Instructions/Certification_Procedures/Small_Animal_Exports/index.htm

VAT Tribunal Case V20519: Gables Farm Dogs and Cats Home *versus* HMRC 04/01/2008: http://financeandtax.decisions.tribunals.gov.uk//Aspx/view.aspx?id=3683

Chapter 21

Law and shelter medicine

Dominic Sullivan and Trevor Cooper

This chapter and QRGs 21.1 and 21.2 reflect the legal framework within which companion animal welfare organizations operate in the UK. At the time of writing, the UK is still part of the European Union. Veterinary surgeons (veterinarians) working outside the UK should refer to local legislation.

Framework and statutory purpose

Companion animal welfare organizations vary in size and structure. Many will be **registered** charities: depending on where they operate, these organizations will be registered with and regulated by the Charity Commission in England and Wales, the Office of the Scottish Charity Regulator or the Charity Commission for Northern Ireland, and will be established for the statutory purpose of advancing animal welfare. The charitable **objects** of each organization describe the purpose for which the charity is established in more detail and give an indication of the way in which the organization works to advance animal welfare.

There is an annual income limit below which it is not possible to register as a registered charity, and so smaller organizations operate outside this regulation (see Chapter 20).

Who is the client?

When a veterinary surgeon is instructed by a charity, the client will, ultimately, be the trustees of the charity in question. Trustees are legally responsible for directing the affairs of charities. They have to maintain control of charitable funds but are also subject to a legal and regulatory duty to use these funds reasonably and only in furtherance of the charity's objects. This is sometimes known as the **duty of prudence**.

All animal welfare charities, large and small, have to balance their resources and generally want to be able to help as many animals as possible. It can be difficult for all concerned to get the balance right between the treatment of an individual animal and the treatment of as many animals as possible, and such decisions can be highly emotive (see Chapter 3).

Charities with branches

Some of the larger companion animal welfare charities have branches throughout the country, which are often run by local volunteers. There are two main types of branch structure:

- **Federated** – local branches are separate legal entities from the national charity. They will be registered charities in their own right and will operate under the umbrella of the national charity. In these cases, the clients are likely to be the trustees of the local registered charity
- **Unfederated** – local branches are not separate legal entities from the national charity. They are governed by the constitution of the national charity and act on delegated authority from the trustees of the national charity. In these cases, the clients are the trustees of the national charity; the local branch acts with delegated authority to enter into contracts for veterinary services on behalf of the charity.

In either case, veterinary treatment is paid for out of charitable funds, and branches are generally subject to national policies, procedures and guidelines issued by the national charity. These policies are aimed at ensuring the welfare of all animals in a charity's care and are also designed to protect the charity's trustees, staff and volunteers from criminal liability for breach of the duty of care imposed upon them by the UK Animal Welfare Acts (discussed later in this chapter).

If it is unclear who the client is, or if confirmation is necessary that a local representative has authority, it is advisable to have a contact within the organization who can clarify such issues. When animals are signed over to charities, the charities acquire ownership. Authority to provide consent for veterinary treatment is generally delegated by the trustees of charities to local staff and volunteers, but it is nonetheless important to make sure that the person instructing the veterinary surgeon has the requisite authority to do so, and the authority, when appropriate, to sign consent forms for specific procedures.

Clinical records

Owners who relinquish their pet to a charity should be asked to sign an acceptance form, which confirms that ownership of the animal passes to the charity. Owners are generally asked to disclose details of their veterinary practice and any existing health issues the animal has. However, these details are not always forthcoming, and even if they are, the original owner must give permission for the clinical records to be made available.

The Royal College of Veterinary Surgeons (RCVS) Code of Professional Conduct for Veterinary Surgeons states that: 'Copies [of clinical and client records] with a relevant clinical history should be passed on request to a colleague taking over the case.'

When a veterinary surgeon is instructed by a charity to examine an animal, it is advisable to obtain the clinical records if possible. If the details of the previous owner's practice have not been requested or disclosed, this should be noted in the records of the charity's veterinary practice. If an illness that was not apparent while an animal was in the charity's care manifests itself after the animal has been rehomed, it is very helpful to have the full clinical history.

Third-party veterinary fees

The duty of prudence to which charities are subject also has to be borne in mind in various situations.

- Charities are occasionally asked to pay for veterinary treatment because the animal's owner (the 'third party' in this context) cannot afford the cost of the treatment. Charities have to exercise caution in these situations because most (but not all) animal welfare charities are established exclusively for the statutory charitable purpose of the advancement of animal welfare and not the prevention or relief of poverty, which is a distinct charitable purpose. Such payments could, thus, fall well outside the charitable objects of many animal welfare charities.
- However, some charities do pay for, or contribute towards, the cost of veterinary treatment in these circumstances because they have the power to do so under their constitutions. If a veterinary surgeon is told by a third party that a charity has agreed to pay for the treatment of their animal, it is important to check with the charity that it has agreed to do so and that it has the power to do so.
- If instructed by a charity to provide treatment for an animal that is owned by a third party, again, veterinary surgeons should make sure (if necessary by contacting the charity's head office) that the charity has the power to pay for, or contribute towards, the cost of the treatment on behalf of the owner.
- Similarly, animal welfare charities are sometimes asked to pay for veterinary treatment for animals presented to a veterinary surgeon by someone other than the animal's owner. A typical scenario might be a road traffic accident in which the identity of the animal's owner is not known or apparent. Again, animal welfare charities have to be careful in these situations. By instructing a veterinary surgeon to carry out treatment, the charity enters into a contract with the veterinary practice and is responsible for payment of the fees. If an owner is subsequently located, the charity can ask for a donation from the owner but cannot compel the owner to pay the bill, as the owner did not consent to the animal's treatment and has no contract with the veterinary practice. The situation in respect of stray dogs and cats is dealt with in QRGs 21.1 and 21.2, respectively.
- When a charity homes an animal with a pre-existing medical condition that the charity knows of, it will sometimes enter into a contractual agreement with the adopter to continue paying for ongoing treatment for that condition. These arrangements should be recorded in writing by the charity and have been agreed and signed off by those with appropriate authority to enter into such arrangements on behalf of

the charity. To avoid any misunderstandings, if a veterinary surgeon is instructed by someone who has entered into an agreement of this nature with a charity, it is advisable to ask for a copy of the paperwork provided by the charity and to keep this with the clinical records. If there is no paperwork, the charity should be contacted for confirmation that it has agreed to pay for treatment and, if it has, the charity should be asked to provide details of any restrictions on the types of treatment covered and any budgetary limits. Often, expensive drugs, prescription food or referrals will not be covered by the ongoing treatment agreement, or there may be a requirement to write a prescription for medication so it can be obtained at a reduced rate via specific arrangements made by the charity.

Unless these 'third-party' arrangements are properly documented and clearly understood by everyone concerned, they can give rise to misunderstandings and can also occupy a somewhat 'grey area' in terms of the charitable purposes and objects of animal welfare charities.

Animal welfare legislation

Unlike commercial boarding establishments and pet shops, companion animal welfare establishments are not currently subject to inspection and licensing by local authorities. However, they do have to comply with various other laws, including those in relation to planning, health and safety, and the environment in relation to statutory nuisances, such as noise and smell.

There are Animal Welfare Acts in each of the UK jurisdictions: these are the Animal Welfare Act 2006, which applies in England and Wales, the Animal Health and Welfare (Scotland) Act 2006 and the Welfare of Animals Act (Northern Ireland) 2011. The legislation in each jurisdiction contains very similar provisions, but there are minor differences in some respects. For example, in Scotland and Northern Ireland abandonment is retained as a separate offence, whereas in England and Wales this is covered by the duty to ensure welfare.

The legislation applies to **protected animals**; these are animals that are 'of a kind commonly domesticated in the British Islands', such as cats and dogs, and it is clear from the explanatory notes to the legislation that this also includes stray dogs and feral cats.

The legislation imposes a duty on owners or keepers to take reasonable steps to ensure that the needs of an animal for which they are responsible are met to the extent required by **good practice**. This includes those who assume responsibility for an animal on a temporary basis, such as veterinary surgeons and workers at animal welfare organizations.

The five 'welfare needs' of an animal include:

- A suitable environment
- A suitable diet
- To be able to exhibit normal behavioural patterns
- To be housed with, or apart from, other animals as appropriate
- To be protected from pain, suffering, injury and disease.

Ownership and duty to ensure welfare

All companion animal welfare charities are subject to UK animal welfare legislation. Charities have a statutory **duty** of care under the respective Animal Welfare Acts in England and Wales, Scotland and Northern Ireland to ensure the welfare of the animals in their care. When animals are signed over to charities by their owners, the trustees of the charity become the legal owners and are, therefore, subject to the duty to ensure welfare (Figure 21.1). The trustees usually delegate the day-to-day care of animals to shelter staff and volunteers. In order to fulfil their duty to ensure welfare, trustees of many charities have clear written policies, procedures and guidance, and provide staff and volunteers with appropriate training (see Chapter 20). This also acts as protection for trustees, staff and volunteers against criminal liability for any breach of the duty of care.

The legislation contains powers to make Codes of Practice and there are now Codes of Practice for the welfare of cats and dogs in England, Wales, Scotland and Northern Ireland. The respective Codes of Practice can be used by the courts as evidence of what constitutes good practice.

Charities will not always own all of the animals in their care. In the case of stray animals, the question of ownership can be quite complex (see QRGs 21.1 and 21.2).

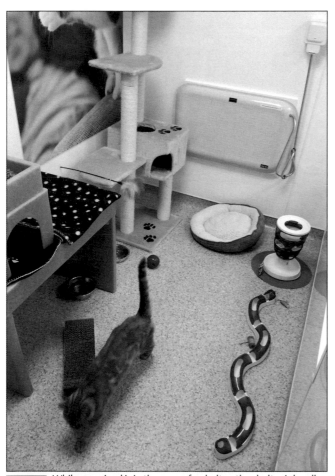

21.1 While an animal is in the care of a shelter, the shelter is legally responsible for meeting all its welfare needs.
(© Cats Protection)

Euthanasia

One of the five welfare needs under animal welfare legislation is the need for an animal to be protected from pain and suffering. The quality of life that an animal has or is likely to have, and the degree of suffering that the animal is experiencing, are welfare issues. In some cases, the only way to achieve this welfare need is by euthanasia. While most charities understand this issue, the decision of whether or not to euthanase an individual animal can be difficult for many charity workers to make. Veterinary surgeons are in a position to assist in these situations (see QRGs 2.1 and 5.2). Most charities will have a policy on euthanasia which should help to ensure this aspect of the duty of care is fulfilled (see Chapter 20).

Mutilation and prohibited procedures

It is an offence under the animal welfare legislation in each UK jurisdiction to carry out a prohibited procedure. The legislation contains powers for the various national authorities to make regulations setting out the procedures that are exempt (i.e. those procedures that are not prohibited), and there are now separate regulations in this respect in England, Scotland, Wales and Northern Ireland (see the list of regulations at the end of this chapter).

Mutilation involves interference with the sensitive tissues or bone structure of an animal other than for therapeutic purposes. Ear tipping of feral cats to identify them as having been neutered is a permitted procedure in England, Wales, Scotland and Northern Ireland (Figure 21.2). Carrying out a prohibited procedure is a criminal offence, and so veterinary surgeons should resist pressure from charities to, for example, remove a cat's teeth as a solution to aggression or to carry out any other prohibited procedure. It is also an offence for those responsible for animals (i.e. the owner/keeper) to permit prohibited procedures to be carried out.

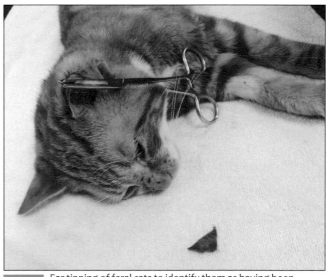

21.2 Ear tipping of feral cats to identify them as having been neutered is a permitted procedure in the UK.
(© Cats Protection)

Docking of dogs' tails

Under the animal welfare legislation in each of the UK jurisdictions, it is an offence to dock a dog's tail other than for therapeutic reasons, except for specific working dogs. Each of the national authorities has power to make regulations in this respect and there are now separate regulations in England, Wales, Northern Ireland and Scotland (see the list of regulations at the end of the chapter). Under this legislation, charities must never allow the docking of tails of dogs in their care, except for therapeutic reasons.

Consumer law and payment for rehomed animals

For animal welfare organizations that aim to rehome the animals in their care, the terms 'rehoming' and 'fostering' are sometimes used. The distinction between these is generally as follows:

- **Rehoming** normally involves the transfer of possession and ownership of the animal from the charity to the new owner
- **Fostering** involves the charity placing an animal in the possession of a 'fosterer' but retaining ownership of the animal. In these situations, the fosterer is merely looking after the animal on behalf of the charity.

Some organizations will accept a donation from the new owner in return for rehoming an animal; the argument is that the donation is freely given and that there is no contract of sale. However, it appears that this argument has not been tested by the courts. By contrast, most of the medium-sized to large companion animal welfare charities now charge an adoption fee and enter into a contract of sale with the new owner, under which both ownership and possession of the animal pass from the charity to the new owner.

It is for the courts to decide, in the circumstances of each case, whether or not a charity is selling an animal 'in the course of a business', in which case consumer law will apply. This phrase has been held to apply to charities even though they do not operate for profit or make a profit when rehoming animals. In other words, when a veterinary surgeon is instructed to provide treatment to animals that a charity aims to rehome, it is sensible to assume that consumer law will apply when the animal is rehomed.

Under consumer law, certain terms are implied in the agreement to rehome an animal. For example, there is an implied term that animals are of 'satisfactory quality'. It may seem strange that animals are regarded as 'goods' for the purposes of consumer law or that consumer law concepts such as 'satisfactory quality' and 'fitness for purpose' should apply to animals; this is because consumer law was not developed with sentient creatures in mind. There is not a great deal of case law on rehoming and consumer law, because the sums of money involved are usually small and so few cases reach the higher courts, in which authoritative decisions are made. However, such case law does exist and indicates that consumer law applies to the rehoming process used by the majority of companion animal welfare charities.

Relevance of consumer law to shelter medicine

The relevance of consumer law to veterinary surgeons instructed by charities is that before rehoming an animal many charities will have the animal examined by a veterinary surgeon and will rely on their professional skill and knowledge when assessing whether the animal is fit for rehoming. Many charities have written rehoming agreements that expressly state that before an animal is rehomed it has been examined by a veterinary surgeon and that, to the best of the charity's knowledge, information and belief, the animal is fit to be rehomed.

Charities will often make it clear in their rehoming agreements that it is impossible to give a guarantee of good health, and that some pre-existing conditions can manifest themselves at a later date or new conditions can develop. However, some charities do not make this clear, and even if they do, that may or may not be a sufficient defence to a claim for misrepresentation and breach of contract under consumer law, if it transpires that the animal had a pre-existing condition, illness or injury.

New owners whose animals turn out to have an undetected health problem are not only likely to be angry and upset that their new pet is sick or injured, but, in some cases, may also want compensation from the charity for the cost of any veterinary treatment incurred in treating the animal. In these circumstances, the charity would have a potential claim against the veterinary surgeon for professional negligence if it were found that the animal was showing clinical signs or indications of illness or injury that could reasonably have been detected prior to rehoming, and the new owner had suffered financial loss as a consequence.

Some charities will ask veterinary surgeons to provide copies of the animal's medical record or complete a medical summary, which they then give to the new owners and, in some cases, to pet insurers, on demand. It is very important for veterinary surgeons acting for charities to ensure that they have brought any existing conditions, behavioural issues, illnesses or injuries to the attention of the charity, and to be satisfied that the charity properly understands this information; charities have to be careful not to misrepresent the health of an animal and so it is very important that they have a clear understanding of any problem. Pet insurance will not cover pre-existing conditions, illness or injury, so it is important that a potential new owner understands what may or may not be covered by pet insurance should they seek to insure the animal.

Thankfully, claims against companion animal welfare charities are rare. However, from time to time a situation will arise in which an animal will manifest a condition, behaviour, illness or injury that may or may not have been pre-existing at the date of rehoming. These situations can be highly emotive, particularly if the animal dies, and they can be very damaging to the reputation of both the charity and the veterinary surgeon in question.

Maintaining clear, accurate and comprehensive case records in accordance with the requirements of the RCVS Code of Professional Conduct for Veterinary Surgeons can make a lot of difference in cases such as these. It is also preferable to have a separate record for each individual animal.

Unlawful types of dog

The law in the UK (Dangerous Dogs Act 1991) prohibits the possession or custody of four types of dog, unless an individual animal has been exempted from the prohibition. These are the Pit Bull Terrier, the Japanese Tosa, the Dogo Argentino and the Fila Brasileiro; the Pit Bull Terrier is the most common in the UK (Figure 21.3). A dog does not have to do anything wrong to be illegal – it is enough that the dog has a substantial number of characteristics of a Pit Bull Terrier or one of the other unlawful types. There is currently no DNA test used for identification, so identification depends on the dog's appearance rather than its parentage. It is generally accepted that dogs cannot be typed until they are at least 9 months old.

This issue is becoming an increasing problem for shelters, which could fall foul of the law for taking in a dog of an unlawful type, even if the organization acted solely in the interests of the dog and was not aware that it was an unlawful type. A criminal offence will be committed by

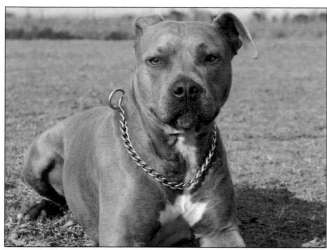

21.3 The Pit Bull Terrier is the most common unlawful dog in the UK.
(Stock image from Stockphotosecrets.com)

the charity as well as any individual who has charge of the dog (although it would be rare for a shelter to be prosecuted, as this would be unlikely to be in the public interest, and in these circumstances non-criminal proceedings can be undertaken in the Magistrates' Court as an alternative). If a shelter rehomes an unregistered Pit Bull Terrier-type dog, then the new owner/keeper will also be committing a criminal offence.

If a veterinary surgeon is asked to treat a dog that they suspect is unlawful, they should bring their concerns to the attention of the shelter immediately. They should urgently seek further advice from a specialist (such as a Dog Legislation Officer from the Police or an expert recommended by the Kennel Club). If the dog is regarded as unlawful, a Magistrates' Court (through either a criminal prosecution or a non-criminal application) may allow it to be exempted from the prohibition and placed on the Index of Exempted Dogs, provided they can be satisfied that the dog would not constitute a danger to public safety. Keeping an exempted dog is subject to stringent conditions, which include that the dog must be neutered, microchipped, muzzled and kept on a lead when in a public place.

The problem for a shelter is that, due to changes to the Exemption Scheme, in England and Wales it is now impossible for a dog to be exempted in an organization's name (though it might still be possible in Northern Ireland and Scotland). Even if the dog can be registered, it is illegal to give the dog away or to sell it, and so rehoming will become especially problematic. A practice has grown up whereby a different keeper can sometimes be nominated to look after the dog on the owner's behalf, but ownership is not transferred. This is a complicated legal area and so anyone who is facing this situation should discuss the options with the Index of Exempted Dogs and/or their solicitor.

Hybrids

Wild cat hybrids and exotic cat species

The Dangerous Wild Animals Act 1976 (DWAA) applies in England, Wales and Scotland. The DWAA requires those keeping dangerous wild animals to obtain a licence from the local authority in order to do so legally. The DWAA originally contained a schedule of wild animals considered to be dangerous, which included all species of Felidae with the sole exception of the domestic cat (*Felis silvestris catus*).

However, partly because of the practice of breeding hybrids between domestic cats and wild cat species, the original DWAA schedule was replaced in 2007 by a revised schedule under the Dangerous Wild Animals Act 1976 (Modification) (No 2) Order 2007. In essence, a licence is required to keep:

* Most species of wild cat, including the Asian leopard cat, the serval and the jungle cat, from which, respectively, hybrid breeds such as Bengals, Savannahs and Chausies are bred (Figure 21.4)
* First-generation (F1) hybrids.

There is no need to obtain a licence to keep:

* Second-generation (F2) or subsequent-generation hybrids
* A number of smaller wild cat species (listed as exceptions in the DWAA schedule) and their purebred offspring and any domestic cat hybrid offspring.

Most cat welfare charities are established to advance the welfare of domestic cats and will not be able to fund treatment for exotic cat species and F1 hybrids out of charitable funds. Exotic cat species and F1 hybrids will have specific husbandry and housing requirements, and cat welfare charities will generally not have the facilities or expertise to take in and care for such cats, and will not hold a licence to do so. It is a criminal offence under the DWAA (as amended) to keep such cats without a licence, and it is a criminal offence to sell (which would include rehoming in return for an adoption fee) such cats to anyone without a licence to keep them.

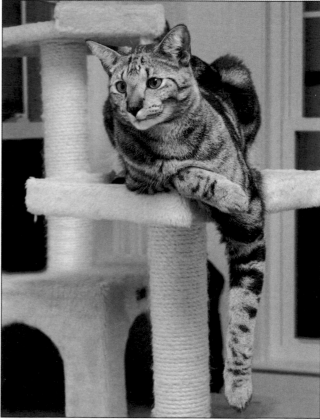

21.4 Wild cat hybrids such as Savannahs (serval cat crossed with domestic cat) can prove challenging for animal welfare organizations.
(Stock image from Stockphotosecrets.com)

In Northern Ireland, the Dangerous Wild Animals (Northern Ireland) Order 2004 applies. All members of the cat family, except for the domestic cat (*F. silvestris catus*), require a licence under this legislation. The Northern Ireland legislation does not explicitly address the question of wild cat hybrids, and it would be up to the local authorities (and ultimately the courts) in Northern Ireland to determine whether or not a licence was required to keep such animals.

Wolf hybrids

Similar legislation applies to wolf hybrids as to wild cat hybrids. If a dog is not *Canis familiaris* (the domestic dog), then it will be regarded as a dangerous wild animal and will need to be licensed. In England, Wales and Scotland, if a dog is crossed with a wolf, the F1 hybrid as well as any F2 hybrid will have to be licensed, but subsequent generations do not. The position in Northern Ireland appears to be that any hybrid will need to be licensed (although this is open to interpretation).

Transportation and travel

Transportation

Under UK animal welfare legislation, all those responsible for animals are subject to the duty to ensure welfare, and this includes welfare during transportation.

In addition, European Council Regulation (EC) No 1/2005 on the Protection of Animals in Transport is implemented in England by the Welfare of Animals (Transport) (England) Order 2006; there is parallel national legislation in Scotland, Wales and Northern Ireland. The Regulation provides that 'No person shall transport animals or cause them to be transported in a way likely to cause undue suffering to them' and sets out various general conditions for the transport of animals, such as the need to keep journey times to a minimum and the need to provide water, food and rest.

One of the general conditions for transport is to ensure that animals are fit for the journey. The technical rules in respect of fitness for transport are set out in Annexe 1 to the Regulation and include a requirement that dogs and cats less than 8 weeks of age should not be considered fit to travel, unless accompanied by their mother. There are, however, situations in which this will not be possible, for example, when orphaned or abandoned puppies and kittens are being transported by animal welfare charities for the purpose of ensuring their welfare.

The Regulation applies only to those engaged in 'economic activity' and does not apply to:

- Transportation of animals not in connection with an economic activity
- Transportation to or from veterinary practices or clinics under veterinary advice
- Journeys where the animal is an individual animal, accompanied by its owner or other responsible person
- Transportation of animals by hobby breeders, provided the income generated does not exceed the expenses of the hobby
- Journeys where the animals are pet animals accompanied by their owner.

The Regulation does not define what constitutes an 'economic activity', but it does explain that 'transport for commercial purposes includes, in particular, transport which directly or indirectly involves or aims at a financial gain'. The Department for Environment, Food and Rural Affairs (Defra) and equivalent bodies in Scotland, Wales and Northern Ireland have produced guidance on implementation of the Regulation in the UK (latest version, February 2011). This guidance indicates that animal welfare charities that do not operate with a view to profit might nevertheless be engaged in economic activities and that the 'focus should be on the particular activity rather than the general purpose or grand plan behind the activity'. In other words, whether or not animal welfare charities fall within the scope of the Regulation appears to depend upon the circumstances and the objectives of the transportation.

Those transporting animals in connection with an economic activity are subject to the following additional requirements under the Regulation:

- Over 65 km and up to 8 hours, it is necessary to hold a valid transporter authorization. Transporter authorizations are issued by the Animal and Plant Health Agency (APHA) (formerly the Animal Health and Veterinary Laboratories Agency) in England, Scotland and Wales, and by the Department of Agriculture and Rural Development (DARDNI) in Northern Ireland, and authorizations last for 5 years
- Over 12 hours, vehicles transporting any species of animal must be inspected and approved.

Guidance notes on animal transporter authorizations and applications for UK transporter authorizations can be downloaded from the respective government websites.

Pet travel and pet passports

Under Regulation (EU) No 576/2013 on the Non-commercial Movement of Pet Animals, dogs, cats and ferrets must be vaccinated against rabies before they can travel to another European Union (EU) country or back into the UK. The requirements for entry into the UK include the animal having:

- An implanted microchip
- A rabies vaccination – it is necessary to wait 21 whole days from the date of the rabies vaccination before travelling from EU or listed countries, and 3 months if travelling from unlisted third countries. Puppies and kittens have to be at least 12 weeks old before vaccination
- A blood test 30 days after vaccination (if returning or travelling from an unlisted third country)
- A pet passport or third country official veterinary certificate (Figure 21.5)
- An *Echinococcus multilocularis* tapeworm treatment (for dogs only).

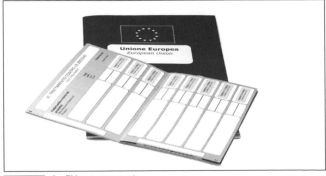

21.5 An EU pet passport.
(Stock image from Stockphotosecrets.com)

Additional import requirements may apply to hybrid breeds (such as Bengal or Savannah cats or Wolfdogs) and advice should be sought from APHA before any such animal travels.

Cats and dogs that have entered the UK illegally

Cats and dogs that have entered the UK without complying with the entry requirements will either be placed in quarantine by the local authority or returned to the country from which they came. In these situations, animal welfare charities are sometimes asked to meet the costs of quarantine and to rehome cats and dogs after the quarantine period. As a rule, charitable funds cannot be used to cover the costs of quarantine if the owners are simply unwilling to pay the fees themselves, and charities would normally only rehome unwanted pets that have been signed over to them.

If a stray or abandoned cat or dog has a microchip with foreign registration details, local authorities may assume that the animal has not entered the country legally and will place it in quarantine. Currently, there is some inconsistency in how Trading Standards offices deal with these situations, and sometimes they declare that the animal does not need to be quarantined. Charities are sometimes contacted by local authorities and presented with the bleak prospect that the animal will be euthanased unless the charity agrees to meet the quarantine costs and subsequently rehome the animal. If charities do become involved, they are obliged to take reasonable steps to locate the owner.

Often, charities are left in a dilemma regarding what to do with these animals in terms of rehoming, particularly if they are not given clear guidance from the authorities. Each charity has to decide on its own policy on this issue, as the law is not clear (see Chapter 20).

Commercial movement between countries in the EU

Anyone travelling with more than five dogs or cats, including rescued animals, falls within the commercial transportation of animals regime (Council Directive 92/65/EEC, the Balai Directive) and will require an Intra Trade Animal Health Certificate (ITAHC). Details of the ITAHC and other requirements that must be met are available from the relevant government websites in each jurisdiction. There is an exception in respect of pets travelling to take part in a competition, show, sporting event or training for such an event, provided that the pets in question are aged over 6 months and written evidence of attendance/registration is provided.

If charities bring animals into the UK from other EU countries, including the Republic of Ireland, for the purpose of rehoming, they cannot use the Pet Travel Scheme (PETS) and must treat the movement as commercial.

The Veterinary Medicines Regulations

Directive 2001/82/EC (as amended) of the European Parliament in relation to veterinary medicinal products is implemented in the UK by the Veterinary Medicines Regulations 2013, which apply throughout the UK.

The Regulations cover the manufacture, authorization, marketing, distribution and post-authorization surveillance of veterinary medicines. The Veterinary Medicines Directorate (VMD) produces Veterinary Medicines Guidance Notes, and the RCVS Code of Professional Conduct for Veterinary Surgeons contains provisions on the classification and responsible use and prescription of veterinary medicines.

The relevant points in relation to shelter medicine are as follows.

- The RCVS Code requires practice premises from which veterinary surgeons supply veterinary medicinal products (except Authorised Veterinary Medicine – General Sales List (AVM-GSL) or over-the-counter medicines) to be registered as **veterinary practice premises**. This includes, among other things, premises 'to which medicines are delivered wholesale, on the authority of one or more veterinary surgeons in practice'. Animal welfare establishments to which veterinary medicines are delivered wholesale must be registered with the RCVS as veterinary practice premises.
- The VMD is responsible for monitoring and inspecting veterinary practice premises. Alternatively, some animal welfare establishments may, if veterinary work is carried out at such premises, be accredited under the RCVS's Practice Standards Scheme.
- Animal welfare establishments that store and use veterinary medicines on site must have in place appropriate policies and procedures for the storage, security, use and disposal of veterinary medicines in order to comply not only with the Veterinary Medicine Regulations, but also with their statutory obligations under animal welfare legislation to ensure the welfare of animals for which they are responsible and their statutory obligations to staff and volunteers under health and safety law.
- Veterinary surgeons who act for animal welfare charities will be involved in the ordering, prescription and supply of veterinary medicines in respect of the animals under their care and treatment. Veterinary surgeons and suitably qualified persons (who are entitled to prescribe or supply certain veterinary medicines under the Veterinary Medicines Regulations) need to take care to satisfy themselves that the person who will use the product is competent to administer it safely and for the use for which it is authorized. Care also has to be taken not to prescribe more than the minimum quantity required for the treatment. It is not acceptable for veterinary surgeons to prescribe on a collective (or 'herd' basis) in the case of cats and dogs in animal welfare establishments. All animals should be checked by a veterinary surgeon before any prescription only medicine – veterinary (POM-V) treatment, including preventive treatments, is prescribed or administered.

Hazardous waste

The Waste Framework Directive (2008/98/EC) is implemented by various waste regulations in England and Wales, Scotland and Northern Ireland. As producers and holders of hazardous waste, animal welfare establishments are required to register with the Environment Agency; classify waste according to the List of Waste or European Waste Catalogue; code, separate and store hazardous waste; and arrange for an authorized business to collect, recycle or dispose of the hazardous waste. It is also necessary to complete the appropriate paperwork and keep records for 3 years.

In addition, cytotoxic drugs are defined as hazardous substances under the Control of Substances Hazardous to Health Regulations 2002 (COSHH) and steps have to be taken in accordance with health and safety law and guidance to protect staff, volunteers and others from any risks in relation to handling cytotoxic drugs.

Statutes

The various statutes that relate to animal welfare and the veterinary treatment of animals in the UK are:

- The Animal Welfare Act 2006
- The Animal Health and Welfare (Scotland) Act 2006
- The Welfare of Animals Act (Northern Ireland) Act 2011
- Animal Health Act 1981
- Veterinary Surgeons Act 1966
- Protection of Animals (Anaesthetics) Acts 1954, 1964 and Amendment Order 1982
- Misuse of Drugs Act 1971.

Regulations

Regulations and associated guidance that relate to veterinary practice in the UK are:

- The Mutilations (Permitted Procedures) (England) (Amendment) Regulations 2010
- The Prohibited Procedures on Protected Animals (Exemptions) (Scotland) Regulations 2017
- The Mutilations (Permitted Procedures) (Wales) (Amendment) Regulations 2017
- The Welfare of Animals (Permitted Procedures by Lay Persons) Regulations (Northern Ireland) 2012

- The Docking of Working Dogs' Tails (England) Regulations 2007
- The Docking of Working Dogs' Tails (Wales) Regulations 2007
- The Welfare of Animals (Docking of Working Dogs' Tails and Miscellaneous Amendments) Regulations (Northern Ireland) 2012
- The Veterinary Medicines Regulations 2013 (and Guidance Notes issued by the Veterinary Medicines Directorate)
- The Misuse of Drugs Regulations 2001
- The Pressure Systems Safety Regulations 2000
- The Ionising Radiations Regulations 1999
- The Control of Substances Hazardous to Health Regulations 2002 (COSHH) (as amended)
- The Waste Framework Directive 2008/98/EC and British Veterinary Association (BVA) Waste Guidelines
- The Waste (England and Wales) (Amendment) Regulations 2012
- The Waste (Scotland) Regulations 2012
- The Waste Regulations (Northern Ireland) 2011.

Useful websites

Animal & Plant Health Agency (APHA):
www.gov.uk/government/organisations/animal-and-plant-health-agency

Association of Lawyers for Animal Welfare:
www.alaw.org.uk

BVA Waste Guidelines:
www.bva.co.uk/Workplace-guidance/Practice-management/Handling-veterinary-waste/

Department of Agriculture Environment and Rural Affairs (DAERA):
www.daera-ni.gov.uk/

RCVS Code of Professional Conduct for Veterinary Surgeons:
www.rcvs.org.uk/advice-and-guidance/code-of-professional-conduct-for-veterinary-surgeons

UK legislation:
www.legislation.gov.uk

Veterinary Medicine Directorate (VMD):
www.gov.uk/government/organisations/veterinary-medicines-directorate

QRG 21.1: Dealing with a stray dog
by Trevor Cooper and Dominic Sullivan

What is a stray?

In general terms, a 'stray' dog is a dog that is at large without a person in charge of it, in either a public place or a private place it is not allowed to be. There are very few feral dogs in the UK (although this is not the case in many other countries) and so it is very likely that for any stray dog in the UK someone has legal responsibility for the dog's welfare. Deliberately allowing a dog to stray is likely to mean that there has been a breach of the duty of care, but most occasions of a dog straying are accidental.

Identification of dogs

Throughout the UK, the law requires that when a dog is in a public place, it must wear a collar, with the name and address of the owner stated either on the collar itself or on a tag attached to the collar. There are limited exemptions from this law, yet prosecutions for failure to comply are rare even though the law is widely ignored. In Northern Ireland, the dog licence has been retained, and so in addition to the requirement to show the owner's information, dogs must also wear a coloured collar tag or disc showing that the dog is licensed. This licence identification tag is issued by the local council and the colour of the tag changes every year.

Tags can be removed or fall off, or an owner can forget to put the dog's collar on or choose to ignore the law. For these reasons, many animal welfare organizations have campaigned for compulsory microchipping of all dogs as a welfare provision, as it will increase the likelihood of a stray dog being returned to its home and increase the speed of that return. Northern Ireland was the first country in the UK to introduce compulsory microchipping, and from 1 January 2013 all dogs aged 8 weeks or more have had to be microchipped before a dog licence can be applied for.

The English government passed the Microchipping of Dogs (England) Regulations 2015, which made it compulsory for all dogs to be microchipped by 6 April 2016, unless a veterinary surgeon certifies that an individual dog's health could be affected adversely by microchipping.

→

QRG 21.1 *continued*

- There is mandatory training for microchip implanters (except for veterinary surgeons, veterinary nurses and others who have 'grandfather rights' – i.e. they can continue to implant microchips without undergoing training).
- Microchips must conform to ISO standards.
- There is a duty to report adverse events to the Veterinary Medicines Directorate (VMD).

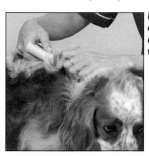

Microchipping of dogs is compulsory in the UK.

With effect from 6 April 2016, in England, Scotland and Wales dogs have also had to be microchipped and registered on a compliant database with the name and address of the keeper, that is, the person with whom the dog normally resides. The breeder (i.e. the owner of the dam that gave birth to the puppy) is regarded as a dog's first keeper, so all dogs have to be microchipped and registered in the name of the breeder before transfer to a new owner/keeper. If a breeder transfers a dog that has not been microchipped they will have committed a criminal offence punishable by a fine of up to £500.

There is an ongoing obligation for a new keeper to keep the database up to date and failure to comply means that the dog is no longer regarded as microchipped. If a keeper has a dog that is not microchipped (or the details are not up to date) they are in breach of the Regulations and an enforcer may serve a 21 day Notice requiring them to comply. Breach of the Notice is a criminal offence punishable by a fine of up to £500.

There are requirements to report an adverse event (if the microchip fails, if the dog has a health condition attributable to the implantation, or if the microchip has migrated) and there are restrictions on who can lawfully implant a microchip in a dog.

As a dog's microchip has to be registered in the name of the person with whom it 'normally' resides, it is unclear when this requirement is triggered for a dog that comes into a shelter or indeed when a foster carer becomes the habitual keeper. As best practice, once a dog has been at a shelter (or with a foster carer) for a month or two, that could well be the tipping point at which the dog has a new 'normal' home and so that is where the dog should be registered.

If a dog is microchipped with a non-ISO-compliant microchip, it will be regarded as not being microchipped, and so, to comply with the Regulations, a second microchip will need to be implanted.

Council responsibilities

In England, Wales and Scotland, every local authority must have an officer who is responsible for dealing with stray dogs, although their duties can be delegated. The council must have a collection service for stray dogs, but some operate only during normal office hours. Outside these hours, where practicable, councils must have an acceptance point where a finder can take a stray dog.

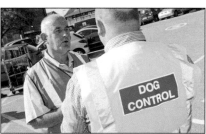

Every local authority must have an officer who is responsible for dealing with stray dogs.

Once a dog has been received by the council, the owner has 7 days to come forward to claim it – the 7 days are calculated from the date of seizure or service of a notice on them. During that period, only urgent treatment should be carried out by a veterinary surgeon, although vaccination and parasite control treatments are acceptable to protect the individual.

If the owner fails to come forward and pay the council's fees within the 7-day period, the council may rehome the dog to a person or a rehoming centre, in which case the original owner's rights are extinguished under Section 149(7) of the Environmental Protection Act 1990. As an alternative to rehoming, the council may have the dog euthanased after the 7 days have elapsed, but Defra guidance to local authorities in England and Wales states that this 'should only be considered after all other avenues have been explored to save the dog by rehoming'. No dog may be disposed of for the purposes of vivisection.

In Northern Ireland, the rules are similar except that an owner has only 5 days to come forward to claim the dog.

There is a requirement for the finder of a stray dog to either return it to the owner, if known, or take it to the council forthwith (in Northern Ireland the finder can also contact the police). If the owner does not claim the dog and pay the due fees within the 7 days (5 days in Northern Ireland), the finder can ask the council if they can have the dog.

If a stray dog is an unregistered Pit Bull Terrier type or one of the other three proscribed types (see the main chapter) the law does not allow such a dog to be given away (or sold) and so it would have to be euthanased after the statutory period has passed if the owner has not come forward to claim it.

Stray dogs and veterinary surgeons

If a council dog warden brings a stray dog to a veterinary practice for treatment, it will be the council that has responsibility for making payment. The dog's health and welfare should be the first consideration. Councils are expected to arrange the treatment of any stray dogs that are injured or require treatment to keep them alive; the costs for such treatment can then be reclaimed from the owner if they come forward to claim the dog. However, if the costs of the treatment are regarded as excessive or if the dog's condition is such that it would be in its best welfare interests to be euthanased, this would be permissible even without waiting the statutory period for the owner to come forward; this would be the council's decision having taken a veterinary surgeon's advice.

If a member of the public or a charity worker brings a stray dog to a veterinary practice, that person or organization will have responsibility for paying for the dog's treatment. The person/organization may say at the outset that they are unable to pay; in such cases, a veterinary surgeon should still provide emergency treatment to ease pain and suffering until the council or the owner can be contacted and further treatment can be discussed. In the meantime, the dog should be scanned for a microchip in the hope that the owner can be traced.

QRG 21.2: Dealing with a stray cat
by Dominic Sullivan and Trevor Cooper

What is a stray?

The term 'stray' cat covers a variety of situations in which a pet cat is no longer living with or being cared for by its owners: it may be lost, abandoned, or, may have strayed from its home. Stray cats need to be distinguished from feral cats; feral cats have not been socialized with people and are discussed below.

The legal position in respect of stray cats differs from that in respect of stray dogs. The Environmental Protection Act 1990, under which owners of stray dogs lose the right to reclaim their dogs after 7 days, does not apply to stray cats.

Ownership

Cats are regarded, in law, as property. A stray cat belongs to its owner, unless it has been abandoned or has been signed over to a third party either by its owner or by someone acting with the owner's authority.

Under common law, the finder of a stray cat may acquire ownership if the owner has intentionally abandoned it. In Scotland, under the Civic Government (Scotland) Act 1982, the finder of a stray cat can acquire ownership of a stray cat after 2 months, if he or she has gained permission from the police to have custody of the cat.

Abandonment

The duty to ensure welfare under the Animal Welfare Act 2006 (and its equivalents in Scotland and Northern Ireland) applies to the 'person responsible for' a cat. Any person responsible for a cat who leaves it without taking reasonable steps to ensure that it is capable of fending for itself, commits an offence. If the cat actually suffers as a result of its abandonment, an offence of causing unnecessary suffering may also be committed. In England and Wales, the duty to ensure welfare replaces the old offence of abandonment. However, in Scotland and Northern Ireland separate offences of abandonment are retained in their respective Animal Welfare Acts.

Possession

The finder of a stray cat acquires rights of possession under common law and is entitled to keep it unless or until the owner demands its return. The common law right to possession is subject to an obligation to take reasonable steps to find the owner if one exists. Most animal welfare charities seek to fulfil this duty by:

- Scanning found stray cats for a microchip
- Posting details on 'Lost and found' pages on the internet or the press
- Making enquiries locally – e.g. how long has the cat been in the area, did it have an owner previously who may have died or moved?
- Putting up posters locally
- Attaching paper collars to stray cats asking the owners to make contact with the finder or charity
- Waiting for a reasonable period of a minimum of 7 days before rehoming stray cats in order to provide the owners with a reasonable period of time in which to claim their pet.

It is important to stress that these are not legal or statutory requirements; they are examples of

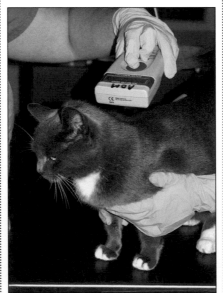

All strays should be thoroughly scanned for a microchip on admission to a shelter or veterinary practice.
(© Cats Protection)

the types of reasonable steps that should normally be taken. In practice, very few cat ownership cases go to court. However, there may be valid reasons why an owner has not come forward within the holding period; these cases can become contentious if the cat has been rehomed. It is advisable for veterinary surgeons to make detailed records of the circumstances in which a stray cat came to be presented for treatment and of any treatment carried out.

The common law right of possession is also subject to a common law duty to ensure the welfare of the cat until its return to the owner.

In addition, the statutory duty to ensure welfare under the Animal Welfare Acts in each UK jurisdiction applies not only to owners but also to anyone who is 'responsible for' a stray cat on either a temporary or a permanent basis; this includes finders, veterinary surgeons and animal welfare charities (see Chapter 21).

Stray cats and veterinary surgeons

Generally speaking, when a stray cat is brought into a veterinary practice, the client will be the person or charity who instructs the veterinary surgeon to carry out treatment, rather than the owner.

If a cat has been abandoned, the finder or charity instructing the veterinary surgeon may have acquired rights of ownership and can give informed consent to treatment. In cases where it is not clear whether or not a stray cat has been abandoned, it is reasonable to assume that the cat may have an owner. In these cases, in the absence of the owner's informed consent, most charities will instruct veterinary surgeons only to carry out urgent and necessary treatments during the 7–14-day holding period. This includes treatment of significant illness or injury and providing analgesia. Vaccination and anti-parasite treatments are permissible to reduce the risk of disease transmission while the cat is in the charity's care.

Non-urgent treatments, such as routine dental work or neutering, should be left for a reasonable ➡

QRG 21.2 *continued*

period (e.g. 7 days) to allow an owner to come forward, as some owners may be annoyed to discover that their cat has been neutered or received other non-urgent treatment without their consent. Although it is difficult to find details of cases of successful prosecutions in the case of neutered cats, anyone who recklessly or intentionally destroys or damages the

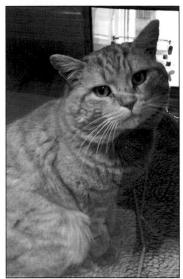

Unneutered strays should not be neutered until reasonable time and effort has been taken to attempt to locate the owner.
(© Cats Protection)

property of another (cats are regarded as 'property for these purposes') commits an offence under the Criminal Damage Act 1971, which applies in England and Wales, or under equivalent legislation in Scotland and Northern Ireland. In addition, if a stray cat is neutered, the owner may have a claim under civil law for damages if the cat was being used for breeding and it can be shown that the owner has suffered financial loss as a consequence.

Euthanasia

It may be necessary to euthanase a stray cat on welfare grounds to prevent suffering. Such decisions should be made in accordance with the RCVS Code of Professional Conduct, which explains the importance of making a full record of the circumstances in which an animal is euthanased without the owner's consent. It may be advisable for the body of a euthanased stray cat to be kept for several days in case an owner comes forward (see QRG 5.2).

Feral cats

Feral cats are cats that have not been socialized with people in the first few weeks of their lives and have had limited or no interaction with people. Feral cats are 'protected

animals' under the Animal Welfare Acts in each of the UK jurisdictions; this is because cats are a species that is commonly domesticated in the UK. It is an offence to cause unnecessary suffering to protected animals, including feral cats. The duty to ensure welfare applies to animals for which 'a person is responsible' on a permanent or temporary basis; consequently, those who feed and look after feral cats might be said to have assumed responsibility for the care of such cats and, if so, may be subject to a duty to ensure their welfare. However, feeding feral cats does not confer ownership on the feeder.

Some cat welfare charities carry out trap-neuter-return (TNR) programmes. While feral cats are in the care of charities or veterinary surgeons for neutering under such programmes, it is prudent to assume that the duty to ensure welfare applies to the charity or veterinary surgeon (see Chapter 4). In Scotland, anyone carrying out TNR work must obtain a licence under the Wildlife and Natural Environment (Scotland) Act 2011 from Scottish Natural Heritage, before releasing feral cats back into the wild after they have been neutered, on the basis that cats (*Felis silvestris catus*) are a non-native species.

Chapter 22

The shelter veterinary team

Shaun Opperman and Rebecca Elmore

An animal shelter is a facility that provides care for homeless, injured, lost or abandoned animals. Shelters vary in size, type (open intake, managed intake, non-euthanasia ('no-kill'), sanctuary, etc.), species admitted and ethos. Depending on these factors, a shelter will perform some or all of the following functions:

- Intake
- Maintenance of the animals under its care
- Reuniting lost animals with their owners
- Veterinary attention
- Behavioural assessment
- Rehoming
- Euthanasia.

Depending on its size and resources, the shelter will employ or utilize people in some or all of these roles:

- Board of trustees
- Directors and other levels of senior management
- Veterinary staff
- Behavioural staff (who may or may not be veterinary professionals)
- Animal welfare assistants/carers
- Administrative support staff
- Volunteers.

Given the nature of shelter work and the sometimes difficult decisions that have to be made on a daily basis, it is vital that all the staff, from the top to the bottom of the organization, understand the values and ethos of the shelter. The management must be robust and a great deal of attention needs to be given to communication within and between the various teams, if all are to work together towards the same aims.

Veterinary services

The shelter must decide at the outset whether to mainly outsource the veterinary work to a private practice/group of practices or directly employ its own clinical staff. There are advantages and disadvantages to both choices.

Outsourcing avoids the inconvenience of recruitment, line management and the administration of annual leave, sickness and many other human resource responsibilities, including disciplinary processes (ultimately, the termination of a contract with a practice may be a simpler and less drawn-out alternative to the handling of complicated disciplinary proceedings). It also relieves the shelter of many of the day-to-day burdens of running a practice and a clinical team. Out-of-hours emergency cover may be similarly outsourced.

However, the veterinary practice must charge for its professional time and services, and will have other clients and work commitments. The practice may have a number of veterinary surgeons (veterinarians) who cover the shelter work, so continuity of care may vary, as may individual experience and competence.

If the shelter chooses the outsourcing route, ideally, a tender should take place in which all local veterinary practices are invited to submit offers. While price is an important consideration, it is just one aspect of any potential contract; of equal or greater importance is the type of service being offered and the ability and willingness of the practice to work to the principles of shelter medicine, which will, in the long run, be more cost-effective. Face-to-face meetings with the short-listed practices will help in this endeavour.

Providing clinical services in house allows for the recruitment of a bespoke veterinary team who are dedicated and loyal to the shelter organization, and familiar with the shelter's values, ethos and policies. With time and training, they will gain invaluable experience in shelter medicine and will develop stronger relationships with the lay staff in the organization (Figure 22.1).

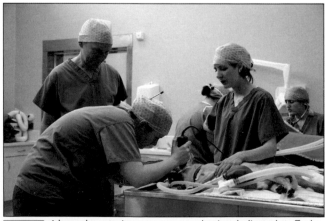

22.1 A bespoke veterinary team means having dedicated staff who develop shelter medicine skills and understand the ethos of the organization.
(© Battersea Dogs and Cats Home)

The provision of in-house services will obviously require an initial capital investment in building facilities and equipment, and ongoing costs of maintenance, but should produce savings in the longer term. In addition, having surgical facilities on site reduces the inconvenience and stress to the animals of transportation to and from a private veterinary surgery. Surgical time then effectively becomes an established and known overhead, where the expense is not determined by the complexity or otherwise of the procedure being performed, which is likely to be the case in private practice.

If resources are limited, the decision of whether to provide dedicated in-house services can initially seem complicated or even daunting. Clearly, the smallest shelters will at least start out by outsourcing, but if the shelter grows and the amount of veterinary work increases, there will come a tipping point when the case for having in-house veterinary services becomes financially viable and manageable.

Service level agreements

If outsourcing, it may be beneficial to have a service level agreement with the practice concerned. This will involve some sort of contract between the two parties that sets out to define the scope of veterinary services that can be undertaken and medicines that may be used. Costs will be agreed in advance to cover specified procedures or surgeries, veterinary time, medicines, out-of-hours cover, etc., and so can be tailored to the resources that the shelter has at its disposal. The service level agreement will also cover consent for surgical procedures, sharing of clinical records, any specific policies, such as early neutering, and will outline the arrangements for service review meetings and management of grievances.

Out-of-hours cover may be provided by a different practice. Whether this is the case or not, service level agreements are particularly important in this area, where costs can be high and members of staff from the shelter may not be available to discuss individual cases. It may be appropriate to cap the costs of treatment per animal or at least outline which procedures or treatments may or may not be given.

One of the advantages of outsourcing is that it may largely obviate the need for dispensary management and compliance with medicines legislation on the part of the shelter. However, in the interests of cost efficiency, larger shelters may register their centre(s) with the Veterinary Medicines Directorate as practice premises, which means that they can then have their own medicines delivered, stored, prescribed and dispensed. This will necessitate the usual stock control systems and standard operating procedures (SOPs) to be in place to cover correct storage, recording of batch numbers, etc. It must also be made clear to lay staff working at the shelter that while there may be a supply of medicines on site, they are not permitted to prescribe, as this is clearly the responsibility of the veterinary surgeon charged with the animals' care. The details of any such arrangement will also be covered in the service level agreement.

The shelter team

The team may work on a full- or part-time basis, depending on the size of the shelter and the amount of veterinary work to be undertaken.

Trustees

The trustees are responsible for the governance of the organization, including the financial security and proper use of funds, and budget approval (see Chapter 20). They shape the vision, mission and values of the organization and plan its long-term strategy and direction. The presence of one or more senior veterinary surgeons, ideally from different sectors (e.g. profit-making, non-profit), at this level is helpful. As well as providing a veterinary and welfare context to the development of strategy and running of the shelter, they can also offer valuable support and guidance to any veterinary staff employed by the organization.

Directors

Similarly, it is best practice to have a veterinary director within the senior management team. Indeed, within its Code of Professional Conduct, the Royal College of Veterinary Surgeons (RCVS) strongly recommends that if a veterinary surgeon provides veterinary services on behalf of an organization, then that organization should appoint a senior veterinary surgeon to director or equivalent status within the business or charity. This person would then have overall responsibility for setting clinical policy guidelines, procedures by which medicines are obtained, stored, used and disposed, and procedures for addressing any clients' complaints about the provision of veterinary services. For further information, refer to the sections on 'Veterinary surgeons and the veterinary team' in the RCVS Code of Professional Conduct.

Veterinary surgeons

Veterinary surgeons can perform a large number of varied roles in a shelter setting, which will include at least some of the following:

* Examination of animals at intake
* Preventive medicine – vaccination, worming, flea treatment, microchipping, etc.
* Medical work-ups
* Surgical procedures
* Provision of out-of-hours emergency cover
* Euthanasia
* Behavioural advice
* Rehoming advice
* Outpatient service to rehomed animals
* Advise on hygiene, husbandry and infection control
* Develop policy guidelines and written SOPs
* Provide advice and training for clinical and non-clinical staff
* Advise on kennel design, building projects, etc.
* Set budgets
* Media work, both for internal communications and external communications (written, radio, television, etc.)
* Fundraising
* Liaise with external bodies, such as government (e.g. the Department for Environment, Food and Rural Affairs) to attempt to influence policies that affect shelters.

Some of these roles are self-explanatory; others will be considered in more detail below.

Intake

Where the animal has been brought into the shelter by their owner to be relinquished, the owner should be asked to fill in a form to provide as many relevant details as possible. This should include any significant medical history and the details of their veterinary surgeon(s). The latter is important as owners may forget or fail to disclose important conditions, or be too vague in their descriptions. In addition, it may not be possible to contact them once they have left the premises, and it is not unknown for owners to leave false contact details. If available, a clinical history should be obtained from the veterinary practice as soon as possible. Any vaccination certificates/pet passports or other documentation is also helpful, as is information relating to any overseas travel. Finally, the owner should be questioned with regard to the animal's behaviour. Skilled intake staff will be able to glean vital information from the owner, which may save time and resources on repeated work-ups and improve the chances of finding the right home for the animal (see QRG 11.1).

It may be evident at this point that, due to significant medical or behavioural issues, the animal has little or no chance of finding a home. Depending on the shelter's policy, the animal may be refused entry at this point or the shelter may offer to euthanase the animal, for which the appropriate written consent must be obtained.

If the animal is a stray dog and has spent some time in local authority kennels, again, any relevant veterinary history or treatments should be obtained at this point. Often, in this case, little information will be available about the animal's behaviour, and staff must exercise appropriate caution in handling until a proper behavioural assessment can be made.

Every animal entering the shelter should receive a veterinary clinical examination on admission to check for signs of infectious diseases and/or any problems that require immediate attention (Figure 22.2). At this time, a vaccination should be administered along with preventive parasite control (see Chapter 11). Animals should then be monitored daily by the shelter staff to check for any signs of illness. This should include food and water intake, urination, defecation, demeanour, behaviour, signs of lameness or any other problems. Any signs of illness should be reported and the animals can then be re-examined.

The veterinary team can train the shelter staff how to perform a basic clinical examination including regular weight checks and body condition scoring. This should be performed at least monthly on all shelter animals and recorded on the clinical records. If the animals are housed at the shelter long term, then a full veterinary clinical examination should be carried out every 6 months. If problems have been identified, however, then clinical rechecks should be scheduled more frequently according to the specific animal and condition.

Within an animal shelter, individual animal health and overall population health are interdependent. The shelter veterinary team must regularly monitor the status of individual animals and the population as a whole to allow early detection of problems and prompt intervention. This can be achieved by the veterinary team performing regular site rounds. The animals can then be observed and assessed individually but also *en masse* and, in this way, infectious disease can be monitored in the context of the whole population. If a problem is discovered by these observations, then further preventive measures can be implemented.

Surgical procedures

Ideally, surgical procedures should be performed before adoption (Figure 22.3). Any complications arising will be easier to deal with and, where the outcome of the surgery is uncertain, such as a tumour removal awaiting histopathology results, the rehoming process will be more straightforward once the prognosis is known. Animals that have to return for surgery will also take up more of the shelter veterinary staff's time in terms of the admission and discharge of the outpatient and any follow-up visits. However, there may be occasions where it is more important to get the animal into a new home before the surgery is performed. This may be the case during particularly busy periods when there is a backlog of surgical procedures, or where the surgery has to be delayed (e.g. ovariohysterectomy of a bitch, while waiting for lactation to cease), or if the animal is not coping in the shelter environment. In these cases, where the surgery is minor or at least the outcome is assured, it may be better to rehome the animal first. Foster carers may provide temporary homes during protracted convalescence, for example, after orthopaedic surgery, where it is felt that a new owner may have difficulty providing the appropriate care. In addition, not having thoroughly bonded with a new pet, the new owner may be more likely to return the animal to the shelter in the face of surgical complications. Prior discussion and effective discharge instructions should go some way to reducing this risk, however.

Where possible, it is usually best policy to neuter all animals before adoption to prevent the risk of unplanned pregnancy (see Chapter 6).

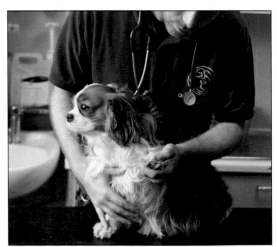

22.2 Every animal should have a thorough clinical examination as soon as possible after arrival at a shelter.
(© Battersea Dogs and Cats Home)

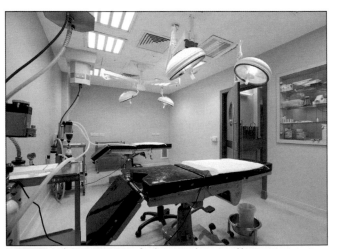

22.3 In-house operating facilities can be a good long-term investment.
(© Battersea Dogs and Cats Home)

Provision for out-of-hours emergency cover

The shelter must make provision for out-of-hours emergency cover in order to provide pain relief and medical attention for animals under its care that are injured or in distress. This would also include appropriate postoperative or inpatient care. This may be covered in house, by a local practice (probably the one that the shelter normally uses in the case of outsourcing) or by a dedicated emergency service clinic. If covered in house, it is helpful to have a veterinary nurse on call as back-up. If not covered in house, then the shelter will need to provide transport to the external clinic.

The main advantages of covering emergency care in house will be ease of access to clinical records and likely familiarity with the patient. In severe cases, the clinician will be in a better position to know when euthanasia may be the preferred option. The suffering of the individual animal, the complexity of the case and various treatment options will be weighed up against the realistic options for rehoming.

The lay staff should also be trained to recognize an emergency that would require out-of-hours treatment and must all be aware of how to contact the out-of-hours veterinary surgeon.

Euthanasia

Apart from performing the procedure itself, the veterinary surgeon is well placed to advise on euthanasia of any of the animals under the care of the shelter. The reasons for euthanasia will vary with the ethos and values of the shelter, but will usually be either for medical, behavioural or legal reasons. Furthermore, in some shelters that have an open intake policy or in local authority kennels, which have a statutory role in collecting strays, euthanasia may also be performed for reasons of space and/or budget. The subject of euthanasia is covered in more detail elsewhere (see QRG 5.2); suffice to say that, being an emotional issue for many of the staff in the shelter, it will have to be sensitively handled. Often the reason will be a mix of medical and temperament issues, which will require close working with the behavioural staff or centre managers. The best approach is for the staff making the decision to be open and clear in their reasoning, taking the time to discuss their decision with lay staff and accepting the need for flexibility in decision-making, and recognizing that there will always be grey areas where staff will look to the veterinary surgeon for guidance.

Rehoming advice

Another role of the veterinary team is to hold a short consultation, before rehoming, with any potential new owner who is interested in an animal with a pre-existing medical condition. With full understanding of the medical condition(s) and what may be required for future management, including any financial implications, the potential owner can assess their own suitability for adopting the animal concerned. If the shelter is using an external practice for veterinary services, this may be more difficult to achieve and so the consultation may have to be done by telephone. Alternatively, this task can be carried out by veterinary nurses or even experienced lay staff where appropriate. Notes should be recorded of any advice given and also that the new owner understands all of the implications of the condition(s) described.

It is also important at this point to identify any potential insurance exclusions relating to a pre-existing condition. Sometimes these may be obscure and so it will be desirable to ensure that the insurance company has a copy of the animal's medical history while at the shelter. The owner can then question the company directly about any exclusions before initiating cover.

Some shelters may offer to see the animal for a period post adoption, say 3 months, to treat, free of charge, any conditions related to the animal's stay that might not have been identified by the shelter team. Alternatively, there may be a written arrangement to cover certain veterinary costs or named conditions for a specified period (carefully worded to avoid future disagreements). Either way, the shelter veterinary team should at least be available for a specified period of time to offer advice to any owner who has post-adoption medical concerns. This provides reassurance to the adopter and a smoother transition for the animal from the shelter to the home (see QRGs 14.1 and 15.1).

Some shelters will have an arrangement with a pet insurance provider to offer several weeks' free medical insurance after rehoming. Obviously, there are sound business reasons behind this offer on the part of the insurance company, but it can also be beneficial to the shelter where a condition has been missed for whatever reason, which might otherwise lead to costly interventions or difficult conversations about returning the animal to the shelter. Encouraging the uptake of insurance also promotes responsible pet ownership.

Veterinary shelter protocols

It is helpful to have a written and accessible set of SOPs covering all the shelter's operational activities (see Chapter 20). Husbandry, hygiene, infection control, etc., all benefit from having clearly defined protocols (Figure 22.4). In turn, having such protocols will facilitate induction, training and supervision of staff and volunteers by the line managers. Ideally, the processes should be

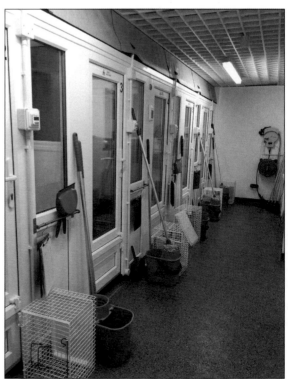

22.4 Husbandry, hygiene and infection control benefit from clearly defined protocols.
(© Cats Protection)

regularly audited; in this way, the SOPs will become 'living' documents that are regularly re-evaluated and, therefore, more credible and relevant to staff, especially if staff are able to provide input.

It is also desirable to have some sort of clinic manual outlining the major protocols for healthcare of animals at the shelter: vaccination, worming, neutering policies, etc. Ideally, these will be evidence-based, but they will also be dependent on budgetary constraints. The clinic manual can also be edited as protocols change, for example, if the shelter grows to take in more animals or more species.

For shelters where more than one clinician provides veterinary care, some thought should be given to consistency of approach. In general practice, this may be less important, as the individual needs and resources of the client will in part determine the approach of the attending veterinary surgeon. However, in the shelter working environment, where the resources must be seen to be fairly deployed, it is reassuring for lay staff if members of the veterinary team are like-minded in their decision-making. If a clinician is seen to deviate from the rest of the team, especially over major treatment decisions or rationale for euthanasia, it will inevitably cause disruption. In this respect, it is advantageous for individual shelters to have a clinic manual that at least covers the common conditions and their favoured treatment protocols. Such a manual can also be useful in securing a more consistent clinical approach from an external practice and may even form part of the service level agreement.

Budget setting

Every shelter, whatever its size or set-up, has to work to a budget, which will depend upon its income and reserves. Although local authorities will receive some central funding for dealing with stray dogs and will use a portion of this to fund kennels (either the local authority's own or those of a shelter that has a contract with the authority to provide this service), shelters are usually funded by charitable income from several sources: legacies, committed giving, fundraising events, sponsorship, etc.

Within the main budget, there will be a separate budget allocated to the veterinary department, and this will be agreed between the chief executive officer/trustees and the veterinary director or head of department, who must then decide on how these funds are best deployed (see Chapter 3).

An example of some of the budget lines might be:

- Salaries (usually the largest part of the budget)
- Drugs
- Vaccines
- Consumables
- Minor equipment
- Maintenance and service contracts
- Laboratory services
- Disposals and crematorium fees
- External private veterinary fees
- Uniform
- Training and continuing professional development (CPD)
- Membership and subscription fees, library.

The shelter should be able to secure appropriate discounts with suppliers where large volumes of drugs and vaccines are used. Where feasible, it may be worth two or more charities joining forces to provide economies of scale in some areas of purchase. Larger charities will have strict

procurement policies, and will go out to tender for the larger contracts.

While sophisticated equipment may be largely unnecessary in the context of shelter medicine, the quality of any equipment purchased should nevertheless be as high as possible (which certainly does not preclude the purchase of second-hand equipment, where real cost savings can be made). Investing in poor-quality dental equipment or surgical kits, for example, is a false economy.

Thought should also be given to the benefits of in house *versus* external provision of laboratory services. There may be apparent cost savings in using external laboratories but there can also be a real benefit to having immediate results to hand in the shelter situation, particularly at intake, where the history of many of the animals is unknown.

Clearly, there is only a finite amount of money that can be spent on the animals in the care of the shelter, and the veterinary team must be conscious of this fact and that there is often a bigger picture to consider. Finding the balance between the needs of the individual and those of the wider population is one of the key challenges of shelter medicine, especially when many staff will naturally focus their concerns on 'the animal in front of them'. There will always be a high demand for shelter resources, and there is no justification for spending an excessive amount of money on one animal and thereby denying valuable resources to the other animals under the care of the shelter, or indeed those outside the shelter waiting to come in. For example, thousands of pounds spent on cataract surgery for an older dog might equally be spent on the vaccination and neutering of many younger animals. For this reason, it is helpful to define a 'scope of service' (see below) so that all staff are aware of the procedures that can be used and medicines that may be prescribed, and those that are beyond the budget of the organization.

Media work

Most shelters will develop an active relationship with various media outlets for several reasons:

- Advertising their animals to get new homes
- Publicizing events
- Fundraising opportunities
- Education and awareness
- Campaigning and influence.

In addition, larger shelters will have an online presence, usually in the form of a website, which may hold a considerable amount of content and be quite complex. Various other social media outlets are also likely to be employed.

Members of the veterinary team will occasionally be called upon to check the details where the shelter is putting out a press release or a story with a veterinary angle, or an educational piece. They may also be asked to do interviews with newspaper journalists, radio or television (Figure 22.5). Some shelters will provide valuable media training for their staff so that they are comfortable in these situations and are not caught out by difficult questioning or an 'off-the-cuff' remark that may prove damaging to the shelter. For the most part, the media are sympathetic to the aims of shelters, and most pieces will be light news stories or fillers, but the interviewee should nevertheless always be mindful that on these occasions they are the spokesperson for their organization and may be quoted as such.

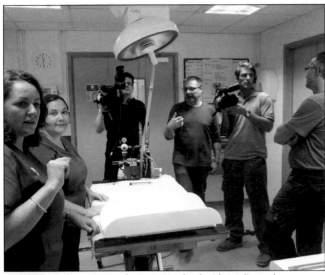

22.5 Shelter vets may become involved with media work.
(© Cats Protection)

Registered or listed veterinary nurses

The registered veterinary nurse (RVN) can perform a number of different roles in a shelter setting, which will include at least some of the following:

* Intake and triage
* Treatments
* Isolation/barrier nursing/intensive care
* Theatre/monitoring general anaesthesia
* Schedule 3 procedures
* Pharmacy/stock management
* Laboratory – in-house blood tests, urine tests, skin scrapes, etc.
* Clinical coach to student veterinary nurses
* Out-of-hours back-up
* Explaining any ongoing medical concerns at the point of rehoming and giving advice after rehoming.

Some shelters are also veterinary nurse training centres. This will often take the form of day-release training with an external provider, and with the team's RVN clinical coaches providing the rest of the training and overseeing portfolio case logs to be written up by the students. This requires considerable resources in terms of staff time and money, but can be good for role development, team structure, morale and recruitment/retention of veterinary nurses.

The RCVS Guide to Professional Conduct provides advice on the duties that RVNs can perform under direction or supervision and, equally, which duties may be performed by student veterinary nurses.

Scope of service

In general practice, the level of care is ultimately determined by the owner's resources and is generally focused on the individual animal. In a shelter situation, the aim will almost certainly be concerned with a population of animals, which in most cases will be stray or unwanted animals in a particular catchment area. This being the case, there is a requirement to decide how best to deploy the limited resources of the shelter to provide the most positive outcomes for that population. Much of the detail

will depend on the type of shelter and the values of the organization, but the principle is the same.

Some of the criteria that are useful for helping to define the scope of veterinary services provided to or within a shelter are:

* Veterinary staff resource and their level of skill and experience
* Budget
* Facilities
* Size of the population to be treated
* Prognosis for recovery and realistic rehoming options after treatment
* Duration of treatment.

The value of having a scope of service, which should ideally be written down and widely communicated, is that by defining the procedures and treatments available to the veterinary team, and by setting limits on these, it creates a framework of care options within which the team works and provides clarity and uniformity to their approach. It also relieves individual members of the team from the stress of having to make difficult treatment decisions, perhaps under pressure from other interested parties, who will themselves gradually learn to accept the boundaries set out by the scope of service. It works best if the rules are not completely rigid, as there are always exceptions, but this should not be an issue, provided there is someone credible in authority whose final decision will be respected. Having a scope of service should not be seen as a lowering of standards of care, rather that it is the best use of the team's clinical skills and experience, balanced with judicious use of resources to achieve the best outcome for as many animals as possible. If the veterinary care is outsourced, then the scope of service will form part of the service level agreement.

The areas to which the scope of service may apply are:

* Medical work-ups – For example, it may be decided that the likelihood of being able to rehome animals with diabetes, epilepsy or certain tumours precludes working these cases up beyond the point of diagnosis
* Screening – This can be expensive and the cost-benefit of screening will always need to be considered. The prevalence and severity of the condition being screened for will be a large part of that consideration; for example, testing for feline leukaemia virus and feline immunodeficiency virus; screening for exotic diseases in pets with a history of overseas travel; screening for *Angiostrongylus* when it may be more effective to simply treat the whole intake population, etc.
* Preventive treatments – For example, the choice of antiparasitic agents
* Medicines available for use – For example, the use of interferon in the treatment of parvovirus
* Surgical treatments – Hip replacement surgery, cataract surgery and similarly complex procedures are likely to be beyond the reach of most shelter budgets
* Access to referral facilities for individual cases – Some referral practices may undertake work at a reduced rate or *pro bono* for charities. Sometimes, staff or volunteers will offer to fundraise for a particular case – while well meaning, this can set a precedent for similar cases in the future, which can be tricky to manage.

Staff morale

In private practice, most patients will have owners who care for them, and so perhaps there can more easily exist a level of detachment between the veterinary surgeon and the animal being presented. In contrast, for the duration of an animal's stay in a shelter, the shelter staff are effectively that animal's owner as well as carer, and this can lead to an enhanced emotional bond between the veterinary staff and the patient. Many of these animals have suffered in very poor circumstances before being presented to a shelter, and it can be extremely rewarding to watch their recovery, both mental and physical, and not least to see them finally placed into a new home where they can be properly cared for. One of the real pleasures for shelter staff is being sent photographs of animals in their new homes – a dog hogging the sofa or a cat sunning itself in the garden – by their proud new owners.

Furthermore, there is a sense of clinical freedom when working in a shelter, in that the clinician is not constrained by an owner's resources, circumstances or beliefs when deciding on treatment choices for their patients. Of course, there are budgetary and ethical restrictions in a shelter, but they will usually be known and largely consistent.

Of course, the flip side is that, as the animal's guardian, the shelter veterinary surgeon is also responsible for the more challenging decisions, be they difficult treatment choices or the decision to euthanase. In private practice, certainly, there is the responsibility that comes with guiding an owner towards what can be, for them, an extremely painful choice, but nevertheless it is ultimately their decision to make. In the shelter environment, while such decisions may be shared with other shelter staff, this responsibility can be quite wearing over time. When other staff actively disagree with veterinary decisions – and there will always be occasions – it can be particularly taxing for the veterinary surgeon and can eventually lead to emotional fatigue and lowered morale. Without effective support, it is all too easy to focus on perceived failures, and the build-up of a blame culture within the shelter becomes a real risk.

It is unavoidable that shelter animals will be euthanased. Medical, behavioural and legal reasons, or just simple overpopulation, will always mean that a large number of unwanted animals cannot be placed into new homes. There are a limited number of kennels, resources and new homes available to match the rate at which stray or abandoned animals are generated in most societies, and euthanasia is one of the inevitable consequences. It cannot be over-stressed how important it is to discuss these issues with staff (and volunteers) before they start work at a shelter, so that they have an understanding of the bigger picture. This process should start with recruitment, but must continue throughout induction and training, and should be part of the culture of the shelter's management. Staff should be given appropriate support, but euthanasia should not be turned into an emotional issue, and the value of compassion, as opposed to sentimentality, should be emphasized.

Deciding which animals to euthanase can be difficult. It is important that the shelter has clear guidelines on euthanasia to assist staff in making their decisions and to reduce the opportunity for disagreement and conflict. Of course, there will always be grey areas in some cases that will divide opinion, but these can be kept to a minimum. The clinician must approach these cases in a fair and consistent manner and not display personal bias. If they are approachable, credible and happy to discuss their reasoning, they are more likely to gain the respect and support of their colleagues. Again, good leadership and management skills are essential if conflict is to be kept to a minimum.

Relationship with local private veterinary surgeries

There will always be a relationship with practices local to the shelter, whether they are the main provider of veterinary services to the shelter or provide only one or another aspect of support, such as emergency out-of-hours cover. Even if the provision of veterinary services is wholly in house, doubtless some of the clients to whom the shelter rehomes animals will use the services of these local practices for their new pets, and so it will be advantageous to all concerned if the relationship is a healthy one, based on a mutual understanding of respective aims and values.

To this end, the following may be helpful:

* Reciprocal visits undertaken by key members of staff to develop awareness and promote understanding
* Face-to-face meetings to build personal relationships. Once these relationships are in place, it will be much easier to iron out any problems that arise in the future. Regular follow-up meetings, perhaps once or twice a year, will help to maintain the relationship and may be a chance to review any service level agreement
* Invitation to the practice team to participate in shelter events
* Encouraging the practice to help fundraise for the shelter and get involved in activities
* Sharing in the shelter's successes
* Sharing and displaying promotional literature
* Collaborating with the practice to develop clinical protocols that are beneficial to animal welfare, e.g. earlier neutering of cats
* Keeping the practice informed on current disease problems at the shelter, e.g. prevalence and severity of 'kennel cough', 'cat 'flu', outbreaks of gastrointestinal disease, etc.
* Ensuring that the shelter's medical records are made available to practices in the event that they take on clients who have adopted from the shelter
* Helping the practice to develop shelter medicine principles so that the practice clinicians understand why, for example, certain tests or medications may not be appropriate.

Record keeping

Veterinary surgeons are required to maintain accurate clinical records for any animal under their care. Computerized systems make the maintenance of these types of records much easier than a handwritten system and also facilitate transfer of clinical records to other practices or insurance companies.

Individual records should have a unique shelter number, the animal's name, species, breed, sex, age, physical description (colour, coat type), microchip number, date of intake, date of departure, source of the animal, reason for entry, any available previous medical/behavioural history, the name and address of a new adopter and a record of anything of significance that relates to the animal once it is on the shelter site. When an animal is adopted, a copy of the records can be forwarded to the new owner's veterinary surgeon.

A challenge arises when veterinary work is outsourced, and that is to what degree the records are duplicated for the benefit of the shelter. Clearly, the acting veterinary surgeon has to keep their own practice records, but the shelter should also keep a record of relevant procedures to enable staff to manage the animals' care and to provide information relevant to potential adopters. If the practice and shelter share the same IT system, then records could be shared electronically, but this is rarely the case, and so a compromise will need to be found. This could be in the form of paper printouts from the practice or handwritten notes, or, in the case of a web-based system, by allowing shelter staff controlled access to veterinary records.

Line management

The shelter environment can be a stressful one in which to work. Many of the decisions made are, at least in part, subjective and may result in an outcome that can be emotional for many members of staff. While there may be sound reasoning behind such decisions, the final say on which animals are admitted to the shelter, which treatments can be given, which animals can be rehomed and, most of all, which animals may be euthanased will often be contentious to some members of staff. This is never more the case than with decisions related to an animal's behaviour, where the degree of subjectivity is seen to be higher.

So, it is extremely important to have a robust line management structure if conflict is to be avoided or at least kept to a minimum. Furthermore, it may seem obvious, but it is equally important that those with the authority to make the more difficult decisions are appropriately skilled and credible in the eyes of the rest of the staff, and that their decisions are supported by the senior management. It can be particularly demoralizing and destabilizing for such decisions to be unfairly undermined by senior management who may lack the skills or experience to do so.

Staff training

All veterinary surgeons must undertake a minimum of 105 hours, and veterinary nurses 45 hours, of CPD over a 3-year rolling period. This is essential to improve the knowledge and expertise of the team. However, there is a cost implication to the shelter and, wherever possible, the training should be sourced as cost-effectively as possible. Cost savings can be made by sharing training with other organizations and by hosting the training in house. Whichever route is taken, all CPD should be targeted at developing and improving the skills and knowledge of the team within the context of the scope of service agreed by the shelter. The Association of Charity Vets provides CPD specifically for this sector.

It is also important that the animal care assistants receive appropriate training, and much of this can be provided by the veterinary team: for example, how to perform a general examination; education around infectious disease control; pregnancy, whelping and neonate care. Providing training in this way is not only cost-effective but will motivate the animal care assistants and help to form strong ties between the veterinary and animal care teams.

Regular staff appraisals with skilled line managers will identify suitable training opportunities to further staff development and increase the knowledge base within the shelter.

Useful websites

Association of Charity Vets:
www. associationofcharityvets.org.uk

RCVS Code of Professional Conduct for Veterinary Surgeons:
www.rcvs.org.uk/advice-and-guidance/code-of-professional-conduct-for-veterinary-surgeons/

RCVS Code of Professional Conduct for Veterinary Nurses:
www.rcvs.org.uk/advice-and-guidance/code-of-professional-conduct-for-veterinary-nurses/

Chapter 23

Working with the non-veterinary shelter team

Lisa Morrow and Runa Hanaghan

Introduction

Veterinary surgeons (veterinarians) will interact with animal shelters on many levels. A veterinary surgeon may see individual animals in a practice setting, they may be contracted to care for groups of animals kept in facilities, such as homing centres or sanctuaries, or they may be employees of the shelter and work in a clinical capacity, an advisory capacity or both. Financial constraints always exist and this is often coupled with a desire to help as many animals as possible. Some shelters are solely volunteer run, some are mainly operated by staff and others utilize a combination of the two to achieve their aims.

Groups of people working within a shelter or in a charitable capacity may be any of the following:

* Shelter manager, reception staff, administrators, fundraisers, volunteers
* Direct animal care staff, volunteer fosterers
* Trainers and behaviourists
* Physiotherapists
* Alternative therapists
* Educators.

This list is not exhaustive; staff and volunteers may have qualifications in other areas and dedicate some of their time to helping out in whatever capacity they can.

The motivation to help in these organizations should ideally be founded on goodwill and a common purpose – to improve animal welfare, particularly for those animals they care for.

Individuals will have their own ethical views and perspectives (see Chapter 2). Some shelter workers may struggle with aspects of pragmatism and the bigger picture, as they may be more strongly focussed on the individual animal they are caring for. It is vital to build a trusting relationship with them, listen to them and have empathy for their point of view.

Animal hoarding may be encountered when working with rescue organizations. The veterinary profession helps in identifying and managing these situations (see QRG 23.1). Although hoarding can initially be motivated by goodwill, once the situation is out of hand, then support and assistance are needed. Identifying these problems early can ensure that good animal welfare is maintained.

Whatever the types of people or the types of roles that are involved, it is important to know the aims and structure of the organization in order to have a clear idea of how decisions are made and who is the appropriate person to speak to in a particular circumstance. A full appreciation of the roles and responsibilities of the people working at a particular shelter is helpful because it improves understanding of the pressures that the workers are under and what their motivations might be.

The role of the veterinary surgeon, the aims and structure of the organization and the role of the person or people the vet is working with, will impact on the type of relationship that develops and how this is managed.

This chapter provides some general guidance on managing relationships with people working in animal shelters. Specific scenarios are presented as case examples at the end of the chapter to illustrate commonly encountered situations where the relationship between the vet and the shelter workers is instrumental in ensuring that the welfare of the animal(s) is maintained. These may be useful for training purposes.

General principles of managing relationships with the non-veterinary shelter team

Veterinary surgeons working in a shelter need to know the organization's general ethos, aims, structure and any relevant policies and protocols that are in place. It is extremely useful to visit the shelter or fosterer to fully understand the set-up from a practical perspective.

* If the organization has existing veterinary-related policies and protocols in place, use these to guide decision-making. There may be occasions when the motivations and interests of the person presenting the animal vary from those of the organization. Policies and protocols are useful to inform the veterinary surgeon how the organization would like its charitable funds to be spent.
* If the organization does not have veterinary-related policies and protocols in place, work with them to develop these as they will facilitate communication, aid decision-making and, thus, strengthen relationships significantly.
* Make sure all veterinary practice staff or in-house veterinary team are fully informed of the working relationship between the shelter and the practice. This includes staff being aware of the organization's policies

and protocols, as well as arrangements within the practice, for care of these animals. This consistency of care and uniform approach to the animals will be greatly valued by the organization. Occasionally, veterinary staff from the practice providing services to the shelter may be actively involved with the organization as volunteers in their own time. This is valuable to the shelter as it can help provide much needed skilled assistance; however, it can also lead to real or perceived conflicts of interest. These may manifest in several ways. For example, pressure might be put on veterinary staff to provide care or options that may not be appropriate for the case. Conversely, it may be perceived that the veterinary staff are encouraging the shelter to spend more money with the practice than is necessary.

- Be aware that lines of communication may be more complex than in the usual veterinary surgeon-client-patient relationship and that often there is more than one person within the organization who may be involved with decision-making.
- Know each person's role within the organization and their level of authority for making decisions.
- As in general practice, the veterinary advice and information that is given is not always fully understood. This means being patient and clear, avoiding technical terminology when explaining and, in some cases, checking to see how the shelter staff or volunteers are doing after a few days. This can help with increasing knowledge and skills within the shelter.
- Establish a strong relationship with the management of the shelter and maintain good communication at all times.
- Work to establish a relationship based on a mutual interest in the welfare of the animal(s).
- Ask questions and be a good listener to help establish mutual understanding.
- Use coaching techniques to build motivation and confidence and engage in a collaborative manner. This will lead to a relationship with a high level of trust and will help when discussing and making decisions about complex or difficult situations.
- Use veterinary expertise to engender understanding and clarity of the animal's needs to those making decisions on the shelter's behalf.
- Where possible and where it is not already provided by the organization, offer educational talks and hands-on training. Sharing veterinary expertise with the staff or volunteers outside the usual veterinary role is a great way of building two-way relationships. For example, giving a presentation on a topic that may seem straightforward from a veterinary perspective can highlight some of the challenges in the shelter environment and may increase the veterinary surgeon's understanding of how the shelter works (see Chapter 24).
- Participating in fundraising events as a volunteer enhances the team feeling and leads to stronger relationships.

Discussing diagnostic and treatment options

The veterinary surgeon has a key role in facilitating decision-making in relation to diagnostic testing and treatment of animals in the care of shelter organizations. The aim is to provide a balanced view of the options available in relation to both monetary and time resources and animal welfare.

For rehoming organizations, veterinary surgeons need to consider that the animal is in a temporary environment and that the ultimate way to achieve a positive welfare state is to find it a new home as soon as possible. However, the health status of the animal needs to be assessed and any problems addressed before placing it in its new home. With sanctuary organizations, the animal may stay in the facility for the duration of its life or be fostered long term in an individual's home, with ownership retained by the organization. Where a permanent home is not necessarily being sought for the animal, the primary considerations in veterinary treatment are essentially the same as for an animal that will ultimately be rehomed. However, the focus will be on creating and preserving a positive welfare state for the animal in the shelter or long-term fostering environment.

In providing a balanced view of the options available, several points are worth considering:

- When discussing a diagnostic procedure, consider whether it will ultimately change how the animal is treated. It is not necessary to reach a definitive diagnosis in all cases and if the test will merely confirm what is already known, then generally there is no need to perform it. This allows the charitable funds to be used to help more animals (see Chapter 3)
- The relative cost of each option. This is not just the monetary value of the main medical or surgical procedure, but all the associated costs to get the animal to the point where the condition is 'cured' or stabilized to a satisfactory level. This would include things such as:
  - The number of diagnostic procedures that are carried out before choosing a treatment option
  - Any post-treatment testing that may be required (this is often triggered by pre-treatment testing so another reason to carefully consider the need for pre-treatment tests)
  - The overall duration and type of morbidity associated with the option
  - The ability of the organization to manage the case within the shelter (or foster) environment (e.g. recumbent spinal cases, complex fractures with external fixators may be challenging)
  - Possible post-operative complications and the time and money associated with these
  - Recovery time, including the time until the animal would be ready for homing
  - Whether multiple procedures or visits to the veterinary practice will be required
  - Any long-term effects that may affect opportunities for rehoming
  - The effects of long-term confinement on welfare, and how this might limit the ability to help more animals with the available resources.
- Does the animal have other concurrent health or behavioural conditions that might affect long-term prognosis and quality of life? For example, cats with hyperthyroidism and concurrent renal disease have a shorter average survival time
- Whether the option results in the animal still requiring on-going treatment long term or whether there is an option that would result in no further treatment being needed; for example, medical *versus* surgical treatment for feline hyperthyroidism.

See Case examples 1 and 2, which can be used with paid staff or volunteers as a teaching aid.

Euthanasia decisions

Euthanasia is an emotive subject and it is important to have clear guidelines on how decisions are reached. A mutual understanding of everyone's views will make decision-making easier for all concerned. The ethos of the shelter will have a big impact on how euthanasia decisions are handled. In addition, each organization will be dealing with different pressures in relation to demand for intake, average time length of stay, facility size, general health and demographics of the population of animals in the local area, and financial constraints (see Chapter 2, QRG 2.1 and QRG 5.2).

Often people involved in a shelter organization believe that they are, at some level, saving the animals – either by rehoming them or by investing in them in a behavioural or clinical way. As such, euthanasia decisions can be hugely challenging due to the emotional concerns from every part of the organization – from volunteers to experienced staff or managers. The welfare of each animal under the care of the veterinary surgeon is the primary focus and taking the time to talk to key members of the organization to ensure that this is understood will help messages around euthanasia to be handled better by all concerned.

The animal may be presented to the veterinary surgeon by the primary carer who could be a volunteer fosterer or a member of shelter staff. This person may be able to make a decision around euthanasia, or another person in the organization may have the authority for decision-making. It is important to know who has the responsibility for making decisions, and equally important to present findings and recommendations clearly and comprehensively. Even if the person presenting the animal is not authorized to make the decision, they may be the carer as well as the person tasked with relaying the information to the ultimate decision-maker and, as such, they need to be fully informed of the findings and recommendations of the veterinary surgeon.

While the individual shelter organization's perspective on euthanasia will influence the decision-making process, the veterinary surgeon plays an integral role in providing the information and professional opinion to assist in the process. Some organizations rely heavily on veterinary recommendations in relation to euthanasia. Organizational policies and guidelines reduce the pressure of decision-making for the people looking after the animals, but do not change the process involved in coming to the decision. The key considerations when making decisions regarding euthanasia are the current quality of life of the animal, the prospect of an acceptable quality of life being achieved within a reasonable time frame and costs and the prospect of finding an environment where it can thrive in the long term. Managing relationships with the people involved in euthanasia in a shelter environment demands the same high level of clarity and objectivity to assist in making a decision as it does for non-shelter clients. It also requires all the sensitivity and compassion that is given to any client and their animal. People working in animal shelters will experience euthanasia more than the average member of the general public, and veterinary surgeons have a role in helping them understand the context of why this might be and to help them with any questions or concerns this may raise for them. Veterinary surgeons can increase people's understanding of this issue and support them in coping with the immediate and long-term effects it may have (see Case example 3).

Dealing with non-compliance with veterinary advice

This situation may arise in relation to advice given for the care of an individual patient or advice on operational changes recommended as a result of disease in a group of animals. In addressing non-compliance, the veterinary surgeon needs to understand why the shelter staff member/ volunteer is being non-compliant and provide them with the reasoning behind the veterinary recommendations. It is good to discuss the various viewpoints; ultimately, the aim is to align all perspectives for the benefit of the animal. Showing the shelter worker that the veterinary surgeon has the best interest of the animal in mind can be an effective approach. In cases of non-compliance with veterinary advice, the veterinary surgeon will also need to bring the issue to the attention of the person's manager; there may be factors that they have not taken into account so it is important to get the manager's perspective.

Many staff may be familiar with veterinary medications and will also know how the veterinary surgeons commonly treat various conditions. There is a risk that they may make decisions themselves on what medications to use without consulting a veterinary professional. This may be in order to save the costs involved in presenting the animal to a veterinary surgeon; however, this is a breach of the legislation surrounding prescribing. Discussions and guidance on how to manage this can be valuable, particularly as the shelter may have access to unused medications on site. Verbal prescriptions may be acceptable as long as the veterinary surgeon is confident that the person receiving the verbal prescription can safely dispense and administer the medication; in such circumstances details of the verbal prescription and advice should be added to the clinical notes.

One of the most difficult things to explain from the consulting room is barrier nursing and managing infectious disease. It is much easier to provide advice on these issues if the veterinary surgeon is familiar with the facility's setup and protocols. Often shelter workers have a good working knowledge of biosecurity, but this is not always the case and it can be helpful to observe the daily routines at the shelter to see if improvements could be made (see Case example 4).

Conveying medical information that may in turn be passed on to new owners or other carers

When dealing with unowned animals that will be passed on to other people, such as adopters, long-term fosterers or even other carers within the organization, the medical conditions of the animal and the long-term consequences and prognoses of these need to be explained in greater detail than with some owners.

Some key points to consider include:

- Shelter workers need to have an excellent understanding of the situation in order to be able to pass on information to third parties (e.g. prospective adopters) accurately
- In some cases it may be useful for a veterinary professional to have a discussion with the prospective owner, especially where conditions or treatments are complex (e.g. with diabetic animals)

- Recognize that there will be a wide range of knowledge and understanding among individuals
- If not already provided by the organization, training sessions to educate the shelter workers on common situations and conditions can greatly increase their understanding and improve their ability to pass on information
- Explain the medical information clearly and simply and avoid using highly technical language
- Check the shelter worker's understanding
- Documentation, such as a summary of the animal's medical history or a copy of the medical record, should be provided so that the shelter worker can read it and pass it on to a new owner or other carer. This is also important to show that the organization has been responsible in its assessment of the animal before rehoming, as this can significantly reduce veterinary issues post homing
- If an animal has a specific medical condition, it is a good idea to provide information sheets or leaflets on the condition or direct the shelter worker/carer to a good website. This is for the carer's benefit, but also means that they can pass the information on to anyone else taking responsibility for the animal
- Many organizations now provide free veterinary insurance on adoption. People working with such organizations must be aware of the implications that a recently treated or ongoing medical condition might have on future insurance cover and exclusions and they need to be able to explain this to the adopter.

Further advice and useful websites

Larger charities may have veterinary departments who are happy to discuss their approach to situations that can happen and offer advice. The following list is not exhaustive: Cats Protection, Dogs Trust, RSPCA, PDSA, Blue Cross, Battersea.

Animal Hoarding websites:
http://vet.tufts.edu/hoarding/
http://icatcare.org/advice/cats-and-human-health/hoarding-overwhelmed-care-giver

---

Case example 1: A Golden Retriever with a persistent cough

Mabel, an 11-year-old Golden Retriever, is in the care of a sanctuary organization that is run as a two-person organization without written policies and protocols. Mabel has been in the care of the sanctuary for 6 months. When she first arrived, she was in quite a poor state and had a pyometra and mammary gland tumours which were treated. She has been noted as coughing a lot recently. On clinical examination, increased lung sounds are heard, but otherwise she is in good body condition and her heart sounds normal. The veterinary surgeon discusses the situation with Mabel's carer and proposes a geriatric blood panel. Alongside this, before the test results are available, a course of antibiotics and a non-steroidal anti-inflammatory drug are prescribed to see if this might improve the dog's coughing.

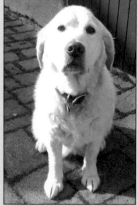

Mabel, an 11-year-old Golden Retriever, presented with a persistent cough.

At her check-up a week later, the dog has improved a little. The biochemistry and haematology results were within normal limits apart from a mild hypercalcaemia and a mild non-regenerative anaemia. The differential diagnoses are foreign body inhalation, pneumonia and neoplasia, with neoplasia at the top of the list. Further diagnostic options discussed are radiography, bronchiolar lavage (BAL) and even computerized tomography (CT). The main concerns are that some tumours are not always easy to detect on plain radiographs and that a BAL is an invasive procedure. A CT scan is costly but would detect neoplasia and foreign bodies would be enhanced enabling a thoracotomy to proceed more accurately.

On discussion with the person in charge, it becomes apparent that the santuary would not be able to manage Mabel postoperatively and that they would not proceed to thoracotomy even if a foreign body had been discovered. Radiography or BAL would now be more appropriate and would essentially rule in or out treatable options. In the course of the discussions, it is also revealed that no matter what condition is found, the sanctuary workers would not consider euthanasia at this stage as they believe the dog is still comfortable and has a good quality of life. The consensus is that further diagnostic testing would not necessarily be of benefit, especially as there is a strong suspicion of neoplasia.

Monitoring of Mabel's quality of life is important and the veterinary surgeon provides the carers with guidance for objective assessment of this. Medical treatment is continued for the time being and a plan for follow-up visits is provided. At some stage euthanasia will need to be considered on welfare grounds and it is explained that this should be before Mabel's welfare becomes compromised by the illness.

DISCUSSION

In a case like this where there are various options available to diagnose the problem, careful questioning and in-depth conversation with the carer of the animal about their perspective and their ability to manage the situation are extremely useful in coming to a decision on how best to approach treatment. The decision is made in the animal's best interest and assists the organization to spend its limited funds wisely. In this case, the discussion with the carer has made it clear that doing any further testing would not change how Mabel is treated, and the money is better spent on treatment and monitoring the condition, in order to ensure her quality of life is maintained. In addition, having a discussion about euthanasia before the need is apparent will prepare the carer for this possibility and ultimately make it easier for the decision to be made when the time comes (see Chapter 2).

Case example 2: A 5-year-old cat with a fractured femur

Lucky is a 5-year-old cat that was relinquished to the care of a rehoming organization as the owner was unable to pay for veterinary treatment for a suspected fractured leg. Not much is known about the cat's history and the previous veterinary surgeon is contacted to obtain the clinical notes and radiographs. The radiographs reveal a transverse fracture in the distal third of the right femur with possible bone fragmentation near the fracture site, and the notes report some crepitus on palpation of the femur under sedation. The volunteer fosterer who is looking after the cat remarks that Lucky is urinating and defecating normally and has a good appetite.

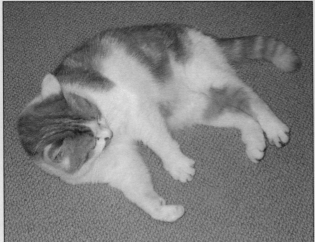

Lucky, a 5-year-old cat, presented with a fractured femur.

The veterinary surgeon discusses initial consider-ations, such as type of fracture, concurrent conditions and any potential anaesthesia issues. A selection of treatment options is presented: pin only, pin and plate, external fixator or amputation. Each option is then dis-cussed in the context of the cat and its current situation: it is in the care of a shelter, has a painful condition that must be treated surgically, and has a good prognosis for a good quality of life in a home environment once the problem is treated.

The fosterer is quite anxious and flustered about what to do as she is not really medically-minded, nor is she in a position to make the decision or authorize treatment beyond the basic examination. She knows the charity's financial resources are not great at the moment as fundraising has been slow and the organization has recently had to pay some expensive veterinary bills. To help the fosterer, and to hopefully expedite a decision, a 'decision table' is provided for the fosterer to take to the person who is authorised to make treatment decisions. The cat is kept at the veterinary clinic until a decision can be made.

Consideration	Treatment option			
	Pin only	Pin and plate	External fixator	Amputation
Monetary cost	++	+++	++++	+
Overall pain and discomfort that needs to be managed (pre- and postoperatively)	++	++	++++	+
Possibility of postoperative complications or repeated treatments	++	++	++++	+
Possible long-term effects or ongoing problems	+++	+++	++	+
Time for the animal to become fit to rehome	+++	++	++++	+

Decision table outlining the treatment options for a cat with a fractured femur. (+ = low; ++++ = high)

DISCUSSION

The initial management of this case is the same as for any client – to give a veterinary assessment, present treatment options and ultimately achieve a decision and informed consent. The additional considerations with this cat are that it is unowned and has been presented by a person who has little medical understanding and does not have the authority to make treatment decisions. The decision table illustrates the treatment options available and outlines considerations that need to be taken into account when reaching a decision. This table can be used by the veterinary surgeon to guide the decision-maker, allowing them to be confident that the decision they make is in the best interests of the animal and the organization. Amputation was chosen as the most appropriate treatment in this situation.

Case example 3: A 1-year-old cat with a spinal injury

Smooch is a 1-year-old cat that was hit by a car in front of a volunteer from a local rehoming organization. Initial presentation indicates abrasions on her head and tail and Horner's syndrome. She is unable to walk or support her weight and her tail is flaccid. Spinal reflexes are absent in the hind limbs. Deep pain sensation is intact, anal tone appears weak to normal and a perineal reflex is present. Survey radiographs reveal a fractured pelvis and a subluxated coccygeal vertebra. The diaphragm and bladder appear intact. She is given analgesia and sent to the homing facility to be monitored because there are indications of some nerve function in the hind end, but it is not yet known whether she can voluntarily urinate and defecate; good nursing care will be required while this assessment is being made. The shelter's policy on cases like this is to opt for euthanasia if voluntary urination and defecation is not achieved. The difficulty is knowing how long to give the cat to regain this function. To some degree it depends on the individual case, but there needs to be a steady improvement over time.

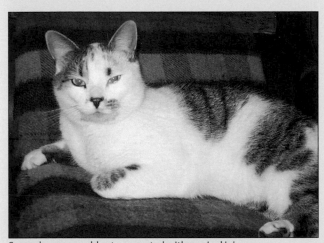

Smooch, a 1-year-old cat, presented with a spinal injury.

It is agreed between the veterinary surgeon and the shelter manager that the cat will be assessed weekly and that if function is not regained by 4 weeks, serious consideration must be given to euthanasia. The centre is largely volunteer-run and has many experienced carers working there. The veterinary surgeon trains a number of the carers to express Smooch's bladder and also teaches them how to do some passive physiotherapy on the hind limbs to keep the muscles active and help with the recovery.

Weekly veterinary assessments show gradual improvement. After each assessment the cat's progress is discussed and the veterinary surgeon is always careful to try to give a realistic (guarded) prognosis and make sure that everyone is aware there is a time limit on how long this cat can remain in the state it is in. Despite this, there is much expectation and hope that Smooch will get better. The Horner's syndrome resolves, the wounds heal well, the cat is bright and alert, is eating and defecating well, and has even made attempts to stand up. There are no issues with urine scald as the carers work hard to rehabilitate her. When Smooch is examined 4 weeks after the accident, she is still unable to urinate on her own. It is time for that conversation about euthanasia. The topic is broached with the manager initially, in the knowledge that extensive discussion with all the volunteers will also be necessary. Discussion with the manager occurs first because she is the one with the authority to make the decision. In addition, the manager and the veterinary surgeon can work together to address the concern that is likely to occur when the decision to euthanase is announced. The veterinary surgeon feels a lot of pressure not to recommend euthanasia; however, the veterinary surgeon and the manager have always been in agreement about the best approach and together they will come up with a plan on how best to manage the volunteers' understandable grief in losing Smooch.

The manager understands that it was agreed to give Smooch four weeks; however, she is concerned that the staff are highly attached to Smooch and wonders whether she can be given another week or two to get better. While agreeing that this would make life easier today, the veterinary surgeon explains that ultimately this would just be delaying the inevitable. Speaking to the volunteers, the veterinary surgeon explains that Smooch has been given time to get better; however, she has not regained the ability to urinate on her own. Long-term confinement with constant intervention is not optimal welfare for a cat and is a quality-of-life issue. The manager gives each volunteer the opportunity to say good-bye if they want and asks if there is anyone who particularly wants to be there when the euthanasia is performed.

DISCUSSION

In these complicated euthanasia situations, there may be a wide range of views and concerns within the team looking after the animal. The animal may appear to be doing very well but the veterinary surgeon needs to help the shelter workers understand that this is a welfare issue in the long term.

It is critical from the outset to explain that if there is not an improvement then euthanasia decisions may ultimately need to be made and it is helpful to set time frames for this. This process is dealt with every week in veterinary practice; however, in the case of a facility with multiple carers it can be a little more complex to manage. A good working relationship with a like-minded manager, coupled with open dialogue will allow the various views to be expressed and people realize that not everyone feels the same way. This can be very helpful in managing the situation.

Integration into the team will ensure all staff and volunteers are comfortable with approaching the veterinary surgeon if they have concerns. Careful handling of a sensitive situation like this can strengthen that relationship even though it is a very difficult process and an emotive time for all.

Case example 4: A litter of puppies with parvovirus

A litter of four puppies is presented to a veterinary surgeon a week after entry into a dog shelter that operates out of two kennel blocks within a boarding kennel. The puppies are suffering from parvovirus and are admitted to the isolation facility within the veterinary practice. Two of the puppies in the litter die and the other two are treated successfully and return to the facility with instructions that they should be put in the isolation kennel and monitored. Four days after the puppies return to the kennel, another litter of puppies that have been in the centre for 3 weeks present with signs of parvovirus and need to be treated at the practice. All of these puppies die. Full outbreak procedures are initiated and the facility is shut to the public.

The facility manager returns from holiday the next day. On investigation, they find out that a staff member, Jodie, had put the recovered litter of puppies into a general kennel because they were short staffed and had wanted to avoid all the extra work involved with isolation. Jodie had cleaned the kennels of both litters and spent some time socializing them, and it is believed this is how transmission occurred. On questioning Jodie, it becomes clear that she did not follow the veterinary surgeon's instructions or the centre's strict protocols for isolation and movement around the facility. Jodie is reprimanded for not following the veterinary surgeon's advice and is asked to review the organization's written protocols. The next day she volunteers to come to the practice to pick up the dam of the litter that died and asks to speak with the veterinary surgeon. Jodie apologizes and says that she should have known better, but she was stressed and overwhelmed. She did not realize how easy it was for parvovirus to spread and thought that once the animal recovered it could not infect others. At the time, she thought the veterinary surgeon was being a bit 'over the top' in asking her to keep the recovered puppies isolated from others. The veterinary surgeon sympathizes with Jodie, as sometimes the pressures of work in the shelter can be great and people do make mistakes. The veterinary surgeon seeks reassurance that she understands how parvovirus is transmitted. The veterinary surgeon also asks Jodie to think about whether there is anything that they can do to prevent this happening again.

DISCUSSION

In a facility that has employees, generally the manager of the facility will deal with issues of non–compliance with veterinary advice; however, it is often useful for the veterinary surgeon to also speak with the person involved. This helps to air the issues and allows the relationship between the veterinary surgeon and non-compliant person to continue positively. The veterinary surgeon's role is to encourage and educate the worker on why compliance is important and to educate on any specific veterinary detail relevant to the issue. It also helps the veterinary surgeon to understand the pressure on the shelter staff. When volunteers are involved, there may or may not be a line of support within the organization for addressing non-compliance and so, in the interest of the welfare of the animals involved, it becomes even more beneficial when the veterinary surgeon has the opportunity to explain the issues, including the rationale behind recommendations and this may highlight the need for further training.

QRG 23.1: Hoarding
by Vicky Halls

Definition of an 'animal hoarder'

A person who hoards animals is someone who accumulates animals and fails to provide minimum standards of care in terms of food, hygiene and health. The number of animals may vary. An animal hoarder will not seek treatment for sick animals or respond appropriately to their starvation or even death. Hoarders also neglect their own health and well being.

Almost every type of animal can be a victim of hoarding; however, cats are common as they are easily available, breed rapidly and can be concealed more effectively than dogs. In most situations, hoarders tend to concentrate on one species. Research shows that a significant majority of hoarders are female.

Hoarders may potentially be pet owners, breeders or people who work under the general umbrella of 'rescue', either as individuals or as part of a larger established organization.

The *Diagnostic and Statistical Manual of Mental Disorders* (DSM-5) classifies the hoarding of inanimate objects as 'Hoarding Disorder' under 'Obsessive-Compulsive and Related Disorders', with animal hoarding as a special manifestation.

Characteristics of animal hoarders may include

- Hoarders of inanimate objects.
- Non-functional utilities in the premises (plumbing, heating, electricity).
- A childhood characterized by chaotic, inconsistent, unstable parenting.
- Anthropomorphic attitude to animals.
- Perceive themselves as 'rescuers'.
- Belief that no one else cares better than them.
- An intense love of animals.
- Belief that they possess special abilities to communicate with animals.
- Recidivism – they will 'reoffend' and acquire more animals if a welfare intervention takes place and animals are removed but their mental health issues are not treated.

Subcategories of animal hoarder

Animal hoarders tend to fall into three categories, each having its own unique characteristics and requiring specific interventions. These categories are:

- Overwhelmed caregiver
- Rescue hoarder
- Exploiter hoarder.

Overwhelmed caregiver

Aids to identification:

- Some awareness of the difficulty of their situation
- Acquire their animals in a passive way (stray cats, unwanted animals, etc.)
- Numbers start at a manageable level but soon get out of hand, often triggered by a change in personal circumstances or a traumatic life experience
- Difficulties in problem-solving and finding a solution for their predicament
- Social isolation
- Animals seen as family members, providing emotional support
- Self-esteem directly linked to the possession of ever-increasing numbers of animals
- Fewer issues with public health or environmental authorities
- Most likely subcategory of animal hoarder to be receptive to intervention and assistance by an animal welfare organization.

Rescue hoarder

Aids to identification:

- Mission to save animals soon becomes an unavoidable compulsion
- Acquisition of animals is active, through advertising and promoting their 'rescue' status
- Possesses an extensive network of 'enablers' who see their efforts as worthy and the act of an animal lover
- Concept of rescuing animals to find homes soon becomes replaced by 'rescue' only
- Belief that they are the only ones who can provide the right level of care
- Not as likely to live with the animals if they operate a remote 'shelter'.

Exploiter hoarder

Aids to identification:

- Sociopathic characteristics, lacking empathy for humans and animals
- Indifferent to the harm they are causing
- Reject any concern or offer of assistance from outsiders
- Employ manipulative, controlling and cunning tactics to avert suspicion
- Adopt the role of expert
- Show no guilt or remorse if prosecuted for their acts of cruelty
- Least likely category to respond to animal welfare interventions.

Consequences of animal hoarding

- Disease associated with overcrowding and poor nutrition.
- Congenital and hereditary diseases, associated with interbreeding in animals that remain unneutered.
- Indiscriminate breeding, adding a further burden to the group.
- Environmental health issues:
  - Fleas, ringworm, *Cheyletiella* and other zoonotic diseases
  - Faecal contamination
  - High levels of ammonia in the air due to the volume of urine present.

Spotting the warning signs

The owner of multiple animals

Individuals may accumulate a large number of animals but care for them to a high standard by providing veterinary care and ensuring all members are neutered or prevented from indiscriminate mating. However, these situations can deteriorate, together with the mental health of the owner, and easily become overwhelming. Veterinary surgeons in practice may often be in a position to pick up the warning signs, which include:

- Owners of multiple animals no longer visit their veterinary practice

QRG 23.1 continued

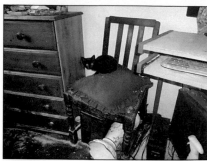

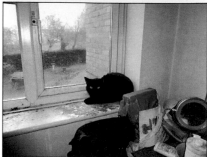

An environment heavily contaminated with matted fur, urine and faeces.
(© Cats Protection)

- Animals are rarely presented for diseases of old age
- Animals are presented only for trauma or infectious disease
- Requests for medication without presenting the animal for examination
- Owner gives vague replies to questions regarding the number of animals owned
- Owner claims to have 'just found' a cat.

The hoarding environment

Evidence of hoarding activity can clearly be seen from the outside of the property:

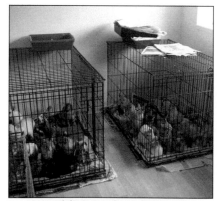

Keeping such large numbers of kittens in cages suggests that this owner is attempting to cope but may be feeling overwhelmed.
(Reproduced with permission from the RSPCA)

- Evidence of hoarding of objects, newspapers, rubbish in the house or in the front garden
- Property in disrepair
- Strong smells from the house; large numbers of flies at the windows
- Owner of the property is rarely seen and considered 'reclusive' by neighbours
- Owner reluctant to allow people into the property
- Evidence that stray or feral cats are being fed at or near the property
- Large number of cats in the vicinity
- Excessive noise from barking dogs from within the property or garden.

All hoarding cases deteriorate and numbers of animals increase with time, so the earlier an intervention takes place, the more likely the situation is to be resolved satisfactorily.

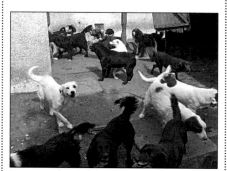

Large numbers of dogs can represent a significant noise nuisance.
(Reproduced with permission from the RSPCA)

Working with hoarders

The most effective solution to animal hoarding is to intervene early, offering support and guidance when the need for it is acknowledged – that is, at the stage when the hoarder could be categorized as an 'overwhelmed caregiver'.

Members of the veterinary team are particularly well placed to provide assistance at this stage, as there is a likelihood that a relationship of trust exists if the owner is a client, and they may, therefore, be receptive to a sensitive and helpful intervention. Overwhelmed caregivers will devote great energy to providing justification and excuses in an attempt to normalize their behaviour and enforce their good intentions. The most effective support the veterinary team can provide will be effective only if the owner feels they are not being judged or criticized for their actions. Various conditions need to exist for this to happen. Namely, the veterinary surgeon involved needs to be:

- Empathic (make every attempt to explore the situation from the owner's perspective)
- Genuine (real desire to help and to avoid appearing patronizing)
- Non-judgemental (potentially suspend their own thoughts and beliefs in order to effect change)
- Practical (offer solutions that appear reasonable to the owner and predictive of a positive outcome)
- Respectful (the client feels valued throughout and is, therefore, less likely to be defensive and uncooperative).

Assistance at this stage will include treatment of any veterinary conditions, neutering and rehoming with the owner's written consent, and monitoring over time to ensure they have developed appropriate strategies for managing a finite and reasonable population of animals in line with the individual's circumstances. It is essential to keep records of all conversations and interventions when working directly with hoarders, including photographs where appropriate, and comprehensive veterinary notes. As hoarding is considered a mental health issue, a comprehensive 'paper trail' of this kind is essential as there may be confusion on the part of the overwhelmed caregiver regarding events. Other agencies, such as Social Services, may need to be contacted.

Dealing with complaints regarding animal hoarding

If an intervention at an early stage has failed, or the situation is judged to be too extreme to consider providing assistance of this kind, it is necessary to bring the case to the attention of the relevant animal welfare organization. The veterinary team may find that this report will include input potentially from many sources: the owner (hoarder), family, friends, 'enablers', neighbours, social and environmental agencies, and other animal charities and welfare organizations. Any complaint regarding cruelty or neglect will be dealt with by the Royal Society ➡

QRG 23.1 *continued*

for the Prevention of Cruelty to Animals (RSPCA) (in England and Wales) or Scottish SPCA (in Scotland) (see Chapter 21). In Northern Ireland, enforcement of the welfare of animals is the responsibility of the local authorities Animal Welfare Officers.

Advice, assistance and support are given at this stage by the relevant animal welfare organization, together with any liaison with police, environmental health and social services. If reasonable improvements are not made within an agreed timescale, then the following procedure will take place:

- Animals are removed from the hoarder's premises
- Evidence is gathered (video and photographic)

- Records are kept of all animals (species, breed, sex)
- A welfare assessment is carried out for each animal
- Post-mortem examinations are done, if necessary
- Veterinary reports are produced
- Prosecution may be considered.

If as a result of the intervention consent is given to neuter and return animals, particularly cats, it is sensible for this to be carried out by veterinary or welfare teams experienced with feral or unsocialized cats, as the equipment and type of handling required are often similar.

When animals are signed over, many are considered to be unsuitable for rehoming due to disease or lack of early socialization and habituation to a normal domestic lifestyle. In these cases, euthanasia is frequently the

appropriate welfare option. However, there are instances in which the animals will benefit from rehoming and go on to lead normal lives. There are no specific criteria that indicate suitability and each situation must be assessed on a case-by-case basis.

References and further reading

American Psychiatric Association (2013) Hoarding disorder. In: *Diagnostic and Statistical Manual of Mental Disorders, 5th edn*, pp. 247–251. American Psychiatric Association Publishing, Washington DC

Arluke A and Killeen C (2009) *Inside Animal Hoarding: The Case of Barbara Erickson and Her 552 Dogs*. Purdue University Press, West Lafayette

Useful websites

Cummings School of Veterinary Medicine at Tufts University-Hoarding of Animals Research Consortium:
http://vet.tufts.edu/hoarding

QRG 23.2: Non-accidental injury

by Paula Boyden and Alexandra Brower

Abuse comes in many forms. The key categories that apply to animals, children and vulnerable adults are physical, sexual and emotional abuse, and neglect. These comprise a range of forms of abuse, including abandonment, hoarding, fighting, and intentional trauma or so-called non-accidental injury – beating, kicking, stamping, stabbing, throwing, burning, choking, suffocating, drowning, hanging, torture, mutilation, poisoning, shooting and vehicular trauma.

In the UK, the law makes no distinction between acts of omission (neglect) and acts of commission (direct acts of cruelty). The offence is considered the same and will attract the same sentence. The role of the veterinary surgeon in such cases is not to prove abuse but to report concerns accordingly. The following sections focus on the legislation and procedures followed in the UK. If practising outside the UK, one should be aware that clarifying intent may become a critical point in framing legal proceedings following abuse investigations; thus, veterinary surgeons should always have a clear understanding of the legal practices in their jurisdiction before taking any

action, and should seek advice from the relevant professional and legal bodies as necessary (see Chapter 21).

Responsibilities

Veterinary surgeons in the UK are not mandated to report cases of suspected abuse; however, readers are urged to consider their moral and ethical responsibilities in this regard. A veterinary surgeon's primary responsibility is to the animals under his/her care. The veterinary surgeon is not expected to prove abuse, but to provide evidence to the courts where required. Where abuse is a serious concern, and for questions about legal and professional obligations, the veterinary surgeon should first contact the Royal College of Veterinary Surgeons (RCVS) Professional Conduct Department before reporting to the relevant welfare organization (www.rcvs.org. uk/advice-and-guidance). If this is not possible, for example, out of hours, then contemporaneous notes should be kept.

There is always concern about client confidentiality (although if an animal is in the care of a shelter, its

previous owners may be known). This is addressed in the RCVS Code of Professional Conduct and warrants a discussion with the RCVS as described above.

In the UK, investigations are generally undertaken by the appropriate Society for the Prevention of Cruelty to Animals (SPCA); the RSPCA covers England and Wales, Scotland is covered by the Scottish SPCA. In Northern Ireland, concerns about neglect or abuse are the responsibility of local authorities Animal Welfare Officers.

Veterinary practices are encouraged to develop their own protocol in order to handle cases of suspected abuse. In this context this should include discussing findings with the shelter management or, indeed, the shelter having a protocol of its own. The Links Group (www. thelinksgroup.org.uk) has, in conjuction with the BVA Animal Welfare Foundation, developed a guidance document for the veterinary team (www.bva-awf.org. uk/advice-vets/recognising-abuse-animals-humens) which not only provides plenty of advice, but will help in developing an individual protocol. →

QRG 23.2 *continued*

Diagnostic considerations
Be well informed

Veterinary professionals working in the UK should familiarize themselves with the Animal Welfare Acts, the General Data Protection Regulation (GDPR) and relevant civil laws before engaging in cases of potential animal abuse. Veterinary professionals working outside the UK should identify and familiarize themselves with comparable laws for the jurisdiction in which they are practising. Obtaining approval, signatures on requests and detailed contact information before proceeding with diagnostics is essential. This means that consent must be given (from the shelter in this instance) before any diagnostic procedures, such as radiography to identify old, unexplained fractures, can be undertaken.

Documentation as diagnosis

Once a suspicion of abuse has been raised and reported, procedures to document, gather and protect evidence must be followed in tandem with diagnostic procedures. The start of evidence gathering should include a chain of custody form that documents the date, time, location and responsible party for each piece of evidence. Photographic documentation, once expected only for post-mortem examinations, has become standard practice in live animal abuse investigations. In an animal abuse investigation, diagnostic procedures can be equivalent to documentation and evidence gathering. A simple example would be radiography of a fracture where, in a case of intentional trauma, the radiograph provides both the diagnosis and the evidence of the trauma.

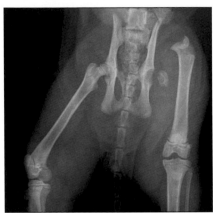

Documentation and diagnosis. Ventrodorsal radiograph of a 5-month-old cat, showing craniodorsal displacement of the left femur relative to the coxofemoral joint.
(Courtesy of Ryane E Englar)

Examination findings outside the norm

Unfortunately, there are no pathognomonic physical indicators for 'abuse', so diagnosis typically relies on a set of consistent physical findings in conjunction with appropriate history and other forms of evidence. That said, veterinary surgeons should be aware that there are physical and behavioural changes in both the animal and the owner consistent with specific types of abuse. The figure below highlights some of the more common physical and behavioural findings in reported cases of abuse, but is by no means comprehensive. Having enough awareness to notice and document these findings is a critical step in addressing cases of animal abuse.

On physical examination, specific areas of the body may require extra attention. The feet can reveal nail and paw pad trauma or hold trace environmental evidence. Abrasions, lacerations and other signs of trauma are commonly found, and relatively easy to identify, on the ears and face. Remember that while the hair coat over the body will hide trauma, it may also hold trace of environmental evidence. Thus, close attention should be paid to examination of the hair and skin over the entire body, and any materials found treated as evidence. This means wearing gloves while examining the animal to avoid contamination, and properly bagging, labelling and recording potential evidence. Findings consistent with some forms of neglect found on routine bloodwork and faecal examination include parasitism, anaemia and hypoproteinaemia. Specific techniques related to veterinary forensics are beyond the scope of this brief introduction, but

Animal ID:			
Organization ID:			
Species:			
Date/Time:	From:	To:	Reason:
(Date)	(Name/Organization)	(Name/Organization)	
(Time)	Signature	Signature	
(Date)	(Name/Organization)	(Name/Organization)	
(Time)	Signature	Signature	
(Date)	(Name/Organization)	(Name/Organization)	
(Time)	Signature	Signature	
(Date)	(Name/Organization)	(Name/Organization)	
(Time)	Signature	Signature	
(Date)	(Name/Organization)	(Name/Organization)	
(Time)	Signature	Signature	
(Date)	(Name/Organization)	(Name/Organization)	
(Time)	Signature	Signature	

Chain of custody form. These forms become part of the medical record and trace the flow of evidence from initial collection through to its use in legal proceedings or its disposal. In their simplest form, they capture the date, time, responsible party and location for each transfer in the history of a sample. They can be critical in legal proceedings if concerns about evidence tampering are presented. →

QRG 23.2 *continued*

Form of abuse	Consistent physical and behavioural changes
Neglect and abandonment	Owner experiencing economic difficulty Animal(s) with unkempt appearance; poor body condition, untreated wounds, flea and tick infestations, etc., without request for a diagnostic examination and treatment Serious illness or injury without request for euthanasia or apparent concern for welfare Dangerous or unsanitary environment Inadequate shelter
Hoarding	See QRG 23.1
Fighting	Characteristic pattern of bite wounds on head, neck and legs Owner indicating treatment of wounds at home
Intentional trauma	History provided not consistent with injuries found Delay in seeking treatment Old injury evident on examination or imaging – rib fractures in particular Repetitive injury Altered (fearful or aggressive) behaviour associated with a particular family member

Common physical and behavioural findings in reported cases of abuse.

are detailed in a number of reference books and publications (see References and further reading), and are presented in continuing education workshops and meetings.

It is important to understand that findings consistent with abuse do not indicate abuse on their own. A good rule of thumb is to seek and identify the cause of any abnormal physical or behavioural finding in a patient, bearing in mind the many findings that can result from abuse.

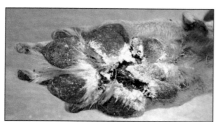

Plantar surface of a dog's paw. In this case, examination of the feet revealed overgrown nails packed with faeces, suggesting that this dog had been kept in a confined area. In addition, the paw pads were coated in a thick white paint. The dog was found in a house with a heavy chain attached to its collar. It had clearly been moved to this location, and no paint was reported in the premises.

The link to abuse of children and vulnerable adults

While there may be no known history for many of the animals in a shelter environment, some at least will have been relinquished. In this regard, it is important that the veterinary surgeon and shelter team are aware of the inter-relationships or 'links' between the abuse of children, vulnerable adults and animals. Domestic abuse can take many forms, and it is possible that animals in a household may well be at risk and part of the cycle of power and control that a perpetrator holds over his/her victims.

> When animals are abused, people are at risk.
> When people are abused, animals are at risk.
>
> Phil Arkow (1996)
> (from Ascione, 2010)

There are pet fostering services available in the UK for victims fleeing domestic abuse, such as the Dogs Trust Freedom Project (www.moretodogstrust.org.uk/freedom-project/freedom-project), which provide short-term care for pets so that victims can flee a violent situation without having to leave their pet behind or relinquish it. Hence, it is important for those dealing with relinquishment to be aware of the 'link', to discuss situations with their colleagues and to offer support/referral where indicated. Pet fostering services in the UK are also provided by the RSPCA, Cats Protection, and Endeavour (previously Paws for Kids). These organizations make up the pet fostering subgroup of the Links Group.

The Links Group is dedicated to promoting communication and cross-reporting between agencies involved in domestic abuse. The group also offers a guidance document for the veterinary team, which can be found, along with further information on fostering services, at www.thelinksgroup.org.uk.

References and further reading

Ascione FR (2010) *The International Handbook of Animal Abuse and Cruelty: Theory, Research, and Application*. Purdue University Press, West Lafayette

Merck MD (2013) *Veterinary Forensics: Animal Cruelty Investigations, 2nd edn*. Wiley-Blackwell, Ames, Iowa

Munro R and Munro HMC (2008) *Animal Abuse and Unlawful Killing: Veterinary Forensic Pathology*. Saunders Elsevier, Edinburgh

Useful websites

Cats Protection Paws Protect: www.cats.org.uk/what-we-do/paws-protect

Dogs Trust Freedom Project: www.moretodogstrust.org.uk/freedom-project/freedom-project

Endeavour (previously Paws for Kids): www.pawsforkids.org.uk/

Raystede Centre for Animal Welfare: www.raystede.org/

RSPCA PetRetreat: www.rspca.org.uk/whatwedo/petretreat

The Links Group Pet Fostering: www.thelinksgroup.org.uk/professionals/pet-fostering-services/

Chapter 24

Training and education in the shelter environment

Karen Hiestand and Emily Newbury

Importance of training and education in the shelter environment

People are drawn to work with animals for many different reasons. In the animal charity sector, and specifically the hands-on shelter environment, many of those employed or working as a volunteer are hugely committed and engaged. However, there can be large variations in their background knowledge, experience, understanding of issues and moral alignment with the shelter's aims. This variability can cause difficulty, not just in day-to-day operations, but also more widely in terms of disagreements over decision-making and direction – for example, a committed volunteer who leans towards an 'animal rights' moral base may find a more utilitarian decision to euthanase an animal deeply distressing (see Chapter 2). The overall dependence of the shelter sector on volunteers presents specific challenges due to volunteer turnover, irregular working hours, a lack of contractual training obligations and reluctance to enforce a training programme that may discourage new starters or be impractical for some (e.g. students on a temporary placement).

While some aspects of hands-on animal care are suitable for on-the-job learning, there is a degree of technical knowledge that is required to successfully underpin good shelter practice. Within the sector, some may believe that experience with pet animals, or experience in a rescue context, constitutes sufficient training for their needs. However, without evidence-based technical knowledge, poor practice and misconceptions can be unintentionally perpetuated. Furthermore, accepted practice in areas such as preventive health strategies, behaviour modification, disinfection, disease treatment options and emerging disease entities will change over time, requiring personnel to be continually updated. Many shelter staff and volunteers are desperately keen to learn for the benefit of the animals they care for and for their own personal development, but they may be limited by the logistical and resource challenges of their working environment.

The consequences of inadequate or out-of-date knowledge include:

* Disease outbreaks
* Animal welfare compromise or death (may be a significant risk, if diseases such as parvovirus are present)
* Financial expense of outbreaks
* Impact on team morale
* Impact on staff and volunteer retention
* Waste of financial resources, e.g. the cost of treatments for diseases may be greater than the cost of prevention; spending on neonatal care rather than neutering pregnant animals
* Public relations repercussions, e.g. from lack of understanding of the law relating to animal ownership.

Planning an educational programme

The earliest stage of planning any educational initiative is to decide what to include and how to present it. Within a single organization, there may be individuals with decades of experience who want to learn more about the details of a particular disease, teenage students on placement who have been given responsibility for cleaning and disinfection, permanent staff with varying levels of knowledge and understanding, and volunteers who work only one or two days a month. Ensuring that all these groups are catered for requires a lot of thought and planning, and ongoing effort.

The dominant method of information delivery in shelters is 'on-the-job' training – this is informal, opportunistic and somewhat reactive, but excellent for rapid induction of new staff and for demonstrating practical skills. However, the experience of each trainee will differ and this method offers limited opportunities for the transmission of detailed technical information. In an ideal world, both new starters and existing staff would be offered a multi-modal education programme that uses a variety of ways to deliver information (visual, verbal, written, experiential, etc.), incorporating the methods most suited to each educational goal and delivered in an engaging manner.

A major limitation to providing training and education is time. Face-to-face training within the shelter can be extremely effective and rewarding, but it is resource-heavy and requires reinforcement for messages to persist. It can be worth investing in specific individuals and upskilling them to create a 'train the trainer' situation where the selected team member can then continue with on-site training for other team members. Other options for the delivery of information include e-learning (an emerging modality in shelter medicine), handbooks, posters, external courses, having a training team based at head office (for larger organizations), etc.

Training may be either curriculum-based or reactive, or a combination of both. The last of these options is preferable as it is impossible to predict every relevant scenario but important to cover a core of vital information. Reactive training may be very effective if the minds of the participants are focused by their awareness of a current disease outbreak or following an unfortunate event. However, as many shelters struggle with staff and volunteer retention, relying on reactive training may result in very irregular coverage of important topics.

It is desirable for shelters to have some written guidelines for common tasks and scenarios. These can be compiled into a handbook and/or disseminated as posters, handouts, reminder e-mails, 'topic of the month' newsletters, etc. This is an excellent opportunity for veterinary involvement, especially with biosecurity and preventive medicine topics, and may act as a prompt for fruitful discussions about current and future practice.

Assessing current training practices

It is worthwhile for veterinary surgeons (veterinarians) who work with shelters to familiarize themselves with each organization's current practice, and with what is and is not working well, when assessing how best to fill in knowledge gaps and correct errors.

While some of the large organizations will have dedicated training officers and access to in-house expertise from veterinary surgeons, nurses, behaviourists etc., many smaller shelters will not. These smaller organizations are extremely dependent on the cumulative knowledge of current and past staff members and advice gleaned from other sources such as the internet. In these circumstances, time pressures and a lack of reliable information may limit both the extent and content of training offered.

What do shelter workers need to know?

As mentioned, there are certain subject areas that are of vital importance in the shelter environment; these will be discussed later in this chapter. However, it is worth briefly considering the progress of training and educational initiatives in related fields, as there may be useful parallels. For example, in the international animal welfare sector, there has been a trend away from didactic educational interventions ('I think you should learn about this') and towards evidence-based, participatory methods ('What are your questions?'; 'What are your current practices?'). This is mirrored in many other fields including human healthcare. To give a veterinary example, Upjohn *et al.* (2012; 2013) carried out an investigation into the health issues of working equids in Lesotho. This work formed part of the planning of an educational programme intended to focus on saddlery, farriery and nutrition. Interestingly, the health priorities identified by the study differed from those originally chosen for inclusion in the intervention.

Applying this approach in the shelter context, it is vital to have an understanding of the current knowledge levels among staff and volunteers to inform the selection of topics and the level of detail presented. For example, the staff/volunteers may be extremely experienced in general cleaning and disinfection, but may be less aware of the concept of fomite spread (see Chapter 9). In that case, time would be better spent discussing less obvious routes of disease transmission rather than revisiting aspects they are already familiar with. Brief interviews with staff members at every level in the organization may help to ascertain their training needs.

Possible topics to cover

When considering what veterinary surgeons may be able to offer shelter workers in terms of training or information provision, perhaps the greatest overall impact can be achieved by starting with biosecurity and preventive medicine.

For example:

- Advising on facility design
- Cleaning regime and disinfectant choice
- Background information about common infectious diseases and options for their management:
    - How diseases are spread, how long they survive on a fomite, common clinical signs and treatments
    - Zoonotic disease – recognition, prevention, management and public health obligations
    - Parasite life cycles and control options
    - The role of vaccination.

Other topics to consider include:

- Safe and appropriate animal handling – not only to improve the welfare of animals in a facility, but also to weave in messages about behaviour and reduce the risk of injuries such as bites and scratches to shelter workers
- Administering medication
- Basics of wound care
- Normal whelping/kittening and neonatal care – a potentially stressful scenario for many shelters (Figure 24.1)
- Dealing with emergencies
- Clear guidance on when veterinary intervention is required
- Nutrition and weight management – especially obesity, considering the confined housing of most animals in shelters and the impact of this on their caloric needs
- Neutering – including why it is important, optimum timing, ethical considerations and how it is performed (this could include inviting workers to observe surgeries)
- Basics of behaviour and ethology, including socialization
- Animal welfare legislation.

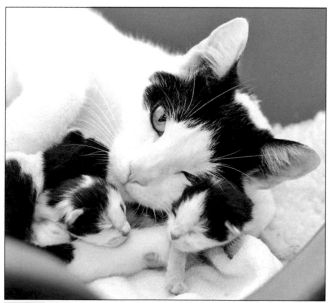

24.1 There are many topics relevant to shelter staff, including neonatal care.
(© Cats Protection)

It is important that appropriate expertise is sought, particularly regarding the last two topics listed above, and that the materials and information presented are suitable and up to date.

What will they do with the information?

Educational interventions generally seek to influence something – people's knowledge, attitudes, beliefs or practices. Although simply imparting information may result in the desired change, this is not always the case, and many factors will play a part. As well as considering the specific audience when devising a training curriculum, the use of technical language and the method of delivery will need to be tailored to their needs. The information that is supplied then has to be digested and retained by the participants; this process will be affected by factors such as their individual learning styles (see below) and levels of engagement. Even if all of the relevant facts are provided to justify a change in practice, this may not occur. Experts in this field have spent decades developing and refining models that seek to account for the major influences upon human behaviour, including social norms (what do others in the shelter do?), the cost to the individual (e.g. in terms of time, money or emotional energy – all of which are under pressure in shelters), practical aspects (e.g. the shelter cannot vaccinate animals at intake if it does not have on-site veterinary cover) and previous habits (Figure 24.2). While these models can never fully represent the decision-making process, they may help to structure thinking when planning an educational programme and prompt consideration of aspects that might otherwise be missed.

Therefore, an ideal shelter educational programme should:

- Engage the target audience
- Provide the required information or experience in a way that is tailored to their needs and the context in which they work
- Be cost-effective – Finances are usually limited in the shelter sector and there are many competing priorities when it comes to spending
- Deal with barriers:
  - To attending training – For example, by arranging 'lunch and learn' sessions, if time during the rest of the day is limited, or using online learning resources
  - To performing a new behaviour – For example, mark buckets to show the line to which they should be filled with water for diluting a specific amount of disinfectant
- Utilize motivators – For example, explaining how improvements in hygiene in the puppy area may reduce cases of diarrhoea and speed up rehoming
- Be appraised for its efficacy – For example, by obtaining feedback, using informal team quizzes to test knowledge
- Have a long-term perspective – For example, consider the frequency of updates/refreshers needed, especially if new staff or volunteers start at the shelter.

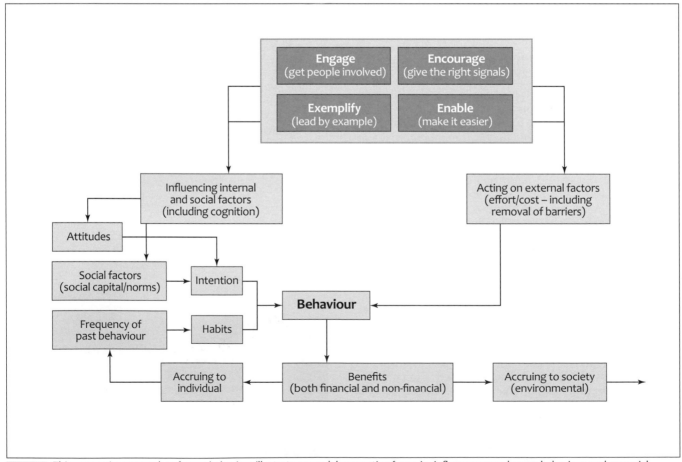

24.2 This composite approach to farmer behaviour illustrates a model accounting for major influences upon human behaviour, such as social factors, attitude and cost, and can be useful for understanding how shelter staff use educational interventions.
(Reproduced with permission from Defra; redrawn after Fishbein and Ajzen, 1975 and Ajzen, 1991)

Publicly available materials

There are many publicly available resources that may be of interest to veterinary and non-veterinary shelter staff (see Figure 24.3 and the Appendix). It is worth noting that some of the content will be influenced by country-specific factors.

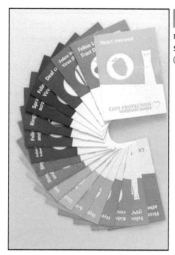

24.3 Many national charities provide educational resources that can be used by shelter staff.
(© Cats Protection)

Training delivery examples

The following case studies are some illustrative examples of training sessions experienced by the authors.

Introducing faecal scoring using 'Poo bingo'
Why?

Dogs at a shelter were frequently affected by diarrhoea but, with frequent staff shift changes, it was difficult to ascertain whether stool quality was improving when it was reported by different people. Faecal scoring was introduced to enable more accurate recording of progress.

How?

The Waltham Faecal Scoring Chart was used. A brief overview of its content and the reasons for using it were given. Then, staff members were then split into small teams and issued bingo grids made up of faecal scoring numbers. Standardized pictures representing different faecal scores were shown, one by one, on the projector, and staff had to call out when they knew what the score was. If they were correct, they could cross the number off their grid until they had three crosses in a row and had won. Prizes were given to the winners.

Results

Following the training session, everyone made an effort to use the faecal scoring system, and laminated copies were provided for reference. After a few weeks, most staff members were using the scoring system in a consistent manner and it greatly helped the monitoring of diarrhoea cases within the shelter. The training was reinforced by actively asking staff to grade a dog's faeces when they reported a case of diarrhoea to the veterinary team.

Teaching veterinary terminology using 'Match the word to the definition'
Why?

Staff members were frequently asked to explain the pre-existing medical conditions of dogs within the shelter when introducing them to potential adopters. This caused stress for both the shelter and veterinary staff, as the terminology was often unfamiliar and adopters would ask questions that the staff members could not answer.

How?

Feedback was sought about the most common veterinary terms and conditions that staff struggled with. In addition, the veterinary surgeons and nurses compiled a list of words they thought would be useful to cover. Terminology and definitions were typed up and printed out, and the printed pages were then cut up to separate the terms from their definitions (e.g. 'carpal valgus' – 'bending outwards of the legs from the wrist joint, usually found in small dogs and rarely a problem'). Staff members were organized into small groups and each group was given the same set of words and definitions. They were given time to try to match them together, using their combined knowledge and experience to reach agreement. Then, the groups came back together to debate and decide on the final pairings.

Results

Staff members were quite proficient at matching words and definitions but the session provided a good opportunity to review certain topics and clarify misunderstandings. In addition to this, a system was instituted by which dogs with complex medical conditions were highlighted with a coloured sticker on their file, indicating that any new owner would need to talk to a veterinary surgeon or nurse about the dog. Finally, the veterinary team wrote brief reviews in accessible language of cases with ongoing medical needs. These were also placed in the dog's file so that adopters could read them and take a copy for future reference.

Other considerations when devising training sessions

- **Breadth *versus* depth:** shelter staff need to know a lot about a few topics, and a little about a lot of topics. The degree of depth with which a topic needs to be approached will depend on the audience; e.g. long-term staff will want and need to know more than casual volunteers, and providing opportunities for their professional development is vital
- **Group size:** if holding an in-person training session, consider whether the topic may be more suitable for whole-group or small-group work
- **Personality dynamics:** when conducting in-person training, it is useful to take the personality dynamics of the group into account and try to provide opportunities for everyone to participate, even if some are more confident than others
- **Learning styles:** the VARK (visual, auditory, read/write and kinaesthetic) questionnaire can be useful to prompt consideration of different types of learners within an organization

- **Combining modalities:** e.g. by following up a training session with a set of review notes, or e-mailing a presentation to all staff for their future reference
- **Feedback from the group:** did the training achieve what was intended? Was it enjoyable? What could be done differently next time to make the training better?

Why should veterinary surgeons get involved?

Veterinary surgeons are in a unique position to influence and provide advice to people – not only to maximize animal welfare but also to assist charity organizations in operating optimally in terms of their resources. Building a strong relationship between practice staff and the workers within a charitable organization is key to allowing open dialogue and to creating avenues for cooperation with staff and volunteer training and guidance (see Chapter 23). Veterinary surgeons' involvement in providing training and information for an organization can significantly enhance the accuracy of knowledge applied in that setting and avoid some of the pitfalls that may be encountered when less appropriate sources are consulted. It can also be very personally rewarding to be involved in a preventive, rather than just problem-solving, capacity.

The bigger picture

An important consideration when providing information to shelter workers is that there is every hope they will pass knowledge on – not just within the organization, but also more widely, to adopters and the general public. This can be an important tool in spreading understanding of appropriate animal care, and is particularly useful for disseminating messages about responsible pet ownership, preventive healthcare and animal behaviour. However, it can also be worthwhile to highlight any differences between the shelter situation and the home environment with regard to some specific aspects of disease prevention and treatment. For example, in the shelter context, biosecurity and infectious disease prevention are commonly considered to be of the utmost importance, due partly to the interplay between stress and immunosuppression. These considerations are lessened in a home environment, where the animal will experience less stress and will most likely be exposed to fewer conspecifics; hence, the specifics of shelter vaccination decisions or parasite control measures may not be transferrable to the home. It is, therefore, important that general principles are well understood, rather than just prescriptive protocols.

Providing information to members of the public

It is ideal if veterinary surgeons engage further with the general public over issues of unwanted animals. Considering avenues to reach audiences both within and outside those normally seen in a clinic setting is important in addressing the root problem of overpopulation.

Key messages to highlight include:

- The scale of the unwanted animal problem
- Benefits of acquiring animals from rescues/shelters rather than other sources
- Responsible ownership.

Many veterinary practices already engage with their community through newsletters and open days, and these are excellent opportunities to consider promoting local shelters and working with them to educate the public. To reach beyond the practice-engaged community, consider working with local community groups and education providers (Figure 24.4). Many organizations already engage in community education initiatives, and volunteering time to participate in these efforts can be both rewarding and effective. Working collaboratively with local animal shelters, and more widely within the community is often not only personally rewarding, but can have knock-on effects for practice marketing and business growth, and may also increase public trust in veterinary surgeons as being primarily devoted to animal welfare.

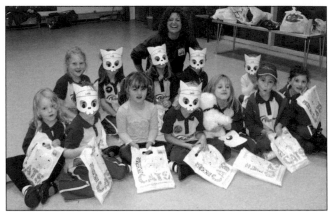

24.4 Engaging with future pet owners.
(© Cats Protection)

References and further reading

Ajzen I (1991) The theory of planned behavior. *Organizational Behavior and Human Decision Processes* **50**, 179–211

Department for Farming and Rural Affairs (2008) *Understanding behaviours in a farming context: bringing theoretical and applied evidence together from across Defra and highlighting policy relevance and implications for future research.* Defra. Available at: http://webarchive.nationalarchives.gov.uk/20130222210253/http://www.defra.gov.uk/statistics/files/defra-stats-foodfarm-environ-obs-research-behavious-aceopaper-nov08.pdf

Fishbein M and Ajzen I (1975) *Belief, attitude, intention and behavior: an introduction to theory and research.* Addison-Wesley, Reading

Upjohn MM, Attwood GA, Lerotholi T, Pfeiffer DU and Verheyen KLP (2013) Quantitative *versus* qualitative approaches: a comparison of two research methods applied to identification of key health issues for working horses in Lesotho. *Preventive Veterinary Medicine* **108**, 313–320

Upjohn MM, Shipton K, Pfeiffer DU *et al.* (2012) Cross-sectional survey of owner knowledge and husbandry practices, tack and health issues affecting working horses in Lesotho. *Equine Veterinary Journal* **44**, 310–318

Useful websites

Waltham Faeces Scoring System:
www.waltham.com/dyn/_assets/_pdfs/resources/FaecesQuality2.pdf

VARK learning styles questionnaire:
http://vark-learn.com/home/

Useful websites and further reading

Section 1: Principles of shelter medicine and population health

Shelter medicine

Useful websites

ASPCA Pro:
www.aspcapro.org

Association of Charity Vets (ACV):
www.associationofcharityvets.org.uk

Association of Shelter Veterinarians:
www.sheltervet.org

Association of Dog and Cat Homes:
www.adch.org.uk/

Battersea Dogs and Cats Home:
www.battersea.org.uk/

BestBETs for Vets:
https://bestbetsforvets.org

Blue Cross:
www.bluecross.org.uk/

BSAVA Library:
www.bsavalibrary.com

BSAVA:
https://www.bsava.com/MyBSAVA/Knowledge-bank/
Practice/Practice-Pack/Module-2

BVA 2009:
https://www.bva.co.uk/Workplace-guidance/Ethical-
guidance/role-of-the-vet-in-treatment-choice/

Cats Protection:
www.cats.org.uk/

Cats Protection information for veterinary surgeons:
www.cats.org.uk/cat-care/vets-info/

Centre for Evidence-based Vet medicine:
www.nottingham.ac.uk/cevm

Dogs Trust:
www.dogstrust.org.uk/

EBVM Learning
http://www.ebvmlearning.org/

National Animal Welfare Trust:
www.nawt.org.uk/

Maddie's fund:
www.maddiesfund.org/

Pet food manufacturers association:
www.pfma.org.uk/

The People's Dispensary for Sick Animals (PDSA):
www.pdsa.org.uk/

RSPCA:
www.rspca.org.uk/home

RCVS Knowledge:
https://knowledge.rcvs.org.uk/quality-improvement/

University of California Davis Koret Shelter Medicine Program:
www.sheltermedicine.com

Scottish Society for the Prevention of Cruelty to Animals (SSPCA):
www.scottishspca.org/

The Ulster Society Prevention Cruelty to Animals (USPCA):
http://uspca.co.uk/

University of Florida Shelter Medicine program:
www.onlinesheltermedicine.vetmed.ufl.edu/

Veterinary Evidence:
www.veterinaryevidence.org/index.php/ve

VetSRev database of veterinary systematic reviews:
https://webapps.nottingham.ac.uk/refbase/

Wood Green:
www.woodgreen.org.uk/

Further reading

Fletcher RH, Fletcher SW and Fletcher GS (2014) *Clinical Epidemiology: The Essentials*. Wolters Kluwer/Lippincott Williams & Wilkins, Philadelphia

Gordis L (2014) *Epidemiology, 5th edn*. Elsevier Saunders, Philadelphia

Miller L and Zawistowski S (2012) *Shelter Medicine for Veterinarians and Staff 2nd edn*, Wiley-Blackwell, Iowa

Newbury S, Blinn MK, Bushby PA, *et al.* (2010) *Guidelines for Standards of Care in Animal Shelters*. www.sheltervet.org/assets/docs/shelter-standards-oct2011-wforward.pdf

Rollin BE (2006) *An Introduction to Veterinary Medical Ethics: Theory and Cases, 2nd edn*. Blackwell Publishing, Oxford

Rothman KJ (2012) Epidemiology: *An Introduction, 2nd edn*. Oxford University Press, Oxford

Salman M (2003) Surveillance and monitoring systems for animal health programs and disease surveys. In: *Animal Disease Surveillance and Survey Systems: Methods and Applications*, ed. M Salman, pp. 3–13. Iowa State Press and Blackwell Publishing, Ames

Sandøe P and Christiansen SB (2008) *Ethics of Animal Use*. Wiley-Blackwell, Oxford

Sandoe P, Corr S and Palmer C (2015) *Companion Animal Ethics*. Wiley-Blackwell, Oxford

Yeates J (2013) *Animal Welfare in Veterinary Practice*. Wiley-Blackwell/UFAW,Oxford

Yeates J (in production) *Companion Animal Care and Welfare*. Wiley-Blackwell, Oxford

Population medicine
Useful websites

Alley Cat Allies:
www.alleycat.org/

Alliance for Contraception in Cats and Dogs (ACC&D):
www.acc-d.org/

Google My Maps:
www.google.com/mymaps

International Companion Animal Management (ICAM) Coalition:
www.icam-coalition.org/resources.html

ISFM guidelines on population management and welfare of unowned domestic cats:
www.icatcare.org/vets/guidelines

Kitten neutering database:
www.kind.cats.org.uk/

Mission Rabies:
www.missionrabies.com/

Oak Tree Animals' Charity, Feral cats and hoarding:
www.oaktreeanimals.org.uk/community/feral-cats-hoarding.html

OIE World Organisation for Animal Health Terrestrial Animal Health Code:
www.oie.int/international-standard-setting/terrestrial-code/

World Health Organization, Rabies:
www.who.int/rabies/animal/dogs/en/

Further reading

Feline Advisory Bureau (2006) *Feral Cat Manual*. International Cat Care, Tisbury

Remfry J (2001) *Ruth Plant, a Pioneer in Animal Welfare*. Jenny Remfry, Barnet

Sutherland WJ (2006) *Ecological Census Techniques, 2nd edn*: a handbook. Cambridge University Press, Cambridge

Section 2: Prevention, management and control of disease in the shelter medicine environment

Shelter design and biosecurity
Useful websites

Chartered Institute of Environmental Health (2013) CIEH *Model Licence: Conditions and Guidance for Cat Boarding Establishments 2013* (updated June 2016):
https://lindec-lu.co.uk/wp-content/uploads/2016/10/CIEH_Model_licence_conditions_and_guidance_cat_boarding_establishments_2013_updated_June_2016.pdf

Chartered Institute of Environmental Health (2016) CIEH Model Licence: Conditions and Guidance for Dog Boarding Establishments 2016:
www.cannockchasedc.gov.uk/sites/default/files/dog_boarding-final_published_version_1_june_2016.pdf

Royal College of Veterinary Surgeons, information regarding veterinary practices:
www.rcvs.org.uk/registration register-of-veterinary-practice-premises/

Royal College of Veterinary Surgeons, Practice Standards Scheme:
www.rcvs.org.uk/practice-standards-scheme/

Universities Federation for Animal Welfare:
www.ufaw.org.uk

United States Humane Society:
www.humanesociety.org

Further reading

Feline Advisory Bureau (2002) *Boarding Cattery Manual*, Feline Advisory Bureau, Tisbury

Key D (2006) *Cattery Design: The Essential Guide to Creating Your Perfect Cattery*. David and Kay Key Kennel & Cattery Design, Chipping Norton

Key D (2008) Kennel Design – *The Essential Guide to Creating Your Perfect Kennels*. David and Kay Key Kennel & Cattery Design, Chipping Norton

Infectious diseases
Useful websites

Advisory Board on Cat Diseases:
www.abcdcatsvets.org

American Animal Hospital Association:
www.aaha.org

American Animal Hospital Association (2011) Canine vaccination guidelines:
www.aaha.org/public_documents/professional/guidelines/caninevaccineguidelines.pdf

American Association of Feline Practitioners:
www.catvets.com

American Association of Feline Practitioners, 2013 AAFP Feline Vaccination Advisory Panel Report:
https://www.catvets.com/guidelines/practice-guidelines/feline-vaccination-guidelines

BVA Animal Welfare Foundation pet travel advice:
www.bva-awf.org.uk/pet-care-advice/pet-travel

Companion Vector-Borne Diseases (Bayer Healthcare):
www.cvbd.org

European Scientific Counsel Companion Animal Parasites (ESCCAP) Guidelines:
www.esccap.org

Europetnet:
www.europetnet.com

FeLV/FIV flowcharts:
www.cats.org.uk/uploads/documents/FIV_FeLV_testing_flowcharts-1117.pdf

International Cat Care:
www.icatcare.org/advice

Koret Shelter Medicine Program:
www.sheltermedicine.com/

Langford Vets Diagnostic Laboratories
www.langfordvets.co.uk/diagnostic-laboratories

PROTECT website:
www.bsava.com/Resources/PROTECT/PROTECT.aspx

University of Glasgow School of Veterinary Medicine information about FIP:
www.gla.ac.uk/schools/vet/cad/researchprojects/fip/fip_about/

University of Glasgow Veterinary Diagnostic Services
www.gla.ac.uk/schools/vet/cad/

World Organisation for Animal Health rabies portal:
www.oie.int/en/animal-health-in-the-world/rabies-portal/

World Small Animal Veterinary Association:
www.wsava.org

Further reading

August JR (2006) *Consultations in Internal Medicine, Vol 5.* Elsevier Saunders, St Louis

August JR (2010) *Consultations in Internal Medicine, Vol 6.* Elsevier Saunders, St Louis

Caveney L, Jones B and Ellis K (2012) *Veterinary Infection, Prevention and Control*. Wiley-Blackwell, Ames

Cooper B, Mullineaux E and Turner L (2011) *BSAVA Textbook of Veterinary Nursing, 5th edn*. BSAVA Publications, Gloucester

Dallas S (1999) *BSAVA Manual of Veterinary Care*. BSAVA Publications, Gloucester

Ettinger SJ and Feldman EC (2010) *Textbook of Veterinary Internal Medicine: Diseases of the Dog and Cat, 7th edn*. Elsevier Saunders, St Louis

Greene C (2013) *Infectious Diseases of the Dog and Cat, 4th edn*. Elsevier Saunders, St. Louis

Jackson HA and Marsella R (2012) *BSAVA Manual of Canine and Feline Dermatology*. BSAVA Publications, Gloucester

Miller L and Hurley K, (2009) *Infectious Disease Management in Animal Shelters*. Wiley-Blackwell, Iowa

Olivry T *et al.* (2015). *Treatment of canine atopic dermatitis: 2015 updated guidelines from the International Committee on Allergic Diseases of Animals (ICADA)*. BMC Vet Res 11: 210 Patel A, Forsythe P and Smith S (2008) *Small Animal Dermatology*. Saunders Elsevier, London

Ramsey I (2014) *BSAVA Small Animal Formulary, 8th edn*. BSAVA Publications, Gloucester

Ramsey I and Tennant B (2001) *BSAVA Manual of Canine and Feline Infectious Diseases*. BSAVA Publications, Gloucester

Scherk MA, Ford RB, Gaskell RM *et al.* (2013) 2013 AAFP Feline Vaccination Advisory Panel Report. *Journal of Feline Medicine and Surgery* **15**, 785–808

Sykes JE (2014) *Canine and Feline Infectious Diseases, 1st edn*. Elsevier Saunders, St Louis

Behaviour
Useful websites

Association of Pet Behaviour Counsellors:
www.apbc.org.uk

The Animal Behaviour and Training Council:
www.abtcouncil.org.uk

Bristol Veterinary School:
www.bristol.ac.uk/vetscience/services/behaviour-clinic/dogbehaviouralsigns/interpretingbehaviour.html

Cat Protection, E-learning:
www.cats.org.uk/learn/e-learning-ufo

Cats Protection/Cat Care/Cat behaviour:
www.cats.org.uk/cat-care/cat-behaviour-hub

Cats Protection, How to introduce cats to dogs:
http://bit.ly/catstodogs

Cats Protection Information Leaflets:
www.cats.org.uk/cat-care/care-leaflets

CCAB Accreditation:
www.asab.org/ccab

Code of practice for the welfare of cats:
www.gov.uk/government/publications/code-of-practice-for-the-welfare-of-cats

Dogs Trust, Dog School classes:
www.dogstrustdogschool.org.uk

Dogs Trust, Sound Therapy for pets:
www.dogstrust.org.uk/help-advice/dog-behaviour-health/sound-therapy-for-pets

PDSA Animal Wellbeing (PAW) Report:
www.pdsa.org.uk/get-involved/our-campaigns/pdsa-animal-wellbeing-report

The Puppy Socialisation Plan:
www.thepuppyplan.com

Low stress handling™ University
https://lowstresshandling.com/

Cattledog Publishing – The legacy of Dr Sophia Yin:
https://drsophiayin.com/blog/entry/free-downloads-posters-handouts-and-more/

Welfare in Dog Training:
www.dogwelfarecampaign.org

Further reading

Bailey G (2008) *The Perfect Puppy, revised edn*. Hamlyn, London

Bradshaw J (2012) *In Defence of Dogs*. Penguin Books, London

Donaldson J (1996) *The Culture Clash, 2nd edn*. James and Kenneth Publishers, Berkeley

Gray J (1971) *The Psychology of Fear and Stress*. McGraw Hill, New York

Horowitz D and Mills D (2009) *BSAVA Manual of Canine and Feline Behavioural Medicine, 2nd edn*. BSAVA Publications, Gloucester

Jensen P *The Behavioural Biology of Dogs*. CAB International, Wallingford, UK

Lindsay SR (2000) *Handbook of Applied Dog Behavior and Training*, Iowa State University Press, Ames

Mech LD and Boitani L (2003) *Wolves: Behavior, Ecology and Conservation*. University of Chicago Press, Chicago

Nicassio-Hiskey N and Alia Mitchell C (2013) *Beyond Squeaky Toys: Innovative Ideas for Eliminating Problem Behaviors and Enriching the Lives of Dogs and Cats*. Smart Pets Press, Lafayette

Pryor K (2002) *Don't Shoot the Dog! The New Art of Teaching and Training, 3rd edn.* Ringpress Book

Rodan I, Sundahl E, Carney H, *et al.* (2011) AAFP and ISFM feline-friendly handling guidelines. *Journal of Feline Medicine and Surgery*, **13(5)**, pp 364-375

Scott JP and Fuller JL (1965) *Genetics and the Social Behavior of the Dog.* University of Chicago Press, Chicago

Serpell J *The Domestic Dog: Its Evolution, Behaviour and Interactions with People*, Cambridge University Press, Cambridge

Turner DC and Bateson P *The Domestic Cats: the biology of its behaviour*, pp. 159-177, Cambridge University Press, Cambridge

Young RJ (2003) *Environmental Enrichment for Captive Animals.* Blackwell Publishing, Oxford

Zulch H and Mills D (2012) *Life Skills for Puppies: Laying the Foundation for a Loving, Lasting Relationship.* Hubble and Hattie, Dorchester

Section 3: Working with people in the shelter environment

Charities
Useful websites

Charity Commission for England and Wales:
www.gov.uk/government/organisations/charity-commission

Charity Commission for Northern Ireland:
www.charitycommissionni.org.uk/

Charity Governance Code:
www.charitygovernancecode.org/en/

National Council of Voluntary Organisations:
www.ncvo.org.uk/

RCVS Code of Professional Conduct for Veterinary Nurses:
www.rcvs.org.uk/advice-and-guidance/code-of-professional-conduct-for-veterinary-nurses/

RCVS Code of Professional Conduct for Veterinary Surgeons:
www.rcvs.org.uk/advice-and-guidance/code-of-professional-conduct-for-veterinary-surgeons/

Scottish Charity Regulator:
www.oscr.org.uk/

VAT Tribunal Case V20519:Gables Farm Dogs and Cats Home *versus* HMRC 04/01/2008:
http://financeandtax.decisions.tribunals.gov.uk//Aspx/view.aspx?id=3683

Further reading

Moynihan A (2015) *The Good Trustee Guide, 6th edn.* National Council of Voluntary Organisations, London

The law
Useful websites

Animal & Plant Health Agency (APHA):
www.gov.uk/government/organisations/animal-and-plant-health-agency

Association of Lawyers for Animal Welfare:
www.alaw.org.uk

British Veterinary Forensic and Law Association:
www.bvfla.org.uk

BVA Waste Guidelines:
www.bva.co.uk/Workplace-guidance/Practice-management/Handling-veterinary-waste/

Department of Agriculture, Environment and Rural Affairs (DAERA):
www.daera-ni.gov.uk/

Department for Environment, Food and Rural Affairs (Defra):
www.gov.uk/government/organisations/department-for-environment-food-rural-affairs

Scottish Government Rural Directorate:
www.gov.scot/Topics/farmingrural/Agriculture/animal-welfare

UK legislation:
www.legislation.gov.uk

Veterinary Medicine Directorate (VMD):
www.gov.uk/government/organisations/veterinary-medicines-directorate

Education
Useful websites

Department for Farming and Rural Affairs (2008) *Understanding behaviours in a farming context: bringing theoretical and applied evidence together from across Defra and highlighting policy relevance and implications for future research.* Defra. Available at: http://webarchive.nationalarchives.gov.uk/20130125181347/http://www.defra.gov.uk/statistics/files/defra-stats-foodfarm-environ-obs-research-behavious-aceopaper-nov08.pdf

VARK learning styles questionnaire: http://vark-learn.com/home/

Waltham Faeces Scoring System: www.waltham.com/dyn/_assets/_pdfs/resources/FaecesQuality2.pdf

Further reading

Fishbein M and Ajzen I (1975) *Belief, attitude, intention and behavior: an introduction of theory and research.* Addison-Wesley, Reading

Non-accidental injury
Useful websites

Cats Protection Paws Protect: www.cats.org.uk/what-we-do/paws-protect

Dogs Trust Freedom Project: www.moretodogstrust.org.uk/freedom-project/freedom-project

Endeavour (previously Paws for Kids): www.pawsforkids.org.uk/

International Veterinary Forensic Science Association: www.ivfsa.org

The Links Group Pet Fostering: www.thelinksgroup.org.uk/professionals/pet-fostering-services/

Raystede Centre for Animal Welfare: www.raystede.org/

RSPCA Pet Retreat: www.rspca.org.uk/whatwedo/petretreat

Further reading

Ascione FR (2010) *The International Handbook of Animal Abuse and Cruelty: Theory, Research, and Application.* Purdue University Press, West Lafayette

Merck MD (2013) *Veterinary Forensics: Animal Cruelty Investigations, 2nd edn.* Wiley-Blackwell, Ames

Munro R and Munro HMC (2008) *Animal Abuse and Unlawful Killing: Veterinary Forensic Pathology.* Saunders Elsevier, Edinburgh

Hoarding
Useful websites

ASPCA animal hoarding resource: https://www.aspca.org/animal-cruelty/animal-hoarding

Cummings School of Veterinary Medicine at Tufts University Hoarding of Animals Research Consortium: http://vet.tufts.edu/hoarding

International Cat Care: http://icatcare.org/advice/cats-and-human-health/hoarding-overwhelmed-care-giver

Further reading

American Psychiatric Association (2013) Hoarding disorder. In: *Diagnostic and Statistical Manual of Mental Disorders, 5th edn.* pp. 247–51. American Psychiatric Association Publishing, Washington DC

Arluke A and Killeen C (2009) *Inside Animal Hoarding: The Case of Barbara Erickson and her 552 Dogs.* Purdue University Press, West Lafayette

Index

Page numbers in *italics* refer to figures
Page numbers in **bold** refer to Quick Reference Guides (QRGs)